Hugo and Russell's
Pharmaceutical Microbiology

EDITED BY

Stephen P Denyer

B Pharm PhD FRPharmS
Welsh School of Pharmacy
Cardiff University
Cardiff

Norman A Hodges

B Pharm PhD MRPharmS
School of Pharmacy and Biomolecular Sciences
Brighton University
Lewes Road
Brighton

Sean P Gorman

BSc PhD MPS
School of Pharmacy
Queen's University Belfast
Medical Biology Centre
University Road
Belfast

SEVENTH EDITION

Blackwell
Science

© 1977, 1980, 1983, 1987, 1992, 1998, 2004 by Blackwell Science Ltd
a Blackwell Publishing company
Blackwell Science, Inc., 350 Main Street, Malden, Massachusetts 02148-5020, USA
Blackwell Publishing Ltd, 9600 Garsington Road, Oxford OX4 2DQ, UK
Blackwell Science Asia Pty Ltd, 550 Swanston Street, Carlton, Victoria 3053, Australia
The right of the Author to be identified as the Author of this Work has been asserted in
accordance with the Copyright, Designs and Patents Act 1988.

First published 1977
Second edition 1980
Third edition 1983
Reprinted 1986
Fourth edition 1987
Reprinted 1989, 1991

Italian edition 1991
Fifth edition 1992
Reprinted 1993, 1994, 1995
Sixth edition 1998
Reprinted 1999, 2000, 2002, 2003
Seventh edition 2004

Library of Congress Cataloging-in-Publication Data
Hugo and Russell's pharmaceutical microbiology / edited by Stephen Denyer, Norman A.
Hodges, Sean P. Gorman. — 7th ed.
    p. cm.
Rev. ed. of: Pharmaceutical microbiology / edited by W.B. Hugo and A.D. Russell.
Includes bibliographical references and index.
    ISBN 0-632-06467-6
  1. Pharmaceutical microbiology.
    [DNLM: 1. Anti-Infective Agents. 2. Technology, Pharmaceutical. QV 250
H895 2004] I. Title: Pharmaceutical microbiology. II. Hugo, W. B. (William
Barry) III. Denyer, S. P. IV. Hodges, Norman A.V,. Gorman, S. P. VI.
Pharmaceutical microbiology.

    QR46.5.P48 2004
    615'.1'01579—dc22

                                                                    2003024264

ISBN 0-632-06467-6

A catalogue record for this title is available from the British Library

Set in Sabon 9.5/12 pt by SNP Best-set Typesetter Ltd., Hong Kong
Printed and bound in the United Kingdom by Ashford Colour Press, Gosport

Commissioning Editor: Maria Khan
Managing Editor: Rupal Malde
Production Editor: Fiona Pattison
Production Controller: Kate Charman

For further information on Blackwell Publishing, visit our website:
http://www.blackwellpublishing.com

Hugo and Russell's
Pharmaceutical Microbiology

Contents

v

Contributors

Dr David Allison
School of Pharmacy and Pharmaceutical
    Sciences
University of Manchester
Oxford Road
Manchester M13 9PL
UK

Dr Rosamund Baird
Visiting Senior Lecturer
School of Pharmacy and Pharmacology
University of Bath
Claverton Down
Bath BA2 7AY
UK

Dr Miguel Cámara
Senior Lecturer in Molecular Microbiology
Institute of Pharmaceutical Sciences
School of Pharmaceutical Sciences
University of Nottingham
Nottingham NG7 2RD
UK

Dr Michael Corbel
National Institute for Biological Standards
    and Control
Blanche Lane
South Mimms
Potters Bar
Hertfordshire EN6 3QG
UK

Professor Stephen Denyer
Welsh School of Pharmacy
Cardiff University
Cardiff CF10 3XF
UK

Professor Roger Finch
Professor of Infectious Diseases
Clinical Sciences Building
University of Nottingham
The City Hospital
Nottingham NG5 1PB
UK

Professor James Ford
School of Pharmacy and Chemistry
Liverpool John Moores University
Byrom Street
Liverpool L3 3AF
UK

Dr James Furr
Welsh School of Pharmacy
Cardiff University
King Edward VII Avenue
Cardiff CF10 3XF
Wales

Professor Peter Gilbert
School of Pharmacy and Pharmaceutical
    Sciences
University of Manchester
Oxford Rd
Manchester M13 9PL
UK

Professor Sean Gorman
Professor of Pharmaceutical Microbiology
School of Pharmacy
The Queen's University of Belfast
Belfast BT9 7BL
Northern Ireland

Dr Mark Gumbleton
Welsh School of Pharmacy
Cardiff University
King Edward VII Avenue
Cardiff CF10 3XF
Wales

Dr Norman Hodges
Principal Lecturer in Pharmaceutical
    Microbiology
School of Pharmacy and Biomolecular
    Sciences
University of Brighton
Lewes Road
Brighton BN2 4GJ
UK

Dr Robert Jones
School of Pharmacy and Biomedical Sciences
University of Portsmouth
St Michael's Building
White Swan Road
Portsmouth PO1 2DT
UK

Dr Kevin Kavanagh
Head of Medical Mycology Unit
Department of Biology
National University of Ireland
Maynooth
Co. Kildare
Ireland

Dr Peter Lambert
Aston Pharmacy School
Aston University
Aston Triangle
Birmingham B4 7ET
UK

Dr Jean-Yves Maillard
School of Pharmacy and Biomolecular
    Sciences
University of Brighton
Lewes Rd
Brighton BN2 4GJ
UK

Dr Tim Paget
Department of Biological Sciences
University of Hull
Hull HU6 7RX
UK

Professor A Denver Russell
Welsh School of Pharmacy
Cardiff University
King Edward VII Avenue
Cardiff CF10 3XF
Wales

Dr Eileen Scott
School of Pharmacy
The Queen's University of Belfast
Belfast BT9 7BL
Northern Ireland

Dr Anthony Smith
Department of Pharmacy and Pharmacology
University of Bath (5 West — 2.18)
Claverton Down
Bath BA2 7AY
UK

Professor JMB (Sandy) Smith
Head of Department of Microbiology
Otago School of Medical Sciences
University of Otago
Dunedin
New Zealand

Dr David Stickler
School of Biosciences
Cardiff University
Main Building
Museum Avenue
PO Box 915
Cardiff CF10 3TL
Wales

Dr Derek Sullivan
Microbiology Research Unit
School of Dental Science
Trinity College
Dublin 2
Ireland

Dr Elaine Underwood
SMA Nutrition
Huntercomb Lane South
Taplow
Maidenhead
Berks SL6 0PH
UK

Dr Sally Varian
Consultant
Ulverston
Cumbria LA12 8PI
UK

Preface to the Seventh edition

We were much honoured to be recommended by Professor A.D. Russell to act as editors for the 7th edition of *Pharmaceutical Microbiology*. All three of us have used this textbook in its various editions throughout our careers as teachers and researchers, and we recognize the important role it fulfils.

As might be anticipated when a new editorial team is in place, a substantial number of changes have been made. Well over half the chapters have new authors or co-authors. We also use Chapter 1 to give a rationale for the scope and content of the book, emphasizing the interrelated character of the discipline of pharmaceutical microbiology. In addition, by combining and reorganizing chapters, by introducing new material and through a revised page format we have tried to provide readers with a distinctive 7th edition.

We must thank our contributors for their willing collaboration in this enterprise, especially Professor Russell for his continuing contributions, and our publishers for their support and expertise.

Finally, this addition is a tribute to the farsightedness of A.D. Russell and W.B. Hugo who took up the challenge in 1977 to produce a popular and concise read for pharmacy students required to study pharmaceutical microbiology. We are delighted that this current edition recognizes these origins by continuing the association with Hugo and Russell in its revised title.

S.P. Denyer
S.P. Gorman
N.A. Hodges

Preface to the First Edition

When we were first approached by the publishers to write a textbook on pharmaceutical microbiology to appear in the spring of 1977, it was felt that such a task could not be accomplished satisfactorily in the time available.

However, by a process of combined editorship and by invitation to experts to contribute to the various chapters this task has been accomplished thanks to the cooperation of our collaborators.

Pharmaceutical microbiology may be defined as that part of microbiology which has a special bearing on pharmacy in all its aspects. This will range from the manufacture and quality control of pharmaceutical products to an understanding of the mode of action of antibiotics. The full extent of microbiology on the pharmaceutical area may be judged from the chapter contents.

As this book is aimed at undergraduate pharmacy students (as well as microbiologists entering the pharmaceutical industry) we were under constraint to limit the length of the book to retain it in a defined price range. The result is to be found in the following pages. The editors must bear responsibility for any omissions, a point which has most concerned us. Length and depth of treatment were determined by the dictate of our publishers. It is hoped that the book will provide a concise reading for pharmacy students (who, at the moment, lack a textbook in this subject) and help to highlight those parts of a general microbiological training which impinge on the pharmaceutical industry.

In conclusion, the editors thank most sincerely the contributors to this book, both for complying with our strictures as to the length of their contribution and for providing their material on time, and our publishers for their friendly courtesy and efficiency during the production of this book. We also wish to thank Dr H.J. Smith for his advice on various chemical aspects, Dr M.I. Barnett for useful comments on reverse osmosis, and Mr A. Keall who helped with the table on sterilization methods.

W.B. Hugo
A.D. Russell

Part 1

Biology of Microorganisms

Chapter 1

Introduction to pharmaceutical microbiology

Stephen Denyer, Norman Hodges and Sean Gorman

1 Microorganisms and medicines

Despite continuing poverty in many parts of the world and the devastating effects of HIV and AIDS infection on the African continent and elsewhere, the health of the world's population is progressively improving. This is reflected in the increase in life expectancy that has been recorded for the great majority of the countries reporting statistics to the World Health Organization over the last 40 years. In Central America, for example, the life expectancy has increased from 55 years in 1960 to 71 years in 2000, and the increase in North (but not sub-Saharan) Africa is even greater, from 47 to 68 years. Much of this improvement is due to better nutrition and sanitation, but improved health care and the greater availability of effective medicines with which to treat common diseases are also major contributing factors. Substantial inroads have been made in the prevention and treatment of cancer, cardiovascular disease and other major causes of death in Western society, and of infections and diarrhoeal disease that remain the big killers in developing countries. Several infectious diseases have been eradicated completely, and others from substantial parts of the world. The global eradication of smallpox in 1977 is well documented, but 2002 saw three of the world's continents declared free of polio, and the prospects are good for the total elimination of polio, measles and Chagas disease.

The development of the many vaccines and other medicines that have been so crucial to the improvement in world heath has been the result of the large investment in research by the major international pharmaceutical companies. This has led to the manufacture of pharmaceuticals becoming one of the most consistently successful and important industries in many countries, not only in the traditional strongholds of North America, Western Europe and Japan but, increasingly, in Eastern Europe, the Indian subcontinent and the Far East. Worldwide sales of medicines and medical devices are estimated to have exceeded $US 401 billion (approximately £250 billion) in 2002, and this figure is rising by 8% per annum. In the UK alone, the value of pharmaceutical exports is currently £10.03 billion each year, a figure that translates to more than £150 000 for each employee in the industry.

The growth of the pharmaceutical industry in recent decades has been paralleled by rising standards for product quality and more rigorous regulation of manufacturing procedures. In order to receive a manufacturing licence, a modern medicine must be shown to be effective, safe and of good quality. Most medicines consist of an active ingredient that is formulated with a variety of other materials (excipients) that are necessary to ensure that the medicine is effective, and remains stable, palatable and safe during storage and use. While the efficacy and safety aspects of the active ingredient are within the domain of the pharmacologist and toxicologist, respectively, many other disciplines contribute to the efficacy, safety and quality of the manufactured product as a whole. Analytical chemists and pharmacists take lead responsibility for ensuring that the components of the medicine are present in the correct physical form and concentration, but quality is not judged solely on the physicochemical properties of the product: microorganisms also have the potential to influence efficacy and safety.

It is obvious that medicines contaminated with potentially pathogenic (disease-causing) microorganisms are a safety hazard, so medicines administered by vulnerable routes (e.g. injections) or to vulnerable areas of the body (e.g. the eyes) are manufactured as sterile products. What is less predictable is that microorganisms can, in addition to initiating infections, cause product spoilage by chemically decomposing the active ingredient or the excipients. This may lead to the product being under-strength, physically or chemically unstable or possibly contaminated with toxic materials. Thus, it is clear that pharmaceutical microbiology must encompass the subjects of sterilization and preservation against microbial spoilage, and a pharmacist with responsibility for the safe, hygienic manufacture and use of medicines must know where microorganisms arise in the environment, i.e. the sources of microbial contamination, and the factors that predispose to, or prevent, product spoilage. In these respects, the pharmaceutical microbiologist has a lot in common with food and cosmetics microbiologists, and there is substantial scope for transfer of knowledge between these disciplines.

Disinfection and the properties of chemicals (biocides) used as antiseptics, disinfectants and preservatives are subjects of which pharmacists and other persons responsible for the manufacture of medicines should have a knowledge, both from the perspective of biocide use in product formulation and manufacture, and because antiseptics and disinfectants are pharmaceutical products in their own right. However, they are not the only antimicrobial substances that are relevant to medicine; antibiotics are of major importance and represent a product category that regularly features among the top five most frequently prescribed. The term 'antibiotic' is used in several different ways: originally an antibiotic was defined as a naturally occurring substance that was produced by one microorganism that inhibited the growth of, or killed, other microorganisms, i.e. an antibiotic was a natural product, a microbial metabolite. More recently the term has come to encompass certain synthetic agents that are usually used systemically (throughout the body) to treat infection. A knowledge of the manufacture, quality control and, in the light of current concerns about resistance of microorganisms, the use of antibiotics, are other areas of knowledge that contribute to the discipline of pharmaceutical microbiology.

Commercial antibiotic production began with the manufacture of penicillin in the 1940s, and for many years antibiotics were the only significant example of a medicinal product that was made using microorganisms. Following the adoption in the 1950s of microorganisms to facilitate the manufacture of steroids and the development of recombinant DNA technology in the last three decades of the 20th century, the use of microorganisms in the manufacture of medicines has gathered great momentum. It led to more than 100 biotechnology-derived products on the market by the new millennium and another 300 or more in clinical trials. While it is true to say that traditionally the principal pharmaceutical interest in microorganisms is that of controlling them, exploiting microbial metabolism in the manufacture of medicines is a burgeoning area of knowledge that will become increasingly important, not only in the pharmacy curriculum but also in those of other disciplines employed in the pharmaceutical industry. Table 1.1 summarizes these benefits and uses of microorganisms in pharmaceutical manufacturing, together with the more widely recognized hazards and problems that they present.

Looking ahead to the early decades of the 21st century, it is clear that an understanding of the physiology and genetics of microorganisms will also become more important, not just in the production of new therapeutic agents but in the understanding of infections and other diseases. Several of the traditional diseases that were major causes of death before the antibiotic era, e.g. tuberculosis and diphtheria, are now re-emerging in resistant form — even in developed countries — adding to the problems posed by infections in which antibiotic resistance has long been a problem, and those like Creutzfeldt–Jakob disease, West Nile virus and severe acute respiratory syndrome (SARS) that have only been recognized in recent years.

Not only has the development of resistance to established antibiotics become a challenge, so too has the ability of microorganisms to take advantage of changing practices and procedures in medicine and surgery. Microorganisms are found almost everywhere in our surroundings and they possess

Table 1.1 Microorganisms in pharmacy: benefits and problems

Benefits or uses	Related study topics	Harmful effects	Study topic
The manufacture of: antibiotics steroids therapeutic enzymes polysaccharides products of recombinant DNA technology	Good manufacturing practice Industrial 'fermentation' technology Microbial genetics	May contaminate non-sterile and sterile medicines with a risk of infection	Non-sterile medicines: Enumeration of microorganisms in the manufacturing environment (environmental monitoring) and in raw materials and manufactured products Identification and detection of specific organisms Sterile medicines: Sterilization methods Sterilization monitoring and validation procedures Sterility testing Assessment and calculation of sterility assurance Aseptic manufacture
Use in the production of vaccines	Quality control of immunological products		
As assay organisms to determine antibiotic, vitamin and amino acid concentrations	Assay methods	May contaminate non-sterile and sterile medicines with a risk of product deterioration	Enumeration, identification and detection as above, plus Characteristics, selection and testing of antimicrobial preservatives
To detect mutagenic or carcinogenic activity	Ames mutagenicity test	Cause infectious and other diseases	Immunology and infectious diseases Characteristics, selection and use of vaccines and antibiotics Use of biocides in infection and contamination control Control of antibiotic resistance
		Cause pyrogenic reactions (fever) when introduced into the body even in the absence of infection	Bacterial structure Pyrogen and endotoxin testing
		Provide a reservoir of antibiotic resistance genes	Microbial genetics

the potential to reproduce extremely rapidly; it is quite possible for cell division to occur every 20 minutes under favourable conditions. These characteristics mean that they can adapt readily to a changing environment and colonize new niches. One feature of modern surgery is the ever-increasing use of plastic, ceramic and metal devices that are introduced into the body for a wide variety of purposes, including the commonly encountered urinary or venous catheters and the less common intra-ocular lenses, heart valves, pacemakers and hip prostheses. Many bacteria have the potential to produce substances or structures that help them to attach to these devices, even while combating the immune system of the body. Thus, colonization often necessitates removal and replacement of the device in question — often leading to great discomfort for the patient and substantial monetary cost to the health-care service. It has recently been estimated that, on average, a hospital-acquired infection results in an extra 14 days in hospital, a 10% increase in the chance of dying and more than £3000 additional expenditure on health care. The development of strategies for eliminating, or at least restricting, the severity or consequences of these device-related infections is a challenge for pharmacists and microbiologists within the industry, and for many other health-care professionals.

In addition to an improved understanding of the mechanisms of antibiotic resistance, of the links between antibiotic resistance and misuse, and of the factors influencing the initiation of infections in the body, our insights into the role of microorganisms in other disease states have broadened significantly in recent years. Until about 1980 it was probably true to say that there was little or no recognition of the possibility that microorganisms might have a role to play in human diseases other than clear-cut infections. In recent years, however, our perception of the scope of microorganisms as agents of disease has been changed by the discovery that *Helicobacter pylori* is intimately involved in the development of gastric or duodenal ulcers and stomach cancer; by the findings that viruses can cause cancers of the liver, blood and cervix; and by the suspected involvement of microorganisms in diverse conditions like parkinsonism and Alzheimer's disease.

Clearly, a knowledge of the mechanisms whereby microorganisms are able to resist antibiotics, colonize medical devices and cause or predispose humans to other disease states is essential in the development not only of new antibiotics, but of other medicines and health-care practices that miminize the risks of these adverse situations developing.

2 The scope and content of the book

Criteria and standards for the microbiological quality of medicines depend upon the route of administration of the medicine in question. The vast majority of medicines that are given by mouth or placed on the skin are non-sterile, i.e. they may contain some microorganisms (within limits on type and concentration), whereas all injections and ophthalmic products must be sterile, i.e. they contain no living organisms. Products for other anatomical sites (e.g. nose, ear, vagina and bladder) are often sterile but not invariably so (Chapter 19). The microbiological quality of non-sterile medicines is controlled by specifications defining the concentration of organisms that may be present and requiring the absence of specific, potentially hazardous organisms. Thus the ability to identify the organisms present, to detect those that are prohibited from particular product categories and to enumerate microbial contaminants in the manufacturing environment, raw materials and finished product are clearly skills that a pharmaceutical microbiologist should possess (Chapters 2–6). So, too, is a familiarity with the characteristics of antimicrobial preservatives that may be a component of the medicine required to minimize the risk of microbial growth and spoilage during storage and use by the patient (Chapters 16 and 17).

For a sterile product the criterion of quality is simple; there should be no detectable microorganisms whatsoever. The product should, therefore, be able to pass a test for sterility, and a knowledge of the procedures and interpretation of results of such tests is an important aspect of pharmaceutical microbiology (Chapter 20). Injections are also subject to a test for pyrogens; these are substances that cause a rise in body temperature when introduced into the body. Strictly speaking, any substance which causes fever following injection is a pyrogen, but in reality the vast majority are of bacterial origin, and it is for this reason that the detection, assay and removal of bacterial pyrogens (endotoxins) are considered within the realm of microbiology (Chapter 19).

Sterile medicines may be manufactured by two different strategies. The most straightforward and preferred option is to make the product, pack it in its final container and sterilize it by heat, radiation or other means (terminal sterilization, Chapter 20). The alternative is to manufacture the product from sterile ingredients under conditions that do not permit the entry of contaminating organisms (aseptic manufacture, Chapters 15 and 21); this latter option is usually selected when the ingredients or physical form of the product render it heat- or radiation-sensitive. Those responsible for the manufacture of sterile products must be familiar with the sterilization or aseptic manufacturing procedures available for different product types, and those who have cause to open, use or dispense sterile products (in a hospital pharmacy, for example) should be aware of the aseptic handling procedures to be adopted in order to minimize the risk of product contamination.

The spoilage of medicines as a result of microbial contamination, although obviously undesirable, has as its main consequence financial loss rather than ill health on the part of the patient. The other major problem posed by microbial contamination of medicines, that of the risk of initiating infection, although uncommon, is far more important in terms of risk to the patient and possible loss of life (Chapters 7 and 16). Infections arising by this means also have financial implications, of course, not only in additional treatment costs but in terms of product recalls, possible litigation and damage to the reputation of the manufacturer.

The range of antimicrobial drugs used to prevent and treat microbial infections is large; for example, a contemporary textbook of antimicrobial chemotherapy lists no fewer than 43 different cephalosporin antibiotics that were already on the market or the subject of clinical trials at the time of publication. Not only are there many antibiotic products, but increasingly, these products really have properties that make them unique. It is far more difficult now than it was, say, 20 years ago, for a manufacturer to obtain a licence for a 'copycat' product, as licensing authorities now emphasize the need to demonstrate that a new antibiotic (or any new medicine) affords a real advantage over established drugs. Because of this range and diversity of products, pharmacists are now far more commonly called upon to advise on the relative merits of the antibiotics available to treat particular categories of infection than was the case hitherto (Chapters 10, 12 and 14). A prerequisite to provide this information is a knowledge not only of the drug in question, but the infectious disease it is being used to treat and the factors that might influence the success of antibiotic therapy in that situation (Chapter 7).

While there was a belief among some commentators a generation ago that infectious disease was a problem that was well on the way to permanent resolution owing to the development of effective vaccines and antibiotics, such complacency has now completely disappeared. Although cardiovascular and malignant diseases are more frequent causes of death in many developed countries, infectious diseases remain of paramount importance in many others, so much so that the five leading infections — respiratory, HIV/AIDS, diarrhoeal disease, tuberculosis and malaria, accounted for 11.5 million deaths in 1999. The confidence that antibiotics would be produced to deal with the vast majority of infections has been replaced by a recognition that the development of resistance to them is likely to substantially restrict their value in the control of certain infections (Chapter 13). Resistance to antibiotics has increased in virtually all categories of pathogenic microorganisms and is now so prevalent that there are some infections and some organisms for which, it is feared, there will soon be no effective antibiotics. It has been estimated that the annual cost of treating hospital-acquired infections may be as high as \$4 billion in the USA alone. The scale and costs of the problem are such that increasing attention is being paid to infection control procedures that are designed to minimize the risk of infection being transmitted from one patient to another within a hospital. The properties of disinfectants and antiseptics, the measurement of their antimicrobial activity and the factors influencing their selection for use in hospital infection control strategies or contamination control in the manufacturing setting are topics with which both pharmacists and industrial microbiologists should be familiar (Chapters 11 and 18).

It has long been recognized that microorganisms are valuable, if not essential, in the maintenance of our ecosystems. Their role and benefits in the carbon and nitrogen cycles in terms of recycling dead plant and animal material and in the fixation of atmospheric nitrogen are well understood. The uses of microorganisms in the food, dairy and brewing industries are also well established, but until the late 20th century advances in genetics, immunology and biotechnology, their benefits and uses in the pharmaceutical industry were far more modest. For many years the production of antibiotics (Chapter 22) and microbial enzyme-mediated production of steroids were the only significant pharmaceutical examples of the exploitation of metabolism of microorganisms. The value of these applications, both in monetary and health-care terms has been immense. Antibiotics currently have an estimated world market value of $25 billion and by this criterion they are surpassed as products of biotechnology only by cheese and alcoholic beverages, but the benefits they afford in terms of improved health and life expectancy are incalculable. The discovery of the anti-inflammatory effects of corticosteroids had a profound impact on the treatment of rheumatoid arthritis in the 1950s, but it was the use of enzymes possessed by common fungi that made cortisone widely available to rheumatism sufferers. The synthesis of cortisone by traditional chemical methods involved 31 steps, gave a yield of less than 0.2% of the starting material and resulted in a product costing, even in 1950s terms, $200 per gram. Exploiting

microbial enzymes reduced the synthesis to 11 steps and the cost rapidly fell to $6 per gram.

Apart from these major applications, however, the uses of microorganisms in the manufacture of medicines prior to 1980 were very limited. Enzymes were developed for use in cancer chemotherapy (asparaginase) and to digest blood clots (streptokinase), and polysaccharides also found therapeutical applications (e.g. dextran—used as a plasma expander). These were of relatively minor importance, however, compared with the products that followed the advances in recombinant DNA technology in the 1970s. This technology permitted human genes to be inserted into microorganisms, which were thus able to manufacture the gene products far more efficiently than traditional methods of extraction from animal or human tissues. Insulin, in 1982, was the first therapeutic product of DNA technology to be licensed for human use, and it has been followed by human growth hormone, interferon, blood clotting factors and many other products. DNA technology has also permitted the development of vaccines which, like that for the prevention of hepatitis B, use genetically engineered surface antigens rather than whole natural virus particles, so these vaccines are more effective and safer than those produced by traditional means (Chapters 9 and 23).

All these developments, together with miscellaneous applications in the detection of mutagenic and carcinogenic activity in drugs and chemicals and in the assay of antibiotics, vitamins and amino acids (Chapter 25), have ensured that the role of microorganisms in the manufacture of medicines is now well recognized, and that a basic knowledge of immunology (Chapter 8), gene cloning and other biotechnology disciplines (Chapter 24) is an integral part of pharmaceutical microbiology.

Chapter 2
Fundamental features of microbiology

Norman Hodges

1 Introduction

Microorganisms differ enormously in terms of their shape, size and appearance and in their genetic and metabolic characteristics. All these properties are used in classifying microorganisms into the major groups with which many people are familiar, e.g. bacteria, fungi, protozoa and viruses, and into the less well known categories like chlamydia, rickettsia and mycoplasmas. The major groups are the subject of individual chapters immediately following this, so the purpose here is not to describe any of them in great detail but to summarize their features so that the reader may better understand the distinctions between them. A further aim of this chapter is to avoid undue repetition of information in the early part of the book by considering such aspects of microbiology as cultivation, enumeration and genetics that are common to some, or all, of the various types of microorganism.

1.1 Viruses, viroids and prions

Viruses do not have a cellular structure. They are particles composed of nucleic acid surrounded by protein; some possess a lipid envelope and associated glycoproteins, but recognizable chromosomes, cytoplasm and cell membranes are invariably absent. Viruses are incapable of independent replication as they do not contain the enzymes necessary to copy their own nucleic acids; as a consequence, all viruses are intracellular parasites and are reproduced using the metabolic capabilities of the host cell. A great deal of variation is observed in shape (helical, linear or spherical), size (20–400 nm) and nucleic acid composition (single- or double-stranded, linear or circular RNA or DNA), but almost all viruses are smaller than bacteria and they cannot be seen with a normal light microscope; instead they may be viewed using an electron microscope which affords much greater magnification.

Viroids (virusoids) are even simpler than viruses, being infectious particles comprising single-stranded RNA without any associated protein. Those that have been described are plant pathogens, and, so far, there are no known human pathogens in this category. Prions are unique as infectious agents in that they contain no nucleic acid. A prion is an atypical form of a mammalian protein that can interact with a normal protein molecule and cause it to undergo a conformational change so that it, in turn, becomes a prion and ceases its normal function. Prions are the agents responsible for transmissible spongiform encephalopathies, e.g. Creutzfeldt–Jakob disease (CJD) and bovine spongiform encephalopathy (BSE). They are the simplest and most recently recognized agents of infectious disease, and are important in a pharmaceutical context owing to their extreme resistance to conventional sterilizing agents like steam, gamma radiation and disinfectants (Chapter 18).

1.2 Prokaryotes and eukaryotes

The most fundamental distinction between the various microorganisms having a cellular structure (i.e. all except those described in section 1.1 above) is their classification into two groups—the prokaryotes and eukaryotes—based primarily on their cellular structure and mode of reproduction. Expressed in the simplest possible terms, prokaryotes are the bacteria and archaea (see section 1.2.1), and eukaryotes are all other cellular microorganisms, e.g. fungi, protozoa and algae. The crucial difference between these two types of cell is the possession by the eukaryotes of a true cell nucleus in which the chromosomes are separated from the cytoplasm by a nuclear membrane. The prokaryotes have no true nucleus; they normally possess just a single chromosome that is not separated from the other cell contents by a membrane. Other major distinguishing features of the two groups are that prokaryotes are normally haploid (possess only one

copy of the set of genes in the cell) and reproduce asexually; eukaroyotes, by contrast, are usually diploid (possess two copies of their genes) and normally have the potential to reproduce sexually. The capacity for sexual reproduction confers the major advantage of creating new combinations of genes, which increases the scope for selection and evolutionary development. The restriction to an asexual mode of reproduction means that the organism in question is heavily reliant on mutation as a means of creating genetic variety and new strains with advantageous characteristics, although many bacteria are able to receive new genes from other strains or species (see section 6.1 and Chapter 3). Table 2.1 lists some distinguishing features of the prokaryotes and eukaryotes.

1.2.1 Bacteria and archaea

Bacteria are essentially unicellular, although some species arise as sheathed chains of cells. They possess the properties listed under prokaryotes in Table 2.1, but, like viruses and other categories of microorganisms, exhibit great diversity of form, habitat, metabolism, pathogenicity and other characteristics. The bacteria of interest in pharmacy and medicine belong to the group known as the

Table 2.1 Distinguishing features of prokaryotes and eukaryotes

Characteristic	Eukaryotes	Prokaryotes
Size	Normally > 10 μm	Typically 1–5 μm
Location of chromosomes	Within a true nucleus separated from the cytoplasm by a nuclear membrane	In the cytoplasm, usually attached to the cell membrane
Nuclear division	Exhibit mitosis and meiosis	Mitosis and meiosis are absent
Nucleolus	Present	Absent
Reproduction	Asexual or sexual reproduction	Normally asexual reproduction
Chromosome number	>1	1
Mitochondria and chloroplasts	May be present	Absent
Cell membrane composition	Sterols present	Sterols absent
Cell wall composition	Cell walls (when present) usually contain cellulose or chitin but not peptidoglycan	Walls usually contain peptidoglycan
Ribosomes	Cytoplasmic ribosomes are 80S	Ribosomes are smaller, usually 70S
Flagella	Structurally complex	Structurally simple
Pili	Absent	Present
Fimbriae	Cilia	Present
Storage compounds	Poly-β-hydroxybutyrate absent	Poly-β-hydroxybutyrate often present

eubacteria. The other subdivision of prokaryotes, the archaea, have little or no pharmaceutical importance and largely comprise organisms capable of living in extreme environments (e.g. high temperatures, extreme salinity or pH) or organisms exhibiting specialized modes of metabolism (e.g. by deriving energy from sulphur or iron oxidation or the production of methane).

The eubacteria are typically rod-shaped (bacillus), spherical (cocci), curved or spiral cells of approximately 0.5–5.0 μm (longest dimension) and are divided into two groups designated Gram-positive and Gram-negative according to their reaction to a staining procedure developed in 1884 by Christian Gram (see Chapter 3). Although all the pathogenic species are included within this category there are very many other eubacteria that are harmless or positively beneficial. Some of the bacteria that contaminate or cause spoilage of pharmaceutical materials are saprophytes, i.e. they obtain their energy by decomposition of animal and vegetable material, while many could also be described as parasites (benefiting from growth on or in other living organisms without causing detrimental effects) or pathogens (parasites damaging the host). Rickettsia and chlamydia are types of bacteria that are obligate intracellular parasites, i.e. they are incapable of growing outside a host cell and so cannot easily be cultivated in the laboratory. Most bacteria of pharmaceutical and medical importance possess cell walls (and are therefore relatively resistant to osmotic stress), grow well at temperatures between ambient and human body temperature, and exhibit wide variations in their requirement for, or tolerance of, oxygen. Strict aerobes require atmospheric oxygen, but for strict anaerobes oxygen is toxic. Many other bacteria would be described as facultative anaerobes (normally growing best in air but can grow without it) or micro-aerophils (preferring oxygen concentrations lower than those in normal air).

1.2.2 *Fungi*

Fungi are eukaryotes and therefore differ from bacteria in the ways described in Table 2.1 and are structurally more complex and varied in appearance. Fungi are considered to be non-photosynthe-

sizing plants, and the term *fungus* covers both yeasts and moulds, although the distinction between these two groups is not always clear. Yeasts are normally unicellular organisms that are larger than bacteria (typically 5–10 μm) and divide either by a process of binary fission (see section 4.2 and Fig. 2.1a) or budding (whereby a daughter cell arises as a swelling or protrusion from the parent that eventually separates to lead an independent existence, Fig. 2.1b). *Mould* is an imprecise term used to describe fungi that do not form fruiting bodies visible to the naked eye, thus excluding toadstools and mushrooms. Most moulds consist of a tangled mass (mycelium) of filaments or threads (hyphae) which vary between 1 and > 50 μm wide (Fig. 2.1c); they may be differentiated for specialized functions, e.g. absorption of nutrients or reproduction. Some fungi may exhibit a unicellular (yeast-like) or mycelial (mould-like) appearance depending upon cultivation conditions. Although fungi are eukaryotes that should, in theory, be capable of sexual reproduction, there are some species in which this has never been observed. Most fungi are saprophytes with relatively few having pathogenic potential, but their ability to form spores that are resistant to drying makes them important as contaminants of pharmaceutical raw materials, particularly materials of vegetable origin.

1.2.3 *Protozoa*

Protozoa are eukaryotic, predominantly unicellular microorganisms that are regarded as animals rather than plants, although the distinction between protozoa and fungi is not always clear and there are some organisms whose taxonomic status is uncertain. Many protozoa are free-living motile organisms that occur in water and soil, although some are parasites of plants and animals, including humans, e.g. the organisms responsible for malaria and amoebic dysentery. Protozoa are not normally found as contaminants of raw materials or manufactured medicines and the relatively few that are of pharmaceutical interest owe that status primarily to their potential to cause disease.

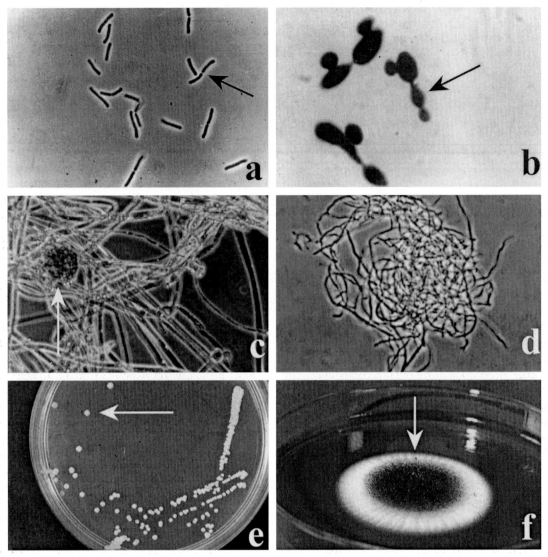

Fig. 2.1 (a) A growing culture of *Bacillus megaterium* in which cells about to divide by binary fission display constrictions (arrowed) prior to separation. (b) A growing culture of the yeast *Saccharomyces cerevisiae* displaying budding (arrowed). (c) The mould *Mucor plumbeus* exhibiting the typical appearance of a mycelium in which masses of asexual zygospores (arrowed) are formed on specialized hyphae. (d) The bacterium *Streptomyces rimosus* displaying the branched network of filaments that superficially resembles a mould mycelium. (e) The typical appearance of an overnight agar culture of *Micrococcus luteus* inoculated to produce isolated colonies (arrowed). (f) A single colony of the mould *Aspergillus niger* in which the actively growing periphery of the colony (arrowed) contrasts with the mature central region where pigmented asexual spores have developed.

2 Naming of microorganisms

Microorganisms, just like other organisms, are normally known by two names: that of the genus (plural = genera) and that of the species. The former is normally written with an upper case initial letter and the latter with a lower case initial letter, e.g. *Staphylococcus aureus* or *Escherichia coli*. These may be abbreviated by shortening the name of the genus provided that the shortened form is unambiguous, e.g. *Staph. aureus, E. coli*. Both the full and the shortened names are printed in *italics* to designate their status as proper names (in old books, theses or manuscripts they might be in roman type but underlined). The species within a genus are sometimes referred to by a collective name, e.g. staphylococci or pseudomonads, and neither these names, nor names describing groups of organisms from different genera, e.g. coliforms, are italicized or spelt with an upper case initial letter.

3 Microbial metabolism

As in most other aspects of their physiology, microorganisms exhibit marked differences in their metabolism. While some species can obtain carbon from carbon dioxide and energy from sunlight or the oxidation of inorganic materials like sulphides, the vast majority of organisms of interest in pharmacy and medicine are described as chemo-heterotrophs — they obtain carbon, nitrogen and energy by breaking down organic compounds. The chemical reactions by which energy is liberated by digestion of food materials are termed catabolic reactions, while those that use the liberated energy to make complex cellular polymers, proteins, carbohydrates and nucleic acids, are called anabolic reactions.

Food materials are oxidized in order to break them down and release energy from them. The term oxidation is defined as the removal or loss of electrons, but oxidation does not invariably involve oxygen, as a wide variety of other molecules can accept electrons and thus act as oxidizing agents. As the oxidizing molecule accepts the electrons, the other molecule in the reaction that provides them is simultaneously reduced. Consequently, oxidation and reduction are invariably linked and such reactions are often termed redox reactions. The term redox potential is also used, and this indicates whether oxidizing or reducing conditions prevail in a particular situation, e.g. in a body fluid or a culture medium. Anaerobic organisms prefer low redox potentials (typically zero to $-200\,mV$ or less) while aerobes thrive in high redox potential environments (e.g. zero to $+200\,mV$ or more).

There are marked similarities in the metabolic pathways used by pathogenic bacteria and by mammals. Many bacteria use the same process of glycolysis that is used by humans to begin the breakdown of glucose and the release of energy from it. Glycolysis describes the conversion of glucose, through a series of reactions, to pyruvic acid, and it is a process for which oxygen is not required, although glycolysis is undertaken by both aerobic and anaerobic organisms. The process releases only a relatively small amount of the energy stored in a sugar molecule, and aerobic microorganisms, in common with mammals, release much more of the energy by aerobic respiration. Oxygen is the molecule at the end of the sequence of respiratory reactions that finally accepts the electrons and allows the whole process to proceed, but it is worth noting that many organisms can also undertake *anaerobic* respiration, which uses other final electron acceptors, e.g. nitrate or fumarate.

As an alternative to respiration many microorganisms use fermentation as a means of releasing more energy from sugar; fermentation is, by definition, a process in which the final electron acceptor is an organic molecule. The term is widely understood to mean the production by yeast of ethanol and carbon dioxide from sugar, but in fact many organisms apart from yeasts can undertake fermentation and the process is not restricted to common sugar (sucrose) as a starting material or to ethanol and carbon dioxide as metabolic products. Many pathogenic bacteria are capable of fermenting several different sugars and other organic materials to give a range of metabolic products that includes acids (e.g. lactic, acetic and propionic), alcohols (e.g. ethanol, propanol, butanediol) and other commercially important materials like the solvents acetone and butanol. Fermentation is, like glycolysis, an anaerobic process, although the term is commonly used in the pharmaceutical and biotechnology industries to describe the manufacture of a wide range of substances by microorganisms where the biochemical process is neither fermentative nor even anaerobic, e.g. many textbooks refer to antibiotic fermentation, but the production vessels are usually vigorously aerated and far from anaerobic.

Microorganisms are far more versatile than mammals with respect to the materials that they can use as foods and the means by which those foods are broken down. Some pathogenic organisms can grow on dilute solutions of mineral salts and sugar (or other simple molecules like glycerol, lactic or pyruvic acids), while others can obtain energy from rarely encountered carbohydrates or by the digestion of proteins or other non-carbohydrate foods. In addition to accepting a wide variety of food materials, many microorganisms can use alternative metabolic pathways to break the food down depending on the environmental conditions, e.g. facultative anaerobes can switch from respiration to fermentation if oxygen supplies are depleted. It is partly this ability to switch to different metabolic pathways that explains why none of the major antibiotics work by interfering with the chemical reactions microorganisms use to metabolize their food. It is a fundamental principle of antibiotic action that the drug must exploit a difference in metabolism between the organism to be killed and the human host; without such a difference the antibiotic would be very toxic to the patient too. However, not only do bacteria use metabolic pathways for food digestion that are similar to our own, many of them would have the ability to switch to an alternative energy-producing pathway if an antibiotic was developed that interfered with a reaction that is unique to bacteria.

The metabolic products that arise during the period when a microbial culture is actually growing are termed primary metabolites, while those that are produced after cell multiplication has slowed or stopped, i.e. in the 'stationary phase' (see Chapter 3), are termed secondary metabolites. Ethanol is a primary metabolite of major commercial importance although it is only produced in large quantities by some species of yeast. More common than ethanol as primary metabolites are organic acids, so it is a common observation that the pH of a culture progressively falls during growth, and many organisms further metabolize the acids so the pH often rises after cell growth has ceased. The metabolites that are found during secondary metabolism are diverse, and many of them have commercial or therapeutic importance. They include antibiotics, enzymes (e.g. amylases that digest starch and proteolytic enzymes used in biological washing powders), toxins (responsible for many of the symptoms of infection but some also of therapeutic value, e.g. botox—the toxin of *Clostridium botulinum*) and carbohydrates (e.g. dextran used as a plasma expander and for molecular separations by gel filtration).

4 Microbial cultivation

The vast majority of microorganisms of interest in pharmacy and medicine can be cultivated in the laboratory and most of them require relatively simple techniques and facilities. Some organisms are parasites and so can only be grown inside the cells of a host species—which often necessitates mammalian cell culture facilities—and there are a few (e.g. the organism responsible for leprosy) that have never been cultivated outside the living animal.

4.1 Culture media

A significant number of common microorganisms are capable of synthesizing all the materials they need for growth (e.g. amino acids, nucleotides and vitamins) from simple carbon and nitrogen sources and mineral salts. Such organisms can grow on truly synthetic (chemically defined) media, but many organisms do not have this capability and need a medium that already contains these biochemicals. Such media are far more commonly used than synthetic ones, and several terms have been used to describe them, e.g. routine laboratory media, general purpose media and complex media. They are complex in the sense that their precise chemical composition is unknown and is likely to vary slightly from batch to batch. In general, they are aqueous solutions of animal or plant extracts that contain hydrolysed proteins, B-group vitamins and carbohydrates.

Readily available and relatively inexpensive sources of protein include meat extracts (from those parts of animal carcasses that are not used for human or domestic animal consumption), milk and soya. The protein is hydrolysed to varying degrees to give peptones (by definition not coagulable by heat or ammonium sulphate) or amino acids. Trypsin or other proteolytic enzymes are preferred to acids as a means of hydrolysis because acids cause more amino acid destruction; the term 'tryptic' denotes the use of the enzyme. Many microorganisms require B-group vitamins (but not the other water- or fat-soluble vitamins required by mammals) and this requirement is satisfied by yeast extract. Carbohydrates are used in the form of starch or sugars, but glucose (dextrose) is the only sugar regularly employed as a nutrient. Microorganisms differ in terms of their ability to ferment various sugars and their fermentation patterns may be used as an aid in identification. Thus, other sugars included in culture media are normally present for these diagnostic purposes rather than as carbon and energy sources. Sodium chloride may be incorporated in culture media to adjust osmotic pressure, and occasionally buffers are added to neutralize acids that result from sugar metabolism. Routine culture media may be enriched by the addition of materials like milk, blood or serum, and organisms that need such supplements in order to grow are described as 'exacting' in their nutritional requirements.

Culture media may be either liquid or solid; the latter term describes liquid media that have been gelled by the addition of agar, which is a carbohydrate extracted from certain seaweeds. Agar at a concentration of about 1–1.5% w/v will provide a firm gel that cannot be liquefied by the enzymes normally produced during bacterial growth (which is one reason it is used in preference to gelatin). Agar is unusual in that the melting and setting temperatures for its gels are quite dissimilar. Fluid agar solutions set at approximately 40°C, but do not reliquefy on heating until the temperature is in excess of 90°C. Thus agar forms a firm gel at 37°C which is the normal incubation temperature for many pathogenic organisms (whereas gelatin does not) and when used as a liquid at 45°C is at a sufficiently low temperature to avoid killing microorganisms — this property is important in pour plate counting methods (see section 5).

In contrast to medium ingredients designed to support microbial growth, there are many materials commonly added to selective or diagnostic media whose function is to restrict the growth of certain types of microorganism while permitting or enhancing the growth of others. Examples include antibacterial antibiotics added to fungal media to suppress bacterial contaminants, and bile to suppress organisms from anatomical sites other than the gastrointestinal tract. Many such additives are used in media for organism identification purposes, and these are considered further in subsequent chapters. The term enrichment sometimes causes confusion in this context. It is occasionally used in the sense of making a medium nutritionally richer to achieve more rapid or profuse growth. Alternatively, and more commonly, an enrichment medium is one designed to permit a particular type of organism to grow while restricting others, so the one that grows increases in relative numbers and is 'enriched' in a mixed culture.

Solid media designed for the growth of anaerobic organisms usually contain non-toxic reducing agents, e.g. sodium thioglycollate or sulphur-containing amino acids; these compounds create redox potentials of −200 mV or less and so diminish or eliminate the inhibitory effects of oxygen or oxidizing molecules on anaerobic growth. The inclusion of such compounds is less important in liquid media where a sufficiently low redox potential may be achieved simply by boiling; this expels dissolved oxygen, which in unstirred liquids, only slowly resaturates the upper few millimetres of liquid. Redox indicators like methylene blue or resazurin may be incorporated in anaerobic media to confirm that a sufficiently low redox potential has been achieved.

Media for yeasts and moulds often have a lower pH (5.5–6.0) than bacterial culture media (7.0–7.4). Lactic acid may be used to impart a low pH because it is not, itself, inhibitory to fungi at the concentrations used. Some fungal media that are intended for use with specimens that may also contain bacteria may be supplemented with antibacterial antibiotics, e.g. chloramphenicol or tetracyclines.

4.2 Cultivation methods

Most bacteria and some yeasts divide by a process of binary fission whereby the cell enlarges or elongates, then forms a cross-wall (septum) that separates the cell into two more-or-less equal compartments each containing a copy of the genetic material. Septum formation is often followed by constriction such that the connection between the two cell compartments is progressively reduced (see

Fig. 2.1a) until finally it is broken and the daughter cells separate. In bacteria this pattern of division may take place every 25–30 minutes under optimal conditions of laboratory cultivation, although growth at infection sites in the body is normally much slower owing to the effects of the immune system and scarcity of essential nutrients, particularly iron. Growth continues until one or more nutrients is exhausted, or toxic metabolites (often organic acids) accumulate and inhibit enzyme systems. Starting from a single cell many bacteria can achieve concentrations of the order of 10^9 cells ml^{-1} or more following overnight incubation in common liquid media. At concentrations below about 10^7 cells ml^{-1} culture media are clear, but the liquid becomes progressively more cloudy (turbid) as the concentration increases above this value; turbidity is, therefore, an indirect means of monitoring culture growth. Some bacteria produce chains of cells, and some elongated cells (filaments) that may exhibit branching to produce a tangled mass resembling a mould mycelium (Fig. 2.1d). Many yeasts divide by budding (see section 1.2.3 and Fig. 2.1b) but they, too, would normally grow in liquid media to produce a turbid culture. Moulds, however, grow by extension and branching of hyphae to produce a mycelium (Fig. 2.1c) or, in agitated liquid cultures, pellet growth may arise.

When growing on solid media in Petri dishes (often referred to as 'plates') individual bacterial cells can give rise to colonies following overnight incubation under optimal conditions. A colony is simply a collection of cells arising by multiplication of a single original cell or a small cluster of them (called a colony-forming unit or CFU). The term 'colony' does not, strictly speaking, imply any particular number of cells, but it is usually taken to mean a number sufficiently large to be visible by eye. Thus, macroscopic bacterial colonies usually comprise hundreds of thousands, millions or tens of millions of cells in an area on a Petri dish that is typically 1–10 mm in diameter (Fig. 2.1e). Colony size is limited by nutrient availability and/or waste product accumulation in just the same way as cell concentration in liquid media. Colonies vary between bacterial species, and their shapes, sizes, opacities, surface markings and pigmentation may all be characteristic of the species in question, so these properties may be an aid in identification procedures (see Chapter 3).

Anaerobic organisms may be grown on Petri dishes provided that they are incubated in an anaerobic jar. Such jars are usually made of rigid plastic with airtight lids, and Petri dishes are placed in them together with a low temperature catalyst. The catalyst, consisting of palladium-coated pellets or wire, causes the oxygen inside the jar to be combined with hydrogen that is generated by the addition of water to sodium borohydride; this is usually contained in a foil sachet that is also placed in the jar. As the oxygen is removed, an anaerobic atmosphere is achieved and this is monitored by an oxidation reduction (redox) indicator; resazurin is frequently used, as a solution soaking a fabric strip.

Yeast colonies often look similar to those of bacteria, although they may be larger and more frequently coloured. The appearance of moulds growing on solid microbiological media is similar to their appearance when growing on common foods. The mould colony consists of a mycelium that may be loosely or densely entangled depending on the species, often with the central area (the oldest, most mature region of the colony) showing pigmentation associated with spore production (Fig. 2.1f). The periphery of the colony is that part which is actively growing and it is usually non-pigmented.

4.3 Planktonic and sessile growth

Bacteria growing in liquid culture in the laboratory usually exist as individual cells or small aggregates of cells suspended in the culture medium; the term planktonic is used to describe such freely suspended cells. In recent years, however, it has become recognized that planktonic growth is not the normal situation for bacteria growing in their natural habitats. In fact, bacteria in their natural state far more commonly grow attached to a surface which, for many species, may be solid, e.g. soil particles, stone, metal or glass, or for pathogens an epithelial surface in the body, e.g. lung or intestinal mucosa. Bacteria attached to a substrate in this way are described as sessile, and are said to exhibit the biofilm or microcolony mode of growth.

Planktonic cells are routinely used for almost all the testing procedures that have been designed to assess the activity of antimicrobial chemicals and processes, but the recognition that planktonic growth is not the natural state for many organisms prompted investigations of the relative susceptibilities of planktonic- and biofilm-grown cells to antibiotics, disinfectants and decontamination or sterilization procedures. In many cases it has been found that planktonic and sessile bacteria exhibit markedly different susceptibilities to these lethal agents, and this has prompted a reappraisal of the appropriateness of some of the procedures used (see Chapters 11 and 13).

5 Enumeration of microorganisms

In a pharmaceutical context there are several situations where it is necessary to measure the number of microbial cells in a culture, sample or specimen:

• when measuring the levels of microbial contamination in a raw material or manufactured medicine
• when evaluating the effects of an antimicrobial chemical or decontamination process
• when using microorganisms in the manufacture of therapeutic agents
• when assessing the nutrient capability of a growth medium.

In some cases it is necessary to know the total number of microbial cells present, i.e. both living and dead, e.g. in vaccine manufacture dead and living cells may both produce an immune response, and in pyrogen testing both dead and living cells induce fever when injected into the body. However, in many cases it is the number or concentration of *living* cells that is required. The terminology in microbial counting sometimes causes confusion. A *total count* is a counting procedure enumerating both living and dead cells, whereas a *viable count*, which is far more common, records the living cells alone. However, the term *total viable count* (TVC) is used in most pharmacopoeias and by many regulatory agencies to mean a viable count that records all the different species or types of microorganism that might be present in a sample.

Table 2.2 lists the more common counting methods available. The first three traditional methods of viable counting all operate on the basis that a living cell (or a small aggregate or 'clump' of cells) will give rise to a visible colony when introduced into or onto the surface of a suitable medium and incubated. Thus, the procedure for pour plating usually involves the addition of a small volume (typically 1.0 ml) of sample (or a suitable dilution thereof) into molten agar at 45°C which is then poured into empty sterile Petri dishes. After incubation the resultant colonies are counted and the total is multiplied by the dilution factor (if any) to give the concentration in the original sample. In a surface spread technique the sample (usually 0.1–0.25 ml) is spread over the surface of agar which has

Table 2.2 Traditional and rapid methods of enumerating cells

Traditional methods		Rapid methods (Indirect viable counts)
Viable counts	Total counts	
1 Pour plate (counting colonies *in* agar)	**1** Direct microscopic counting (using Helber or haemocytometer counting chambers)	**1** Epifluorescence (uses dyes that give characteristic fluorescence only in living cells) often coupled to image analysis
2 Surface spread or surface drop (Miles Misra) methods (counting colonies on agar surface)	**2** Turbidity methods (measures turbidity (opacity) in suspensions or cultures)	**2** Adenosine triphosphate (ATP) methods (measures ATP production in living cells using bioluminescence)
3 Membrane filter methods (colonies growing on membranes on agar surface)	**3** Dry weight determinations	**3** Impedance (measures changes in resistance, capacitance or impedance in growing cultures)
4 Most probable number (counts based on the proportion of liquid cultures growing after receiving low inocula)	**4** Nitrogen, protein or nucleic acid determinations	**4** Manometric methods (measure oxygen consumption or CO_2 production by growing cultures)

previously been dried to permit absorption of the added liquid. The Miles Misra (surface drop method) is similar in principle, but several individual drops of culture are allowed to spread over discrete areas of about 1 cm diameter on the agar surface. These procedures are suitable for samples that are expected to contain concentrations in excess of approximately 100 CFU ml^{-1} so that the number of colonies arising on the plate is sufficiently large to be statistically reliable. If there are no clear indications of the order of magnitude of the concentration in the sample, it is necessary to plate out the sample at each of two, three or more (decimal, i.e. 10-fold) dilutions so as to obtain Petri dishes with conveniently countable numbers of colonies (usually taken to be 30–300 colonies).

If 30 is accepted as the lowest reliable number to count and a pour plate method uses a 1.0-ml sample, it follows that the procedures described above are unsuitable for any sample that is expected to contain <30 CFU ml^{-1}, e.g. water samples where the count may be 1 CFU ml^{-1} or less. Here, membrane filter methods are used in which a large, known volume of sample is passed through the membrane which is placed, without inversion, on the agar surface. Nutrients then diffuse up through the membrane and allow the retained cells to grow into colonies on it just as they would on the agar itself.

Some of the relative merits of these procedures are described in Table 2.3.

Most probable number (MPN) counts may be used when the anticipated count is relatively low, i.e. from <1 up to 100 microorganisms per ml. The procedure involves inoculating multiple tubes of culture medium (usually three or five) with three different volumes of sample, e.g. three tubes each inoculated with 0.1 ml, three with 0.01 ml and three with 0.001 ml. If the concentration in the sample is in the range indicated above, there should be a proportion of the tubes receiving inocula in which no microorganisms are present; these will remain sterile after incubation, while others that received inocula actually containing one or more CFU show signs of growth. The proportions of positive tubes are recorded for each sample volume and the results are compared with standard tables showing the MPN of organisms per ml (or per 100 ml) of original sample. The procedure is more commonly used in the water, food and dairy industries than in the pharmaceutical industry, nevertheless it is a valid technique described in pharmacopoeias and appropriate for pharmaceutical materials, particularly water.

Turbidity measurements are the most common means of estimating the total numbers of bacteria present in a sample. Measuring the turbidity using a

Table 2.3 The relative merits of the common viable counting procedures

Counting method	Advantages	Disadvantages
Pour plate	Requires no pre-drying of the agar surface Will detect lower concentrations than surface spread/surface drop methods	Very small colonies of strict aerobes at the base of the agar may be missed Colonies of different species within the agar appear similar —so it is difficult to detect contaminants
Surface spread and surface drop methods	Surface spread often gives larger colonies than pour plates—thus they are easier to count Easier to identify contaminants by appearance of the colonies	Agar surface requires pre- drying to absorb sample Possibility of confluent growth, particularly with moulds, masking individual colonies
Membrane filtration	If necessary, will detect lower concentrations than other methods Antimicrobial chemicals in the sample can be physically removed from the cells	Viscous samples will not go through the membrane and particulate samples may block the membrane thereby restricting filtration capacity

spectrophotometer or colorimeter and reading the concentration from a calibration plot is a simple means of standardizing cell suspensions for use as inocula in antibiotic assays or other tests of anti-microbial chemicals. Fungi cannot readily be handled in this way because the suspension may not be uniform or may sediment in a spectrophotometer cuvette. Consequently, dry weight determinations on known volumes of culture are an alternative means of estimating fungal biomass. Direct microscopic counting may be an appropriate method for bacteria, yeasts and fungal spores but not for moulds, and indirect measures of biomass like assays of insoluble nitrogen, protein or nucleic acids are possible for all cell types, but rarely used outside the research laboratory.

Most of the traditional methods of viable counting suffer from the same limitations:
• relatively labour intensive
• not easy to automate
• slow, because they require an incubation period for colonies to develop or liquid cultures to become turbid
• may require relatively large volumes of culture media, many Petri dishes and a lot of incubator space.

For these reasons much interest and investigative effort has been invested in recent years in the use of so-called 'rapid' methods of detecting and counting microorganisms (see also Chapter 3). These methods enumerate viable organisms — usually bacteria and yeasts rather than moulds — in a matter of hours and eliminate the 24–48-hour (or longer) incubation periods that are typical of traditional procedures. The rapid methods employ various means of indirect detection of living cells, but the following operating principles are the most common:
• Epifluorescent techniques use fluorescent dyes that either exhibit different colours in living and dead cells (e.g. acridine orange) or appear colourless outside the cell but become fluorescent when absorbed and subjected to cellular metabolism (e.g. fluorescein diacetate).
• Living cells generate adenosine triphosphate (ATP) that can readily be detected by enzyme assays, e.g. luciferin emits light when exposed to firefly luciferase in the presence of ATP; light emission can be measured and related to bacterial concentration.
• The resistance, capacitance or impedance of a culture medium changes as a result of bacterial or yeast growth and metabolism, and these electrical properties vary in proportion to cell concentration.
• Manometric techniques are appropriate for monitoring the growth of organisms that consume or produce significant quantities of gas during their metabolism, e.g. yeasts or moulds producing carbon dioxide as a result of fermentation.

These methods are fast, readily automated and eliminate the need for numerous Petri dishes and incubators. On the other hand they require expensive equipment, have limitations in terms of detection limits and may be less readily adapted to certain types of sample than traditional methods. Furthermore, there are problems in some cases with reconciling the counts obtained by rapid methods and by traditional means. The newer techniques may detect organisms that are metabolizing but not capable of reproducing to give visible colonies, so may give values many times higher than traditional methods; this has contributed to the caution with which regulatory authorities have accepted the data generated by rapid methods. Nevertheless, they are becoming more widely accepted and are likely to become an integral part of enumeration procedures in pharmaceutical microbiology in the foreseeable future.

6 Microbial genetics

The nature of the genetic material possessed by a microbial cell and the manner in which that genetic material may be transferred to other cells depends largely upon whether the organism is a prokaryote or a eukaryote (see section 1.2).

6.1 Bacteria

The genes essential for growth and metabolism of bacteria are normally contained on a chromosome of double-stranded DNA, which is in the form of a covalently closed circle (and so designated ccc ds DNA). Additional genes that usually just confer upon the cell a survival advantage under certain circumstances may also be contained upon plasmids; these are usually similar in structure to chromosomes but much smaller and replicate independently (Chapters 3 and 13). The total complement of genes possessed by a cell, i.e. those in the chromosome, plasmid(s) and any received from other sources, e.g. bacteriophages (bacterial viruses), is referred to as the genome of the cell.

Typically bacterial chromosomes are 1 mm or more in length and contain about 1000–3000 genes. As many bacterial cells are approximately 1 µm long, it is clear that the chromosome has to be tightly coiled in order to fit in the available volume. Although all the genes are contained on a single chromosome (rather than being distributed over two or more), it is possible for a cell to contain several *copies* of that chromosome at any one time. Usually there are multiple copies during periods of rapid cell division, but some species seem to have many copies all the time. The mechanisms by which bacterial genes may be transferred from one organism to another are described in Chapter 3.

Plasmids usually resemble chromosomes except that they are approximately 0.1–1.0% of the size of a bacterial chromosome, and there are a few that are linear rather than circular. Plasmid genes are not essential for the normal functioning of the cell but may code for a property that affords a survival advantage in certain environmental conditions; bacteria possessing the plasmid in question would therefore be selected when such conditions exist. Properties which can be coded by plasmids include the ability to utilize unusual sugars or food sources, toxin production, production of pili that facilitate the attachment of a cell to a substrate (e.g. intestinal epithelium) and antibiotic resistance. A cell may contain multiple copies of any one plasmid and may contain two or more different plasmids. However, some plasmid combinations cannot co-exist inside the same cell and are said to be incompatible; this phenomenon enables plasmids to be classified into incompatibility groups.

Plasmids replicate independently of the chromosome within the cell, so that both daughter cells contain a copy of the plasmid after binary fission. Plasmids may also be passed from one cell to another by various means (Chapter 3). Some plasmids exhibit a marked degree of host specificity and may only be transmitted between different strains of the same species, although others, particularly those commonly found in Gram-negative intestinal bacteria, may cross between different species within a genus or between different genera. Conjugative (self-transmissible) plasmids code for genes that facilitate their own transmission from one cell to another by the production of pili. These sex pili initially establish contact between the two cells and then retract, drawing the donor and recipient cells together until membrane fusion occurs.

6.2 Eukaryotes

Eukaryotic microorganisms (yeasts, moulds, algae and protozoa) possess a nucleus that normally contains one or more pairs of linear chromosomes, in which the ds DNA is complexed with protein. The cells may divide asexually and the nucleus undergoes mitosis—a sequence of events by which the nucleus and the chromosomes within it are replicated to give copies identical to the originals. Most eukaryotes also have the potential for sexual reproduction during which the nucleus undergoes meiosis, i.e. a more specialized form of nuclear and chromosome division creating new gene combinations, so the offspring differ from the parents. Despite this potential, there are some eukaryotic cells, particularly fungi, in which a sexual stage in the life cycle has never been observed. Many eukaryotic microorganisms possess plasmids, and some fungal plasmids are based on RNA instead of DNA.

6.3 Genetic variation and gene expression

Microorganisms may adapt rapidly to new environments and devise strategies to avoid or negate stressful or potentially harmful circumstances. Their ability to survive adverse conditions may result from the organism using genes it already possesses, or by the acquisition of new genetic information. The term 'genotype' describes the genetic composition of an organism, i.e. it refers to the genes that the organism possesses, regardless of whether they are expressed or not. It is not uncommon for a microbial cell to possess a particular gene but not to express it, i.e. not to manufacture the protein or enzyme that is the product of that gene, unless or until the product is actually required; this is simply a mechanism to avoid wasting energy. For example, many bacteria possess the genes that code for β-lactamases; these enzymes hydrolyse and inactivate β-lactam antibiotics (e.g. penicillins). In many organisms β-lactamases are only produced in response to the presence of the antibiotic. This form of non-genetic adaptation is termed *phenotypic* adaptation, and there are many situations in which bacteria adopt a phenotypic change to counter environmental stress. But microorganisms may also use an alternative strategy of *genetic* adaptation, by which they acquire new genes either by mutation or conjugation (Chapter 3); subsequently, a process of selection ensures that the mutant organisms that are better suited to the new environment become numerically dominant.

In bacteria, mutation is an important mechanism by which resistance to antibiotics and other antimicrobial chemicals is achieved, although the receipt of entirely new genes directly from other bacteria is also clinically very important. Spontaneous mutation rates (rates not influenced by mutagenic chemicals or ionizing radiation) vary substantially depending on the gene and the organism in question, but rates of 10^{-5}–10^{-7} are typical. These values

mean that, on average, a mutant arises once in every 100 thousand to every 10 million cell divisions. Although these figures might suggest that mutation is a relatively rare event, the speed with which microorganisms can multiply means, for example, that mutants exhibiting increased antibiotic resistance can arise quite quickly during the course of therapy.

7 Pharmaceutical importance of the major categories of microorganisms

Table 2.4 indicates the ways in which the different types of microorganism are considered relevant in pharmacy. The importance of viruses derives exclusively from their pathogenic potential. Because of their lack of intrinsic metabolism viruses are not susceptible to antibiotics, and the number of effective synthetic antiviral drugs is limited. Partly for these reasons, viral infections are among the most serious and difficult to cure, and of all the categories of microorganism, only viruses appear in (the most serious) Hazard Category 4 as classified by the Advisory Committee on Dangerous Pathogens. Because they are not free-living, viruses are

Table 2.4 Pharmaceutical importance of the major categories of microorganisms

Type of organism	Pharmaceutical relevance				
	Contamination or spoilage of raw materials and medicines	Pathogens	Resistance to antibiotics and biocides	Resistance to sterilizing agents and processes	Used in the manufacture of therapeutic agents
Viruses		+			
Prions	+	+		+	
Bacteria					
Gram-negative	+	+	+		+
Gram-positive	+	+	+	+ (spores)	+
Mycobacteria		+	+		
Streptomycetes		+			+
Chlamydia		+			
Rickettsia		+			
Mycoplasma					
Fungi					
Yeasts	+	+	+		+
Moulds	+	+	+		+
Protozoa		+			

incapable of growing on manufactured medicines or raw materials, so they do not cause product spoilage, and they have no synthetic capabilities that can be exploited in medicines manufacture. Viruses are relatively easy to destroy by heat, radiation or toxic chemicals, so they do not represent a problem from this perspective. In this, they contrast with prions; while some authorities would question the categorization of these infectious agents as microorganisms, they are included here because of their undoubted ability to cause, as yet incurable, fatal disease, and their extreme resistance to lethal agents. Pharmacists and health-care personnel in general should be aware of the ability of prions to easily withstand sterilizing conditions that would be satisfactory for the destruction of all other categories of infectious agent.

There are examples of bacteria that are important in each of the different ways indicated by the column headings of Table 2.4. Many of the medically and pharmaceutically important bacteria are pathogens, and some of these pathogens are of long-standing notoriety as a result of their ability to resist the activity of antibiotics and biocides (disinfectants, antiseptics and preservatives). In addition to these long-established resistant organisms, other bacteria have given more recent cause for concern including methicillin-resistant *Staphylococcus aureus*, vancomycin-resistant enterococci and multiply resistant *Mycobacterium tuberculosis* (Chapter 13). While penicillin and cephalosporin antibiotics are produced by fungal species, the majority of the other categories of clinically important antibiotics are produced by species of bacteria, notably streptomycetes. In addition, a variety of bacteria are exploited commercially in the manufacture of other medicines including steroids, enzymes and carbohydrates. The ability of bacteria to grow on diverse substrates ensures that their potential as agents of spoilage in manufactured medicines and raw materials is well recognized, and the ability of many species to survive drying means that they survive well in dust and so become important as contaminants of manufactured medicines. The ability to survive not only in dry conditions but in other adverse environments (heat, radiation, toxic chemicals) is well exemplified by bacterial spores,

and their pre-eminence at or near the top of the 'league table' of resistance to lethal agents has resulted in spores acting as the indicator organisms that have to be eliminated in most sterilization processes.

Like bacteria, fungi are able to form spores that survive drying, so they too arise commonly as contaminants of manufactured medicines. However, the degree of resistance presented by the spores is usually less than that exhibited by bacteria, and fungi do not represent a sterilization problem. Fungi do not generally create a significant infection hazard either; relatively few fungal species are considered major pathogens for animals that possess a fully functional immune system. There are, however, several fungi which, while representing little threat to immunocompetent individuals, are nevertheless capable of initiating an infection in persons with impaired immune function; the term opportunist pathogens is used to describe microorganisms (of all types) possessing this characteristic. In this context it is worth noting that the immunocompromised represent an increasingly large group of patients, and this is not just because of HIV and AIDS. Several other conditions or drug treatments impair immune function, e.g. congenital immunodeficiency, cancer (particularly leukaemia), radiotherapy and chemotherapy, the use of systemic corticosteroids and immunosuppressive drugs (often following tissue or organ transplants), severe burns and malnutrition.

Protozoa are of significance largely owing to the pathogenic potential of a few species. Because protozoa do not possess cell walls they do not survive drying well (unless in the form of cysts), so they are not a problem in the manufacturing environment — and even the encysted forms do not display resistance to sterilizing processes to match that of bacterial spores. It should be noted that protozoal infections are not currently a major problem to human health in temperate climates, although they are more troublesome in veterinary medicine and in the tropics. There are concerns that the geographical ranges of protozoal infections like malaria may extend substantially if current fears about global warming translate into reality.

Chapter 3

Bacteria

David Allison and Peter Gilbert

1 Introduction

The smallest free-living microorganisms are the prokaryotes, comprising bacteria and archaea (see Chapter 2). Prokaryote is a term used to define cells that lack a true nuclear membrane; they contrast with eukaryotic cells (e.g. plants, animals and fungi) that possess a nuclear membrane and internal compartmentalization. Indeed, a major feature of eukaryotic cells, absent from prokaryotic cells, is the presence in the cytoplasm of membrane-enclosed organelles. These and other criteria differentiating eukaryotes and prokaryotes are shown in Table 2.1.

Bacteria and archaea share many traits and it was not until the early 1980s that differences first became evident from analyses of gene sequences. One major difference is the composition of cell walls. A more striking contrast is in the structure of the lipids that make up their cytoplasmic membranes. Differences also exist in their respective patterns of metabolism. Most archaea are anaerobes, and are often found inhabiting extreme environments. It is possible that their unusual membrane structure gives archaeal cells greater stability under extreme conditions. Of notable interest is the observation that no disease-causing archaea have yet been identified. The vast majority of prokaryotes of medical and pharmaceutical significance are bacteria.

Bacteria represent a large and diverse group of microorganisms that can exist as single cells or as cell clusters. Moreover, they are generally able to carry out their life processes of growth, energy generation and reproduction independently of other cells. In these respects they are very different to the cells of animals and plants, which are unable to live alone in nature and can exist only as part of a multicellular organism. They are capable of growing in a range of different environments and can not only cause contamination and spoilage of many pharmaceutical products but also a range of different diseases. For this reason only bacteria will be referred to throughout the remainder of this chapter.

1.1 Bacterial diversity and ubiquity

Bacterial diversity can be seen in terms of variation in cell size and shape (morphology), adaptation to environmental extremes, survival strategies and metabolic capabilities. Such diversity allows bacteria to grow in a multiplicity of environments ranging from hot sulphur springs (65°C) to deep freezers (−20°C), from high (pH 1) to low (pH 13) acidity and high (0.7 M) to low osmolarity (water). In addition, they can grow in both nutritionally rich (compost) and nutritionally poor (distilled water) situations. Hence, although each organism is uniquely suited to its own particular environmental niche and rarely grows out of it, the presence of bacteria may be considered ubiquitous. Indeed, there is no natural environment that is free from bacteria. This ubiquity is often demonstrated by terms used to describe organisms that grow and/or survive in particular environments. An example of such descriptive terminology is shown in Table 3.1.

2 Bacterial ultrastructure

2.1 Cell size and shape

Bacteria are the smallest free-living organisms, their size being measured in micrometres (microns). Be-

Table 3.1 Descriptive terms used to describe bacteria

Descriptive term	Adaptive feature
Psychrophile	Growth range −40°C to +20°C
Mesophile	Growth range +20°C to +40°C
Thermophile	Growth range +40°C to +85°C
Thermoduric	Endure high temperatures
Halophile	Salt-tolerant
Acidophile	Acid-tolerant
Aerobe	Air (oxygen) requiring
Obligate anaerobe	Air (oxygen) poisoned
Autotroph	Utilizes inorganic material
Heterotroph	Requires organic material

cause of this small size a microscope affording a considerable degree of magnification (×400–1000) is necessary to observe them. Bacteria vary in size from a cell as small as 0.1–0.2 μm in diameter to those that are >5 μm in diameter. Bacteria this large, such as *Thiomargarita namibiensis*, are extremely rare. Instead, the majority of bacteria are 1–5 μm long and 1–2 μm in diameter. By comparison, eukaryotic cells may be 2 μm to > 200 μm in diameter. The small size of bacteria has a number of implications with regard to their biological properties, most notably increased and more efficient transport rates. This advantage allows bacteria far more rapid growth rates than eukaryotic cells.

While the classification of bacteria is immensely complex, nowadays relying very much on 16S ribosomal DNA sequencing data, a more simplistic approach is to divide them into major groups on purely morphological grounds. The majority of bacteria are unicellular and possess simple shapes, e.g. round (cocci), cylindrical (rod) or ovoid. Some rods are curved (vibrios), while longer rigid curved organisms with multiple spirals are known as spirochaetes. Rarer morphological forms include the actinomycetes which are rigid bacteria resembling fungi that may grow as lengthy branched filaments; the mycoplasmas which lack a conventional peptidoglycan (murein) cell wall and are highly pleomorphic organisms of indefinite shape; and some miscellaneous bacteria comprising stalked, sheathed, budded and slime-producing forms often associated with aquatic and soil environments.

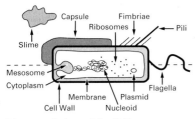

Fig. 3.1 Diagram of a bacterial cell. Features represented above the dotted line are only found in some bacteria, whereas those below the line are common to all bacteria.

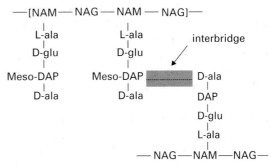

Fig. 3.2 Structure of *Escherichia coli* peptidoglycan.

Often bacteria remain together in specific arrangements after cell division. These arrangements are usually characteristic of different organisms and can be used as part of a preliminary identification. Examples of such cellular arrangements include chains of rods or cocci, paired cells (diplococci), tetrads and clusters.

2.2 Cellular components

Compared with eukaryotic cells, bacteria possess a fairly simple base cell structure, comprising cell wall, cytoplasmic membrane, nucleoid, ribosomes and occasionally inclusion granules (Fig. 3.1). Nevertheless it is important for several reasons to have a good knowledge of these structures and their functions. First, the study of bacteria provides an excellent route for probing the nature of biological processes, many of which are shared by multicellular organisms. Secondly, at an applied level, normal bacterial processes can be customized to benefit society on a mass scale. Here, an obvious example is the large-scale industrial production (fermentation) of antibiotics. Thirdly, from a pharmaceutical and health-care perspective, it is important to be able to know how to kill bacterial contaminants and disease-causing organisms. To treat infections antimicrobial agents are used to inhibit the growth of bacteria, a process known as antimicrobial chemotherapy. The essence of antimicrobial chemotherapy is selective toxicity (Chapters 10, 12 and 14), which is achieved by exploiting differences between the structure and metabolism of bacteria and host cells. Selective toxicity is, therefore, most efficient when a similar target does not exist in the host. Examples of such targets will be noted in the following sections.

2.2.1 Cell wall

The bacterial cell wall is an extremely important structure, being essential for the maintenance of the shape and integrity of the bacterial cell. It is also chemically unlike any structure present in eukaryotic cells and is therefore an obvious target for antibiotics that can attack and kill bacteria without harm to the host (Chapter 12).

The primary function of the cell wall is to provide a strong, rigid structural component that can withstand the osmotic pressures caused by high chemical concentrations of inorganic ions in the cell. Most bacterial cell walls have in common a unique structural component called peptidoglycan (also called murein or glycopeptide); exceptions include the mycoplasmas, extreme halophiles and the archaea. Peptidoglycan is a large macromolecule containing glycan (polysaccharide) chains that are cross-linked by short peptide bridges. The glycan chain acts as a backbone to peptidoglycan, and is composed of alternating residues of N-acetyl muramic acid (NAM) and N-acetyl glucosamine (NAG). To each molecule of NAM is attached a tetrapeptide consisting of the amino acids L-alanine, D-alanine, D-glutamic acid and either lysine or diaminopimelic acid (DAP). This glycan tetrapeptide repeat unit is cross-linked to adjacent glycan chains, either through a direct peptide linkage or a peptide interbridge (Fig. 3.2). The types and numbers of cross-linking amino acids vary from organism to organism. Other unusual features of the

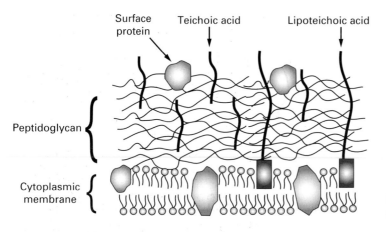

Fig. 3.3 Structure of the Gram-positive cell wall.

cell wall that provide potential antimicrobial targets are DAP and the presence of two amino acids that have the D-configuration.

Bacteria can be divided into two large groups, Gram-positive and Gram-negative, on the basis of a differential staining technique called the Gram stain. Essentially, the Gram stain consists of treating a film of bacteria dried on a microscope slide with a solution of crystal violet, followed by a solution of iodine; these are then washed with an alcohol solution. In Gram-negative organisms the cells lose the crystal violet–iodine complex and are rendered colourless, whereas Gram-positive cells retain the dye. Regardless, both cell types are counter-stained with a different coloured dye, e.g. carbol fuchsin, which is red. Hence, under the light microscope Gram-negative cells appear red while Gram-positive cells are purple. These marked differences in response reflect differences in cell wall structure. The Gram-positive cell wall consists primarily of a single type of molecule whereas the Gram-negative cell wall is a multilayered structure and quite complex.

The cell walls of Gram-positive bacteria are quite thick (20–80 nm) and consist of between 60% and 80% peptidoglycan, which is extensively cross-linked in three dimensions to form a thick polymeric mesh (Fig. 3.3). Gram-positive walls frequently contain acidic polysaccharides called teichoic acids; these are either ribitol phosphate or glycerol phosphate molecules that are connected by phosphodiester bridges. Because they are negatively charged, teichoic acids are partially responsible for the negative charge of the cell surface as a whole. Their function may be to effect passage of metal cations through the cell wall. In some Gram-positive bacteria glycerol–teichoic acids are bound to membrane lipids and are termed lipoteichoic acids. During an infection, lipoteichoic acid molecules released by killed bacteria trigger an inflammatory response. Cell wall proteins, if present, are generally found on the outer surface of the peptidoglycan.

The wall, or more correctly, envelope of Gram-negative cells is a far more complicated structure (Fig. 3.4). Although they contain less peptidoglycan (10–20% of wall), a second membrane structure is found outside the peptidoglycan layer. This outer membrane is asymmetrical, composed of proteins, lipoproteins, phospholipids and a component unique to Gram-negative bacteria, lipopolysaccharide (LPS). Essentially, the outer membrane is attached to the peptidoglycan by a lipoprotein, one end of which is covalently attached to peptidoglycan and the other end is embedded in the outer membrane. The outer membrane is not a phospholipid bilayer although it does contain phospholipids in the inner leaf, and its outer layer is composed of LPS, a polysaccharide–lipid molecule. Proteins are also found in the outer membrane, some of which form trimers and traverse the whole membrane and in so doing form water-filled channels or porins through which small molecules can pass. Other

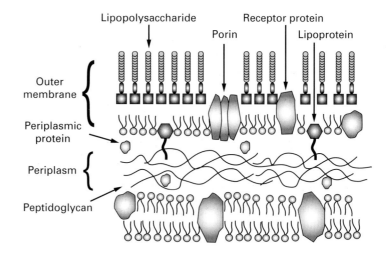

Fig. 3.4 Structure of the Gram-negative cell envelope.

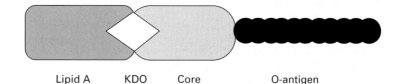

Fig. 3.5 Schematic representation of lipopolysaccharide (LPS).

proteins are found at either the inner or outer face of the membrane.

The LPS (Fig. 3.5) is an important molecule because it determines the antigenicity of the Gram-negative cell and it is extremely toxic to animal cells. The molecule consists of three regions, namely lipid A, core polysaccharide and O-specific polysaccharide. The lipid A portion is composed of a disaccharide of glucosamine phosphate bound to fatty acids and forms the outer leaflet of the membrane. It is the lipid A component that is responsible for the toxic and pyrogenic properties of Gram-negative bacteria. Lipid A is linked to the core polysaccharide by the unique molecule ketodeoxyoctonate (KDO), and at the other end of the core is the O-polysaccharide (O-antigen), which usually contains six-carbon sugars as well as one or more unusual deoxy sugars such as abequose.

Although the outer membrane is relatively permeable to small molecules, it is not permeable to enzymes or large molecules. Indeed, one of the major functions of the outer membrane may be to keep certain enzymes that are present outside the cytoplasmic membrane from diffusing away from the cell. Moreover, the outer membrane is not readily penetrated by hydrophobic compounds and is, therefore, resistant to dissolution by detergents.

The region between the outer surface of the cytoplasmic membrane and the inner surface of the outer membrane is called the periplasm. This occupies a distance of about 12–15 nm, is gel-like in consistency and, in addition to the peptidoglycan, contains sugars and an abundance of proteins including hydrolytic enzymes and transport proteins. Table 3.2 summarizes the major differences in wall composition between Gram-positive and Gram-negative cells.

2.2.2 Cytoplasmic membrane

Biochemically, the cytoplasmic membrane is a fragile, phospholipid bilayer with proteins distributed randomly throughout. These are involved in the various transport and enzyme functions

Table 3.2 Gram-positive and Gram-negative cell wall composition

Feature	Gram-positive cells	Gram-negative cells
Peptidoglycan	60–80%	10–20%
Teichoic acid	Present	Absent
Lipoteichoic acid	Present	Absent
Lipoprotein	Absent	Present
Lipopolysaccharide	Absent	Present
Protein	c. 15%	c. 60%
Lipid	c. 2%	c. 20%

associated with the membrane. A major difference in chemical composition between prokaryotic and eukaryotic cells is that eukaryotes have sterols in their membranes (e.g. cholesterol) whereas prokaryotes do not. The cytoplasmic membrane serves many functions, including transport of nutrients, energy generation and electron transport; it is the location for regulatory proteins and biosynthetic proteins, and it acts as a semi-permeable selectivity barrier between the cytoplasm and the cell environment.

Invaginations of the cytoplasmic membrane are referred to as mesosomes. Those that form near the septum of Gram-positive cells serve as organs of attachment for the bacterial chromosome.

2.2.3 Cytoplasm

The cytoplasm consists of approximately 80% water and contains enzymes that generate ATP directly by oxidizing glucose and other carbon sources. The cytoplasm also contains some of the enzymes involved in the synthesis of peptidoglycan subunits. Ribosomes, the DNA genome (nucleoid) and inclusion granules are also found in the cytoplasm.

2.2.4 Nucleoid

The bacterial chromosome exists as a singular, covalently closed circular molecule of double-stranded DNA comprising approximately 4600 kilobase pairs. It is complexed with small amounts of proteins and RNA, but unlike eukaryotic DNA,

is not associated with histones. The DNA, if linearized, would be about 1 mm in length. In order to package this amount of material the cell requires that the DNA is supercoiled into a number of domains (c. 50) and that the domains are associated with each other and stabilized by specific proteins into an aggregated mass or nucleoid. The enzymes, topoisomerases, that control topological changes in DNA architecture are different from their eukaryotic counterparts (which act on linear chromosomes) and therefore provide a unique biochemical target for antibiotic action.

2.2.5 Plasmids

Plasmids are relatively small, circular pieces of double-stranded extrachromosomal DNA. They are capable of autonomous replication and encode for many auxiliary functions that are not usually necessary for bacterial growth. One such function of great significance is that of antibiotic resistance (Chapter 13). Plasmids may also transfer readily from one organism to another, and between species, thereby increasing the spread of resistance.

2.2.6 Ribosomes

The cytoplasm is densely packed with ribosomes. Unlike eukaryotic cells these are not associated with a membranous structure; the endoplasmic reticulum is not a component of prokaryotic cells. Bacterial ribosomes are 70S in size, comprising two subunits of 30S and 50S. This is smaller than eukaryotic ribosomes, which are 80S in size (40S and 60S subunits). Differences will therefore exist in the size and geometry of RNA binding sites.

2.2.7 Inclusion granules

Bacteria occasionally contain inclusion granules within their cytoplasm. These consist of storage material composed of carbon, nitrogen, sulphur or phosphorus and are formed when these materials are replete in the environment to act as repositories of these nutrients when limitations occur. Examples include poly-β-hydroxybutyrate, glycogen and polyphosphate.

2.3 Cell surface components

The surface of the bacterial cell is the portion of the organism that interacts with the external environment most directly. As a consequence, many bacteria deploy components on their surfaces in a variety of ways that allow them to withstand and survive fluctuations in the growth environment. The following sections describe a few of these components that are commonly found, although not universally, that allow bacteria to move, sense their environment, attach to surfaces and provide protection from harsh conditions.

2.3.1 Flagella

Bacterial motility is commonly provided by flagella, long (c. 12 μm) helical-shaped structures that project from the surface of the cell. The filament of the flagellum is built up from multiple copies of the protein flagellin. Where the filament enters the surface of the bacterium, there is a hook in the flagellum, which is attached to the cell surface by a series of complex proteins called the flagellar motor. This rotates the flagellum, causing the bacterium to move through the environment. The numbers and distribution of flagella vary with bacterial species. Some have a single, polar flagellum, whereas others are flagellate over their entire surface (peritrichous); intermediate forms also exist.

2.3.2 Fimbriae

Fimbriae are structurally similar to flagella, but are not involved in motility. While they are straighter, more numerous and considerably thinner and shorter (3 μm) than flagella, they do consist of protein and project from the cell surface. There is strong evidence to suggest that fimbriae act primarily as adhesins, allowing organisms to attach to surfaces, including animal tissues in the case of some pathogenic bacteria, and to initiate biofilm formation. Fimbriae are also responsible for haemagglutination and cell clumping in bacteria. Among the best characterized fimbriae are the type I fimbriae of enteric (intestinal) bacteria.

2.3.3 Pili

Pili are morphologically and chemically similar to fimbriae, but they are present in much smaller numbers (< 10) and are usually longer. They are involved in the genetic exchange process of conjugation (section 6.3).

2.3.4 Capsules and slime layers

Many bacteria secrete extracellular polysaccharides (EPS) that are associated with the exterior of the bacterial cell. The EPS is composed primarily of c. 2% carbohydrate and 98% water, and provides a gummy exterior to the cell. Morphologically, two extreme forms exist: capsules, which form a tight, fairly rigid layer closely associated with the cell, and slimes, which are loosely associated with the cell. Both forms function similarly, to offer protection against desiccation, to provide a protective barrier against the penetration of biocides, disinfectants and positively charged antibiotics, to protect against engulfment by phagocytes and protozoa and to act as a cement binding cells to each other and to the substratum in biofilms. One such polymer that performs all these functions is alginate, produced by *Pseudomonas aeruginosa*. Bacterial EPS such as alginate and the high molecular weight dextrans produced by *Leuconostoc mesenteroides* may be harvested and used as pharmaceutical aids, surgical dressings and drug delivery systems.

2.3.5 S-layers

Many bacteria produce a cell surface layer composed of a two-dimensional paracrystalline array of proteins termed S-layers. These show various symmetries and can associate with a variety of cell wall structures. Although their true function is currently unknown it is likely that they will act to a certain extent as an external permeability barrier.

3 Biofilms

Any surface, whether it is animate or inanimate, is of considerable importance as a microbial habitat owing to the adsorption of nutrients. As such, a nutrient-rich micro-environment is produced in a nutrient-poor macro-environment whenever a surface–liquid interface exists. Consequently, microbial numbers and activity are usually much greater on a surface than in suspension. Hence, in many natural, medical and industrial settings bacteria attach to surfaces and form multilayered communities called biofilms. These commonly contain more than one species of bacteria, which co-operatively exist together as a functional, dynamic consortium. Biofilm formation usually begins with pioneer cells attaching to a surface, either through the use of specific adhesins such as fimbriae, or non-specifically by EPS. Once established, these cells grow and divide to produce microcolonies, which with time, eventually coalesce to produce a biofilm. A key characteristic of biofilms is the enveloping of the attached cells in EPS. Biofilms help trap nutrients for growth of the enclosed cells and help prevent detachment of cells on surfaces in flowing systems.

Biofilms have a number of significant implications in medicine and industry. In the human body the resident cells within the biofilm are not exposed to attack by the immune system and in some instances can exacerbate the inflammatory response. An example of this type is shown by the growth of *P. aeruginosa* as an alginate-enclosed biofilm in the lungs of cystic fibrosis patients. Bacterial biofilms are also profoundly less susceptible to antimicrobial agents than their free-living, planktonic counterparts. As a consequence, bacterial biofilms that form on contaminated medical implants and prosthetic devices, manufacturing surfaces or fluid conduit systems are virtually impossible to eliminate with antibiotics or biocides. In these situations antimicrobial resistance occurs as a population or community response.

4 Bacterial sporulation

In a few bacterial genera, notably *Bacillus* and *Clostridium*, a unique process takes place in which the vegetative cell undergoes a profound biochemical change to give rise to a specialized structure called an endospore or spore (Fig. 3.6). This process of sporulation is not part of a reproductive cycle,

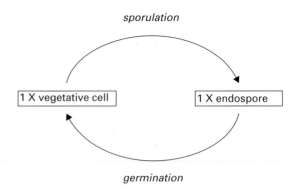

Fig. 3.6 Bacterial sporulation and germination.

but the spore is a highly resistant cell that enables the producing organism to survive in adverse environmental conditions such as lack of moisture or essential nutrients, toxic chemicals, radiation and high temperatures. Because of their extreme resistance to radiation, ethylene oxide and heat, all sterilization processes for pharmaceutical products have been designed to destroy the bacterial spore (Chapter 20). Removal of the environmental stress may lead to germination of the spore back to the vegetative cell form.

4.1 Endospore structure

Endospores are differentiated cells that possess a grossly different structure to that of the parent vegetative cell in which they are formed. The structure of the spore is much more complex than that of the vegetative cell in that it has many layers surrounding a central core (Fig. 3.7). The outermost layer is the exosporium composed of protein; within this are the spore coats, which are also proteinaceous but with a high cysteine content, the cortex that consists of loosely cross-linked peptidoglycan and the central core that contains the genome. Characteristic of the spore is the presence of dipicolinic acid and high levels of calcium ions which complex together. The core is also partially dehydrated, containing only 10–30% of the water content of the vegetative cells. Dehydration has been shown to increase resistance to both heat and chemicals. In addition, the pH of the core is about 1 unit lower than the cytoplasm of the vegetative cell and contains high levels of core-specific proteins that

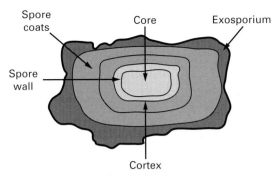

Fig. 3.7 Diagram of endospore structure.

bind tightly to the DNA and protect it from potential damage. These core-specific proteins also function as an energy source for the outgrowth or germination of a new vegetative cell from the endospore.

4.2 Endospore formation

During endospore formation the vegetative cell undergoes a complex series of biochemical events in cellular differentiation, and many genetically directed changes in the cell that underpin the conversion occur in a series of distinct stages. Sporulation requires that the synthesis of some proteins involved in vegetative cell function cease and that specific spore proteins are made. This is accomplished by activation of a variety of spore-specific genes such as *spo* and *ssp*. The proteins coded by these genes catalyse a series of events leading ultimately to the production of a dry, metabolically inert but extremely resistant endospore. The whole process can take only a matter of hours to complete under optimal conditions.

4.3 Endospore germination

Although endospores can lie dormant for decades, they can revert back to a vegetative cell very rapidly. Activation of the process may occur through removal of the stress-inducer that initiated sporulation. During germination loss of resistance properties occurs along with a loss of calcium dipicolinate and cortex components, and degradation of the core-specific proteins. Outgrowth occurs, involving water uptake and synthesis of new RNA, proteins and DNA until eventually, after a matter of minutes, the vegetative cell emerges from the fractured spore coat and begins to divide again.

5 Bacterial toxins

Although bacteria are associated with disease, only a few species are disease-producing or pathogenic (Chapter 7). Of greater concern are those organisms that, if presented with the correct set of conditions, can cause disease, i.e. opportunist pathogens. Examples include *Staphylococcus epidermidis*, a beneficial organism when present on the skin (its normal habitat) yet potentially fatal if attached to a synthetic heart valve, and *P. aeruginosa*, a non-pathogenic environmental organism but again potentially lethal in immunocompromised patients.

The pathogens cause host damage in a number of ways. In most cases pathogens produce a variety of molecules or factors that promote pathogenesis, among which are the toxins: products of bacteria that produce immediate host cell damage. Toxins have been classified as either endotoxin, i.e. cell wall-related, or exotoxin, products released extracellularly as the organism grows.

Endotoxin is the lipid A component of LPS (see section 2.2.1). It possesses multiple biological properties including the ability to induce fever, initiate the complement and blood cascades, activate β lymphocytes and stimulate production of tumour necrosis factor. Endotoxin is generally released from lysed or damaged cells. Care must be taken to eliminate or exclude such heat-resistant material from parenteral products and their delivery systems through a process known as depyrogenation (Chapter 20).

Most exotoxins fall into one of three categories on the basis of their structure and activities. These are the A-B toxins, the cytolytic toxins and the superantigen toxins. The A-B toxins consist of a B subunit that binds to a host cell receptor, covalently bound to the A subunit that mediates the enzymic activity responsible for toxicity. Most exotoxins (e.g. diphtheria toxin, cholera toxin) are of the A-B category. The cytolytic toxins such as haemolysins and phospholipases do not have separable A and B portions but work by enzymically attacking cell constituents, causing lysis. The superantigens also lack an A-B type structure and act by stimulating large numbers of immune response cells to release cytokines, resulting in a massive inflammatory reaction. An example of this type of reaction is *Staphylococcus aureus*-mediated toxic shock syndrome.

6 Bacterial reproduction and growth kinetics

6.1 Multiplication and division cycle

The majority of bacterial cells multiply in number by a process of binary fission. That is, each individual will increase in size until it is large enough to divide into two identical daughter cells. At the point of separation each daughter cell must be capable of growth and reproduction. While each daughter cell will automatically contain those materials that are dispersed throughout the mother cell (mRNA, rRNA, ribosomes, enzymes, cytochromes, etc.), each must also carry at least one copy of the chromosome. The bacterial chromosome is circular and attached to the cytoplasmic membrane where it is able to uncoil during DNA replication. The process of DNA replication proceeds at a fixed rate dependent upon temperature, therefore the time taken to copy an entire chromosome depends on the number of base pairs within it and the growth temperature. For *Escherichia coli* growing at 37°C replication of the chromosome will take approximately 45 minutes. These copies of the chromosome must then segregate to opposite sides of the cell before cell division can proceed. Division occurs in different ways for Gram-positive and Gram-negative bacteria. Gram-negative cells do not have a rigid cell wall and divide by a process of constriction followed by membrane fusion. Gram-positive cells, on the other hand, having a rigid cell wall, must develop a cross-wall (see Fig. 2.1a) that divides the cell into two equal halves. Constriction and cross-wall formation takes approximately 15 minutes to complete. DNA replication, chromosome segregation (C-phase) and cell division (D-phase) occur sequentially in slow-growing cells with generation times of

greater than 1 hour and are the final events of the bacterial cell cycle. Cells are able to replicate faster than once every hour by initiating several rounds of DNA replication at a time. Thus partially replicated chromosomes become segregated into the newly formed daughter cells. In this fashion it is possible for some organisms growing under their optimal conditions to divide every 15–20 minutes. Rod-shaped organisms maintain their diameter during the cell cycle and increase their mass and volume by a process of elongation. When the length of the cell has approximately doubled then the division/constriction occurs centrally. Coccal forms increase in size by radial expansion with the division plane going towards the geometric centre. In some genera the successive division planes are always parallel. Under such circumstances the cells appear to form chains (i.e. streptococci). In staphylococci successive division planes are randomized, giving dividing clusters of cells the appearance of a bunch of grapes. Certain genera, e.g. *Sarcina*, rotate successive division planes by 90° to form tetrads and cubical octets. The appearance of dividing cells under the microscope can therefore be a useful initial guide to identification.

6.2 Population growth

When placed in favourable conditions populations of bacteria can increase at remarkable rates, given that each division gives rise to two identical daughter cells, then each has the potential to divide again. Thus cell numbers will increase exponentially as a function of time. For a microorganism growing with a generation time of 20 minutes, one cell will have divided three times within an hour to give a total of eight cells. After 20 hours of continued division at this rate then the accumulated mass of bacterial cells would be approximately 70 kg (the weight of an average man). Ten hours later the mass would be equivalent to the combined body weight of the entire population of the UK. Clearly this does not happen in nature, rather the supply of nutrients becomes exhausted and the organisms grow considerably more slowly, if at all.

The time interval between one cell division and the next is called the generation time. When considering a growing culture containing thousands of cells, a mean generation time is usually calculated. As one cell doubles to become two cells, which then multiply to become four cells and so on, the number of bacteria n in any generation can be expressed as:

1st generation $n = 1 \times 2 = 2^1$
2nd generation $n = 1 \times 2 \times 2 = 2^2$
3rd generation $n = 1 \times 2 \times 2 \times 2 = 2^3$
xth generation $n = 1 \times 2^x = 2^x$

For an initial population of N_o cells, as distinct from one cell, at the xth generation the cell population will be:

$$N = N_o \times 2^x$$

where N is the final cell number, N_o the initial cell number and x the number of generations. To express this equation in terms of x, then:

$$\text{Log } N = \log N_o + x \log 2$$

$$\text{Log } N - \log N_o = x \log 2$$

$$x = \frac{\log N - \log N_o}{\log 2} = \frac{\log N - \log N_o}{0.301}$$

$$x = 3.3(\log N - \log N_o)$$

The actual generation time is calculated by dividing x into t where t represents the hours or minutes of exponential growth.

6.2.1 Growth on solid surfaces

If microorganisms are immobilized on a solid surface from which they can derive nutrients and remain moist, cell division will cause the daughter cells to form a localized colony. In spite of the small size of the individual organisms, colonies are easily visible to the naked eye. Indeed microbial growth can often be seen on the tonsils of an infected individual or as colonies on discarded or badly stored foods. In the laboratory solidified growth media are deployed to separate different types of bacteria and also as an aid to enumerating viable cell numbers. These media comprise a nutrient soup (broth) that has been solidified by the addition of agar (see Chapter 2). Agar melts and dissolves in boiling water but will not resolidify until the temperature is below 45°C. Agar media are used in the laboratory either poured as a thin layer into a covered dish

(Petri dish) or contained within a small, capped bottle (slant). If suspensions of different species of bacteria are spread onto the surface of a nutrient agar plate then each individual cell will produce a single visible colony. These may be counted to obtain an estimate of the original number of cells. Different species will produce colonies of slightly different appearance, enabling judgements to be made as to the population diversity. The colour, size, shape and texture of colonies of different species of bacteria vary considerably and form a useful diagnostic aid to identification. Transfer of single colonies from the plate to a slant enables pure cultures of each organism to be maintained, cultured and identified.

6.2.2 Growth in liquids

When growing on a solid surface the size of the resultant colony is governed by the local availability of nutrients. These must diffuse through the colony. Eventually growth ceases when the rate of consumption of nutrients exceeds the rate of supply. When grown in liquids the bacteria, being of colloidal dimension and sometimes highly motile, are dispersed evenly through the fluid. Nutrients are therefore equally available to all cells. When considering growth of bacterial populations in liquids it is necessary to consider whether the environment is closed or open with respect to the acquisition of fresh nutrient. Closed systems are typified by batch culture in closed glass flasks. In these waste products of metabolism are retained and all the available nutrients are present at the beginning of growth. Open systems on the other hand have a continual supply of fresh nutrients and removal of waste products.

6.2.2.1 Liquid batch culture (closed)

Figure 3.8 shows the pattern of population growth obtained when a small sample of bacteria is placed within a suitable liquid growth medium held in a glass vessel. As the increase in cell numbers is exponential (1, 2, 4, 8, 16, etc.) then during active growth a logarithmic plot of cell number against time gives a straight line (B). This period is often referred to as the logarithmic growth phase, during which the generation or doubling time may be calculated from the slope of the line. However, the

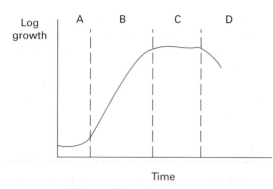

Fig. 3.8 Typical bacterial growth curve in closed batch liquid culture. (A) Lag or adaptive phase; (B) logarithmic or exponential phase; (C) stationary phase; (D) decline phase.

exponential phase is preceded by a lag period (A), during which time the inoculum adapts its physiology to that required for growth on the available nutrients. As growth proceeds nutrients are consumed and waste materials accumulate. This has the effect of reducing the rate of growth (late logarithmic phase) towards an eventual halt (stationary phase, C). Starvation during the stationary phase will eventually lead to the death of some of the cells and adaptation to a dormant state in others (decline phase, D). Patterns of growth such as this occur within inadequately preserved pharmaceutical products, in water storage tanks and in industrial fermentations.

6.2.2.2 Growth in open culture

Except under circumstances of feast–famine, growth of bacteria in association with humans and in our environment is subject to a gradual but continuous provision of nutrients and a dilution of waste products. Under such circumstances the rate of growth of bacteria is governed by the rate of supply of nutrients and the population size. Accordingly, bacteria in our gastrointestinal tracts receive a more or less continuous supply of food and excess bacteria are voided with the faeces (indeed bacteria make up > 90% of the dry mass of faeces). In many situations the bacteria become immobilized, as a biofilm, upon a surface and extract nutrients from the bulk fluid phase.

6.3 Growth and genetic exchange

For many years it was thought that bacteria, dividing by binary fission, had no opportunity for the exchange of genetic material and could only adapt and evolve through mutation of genes. This is not only untrue but masks the profound ability of bacteria to exchange and share DNA across diverse genera. This is of particular significance because it enables bacterial populations to adapt rapidly to changes in their environment, whether this is related to the appearance of a novel food or to the deployment of antibacterial chemicals and antibiotics. Three major processes of genetic exchange can be identified in bacteria — transformation, transduction and conjugation. Further details of these processes appear in Chapter 13 dealing with the development and spread of antibiotic resistance.

6.3.1 Transformation

In 1928 Griffith noticed that a culture of *Streptococcus pneumoniae* that had mutated to become deficient in capsule production could be restored to its normal capsulate form by incubation with a cell-free filtrate taken from a culture of the normal strain. While this discovery preceded the discovery of DNA as the genetic library and was only poorly understood at the time, it demonstrated the ability of certain types of bacteria to absorb small pieces of naked DNA from the environment that may recombine into the recipient chromosome. The process has become known as transformation and is likely to occur naturally in situations such as septic abscesses and in biofilms where high cell densities are associated with death and lysis of significant portions of the population. Transformation is also exploited in molecular biology as a means of transferring genes between different types of bacteria.

6.3.2 Transduction

Viruses are discussed more fully elsewhere (Chapter 5); however, there is a group of viruses, called bacteriophages, which have bacterial cells as their hosts. These bacteriophages inject viral DNA into the host cell. This viral DNA is then replicated and transcribed at the expense of the host and assembled into new viral particles. Under normal circumstances the host cell becomes lysed in order to release the viral progeny, but in exceptional circumstances, rather than enter a replication cycle the viral DNA becomes incorporated, by recombination, into the chromosome of the bacterium. This is known as a temperate phage. The viral DNA thus forms part of the bacterial chromosome and will be copied to all daughter cells. Temperate phage will become active once again at a low frequency and phasing between temperate and lytic forms ensures the long-term survival of the virus. Occasionally during this transition back to the lytic form the excision of the viral DNA from the bacterial chromosome is inaccurate. The resultant virus may then either be defective, if viral DNA has been lost, or it may carry additional DNA of bacterial origin. Subsequent temperate infections caused by the latter virions will result in this bacterial DNA having moved between cells: a process of gene movement known as transduction. As the host range of some bacteriophages is broad then such processes can move DNA between diverse species.

6.3.3 Conjugation

Conjugation is thought to have evolved through transduction, and relates to the generation of defective viral DNA. This can be transcribed to produce singular viral elements, which cannot assemble or lyse the host cell. Such DNA strands are known as plasmids. They are circular and can either be integrated into the main chromosome, in which case they are replicated along with the chromosome and passed to daughter cells, or they are separate from it and can replicate independently. The simplest form of plasmid is the F-factor (fertility factor); this can be transcribed at the cell membrane to generate an F-pilus within the cell envelope and cells containing an F-factor are designated F^+. The F-pilus is a hollow appendage that is capable of transferring DNA from one cell to another, through a process that is very similar to the injection of viral DNA into a cell during infection. In its simplest form an unassociated F-factor will simply transfer a copy to a recipient cell, and such a transfer process is known as

conjugation. Integration with, and dissociation of, the F-factor with the chromosome occurs randomly. When it is in the integrated form, designated Hfr (high frequency of recombination), then not only can a copy of the plasmid DNA be transferred across the F-pilus but so also can a partial or complete copy of the donor chromosome. Subsequent recombination events incorporate the new DNA into the recipient chromosome.

Just as the excision of temperate viral DNA from the host chromosome could be inaccurate, and lead to additions and deletions from the sequence, so too can the F-factor gather chromosomal DNA as the host cells change from Hfr to F^+. In such instances the plasmid that is formed will transfer not only itself but also this additional DNA into recipient cells. This is particularly significant because the unassociated plasmid can replicate autonomously from the chromosome to achieve a high copy number. It can also be transferred simultaneously to many recipient bacteria. If the transported DNA encoded a mechanism of antibiotic resistance (Chapter 13) it would not be difficult to imagine how whole populations could rapidly acquire the resistance characteristics.

7 Environmental factors that influence growth and survival

The rate of growth of a microbial population depends upon the nature and availability of water and nutrients, temperature, pH, the partial pressure of oxygen and solute concentrations. In many laboratory experiments the microorganisms are provided with an excess of complex organic nutrients and are maintained at optimal pH and temperature. This enables growth to be very rapid and the results visualized within a relatively short time period. Such idealized conditions rarely exist in nature, where microorganisms not only compete with one another for nutrients but also grow under suboptimal conditions. Particular groups of organisms are adapted to survive under particular conditions; thus Gram-negative bacteria tend to be aquatic whereas Gram-positive bacteria tend to prefer more arid conditions such as the skin. The next two sections of this chapter will consider separately the

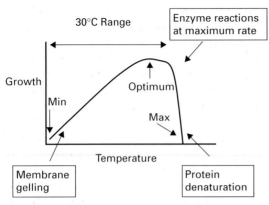

Fig. 3.9 The effect of temperature on bacterial growth.

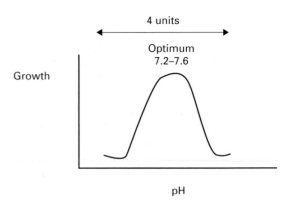

Fig. 3.10 The effect of pH on bacterial growth.

physicochemical factors that affect growth and survival of bacteria, and the availability and nature of the available nutrients.

7.1 Physicochemical factors that affect growth and survival of bacteria

7.1.1 Temperature

Earlier in this chapter various classes of bacteria (thermophile, mesophile, etc.) were described according to the range of temperatures under which they could grow. The majority of bacteria that have medical or pharmaceutical significance are mesophiles and have optimal growth temperatures between ambient and body temperature (37°C). Individual species of bacteria also have a range of temperatures under which they can actively grow and multiply (permissive temperatures). For every organism there is a minimum temperature below which no growth occurs, an optimum temperature at which growth is most rapid and a maximum temperature above which growth is not possible (Fig. 3.9). As temperatures rise, chemical and enzymic reactions within the cell proceed more rapidly, and growth becomes faster until an optimal rate is achieved. Beyond this temperature certain proteins may become irreversibly damaged through thermal lysis, resulting in a rapid loss of cell viability.

The optimum temperature for growth is much nearer the maximum value than the minimum and the range of the permissive temperatures can be quite narrow (3–4°C) for obligate pathogens yet broad (10–20°C) for environmental isolates, reflecting the range of temperatures that they are likely to encounter in their specialized niches. If the temperature exceeds the permissive range then provided that lethal temperatures are not achieved (c. 60°C for most Gram-negative mesophiles) the organisms will survive but not grow. Temperatures of 105°C and above are rapidly lethal and can be deployed to sterilize materials and products. Generally bacteria are able to survive temperatures beneath the permissive range provided that they are gradually acclimatized to them.

7.1.2 pH

As for temperature, each individual microorganism has an optimal pH for growth and a range about that optimum where growth can occur albeit at a slower pace. Unlike the response to temperature, pH effects on growth are bell-shaped (Fig. 3.10), and extremes of pH can be lethal. Generally those microorganisms that have medical or pharmaceutical significance have pH growth optima of between 7.4 and 7.6 but may grow suboptimally at pH values of 5–8.5. Thus growth of lactobacilli within the vaginal vault reduces the pH to approximately 5.5 and prevents the growth of many opportunist pathogens. Accordingly, the pH of a pharmaceutical preparation may dictate the range of microorganisms that could potentially cause its spoilage.

7.1.3 Water activity/solutes

Water is essential for the growth of all known forms of life. Gram-negative bacteria are particularly adapted to an existence in, and are able to extract trace nutrients from, the most dilute environments. This adaptation has its limitations because the Gram-negative cell envelope cannot withstand the high internal osmotic pressures associated with rapid re-hydration after desiccation and the organisms are unable to grow in the presence of high concentrations of solute. The availability of water is reflected in the water activity of a material or liquid. Water activity (Aw) is defined as the vapour pressure of water in the space above the material relative to the vapour pressure above pure water at the same temperature and pressure. Pure water by definition has an Aw of 1.00. Pharmaceutical creams might have Aw values of 0.8–0.98, whereas strawberry jam might have an Aw of c. 0.7. Generally Gram-negative bacteria cannot grow if the Aw is below 0.97, whereas Gram-positive bacteria can grow in materials with Aw of 0.8–0.98 and can survive re-hydration after periods of desiccation, hence their dominance in the soil. Yeasts and moulds can grow at low Aw values, hence their appearance on moist bathroom walls and on the surface of jam. The water activity of a pharmaceutical product can markedly affect its vulnerability to spoilage contaminants (see Chapter 16).

7.1.4 Availability of oxygen

For many aerobic microorganisms oxygen acts as the terminal electron acceptor in respiration and is essential for growth. Alternate terminal electron acceptors are organic molecules whose reduction leads to the generation of organic acids such as lactic acid. They can sometimes be utilized under conditions of low oxygen or where carbon substrate is in excess (fermentation), and highly specialized groups of microorganisms can utilize inorganic materials such as iron as electron acceptors (e.g. iron-sulphur bacteria). Different groups of organisms therefore vary in their dependence upon oxygen. Paradoxically there are many bacteria for which oxygen is highly toxic (obligate anaerobes), so the presence or absence of oxygen within a nutrient environment can profoundly affect both the rate and nature of the microbial growth obtained. Strongly oxygen-dependent bacteria will tend to grow as a thin pellicle on the surfaces of liquid media where oxygen is most available. Special media and anaerobic chambers are required to grow obligate anaerobes within the laboratory, yet such organisms persist and actively grow within the general environment. This is because the close proximity of strongly aerobic cells and anaerobes will create an anoxic micro-environment in which the anaerobe can flourish. This is particularly the case for the mouth and gastrointestinal tract where obligate anaerobes such as *Bacteroides* and *Fusobacter* can be found in association with strongly aerobic streptococci.

The inability of oxygen to diffuse adequately into a liquid culture is often the factor that causes an onset of stationary phase, so culture density is limited by oxygen demand. The cell density at stationary phase can often be increased, therefore, by shaking the flask or providing baffles. Diffusion of oxygen may also be a factor limiting the size of bacterial colonies formed on an agar surface.

7.2 Nutrition and growth

Bacteria vary considerably in their requirements for nutrients and in their ability to synthesize for themselves various vitamins and growth factors. Clearly the major elemental requirements for growth will match closely the elemental composition of the bacteria themselves. In this fashion there is a need for the provision of carbon, nitrogen, water, phosphorus, potassium and sulphur with a minor requirement for trace elements such as magnesium, calcium, iron, etc. The most independent classes of bacteria are able to derive much of their nutrition from simple inorganic forms of these elements. These organisms are called chemolithotrophs and can even utilize atmospheric carbon dioxide and nitrogen as sources of carbon and nitrogen. Indeed, such bacteria are, in addition to the green plants and algae, a major source of organic molecules and so they are more beneficial than problematic to man. The majority of bacteria require a fixed carbon source, usually in the form of a sugar, but this may also be obtained from complex organic molecules such as benzene, paraffin waxes and proteins. Nitrogen can generally be obtained from ammonium ions but is also available by deamination of amino acids, which can thus provide both carbon and nitrogen sources simultaneously. Many classes of bacteria are auxotrophic and can grow on simple sugars together with ammonium ions, a source of potassium and trace elements. Such bacteria can synthesize for themselves all the amino acids and ancillary factors required for growth and division. These bacteria, e.g. pseudomonads and *Achromobacter* species, are generally free-living environmental strains but they can sometimes cause infections in immunocompromised people. In the laboratory they can be grown in simple salts media with few, if any, complex supplements. The rate of growth of such organisms depends not only on temperature and pH but also on the nature of the carbon and nitrogen sources. Thus, a faster rate of growth is often obtained when glucose or succinate is the carbon source rather than lactose or glycerol, and when amino acids are provided as sources of nitrogen rather than ammonium salts. If faced with a choice of carbon and nitrogen sources then the bacteria will adapt their physiology to the preferred substrate and only when this is depleted will they turn their attention to the less preferred substrate. Growth in liquid cultures with dual provision of substrate such as this is often characterized by a second lag phase during the logarithmic growth period while this adaptation takes place. This is called diauxic growth (Fig. 3.11).

As the association between bacteria and higher life forms becomes closer then more and more preformed biosynthetic building blocks become available without the need to synthesize them from their basic elements. Thus a pathogenic organism growing in soft tissues will have available to it glucose and metal ions from the blood and a whole plethora of amino acids, bases, vitamins, etc. from lysed tissue cells. While most bacteria will utilize these when they are available, a number of bacteria that have become specialized pathogens have lost their ability to synthesize many of these chemicals and so cannot grow in situations where the chemicals are not provided in the medium. Consequently many pathogens require complex growth media if they are to be cultured *in vitro*.

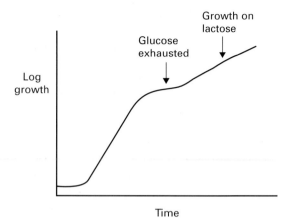

Fig. 3.11 Diauxic growth on a mixture of glucose and lactose.

All that has been discussed earlier about the physicochemical and nutritional constraints on bacterial growth has been based on laboratory studies. By definition, the only bacteria that we can describe in this way are those that can be cultured artificially. It cannot be overstated that a majority of bacterial species and genera cannot be cultured in the laboratory. In the past the presence of such nonculturable bacteria has been attributed to dead, moribund cells. With the advent of modern molecular tools, however, it has now been realized that these organisms are viable. By amplifying their DNA and sequence mapping, the genetic relationship of such bacteria to the culturable ones can be demonstrated and whole new families of hitherto unrecognized bacteria are being identified. It is possible that in the future many disease states currently thought to have no microbiological involvement could be identified as being of bacterial origin. A recent example of this has been the association of *Helicobacter pylori* with gastric ulcers and gastric cancers.

8 Detection, identification and characterization of organisms of pharmaceutical and medical significance

There are many situations in which microorganisms must not only be detected and enumerated but where they must also be identified either to make a specific diagnosis of infection or to ensure the absence of specified bacteria from certain types of product. In such circumstances various cultural approaches are available that deploy enrichment and selection media. Once a microorganism has been isolated in pure culture, usually from a single colony grown on an agar plate, then further characterization may be made by the application of microscopy together with some relatively simple biochemical tests. Over the last 20 years the biochemical characterization of individual organisms has become simplified by the introduction of rapid identification systems. In recent years molecular approaches have enabled identification of organisms without the need to culture them.

8.1 Culture techniques

Conventional approaches to microbiological examination of specimens require that they be cultured to assess the total numbers of specific groups of microorganisms or to determine the presence or absence of particular named species. The majority of samples taken for examination contain mixtures of different species, so simple plating onto an agar surface may fail to detect an organism that is present at < 2 % of the total viable population. Various enrichment culture techniques may therefore be deployed to detect trace numbers of particular pathogens, prior to confirmatory identification.

8.1.1 Enumeration

The simplest way in which to enumerate the microorganisms that contaminate an object or liquid sample is to dilute that sample to varying degrees and inoculate the surface of a pre-dried nutrient agar with known volumes of those dilutions (see Chapter 2). Individual viable bacteria that are able to grow on the nutrients provided and under the conditions of incubation will produce visible colonies that can be counted and the numbers related back to the original sample. Such counting procedures are often lengthy and tedious, the number of colonies formed might not relate to the viable number of cells, as clumps of cells will only produce a single colony and they will only detect a particular subset of the viable bacteria present in the sample

that can grow under the chosen conditions. Accordingly a variety of different media and cultural conditions are deployed to enumerate different categories of organism.

A number of techniques are currently being developed in order speed up the enumeration process, although some of these rapid enumeration techniques indirectly measure the most probable number of viable cells.

8.1.1.1 Enumeration media
Enumeration media will only ever culture a subset of cells towards which the medium and incubation conditions are directed. Thus, simple salts media with relatively simple sugars as carbon sources and trace levels of amino acids are often used to enumerate bacteria associated with water (e.g. R2A medium). Such plates may be incubated under aerobic or anaerobic conditions at a range of temperatures. Different temperatures will select for different subsets of cells, therefore any description of a viable bacterial count must specify the incubation conditions. In medical microbiology temperatures akin to the human body are often deployed because only those bacteria able to grow at such temperatures are likely to cause infection. However, psychrophilic Gram-negative bacteria (growing in water at 10°C) can be a major source of bacterial pyrogen, so a variety of incubation temperatures are often used in monitoring pharmaceutical waters and products. Highly nutritious media, e.g. blood agar, are also used as enumeration media. This is particularly the case when looking for microorganisms such as staphylococci that are usually found in association with animals and man. Such agar plates may be deliberately exposed to air (settle plates) and the number of colonies formed related to the bacteria content of a room. In the pharmaceutical industry microbiological monitoring will generally report the total aerobic count and, less commonly, the total anaerobic counts obtained on a moderately rich medium such as tryptone soya agar. Sometimes inhibitors of bacterial growth (e.g. Rose Bengal) can be added to a medium in order to select for moulds.

8.1.1.2 Rapid enumeration techniques
The detection and quantification of components of

bacterial cells is considerably faster than those approaches requiring the growth of colonies, and estimates of total viable cell number can thereby be obtained within minutes rather than hours and days.

Some of the rapid methods that have been used for bacteria and other microorganisms, e.g. bioluminescence, epifluorescence and impedance techniques, have been described in Chapter 2, but there are other rapid methods that have found more limited application; these will be considered here. In the examination of pharmaceutical waters and aqueous pharmaceutical products electronic particle counters, e.g. Coulter counters, can be used to determine bacterial concentration, although these instruments do not discriminate between living and dead cells. Similar counters are available that are able to analyse particles found in air. Other rapid techniques aim to detect microbial growth rather than to visualize individual cells and colonies. As bacteria grow in liquid culture they not only alter the conductivity of the culture (see Chapter 2), they also generate small quantities of heat. The time taken to detect this heat can be directly related to the numbers of viable cells present by means of microcalorimeters. Once again this is a considerable improvement over conventional culture, but unlike particle counting and bioluminescence can only detect those organisms that are able to grow in the chosen medium.

None of the rapid techniques are able to isolate individual organisms. They do not therefore aid in the characterization or identification of the contaminants.

8.1.2 Enrichment culture

Enrichment cultures are intended to increase the dominance of a numerically minor component of a mixed culture such that it can be readily detected on an agar plate. Enrichment media are always liquid and are intended to provide conditions that are favourable for the growth of the desired organism and unfavourable for the growth of other likely isolates. This can be achieved either through manipulation of the pH and tonicity of the medium or by the inclusion of chemicals that inhibit the growth of unwanted species. Thus, MacConkey broth contains bile salts that will inhibit the growth of non-enteric bacteria and may be used to enrich for Enterobacteriaceae. Several serial passages through enrichment broths may be made, and after enrichment it is not possible to relate the numbers of organisms detected back to that in the original sample.

8.1.3 Selective media

Selective media are solidified enrichment broths, so again they are intended to suppress the growth of particular groups of bacteria and to allow the growth of others. The methods of creating this situation are the same as for enrichment broths. Thus mannitol salts agar will favour the growth of micrococci and staphylococci, and cetrimide agar will favour the growth of pseudomonads. The use of selective media is an adjunct to characterizing the nature of contaminants. Counts of colonies obtained on selective solid media are often documented as presumptive counts, so for example, colonies formed on a MacConkey agar (containing bile salts) might be cited as a presumptive coliform count.

8.1.4 Identification media (diagnostic)

Identification media contain nutrients and reagents that indicate, usually through some form of colour formation, the presence of particular organisms. This enables them to be easily detected against a background of other species. In this fashion inclusion of lactose sugar and a pH indicator into MacConkey agar facilitates the identification of colonies of bacteria that can ferment lactose. Fermentation leads to a reduction in pH within these colonies and can be detected by an acid shift in the pH indicator, usually to red. Lactose-fermenting coliforms (*Escherichia* spp., *Klebsiella* spp.) can therefore be easily distinguished from non-fermentative coliforms (*Salmonella* spp., *Shigella* spp.). Similarly, the inclusion of egg-yolk lecithin into an agar gives it a cloudy appearance that clears around colonies of organisms that produce lecithinase (a virulence factor in staphylococci). While there are numerous types of selective and diagnostic media available, they can only be used as a guide to identification, but microscopy and biochemical or genetic characterization are much more definitive.

8.2 Microscopy

Observation of stained and wet preparations of clinical specimens (blood, pus, sputum) and isolated pure cultures of bacteria from the manufacturing environment provides rapid and essential information to guide further identification. The application of simple stains such as the Gram stain can divide the various genera of bacteria into two convenient broad groups. The size and shapes of individual cells and their arrangement into clusters, chains and tetrads will also guide identification, as will specific stains for the presence of endospores, capsules, flagella and inclusion bodies. Examination of wet preparations can give an indication as to the motility status of the isolate, and these procedures all represent an important first stage in the identification process.

8.3 Biochemical testing and rapid identification

The differing ability of bacteria to ferment sugars, glycosides and polyhydric alcohols is widely used to differentiate the Enterobacteriaceae and in diagnostic bacteriology generally. Fermentation can be indicated by pH changes in the medium with or without gas production visualized by the collection of bubbles in inverted tubes. More specialized media examine the ability of certain strains to oxidize or reduce particular substrates. There are many

Table 3.3 Examples of some pharmaceutically useful bacteria

Organism	Characteristics	Pharmaceutical relevance
Actinomyces spp.	Gram-positive, filamentous rods	Antibiotic production
Bacillus stearothermophilus	Gram-positive rod, aerobic, spore-former	Used to validate and monitor moist heat sterilization processes
Bacillus subtilis	Gram-positive rod, aerobic, spore-former	Used to validate and monitor dry heat and ethylene oxide sterilization processes
Bacillus pumilus	Gram-positive rod, aerobic, spore-former	Used to validate and monitor radiation sterilization processes
Bordetella pertussis	Gram-negative rod, aerobe	Vaccine against whooping cough
Brevundimonas (formerly *Pseudomonas*) *diminuta*	Gram-negative, micro-aerobic rod	0.22-μm filter challenge test
Clostridium sporogenes	Gram-positive rod, anaerobe, spore-former	Used to confirm anaerobic growth conditions
Clostridium tetani	Gram-positive rod, anaerobe, spore-former	Vaccine against tetanus
Corynebacterium diphtheriae	Gram-positive rod, aerobe	Vaccine against diphtheria
Escherichia coli	Gram-negative enteric rod, facultative anaerobe	Kelsey-Sykes disinfectant capacity test Preservative limit test
Haemophilus influenzae type b	Gram-negative rod, aerobe	Vaccine against Hib infections
Leuconostoc mesenteroides	Gram-positive rod	Dextran production
Neisseria meningitidis	Gram-negative cocci, aerobic	Vaccine against meningitis C
Pseudomonas aeruginosa	Gram-negative, micro-aerobic rod	Alginate production Kelsey-Sykes disinfectant capacity test
Proteus vulgaris	Gram-negative, aerobic rod	Kelsey-Sykes disinfectant capacity test
Salmonella typhi	Gram-negative enteric rod, facultative anaerobe	Chick Martin/Rideal Walker disinfectant coefficient test
Staphylococcus aureus	Gram-positive, aerobic cocci	Kelsey-Sykes disinfectant capacity test Preservative limit test

Table 3.4 Examples of some pharmaceutically problematic bacteria

Organism	Characteristics	Pharmaceutical relevance
Bacteroides fragilis	Gram-negative enteric rod, anaerobe	Wound infections
Bordetella pertussis	Gram-negative rod, aerobe	Causative agent of whooping cough
Campylobacter jejuni	Gram-negative enteric spiral rod, micro-aerophilic	Severe enteritis
Clostridium tetani	Gram-positive rod, anaerobe, spore-former	Causative agent of tetanus
Corynebacterium diphtheriae	Gram-positive rod, aerobe	Causative agent of diphtheria
Escherichia coli	Gram-negative enteric rod, facultative anaerobe	Food poisoning, severe enteritis
Haemophilus influenzae	Gram-negative rod, aerobe	Causative agent of infantile meningitis and chronic bronchitis
Legionella pneumophila	Gram-negative rod, aerobic	Causative agent of Legionnaire's disease
Mycobacterium tuberculosis	Gram-positive, acid-fast rod, aerobe	Causative agent of tuberculosis Disinfectant resistance Intracellular pathogen
Pseudomonas aeruginosa	Gram-negative, micro-aerobic rod	General environmental contaminant Quintessential opportunist pathogen High resistance to antibiotics and biocides Biofilm-former
Salmonella spp.	Gram-negative enteric rods, facultative anaerobes	Varying degrees of food poisoning, typhoid fever
Staphylococcus aureus	Gram-positive, aerobic, catalase-positive cocci	Skin contaminant Food poisoning Toxic shock syndrome Pyogenic infections
Staphylococcus epidermidis	Gram-positive, aerobic, catalase-positive cocci	Implanted medical device/prosthetic device contaminant Biofilm-former
Streptococcus spp.	Gram-positive, aerobic, catalase-negative cocci	Causative agents of tonsilitis and scarlet fever

hundreds of individual biochemical tests available that each separately seek the presence of a particular enzyme or physiological activity. Taxonomic studies have led to the recognition that certain of these tests in combination characterize particular species of bacteria. Various manuals such as *Bergey's Manual* and Cowan and Steele's *Manual for the Identification of Medically Important Bacteria* provide a logical and sequential framework for the conduct of such tests. Identification of particular species and genera by such processes is time-consuming, expensive and may require numerous media and reagents.

This process has become simplified in recent years by the development of rapid identification methods and kits. The latter often use multi-well microtitration plates that can be inoculated in a single operation either with an inoculated wire or with a suspension of a pure culture. Each individual well contains the medium and reagents for the conduct of a single biochemical test. Identification kits vary in their complexity and also in the precision of the identification made. Simple kits may perform only 8–15 tests, more complex ones are capable of performing 96 simultaneous biochemical evaluations. Scoring of each test and entry into a computer database then allows the pattern of test results to be compared with a large panel of organisms and a probability of identity calculated. As different sets of tests will be required for different classes of bacteria, guidance as to the initial choice of kit is given on the basis of the Gram stain reaction, and the results of oxidase and catalase tests performed directly on isolated colonies. In large diagnostic laboratories and in quality assurance laboratories automated systems are deployed that can inoculate, incubate and analyse hundreds of individual samples at a time.

8.4 Molecular approaches to identification

The need to identify microorganisms rapidly has led to the development of a number of molecular identification and characterization tools. These have not yet become routinely adopted in the analytical or diagnostic laboratory but will probably do so in the future. One such technique isolates and amplifies 16S ribosomal DNA and, following sequencing of the bases, compares this with known sequences held in a reference library. This approach enables phylogenetic relationships to be derived even for those bacteria that have not previously been identified. Other systems examine the patterns of key constituents of the cells such as fatty acids and assign identities based on similarity matches to known reference cultures.

Molecular approaches can be of particular use when attempting to detect a particular species. Thus gene probes carrying fluorescent dyes can be used in hybridization procedures with the collected clinical material. Examination under the fluorescent microscope will show the targeted organism as fluorescent against a background of non-fluorescent organisms.

8.5 Pharmaceutically and medically relevant microorganisms

Microorganisms of medical and pharmaceutical relevance can be broadly classified into those organisms that are harmful or problematic, and those that can be used to our advantage. Some microor-

ganisms, depending on the situation, can fall into both categories. Microorganisms cause some of the most important diseases of humans and animals and they can also be found as major contaminants of pharmaceutical products. On the other hand, many large-scale industrial processes, e.g. antibiotic production, are based on microorganisms, and selected species can be used to test disinfectant efficacy and to monitor sterilization procedures. Tables 3.3 and 3.4 respectively, list examples of some of the more pharmaceutically relevant beneficial and problematic microorganisms. Specific texts should be referred to for more detailed descriptions.

9 Further reading

Buchanan, R. E. & Gibbons, N. E. (1974) *Bergey's Manual of Determinative Bacteriology*, 8th edn. Williams & Wilkins, Baltimore.

Costerton, J. W., Lewandowski, Z., deBeer, D., Caldwell, D., Korber, D. & James, G. (1994) Biofilms, the customised microniche. *Journal of Bacteriology*, **176**, 2137–2142.

Cowan, S. T. (1993) *Cowan and Steel's Manual for the Identification of Medical Bacteria* (eds G. Barrow & R. K. A. Feltham), 3rd edn. Cambridge University Press, Cambridge.

Gould, G. W. (1985) Modification of resistance and dormancy. In: *Fundamental and Applied Aspects of Bacterial Spores* (eds G. J. Dring, D. J. Ellar & G. W. Gould), pp. 371–382. Academic Press, London.

Madigan, M. T., Martinko, J. M. & Parker, J. (2000) *Brock Biology of Microorganisms*, 9th edn. Prentice-Hall, New Jersey.

Murray, P .R., Kobayashi, G. S., Pfaller, M. A. & Rosenthal, K. S. (1994) *Medical Microbiology*, 2nd edn. Mosby-Year Book, London.

Roitt, I. M. (1994) *Essential Immunology*, 8th edn. Blackwell Scientific Publications, Oxford.

Salyers, A. A. & Drew, D. D. (1994) *Bacterial Pathogenesis: A Molecular Approach*. ASM Press, Washington.

Stryer, L. (2002) *Biochemistry*, 5th edn. W. H. Freeman & Co., San Francisco.

Sutherland, I. W. (1985) Biosynthesis and composition of Gram-negative bacterial extracellular and wall polysaccharides. *Annu Rev Microbiol*, **10**, 243–270.

Chapter 4
Fungi

Kevin Kavanagh and Derek Sullivan

1 What are fungi?

Yeasts, such as brewers' yeast, and moulds, such *Penicillium chrysogenum* which produces the antibiotic penicillin, are classified as fungi. Yeast cells tend to grow as single cells that reproduce asexually in a process known as budding, although a minority of species (e.g. *Schizosaccharomyces pombe*) reproduce by fission. Many yeast species are capable of sexual reproduction and the formation of spores. In contrast, moulds grow as masses of overlapping and interlinking hyphal filaments and reproduce by producing masses of spores in a variety of structures. This division between yeasts and moulds based on growth morphology is not clear-cut, as some yeasts can produce hyphae under specific conditions (e.g. *Candida albicans*), while many normally filamentous fungi possess a yeast-like phase at some point in their life cycle. Fungi are eukaryotic organisms, i.e. their cells possess a nuclear membrane, consequently there are many similarities between the biochemistry of fungal cells and human cells. Fungi are widely distributed in nature, occurring as part of the normal flora on the body of warm-blooded animals, as decomposers of organic matter and as animal and plant pathogens. Medically, fungi are an extremely important group of microbes, being responsible for a number of potentially fatal diseases in humans (Table 4.1), but a significant number of fungi are of great benefit to humanity in terms of the production of alcoholic beverages, bread and antibiotics (Table 4.2). Fungi have also been utilized for a range of molecular biological applications.

From a taxonomic point of view the Kingdom fungi can be subdivided into six Classes. The Class Oomycetes contains the mildews and water moulds, the Class Ascomycetes contains the mildews, some moulds and most yeast species (including *Saccharomyces cerevisiae*), the Class Basidiomycetes contains the mushrooms and bracket fungi, the Class Teliomycetes contains the rust fungi (plant pathogens), the Class Ustomycetes contains the smuts (plant pathogens) and the Class Deuteromycetes contains species such as *Aspergillus*, *Fusarium* and *Penicillium* (Fig. 4.1 illustrates the typical septate hyphae of this Class).

2 The structure of the fungal cell

The typical yeast cell is oval in shape and is surrounded by a rigid cell wall, which contains a number of structural polysaccharides and may account for up to 25% of the dry weight of the cell wall (Fig. 4.2). Glucan accounts for 50–60%, mannan for 15–23% and chitin for 1–9% of the dry weight of the wall, respectively, with protein and lipids also

Table 4.1 Examples of fungal diseases and selected causative agents

Type of mycosis	Disease	Species name
Superficial	Pityriasis versicolor	*Malassezia furfur*
	White piedra	*Trichosporon beigelii*
Cutaneous	Tinea pedis (athlete's foot)	*Trichophyton rubrum*
	Onychomycosis (nail infection)	*Trichophyton rubrum*
	Tinea capitis (scalp ringworm)	*Trichophyton tonsurans*
Subcutaneous	Chromoblastomycosis	*Fonsecaea pedrosoi*
	Mycetoma	*Acremonium* spp.
Systemic	Blastomycosis	*Blastomyces dermatitidis*
	Histoplasmosis	*Histoplasma capsulatum*
	Coccidioidomycosis	*Coccidioides immitis*
	Paracoccidioidomycosis	*Paracoccidioides brasiliensis*
Opportunistic	Candidosis (superficial/systemic)	*Candida albicans*
		Candida glabrata
		Candida parapsilosis
	Aspergillosis	*Aspergillus fumigatus*
	Pneumonia	*Pneumocystis carinii*

Table 4.2 Examples of economically important fungi

Fungal species	Application
Filamentous fungi	
Agaricus bisporus	Edible mushroom
Aspergillus, Penicillium spp.	Enzymes (catalase, lipase, amylase)
Aspergillus sp. + *Saccharomyces* sp.	*Sake* (rice wine)
Fusarium graminearum	Single cell protein
Penicillium chrysogenum	Penicillin production
Penicillium notatum	Enzyme (glucose oxidase)
Penicillium roqueforti	Cheese flavouring (Roquefort 'blue' cheese)
Yeasts	
Pichia sp.	Gene expression system
Saccharomyces cerevisiae	Bakers' yeast—bread
	Brewers' yeast—beer, wine, cider, etc.
	Enzyme (invertase)
	Gene expression system
	Dietary supplement

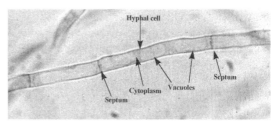

Fig. 4.1 Septate hyphae of *Aspergillus fumigatus*.

present in smaller amounts. The thickness of the cell wall may vary during the life of the cell but the average thickness in the yeast *C. albicans* varies from 100 to 300 nm. Glucan, the main structural component of the fungal cell wall, is a branched polymer of glucose which exists in three forms in the cell, i.e. β-1,6-glucan, β-1,3-glucan and β-1,3,-β-1,6-complexed with chitin. Mannan is a polymer of the sugar mannose and is found in the outer layers of the cell wall. The third principal structural component, chitin, is concentrated in bud scars which are areas of the cell from which a bud has detached. Proteins and lipids are also present in the cell wall and under some conditions may represent up to 30% of the cell wall contents. Mannoproteins form a fibrillar layer that radiates from an internal skeletal layer, which is formed by the polysaccharide component of the cell wall. The innermost layer is rich in glucan and chitin, which provides rigidity to the wall and is important in regulating cell division.

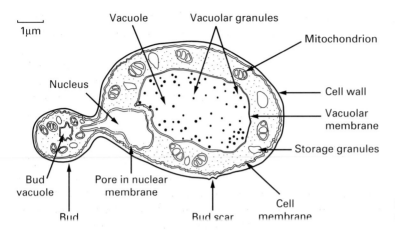

Fig. 4.2 Diagrammatic representation of 'typical' yeast cell.

Labels in figure: Vacuole · Vacuolar granules · Mitochondrion · Nucleus · Cell wall · Vacuolar membrane · Storage granules · Cell membrane · Bud scar · Pore in nuclear membrane · Bud · Bud vacuole · 1μm

Enzymatic or mechanical removal of the cell wall leaves an osmotically fragile protoplast that will burst if not maintained in an osmotically stabilized environment. Incubation of protoplasts in an osmotically stabilized agar growth medium will allow the re-synthesis of the wall and the resumption of normal cellular functions. The ability to generate protoplasts from fungi opens the possibility of fusing these under defined conditions to generate strains with novel biotechnological applications.

The periplasmic space is a thin region that lies directly below the cell wall. It contains secreted proteins that do not penetrate the cell wall and is the location for a number of enzymes required for processing nutrients before entry into the cell. The cell membrane or plasmalemma is located directly below the periplasmic space and is a phospholipid bilayer that contains phospholipids, lipids, protein and sterols. The plasmalemma is approximately 10 nm thick and in addition to being composed of phospholipids also contains globular proteins. The dominant sterol in fungal cell membranes is ergosterol, which is the target of the antifungal agent amphotericin B. Sterols are important components of the plasmalemma and represent regions of rigidity in the fluidity provided by the phospholipid bilayer.

Most of the cell's genome is concentrated in the nucleus, which is surrounded by a nuclear membrane that contains pores to allow communication with the rest of the cell (Fig. 4.2). The nucleus is a discrete organelle and, in addition to being the repository of the DNA, also contains proteins in the form of histones. Yeast chromosomes vary in size from 0.2 to 6 Mb and the number per yeast is also variable, with *S. cerevisiae* having as many as 16 while the fission yeast *Sch. pombe* has as few as 3. In addition to the genetic material in the nucleus the yeast cell often has extrachromosomal information in the form of plasmids. For example, the 2-μm plasmid is present in *S. cerevisiae*, although its function is unclear, and killer plasmids in the yeast *Kluyveromyces lactis* which encode a toxin.

Actively respiring fungal cells possess a distinct mitochondrion, which has been described as the 'power-house' of the cell (Fig. 4.2). The enzymes of the tricarboxylic acid cycle (Kreb's cycle) are located in the matrix of the mitochondrion, while electron transport and oxidative phosphorylation occur in the mitochondrial inner membrane. The outer membrane contains enzymes involved in lipid biosynthesis. The mitochondrion is a semi-independent organelle as it possesses its own DNA and is capable of producing its own proteins on its own ribosomes, which are referred to as mitoribosomes.

The fungal cell contains a vast number of ribosomes, which are usually present in the form of polysomes — lines of ribosomes strung together by a strand of mRNA. Ribosomes are the site of protein biosynthesis. The system that mediates the export of proteins from the cell involves a number of membranous compartments including the Golgi apparatus, the endoplasmic reticulum and the plasmalemma. In addition, the vacuole is employed as a 'storage space' where nutrients, hydrolytic enzymes or metabolic intermediates are retained until required.

3 Medical significance of fungi

Fungi represent a significant group of pathogens capable of causing a range of diseases in humans. While the majority of fungi appear to be harmless to humans it is worth bearing in mind that in the right set of conditions a normally non-pathogenic fungus can cause a clinically relevant problem. In a case of a profoundly immunocompromised individual, a wide range of fungi can present as capable of inducing disease.

The most common fungal pathogens of humans can be divided into three broad classes: the yeasts, the moulds and the dermatophytes. The yeast *C. albicans* is the most frequently encountered human fungal pathogen, being responsible for a wide range of superficial and systemic infections. The superficial infections include oropharyngeal and genital conditions, the former occur predominantly in HIV-positive individuals, geriatric people and premature infants and may arise when a weakened or immature immune system is present. Genital candidosis is very common and approximately 75% of women are affected by vulvovaginal candidosis (VVC) during their life, with a further 5–12% suffering from recurring bouts of infection over a prolonged period of time. Genital candidosis in men is comparatively rare, although it is occasionally seen in alcoholics and diabetics. Candidosis of the skin and fingernails (onychomycosis) may be present in up to 10% of cancer patients. Continually moist, macerated or burnt skin is an ideal environment for the development of cutaneous candidosis.

C. albicans is also responsible for a range of systemic infections and many of these can commence as superficial infections. Infection of the gastrointestinal tract is seen in diabetics, cancer and AIDS patients and the oesophagus is a common site of infection, rendering swallowing difficult. *Candida* infection of the respiratory tract is seen in those with underlying disease (e.g. cancer) or following the insertion of a silicone voice prosthesis. The urinary tract can also be the site of candidosis, which may be due to renal infection, other underlying disease(s) or cystitis. The presence of an indwelling urinary catheter may also predispose to *Candida* infection.

A range of factors is capable of predisposing the individual to superficial or systemic infections. Factors which impair the host's immune system such as the presence of underlying disease (AIDS, cancer, diabetes), the use of immunosuppressive therapy during organ transplantation and broad-spectrum antibiotic therapy can leave the individual susceptible to candidosis. Different stages of life may also predispose to specific types of infection. For example, pregnant women have a higher incidence of vaginal candidosis and premature infants and geriatric individuals are susceptible to oral candidosis due to either immature or faltering immune systems, respectively. Other factors that may predispose to *Candida* infection include the presence of indwelling catheters and skin damage as a result of burns or other trauma.

The mould *Aspergillus fumigatus* is the dominant fungal pulmonary pathogen of humans and generally presents as a problem in those with pre-existing lung disease or damage. In addition to pulmonary infection other sites may be affected including the brain, kidneys and sinuses, depending on the level of immunocompromisation of the individual. Groups particularly susceptible to colonization by *Aspergillus* species include those with cavities as a result of tuberculosis, patients affected with asthma or cystic fibrosis and those with profound immunosuppression due to leukaemia (neutropenia). Aspergillosis presents as a serious problem in patients immunosuppressed in advance of organ transplantation.

Dermatophyte is the term applied to a range of fungi capable of colonizing the skin, nails or hair. The principal dermatophytic fungi are *Trichophyton*, *Microsporum* and *Epidermophyton* species. The most commonly encountered dermatophytic infections are athlete's foot (infection of the foot) and ringworm (fungal infection of the scalp or skin).

4 Fungal species identification methods

The first step in identifying a fungus in clinical samples is to observe the tissue sample microscopically, often in conjunction with specific staining procedures. For instance, addition of potassium hydroxide to the specimen facilitates any fungal elements present to be distinguished from host structures. Tissue samples routinely tested for fungi in the diagnostic laboratory include blood, cerebrospinal fluid, bronchial aspirates and biopsy material, all of which are usually sterile. While microscopic analysis of samples is certainly rapid and inexpensive it is not very sensitive. Consequently, in the diagnostic laboratory samples are routinely inoculated onto agar plates that specifically allow the growth of fungi. A wide variety of media have been developed for the selective growth of fungal species. On these media filamentous fungi are often identifiable to the species level based on their colony morphology following macroscopic and microscopic analysis, with many species having recognizable characteristic hyphal and conidial structures. As *C. albicans* and the recently discovered closely related species *C. dubliniensis* can grow in the yeast or hyphal form, the ability of these species to produce germ-tubes (i.e. hyphae) can easily be tested in the laboratory by incubation of the cells in serum. Similarly these species are also the only members of the genus *Candida* to produce large spore-like structures called chlamydospores on specific media. Identification of other clinically important *Candida* species has been greatly facilitated by the recent introduction of commercially available chromogenic media, which allow the *Candida* species to be distinguished from each other on the basis of colony colour. In addition, *Candida* species can also be identified on the basis of their different nutrient (especially carbohydrate) requirements, which can be assessed using commercial kits. In addition, as in the case of direct microscopic analysis of samples, the levels of fungal elements present in samples taken are often very low and are not present at sufficiently high levels to be detected using culture-based methods. Therefore, in many cases the identity of the agent responsible for causing a fungal infection is only determined once the infection has been cured using empirical treatment. Indeed sometimes the cause of disease is only identified at autopsy.

Clearly, to improve our ability to treat fungal diseases effectively there is a great need to develop techniques that allow the detection and identification of infecting fungal species more quickly. Currently, two areas of research are endeavouring to facilitate this goal. Firstly, it has been proposed that rather than detecting the infecting species it may be more appropriate to monitor the host immune response to specific pathogens. To this end enzyme-linked immunosorbent assay (ELISA)-based tests have been developed to detect antibodies to specific antigens belonging to fungal species. In another recent development molecular biologists are attempting to adapt polymerase chain reaction (PCR)-based methods to detect the nucleic acids of specific fungal species in normally sterile sites. This method in tandem with genome-based microchip technology offers great promise for automated diagnosis. While both ELISA-based and PCR-based technologies have the potential to revolutionize the diagnosis of fungal infections as they are very rapid and accurate, they are still at the experimental stage and are only in use in specialized laboratories.

5 Antifungal therapy

The choice and dose of an antifungal agent will depend on the nature of the condition, whether there are any underlying diseases, the health of the patient and whether antifungal resistance has been identified as compromising therapy. Part of the difficulty in designing effective antifungal agents lies in the fact that fungi are eukaryotic organisms, so agents that will kill fungi may also have a deleterious effect on human tissue. The ideal antifungal drug should target a pathway or process specific to the fungal cell, so reducing the possibility of damaging tissue and inducing unwanted side-effects.

5.1 Polyene antifungal agents

Polyene antifungal agents are characterized by having a large macrolide ring of carbon atoms closed by the formation of an internal ester or lactone (Fig. 4.3). In addition, polyenes have a large number of hydroxyl groups distributed along the macrolide ring on alternate carbon atoms. This combination of highly polar and non-polar regions within the molecule render the polyenes amphiphatic, i.e.

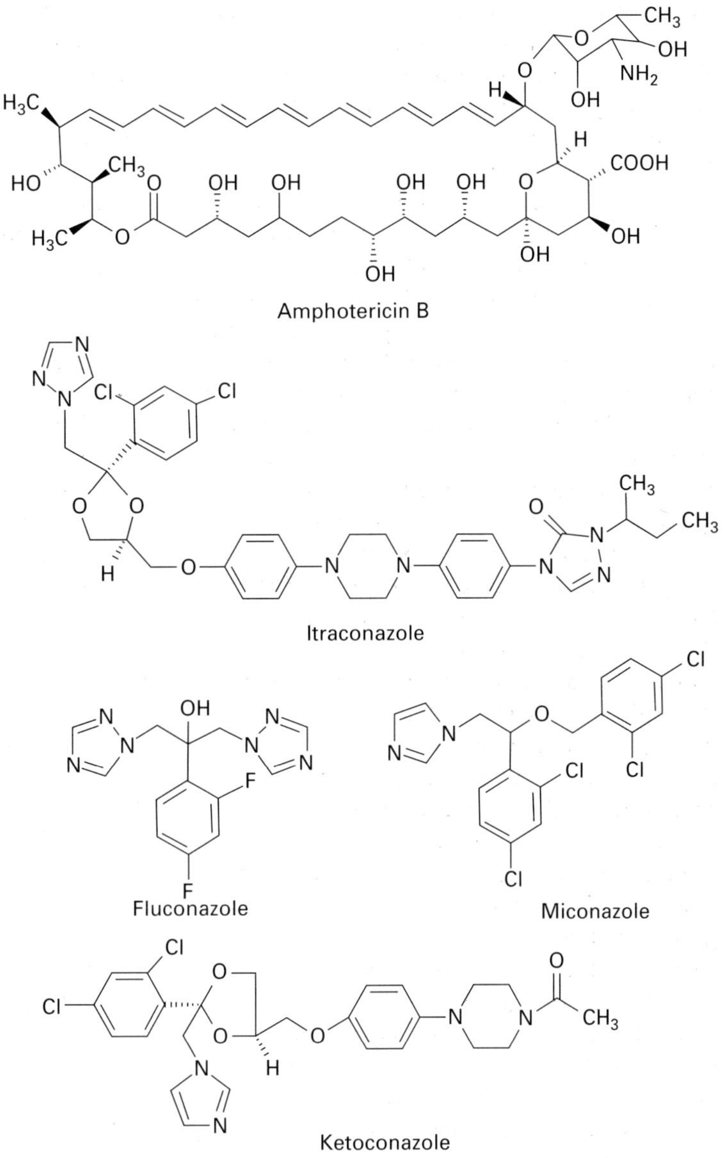

Fig. 4.3 Structures of polyene (amphotericin B) and azole (itraconazole, fluconazole, miconazole and ketoconazole) antifungal agents.

having hydrophobic and hydrophilic regions in the one molecule which assists solubility in lipid membranes.

The principal polyenes are amphotericin B and nystatin. Amphotericin B is produced by the bacterium *Streptomyces nodosus* and its activity is due to the ability to bind ergosterol, which is the dominant sterol in fungal cell membranes, and consequently increases membrane permeability by the formation of pores (Fig. 4.4). The action of ampho-

tericin B seems to rely on the formation of pores through which intracellular contents can escape from the cell. Amphotericin B can lead to renal damage during prolonged antifungal therapy. Amphotericin B is active against a broad range of fungal pathogens and is considered the 'gold standard' against which the activity of other antifungal agents is measured. Due to its renal toxicity amphotericin B tends to be reserved for severe cases of systemic fungal disease, but recent formulations in which the

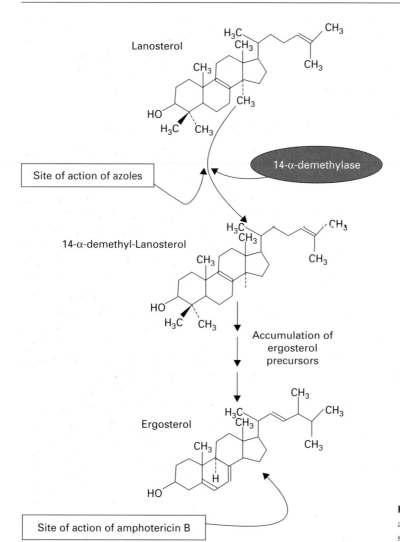

Fig. 4.4 Modes of action of polyene and azole antifungal agents showing sites of action.

drug is encapsulated within liposomes have been shown to be of reduced toxicity.

Nystatin was discovered in 1950 and exhibits the same mode of action as amphotericin B but tends to be of lower solubility, which has restricted its use to the treatment of topical infections. While nystatin was effective for the treatment of conditions such as oral and vaginal candidosis its use has been overtaken by the introduction of azole antifungal drugs.

5.2 Azole antifungal agents

The first generation of azole antifungal agents revo-

lutionized the treatment of mucosal and invasive fungal infections and azoles are still the most widely used group of antifungal agents. The azole derivatives are classified as imidazoles or triazoles on the basis of whether they have two or three nitrogen atoms in the five-membered azole ring (Fig. 4.3). The azoles in current and long-standing clinical use are clotrimazole, miconazole, econazole and ketoconazole, while newer drugs such as itraconazole, fluconazole and voriconazole have important applications in the treatment of systemic infections. Azoles function by interfering with ergosterol biosynthesis by binding to the cytochrome P-450-

mediated enzyme known as 14-α-demethylase (P-450$_{DM}$). This blocks the formation of ergosterol by preventing the methylation of lanosterol (a precursor of ergosterol) (Fig. 4.4), resulting in a reduction in the amount of ergosterol in the fungal cell membrane, which leads to membrane instability, growth inhibition and cell death in some cases. An additional consequence of the block in ergosterol biosynthesis is the build-up of toxic intermediates, which can prove fatal to the cell (see Chapter 12).

Azoles exhibit a broad spectrum of activity *in vitro*, being capable of inhibiting the growth of most *Candida*, *Cryptococcus* and *Aspergillus* species and dermatophytes. Miconazole was the first azole used to treat systemic fungal infections but demonstrated a number of toxic side-effects. Ketoconazole produced high serum concentrations upon oral administration but had poor activity against aspergillosis. In addition, ketoconazole was associated with a range of side-effects which limited its applicability. Newer triazoles such as fluconazole and itraconazole have increased the options for dealing with fungal infections. Fluconazole was introduced for clinical use in 1990, is water-soluble and shows good penetration and deposition into the pulmonary tissues; it also reaches high levels in the cerebrospinal and peritoneal fluids. Fluconazole has proved highly effective in the treatment of infections caused by *C. albicans* but shows limited activity against *Aspergillus*. Itraconazole became available for clinical use in the late 1980s and was the first azole with proven efficacy against *Aspergillus*. Itraconazole is effective in treating severe *Aspergillus* infections and exhibits both fungicidal and fungistatic effects. Upon ingestion itraconazole undergoes extensive hepatic metabolism which yields up to 30 metabolites — a number of which retain antifungal activity. Itraconazole is currently available as an intravenous formulation and is widely used for the treatment of severe *Aspergillus* infection in this form. Fluconazole and itraconazole demonstrate significantly reduced side-effects compared with ketoconazole. Novel azole drugs with increased ability to inhibit the fungal 14-α-demethylase are also becoming available. These agents, which include voriconazole, posaconazole and ravuconazole, have a wider spectrum of activity than fluconazole and it has been suggested that some of them show fungicidal effects with some species (e.g. *Aspergillus* spp.). Voriconazole is one of the newest second generation triazole antifungal drugs and it shows good activity against pulmonary aspergillosis and cerebral aspergillosis.

5.3 Synthetic antifungal agents

Flucytosine is a synthetic fluorinated pyrimidine that has been used as an oral antifungal agent and demonstrates good activity against a range of yeast species and moderate levels of activity against *Aspergillus* species. Two modes of action have been proposed for flucytosine (see Chapter 12). One involves the disruption of protein synthesis by the inhibition of DNA synthesis, while the other possible mode of action is the depletion in the amino acid pools within the cell as a result of inhibition of protein synthesis. In general yeast cells increase in size when exposed to sub-MIC levels of flucytosine and display alterations in their surface morphology, both of which can be interpreted as a result of an imbalance in the control of cellular growth. Many fungi are inherently resistant to flucytosine or develop resistance after a relatively short exposure and resistance has been attributed to alteration in the enzyme (cytosine deaminase) required to process flucytosine once inside the cell or to an elevation in the amount of pyrimidine synthesis. The problem of resistance has limited the use of flucytosine so that now it is generally used in combination with an antifungal agent (e.g. amphotericin B) where it can potentiate the effect of the second agent.

6 Mechanisms of antifungal drug resistance

Resistance to antifungal drugs is becoming an increasingly perplexing problem. This is particularly the case with one of the most widely used antifungal agents, fluconazole. As outlined previously this drug is a fungistatic agent that acts by inhibiting the activity of cytochrome P-450 (lanosterol α-demethylase), an enzyme in the pathway responsible for the synthesis of ergosterol. Inhibition of this enzyme results in decreased ergosterol levels and a build-up of toxic intermediary products, which subsequently leads to aberrant membrane function and stasis of cell growth and division. However, since the widespread introduction of fluconazole during the early 1990s, there have been increasing reports of *Candida* strains that have decreased susceptibility to azole drugs and of infections that are recalcitrant to treatment. In addition, the prevalence of infections caused by *Candida* species that are inherently less susceptible to azoles has increased over the same time period. One of the most important mechanisms of resistance is the overexpression of efflux proteins which act by pumping the drug out of the cell at a rate faster than the drug enters the cell (see Fig. 4.5). Therefore the intracellular concentration of the drug does not reach a level high enough to inhibit the target enzyme. Another resistance mechanism that has been identified is mutation within the gene encoding the cytochrome P-450. These amino acid substitutions do not affect the activity of the enzyme, but the conformation of the enzyme is sufficiently altered to decrease the affinity of the enzyme for the drug, thus the levels of membrane ergosterol are not altered significantly. An alternative resistance mechanism is the overexpression of the gene encoding the target cytochrome enzyme, this results in increased levels of the cytochrome inside the cell, thus countering the effects of the drug. Finally, another resistance mechanism is mutation in genes that encode other proteins involved in the biosynthesis of ergosterol. These mutations prevent the build-up of toxic by-products, thus the inhibitory effects of the azoles are decreased. Very often in azole-resistant clinical isolates of *C. albicans* multiple resistance mechanisms have been identified as contributing to the resistance phenotype, thus it is difficult to determine which are the most important mechanisms (see Fig. 4.5).

Resistance to other antifungal agents such as amphotericin B has been observed less frequently in clinical fungal isolates; however, the molecular basis of this resistance is not currently well understood. To solve the problems associated with antifungal resistance a number of novel azole drugs (e.g. voriconazole) and novel classes of drug (e.g echinocandins) have been developed (see Chapter 12).

7 Some clinically important fungi

7.1 *Candida albicans* — the dominant fungal pathogen

The yeast *C. albicans* is an opportunist fungal pathogen which can be present as a normal part of the body's microflora. *C. albicans* displays a variety of virulence factors which aid colonization and persistence in the body. One of the most important of these factors is the ability to adhere to host tissue using a variety of mechanisms (Fig. 4.6). The importance of adherence may be illustrated by the ability of *C. albicans* to adhere to various mucosal surfaces and to withstand forces that may lead to its removal from the body such as the bathing/washing action of body fluids. A hierarchy exists among *Candida* species indicating that the more common aetiological agents of candidosis (*C. albicans* and *Candida tropicalis*) are more adherent to host tissue *in vitro* than relatively non-pathogenic species such as *C. krusei* and *Candida guilliermondii*.

Adherence to host tissue is achieved by a combination of specific and non-specific mechanisms. Specific adherence mechanisms include ligand–receptor interactions, while non-specific mechanisms include electrostatic forces, aggregation and cell surface hydrophobicity. Non-specific interactions are the primary interaction (occurring over longer distances) involved in the adherence process and are reversible. However, non-specific adherence is consequently deemed irreversible as a result of specific mechanisms that involve the ability of the yeast to recognize a variety of host cell receptors/ligands using cell surface molecules.

C. albicans can exist in two morphologically distinct forms — budding blastospores or hyphae. The yeast can switch between each form and is usually encountered in tissue samples in both morphological forms (Fig. 4.7). The hyphae are capable of thigmotropism (contact sensing), which may aid in finding the line of least resistance between and through layers of cells in tissue. *C. albicans* produces a range of extracellular enzymes that facilitate adherence and/or tissue penetration. Phospholipase A, B, C and lysophospholipase may function to damage host cell membranes and facilitate invasion. *C. albicans* produces a range of acid

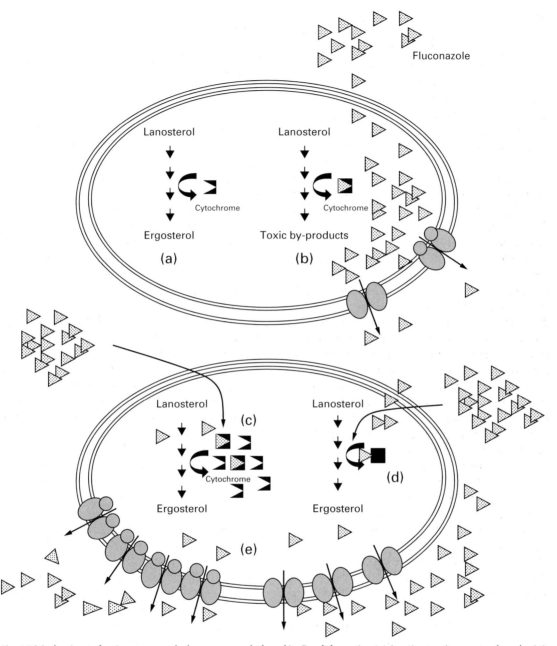

Fig. 4.5 Mechanisms of resistance to azole drugs commonly found in *Candida* species. (a) A major step in ergosterol synthesis is catalysed by the cytochrome P-450 enzyme lanosterol 14α-demethylase. (b) Fluconazole inhibits the activity of cytochrome P-450 enzyme lanosterol 14α-demethylase, which results in a depletion of the ergosterol content of the cell membrane and the build-up of toxic precursors. (c) Overexpression of the gene encoding the lanosterol 14α-demethylase allows enough enzyme activity to enable sufficient ergosterol production. (d) Mutations in the active site of the target enzyme can result in a decreased affinity for the drug without affecting the catalytic activity of the enzyme. (e) Increased expression of the genes encoding specific transmembrane pumps (e.g. *CDR1* and *MDR1*) prevents the accumulation of the drug inside the cell.

proteinases which have been shown to aid adherence and invasion but which also play an important role in the degradation of the immunoglobulins IgG and IgA. The proteinases have a low pH optimum and this may assist the yeast colonization of the vagina, which is a low pH environment. Haemolysin production by *C. albicans* has also been documented and seems to be important in allowing the yeast access to iron released from ruptured red blood cells. An important immune evasion tactic of *C. albicans* is the ability to bind to platelets via fibrinogen-binding ligands, which results in the fungal cell being surrounded by a cluster of platelets.

C. albicans is capable of giving rise to a variety of inter-convertible phenotypes which can be considered as providing an extra dimension to the existing virulence factors associated with this yeast. A number of switching systems have been identified and phenotypic switching may have evolved to compensate for the lack of variation achieved in other organisms that utilize sexual reproduction. Phenotypic switching allows the yeast to exploit micro-niches in the body and alters a variety of factors (e.g. antifungal drug resistance, adherence, extracellular enzyme production), in addition to the actual phenotype and so may be considered as the 'dominant' or 'controlling' virulence factor.

In terms of tissue colonization and invasion, adherence is the initial step in the process. Once the yeast has adhered, enzymes (phospholipase and proteinase) can facilitate adherence by damaging or degrading cell membranes and extracellular proteins. Hyphae may be produced and penetrate layers of cells using thigmotropism to find the line of least resistance. The passage through cells is undoubtedly aided by the production of extracellular enzymes. Once endothelial cells are reached enzymes may assist in the degradation of tissue and allow the yeast to enter the host's bloodstream, where phenotypic switching or coating with platelets may be used to evade the immune system. While in the bloodstream the haemolysin may function to burst blood cells and release iron, which is essential for growth. Escape from the bloodstream involves adherence to the walls of capillaries and passage across the wall.

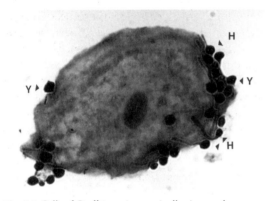

Fig. 4.6 Cells of *C. albicans* (arrows) adhering to a human buccal epithelial cell. Y, yeast cells; H, hyphal cells.

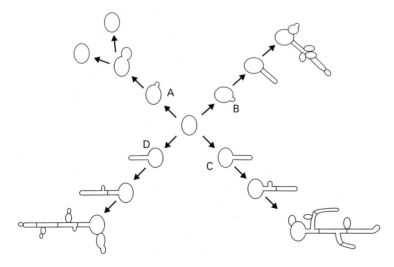

Fig. 4.7 Growth morphologies of *Candida albicans*. (A) Budding morphology; (B) hyphal formation; (C) germ-tube formation leading to hyphal formation; (D) pseudohyphal formation.

7.2 *Aspergillus fumigatus*

Aspergillus fumigatus is a saprophytic fungus that is widely distributed in nature where it is frequently encountered growing on decaying vegetation and damp surfaces. *A. fumigatus* can present as an opportunist pathogen of humans and is the commonest aetiological agent of pulmonary aspergillosis, being responsible for 80–90% of cases. While the incidence of disease due to *Aspergillus* species is less than that due to *Candida*, aspergillosis results in greater mortality rates.

A. fumigatus produces a number of extracellular enzymes that facilitate growth in the lung and dissemination through the body. Phospholipase production has been shown in clinical isolates of this fungus, with optimal production occurring at 37°C. This enzyme plays a critical role in tissue degradation and may facilitate exit of the fungus from the lung into the bloodstream. Fungal proteases are responsible for tissue degradation and neutralization of the immune system and probably evolved to allow the fungus to degrade animal and plant material. Elastin constitutes almost 30% of lung tissue and many *A. fumigatus* isolates display elastinolytic activity, while isolates incapable of elastinase production display reduced virulence in mice. *A. fumigatus* produces two elastinases: a serine protease and a metalloproteinase. Apart from their direct role in tissue degradation *A. fumigatus* proteases (in particular the serine protease) may also function as allergens, which may be important in the induction and persistence of allergic aspergillosis. Local inflammation due to the presence of proteases results in airway damage and *in vitro* studies have shown that proteases are capable of inducing epithelial cell detachment from basement membranes. Such desquamation may partly explain the extent of damage seen in the lungs of asthmatic and cystic fibrosis patients affected with allergic aspergillosis. In addition, proteases induce the release of the pro-inflammatory IL-6 and IL-8 cytokines in cell lines derived from airway epithelial cells, which may induce mucosal inflammatory response and subsequent damage to the surrounding tissue.

The production and secretion of toxins into surrounding tissues by the proliferating fungus is regarded as an important virulence attribute and may facilitate fungal growth in the lung. Gliotoxin is the main toxin produced by *A. fumigatus*, others include helvolic acid, fumigatin and fumagillin. It is believed that toxins play a significant role in facilitating the colonization of the lung by *A. fumigatus*, as they can act to retard elements of the local immunity. Significantly, *Aspergillus* species that do not produce toxins to the same extent as *A. fumigatus* isolates are rarely seen in clinical cases.

7.3 *Histoplasma capsulatum*

Histoplasma capsulatum is a dimorphic fungus that is the cause of histoplasmosis — the most prevalent fungal pulmonary infection in the USA. Histoplasmosis is common among AIDS patients but is also found among infants and geriatric subjects living in endemic areas who may be susceptible to infection because of impaired immune function. The mortality rate among infants exposed to a large dose of *H. capsulatum* may be 40–50%. *H. capsulatum* grows in the mycelial form in soil while in tissue it is encountered as round budding cells. Its natural habitat is soil that has been enriched with the droppings of bats or birds, and disturbance of such soil by natural (e.g. wind) or human (e.g. agriculture) activities releases large numbers of airborne spores that upon inhalation can establish pulmonary infection in individuals or in populations distant from the original source of spores.

After inhalation of *H. capsulatum*, pulmonary macrophages engulf the yeast cells and provide a protected environment for the yeast to multiply and disseminate from the lungs to other tissues. The ability to survive within the hostile environment provided by the macrophage is the key to the success of *H. capsulatum* as a pathogen. Normal individuals who inhale a large number of *H. capsulatum* spores can develop a non-specific flu-like illness associated with fever, chills, headache and chest pains after a 3-week incubation period that resolves without treatment. Chronic pulmonary histoplasmosis is seen in males in the 45–55-year age group who may have been exposed to low levels of spores over a long period of time. The condition is progressive, leads to a loss of lung function and death if untreated.

7.4 *Cryptococcus neoformans*

Cryptococcus neoformans is a capsulate yeast that is most frequently associated with infection in immunocompromised patients, particularly those with AIDS, where meningitis is the most common clinical manifestation. *C. neoformans* is a facultative intracellular pathogen that is capable of surviving and replicating within macrophages and withstanding the lytic activity within these cells. In order to survive within macrophages *C. neoformans* appears to accumulate polysaccharides within a cytoplasmic vesicle. As part of its survival strategy *C. neoformans* also produces melanin, which has the ability to bind and protect against microbicidal peptides. In addition, melaninization may allow the cell to withstand the effects of harmful hydroxyl radicals and so survive in hostile environments. The capsule of *C. neoformans* is a virulence factor in that it protects the cell from the immune response and capsular material (glucuronoxylomannans) induces the shedding of host cell adherence molecules required for the migration of host inflammatory cells to the site of infection, thus explaining the reduced inflammatory response to this yeast.

In immunocompromised patients pulmonary infection can lead to disseminated forms of the disease where the eyes, skin and bones become infected. Cryptococcal meningitis is particularly associated with AIDS patients, where it is a major cause of death. While cryptococcosis may be controlled by antifungal therapy, in AIDS patients there is a danger of relapse unless antifungal therapy is constantly maintained.

7.5 Dermatophytes

The dermatophytes are a group of keratinophilic fungi that can metabolize keratin — the principal protein in skin, nails and hair. Tinea capitis is defined as the infection of the hair and scalp with a dermatophyte, usually *Microsporum canis* or *Trichophyton violaceum*. In Europe and North Africa *T. violaceum* may be responsible for approximately 60% of cases of tinea capitis. This condition is characterized by a mild scaling and loss of hair and in some cases it may be contagious. Tinea corporis is characterized by infection of the skin of the trunk, leg and arms with a dermatophyte and is usually caused by *Trichophyton* spp., *Microsporum* spp. or *Epidermophyton floccosum*. Lesions are itchy, dry and show scaling. Typically lesions retain a circular morphology and the condition is often referred to as 'ringworm'. Tinea cruris is seen where the skin of the groin is infected with a dermatophytic fungus, usually *E. floccosum* or *Trichophyton rubrum*. This condition is highly contagious via fomites (towels, sheets, etc.) and up to 25% of patients show recurrence following antifungal therapy. Tinea pedis presents as infection of the feet with a dermatophyte and is very common and easily contracted. The principal fungi responsible for this condition are *T. rubrum* and *E. floccosum* and the sites of infection may include the webs of the toes, the sides of the feet or the soles of the feet. Tinea manuum is a fungal infection of the hands and can be caused by a range of fungi, most notably *Trichophyton mentagrophytes*. Infection is often seen in association with eczema and can result from transmission of fungi from another infected body site. Tinea unguium is defined as infection of the fingernails or toenails and is often described as onychomycosis, which includes infections due to a range of other fungi, bacteria and nail damage associated with certain disease states (e.g. psoriasis).

8 Antibiotic production by fungi

Perhaps one of the most important discoveries regarding the beneficial use of fungi for humans was the identification in 1929 by Sir Alexander Fleming that an isolate of *Penicillium notatum* produced a substance capable of killing Gram-positive bacteria. This compound was subsequently identified as penicillin and was the first member of the β-lactam class of antibiotics to be discovered. These compounds function by inhibiting peptidoglycan synthesis in bacteria and their use has reduced the importance of the Gram-positive bacteria as a cause of disease. Subsequent to the identification of penicillin production by *P. notatum* a screen revealed that *Penicillium chrysogenum* was a superior producer. Following a series of mutagenic and selection procedures the strain used in conventional fermentations is capable of producing penicillin at a rate of 7000 mg/L compared with the 3 mg/L of Fleming's *P. notatum* isolate. A typical penicillin fermentation yields three types of penicillin, namely F, G and V. The latter can be used directly; however, penicillin G is modified by the action of penicillin acylase to give a variety of semi-synthetic penicillins that show resistance to the action of bacterial penicillinases, which are implicated in conferring antibacterial drug resistance.

The majority of antibiotics obtained from fungi are produced by fermentation and most are secondary metabolites, production of which occurs in the stationary phase and is linked to sporulation. Catabolite repression can inhibit antibiotic production and one way to avoid this is to use low levels of glucose in the fermentation medium or to obtain a mutant that is not catabolite-repressed. The chemical content of the medium must be monitored, as high levels of nitrogen or phosphate (PO_4) retard antibiotic production. One problem that seriously affects the productivity of antibiotic fermentations is feedback inhibition, where the antibiotic builds to high intracellular levels and retards production or kills the cell. One means of reversing this is to introduce low levels of the antifungal agent amphotericin B, which increases membrane permeability, leading to a decrease in intracellular antibiotic levels and a concomitant increase in production.

Antibiotic production can be maximized by optimizing production as a result of random mutagenesis and selection. Another approach has been to fuse or mate high producing strains with good secretors. Rational selection is a process where a chelating agent is introduced into the fermentation to complex all the metal ions present and consequently has a beneficial effect on antibiotic production. More recently genetic manipulation has been employed to express the genes for antibiotic production in another species that has the possibility of producing hybrid antibiotics with novel targets.

9 Genetic manipulation of fungi

Fungi have been utilized for an extensive range of biotechnological applications. The *S. cerevisiae* expression system for producing recombinant protein

has a number of advantages including producing yields of purified secreted protein in the region of 20 mg/L. The yeast has been employed for the production of small hepatitis B surface proteins for use in recombinant hepatitis B vaccines and in the production of several recombinant malarial proteins, again for use in a vaccine. Antimalarial vaccine components produced by *S. cerevisiae* are currently in phase one clinical trials. *S. cerevisiae* has also been employed to produce the interferon class of cytokines, which are important in the treatment of diseases such as AIDS-associated Kaposi's sarcoma, and to prevent re-occurrence of infections in patients suffering from chronic granulomatous disease.

Yeasts are a popular choice for foreign gene expression as they have traditionally been classed as GRAS (generally regarded as safe), are easy to cultivate and are physically robust. From a genetic point of view *S. cerevisiae* is a eukaryotic organism, possesses a small genome and often contains natural plasmids (e.g. 2 µm circle) which can be utilized for transformation. In terms of their use as a molecular biological tool yeast strains can be transformed easily, are generally good secretors of protein, splice introns from animal genes and their RNA polymerase recognizes animal promoters. A number of vectors are utilized for transforming yeast cells and include integrative plasmids (e.g. Yip), independently replicating plasmids (e.g. Yrp) and specialized plasmids (e.g. yeast killer plasmid). Once a yeast has been transformed with a plasmid containing the gene of interest, the gene is transcribed and translated. Post-translation modification (e.g. glycosylation) occurs and secretion involves export of the protein of interest from the cell. As *S. cerevisiae* is not a prolific secretor of foreign protein, superior yeast secretors such as the yeast *Candida maltosa*, *Yarrowia lipolytica* and *Pichia* species have become more routinely employed in recent years.

The ability to enzymically remove fungal cell walls and produce a protoplast has been exploited to generate strains capable of enhanced ethanol production or the metabolism of novel combinations of carbohydrates. Once protoplasts are formed they may be fused by incubation in polyethylene glycol (PEG) and calcium ions, which induces membrane breakdown. Selection of the resulting fusants ensures the isolation of hybrids combining characteristics of both parents. Protoplast fusion has been particularly successful in overcoming sexual incompatibility barriers that exist between fungal species. Protoplast fusion has been utilized to generate strains of *S. cerevisiae* that produce glucoamylase, overproduce the amino acid methionine and ferment xylose to ethanol. Fungal cell transformation is also possible once protoplasts have been isolated.

Fungi have been utilized for thousands of years for the production of various foods and beverages. While these applications are still important, fungi are now being used in novel ways for the production of single cell protein, antibiotics, enzymes and as expression systems for the production and secretion of foreign proteins. Consequently, the continued use of fungi on a wide scale by humans is guaranteed.

10 Further reading

Abu-Salah, K. (1996) Amphotericin B: an update. *Br J Biomed Sci,* 53, 122–133.

Bennett, J. (1998) Mycotechnology: the role of fungi in biotechnology. *J Biotechnol,* 66, 101–107.

Cohen, B. (1998) Amphotericin B toxicity and lethality: a tale of two channels. *Int J Pharmaceut,* 162, 95–106.

Cotter, G. & Kavanagh, K. (2000) Adherence mechanisms of *Candida albicans. Br J Biomed Sci,* 57, 241–249.

Daly, P. & Kavanagh, K. (2001) Pulmonary Aspergillosis: clinical presentation, diagnosis and therapy. *Br J Biomed Sci,* 58, 197–205.

Daum, G., Lees, N. D., Bard, M. & Dickson, R. (1998) Biochemistry, cell biology and molecular biology of lipids of *Saccharomyces cerevisiae. Yeast,* 14, 1471–1510.

Denning, D. (1996) Aspergillosis: diagnosis and treatment. *Int J Antimicrob Agents,* 6, 161–168.

Jennings, D. & Lysek, G. (1999) *Fungal Biology,* 2nd edn. Bios Scientific Publishers, Oxford.

Kavanagh, K. & Whittaker, P. A. (1996) Application of protoplast fusion to the non-conventional yeasts. *Enz Microbiol Technol,* 18, 45–51.

Koltin, Y. & Hitchcock, C. (1997) The search for new triazole antifungal agents. *Curr Opin Chem Biol,* 1, 176–182.

Odds, F. (1996) Resistance of clinically important yeast to antifungal agents. *Int J Antimicrob Agents,* 6, 145–147.

Richardson, M. & Johnson, E. (2000) *The Pocket Guide to Fungal Infection.* Blackwell Science, Oxford.

Stewart, G. (1997) Genetic manipulation of brewer's and distiller's yeast strains. *Food Sci Technol Today,* 11, 181–182.

Sheehan, D., Hitchcock, C. & Sibley, C. (1999) Current and emerging azole antifungal agents. *Clin Microbiol Rev,* 12, 40–79.

Walker, G. (1998) *Yeast Physiology and Biotechnology.* Wiley, Chichester, UK.

Chapter 5

Viruses

Jean-Yves Maillard and David Stickler

1 Introduction

Following the demonstration by Koch and his colleagues that anthrax, tuberculosis and diphtheria were caused by bacteria, it was thought that similar organisms would, in time, be shown to be responsible for all infectious diseases. It gradually became obvious, however, that for a number of important diseases no such bacterial cause could be established. Infectious material from a case of rabies, for example, could be passed through special filters which held back all particles of bacterial size, and the resulting bacteria-free filtrate still proved to be capable of inducing rabies when inoculated into a susceptible animal. The term virus had, up until this time, been used quite indiscriminately to describe any agent capable of producing disease, so these filter-passing agents were originally called filterable viruses. With the passage of time the description 'filterable' has been dropped and the name virus has come to refer specifically to what are now known to be a distinctive group of microorganisms different in structure and method of replication from all others.

2 General properties of viruses

All forms of life—animal, plant and even bacterial—are susceptible to infection by viruses. Three main properties distinguish viruses from their various host cells: size, nucleic acid content and metabolic capabilities.

2.1 Size

Whereas a bacterial cell like a staphylococcus might be 1000 nm in diameter, the largest of the human pathogenic viruses, the poxviruses, measure only 250 nm along their longest axis, and the smallest, the poliovirus, is only 28 nm in diameter. They are mostly, therefore, beyond the limit of resolution of the light microscope and have to be visualized with the electron microscope.

2.2 Nucleic acid content

Viruses contain only a single type of nucleic acid, either DNA or RNA.

2.3 Metabolic capabilities

Virus particles have no metabolic machinery of their own. They cannot synthesize their own protein and nucleic acid from inanimate laboratory media and thus fail to grow on even nutritious media. They are obligatory intracellular parasites, only growing within other living cells whose energy and protein-producing systems they redirect for the purpose of manufacturing new viral components. The production of new virus particles generally results in death of the host cell and as the particles spread from cell to cell (e.g. within a tissue), disease can become apparent in the host.

3 Structure of viruses

In essence, virus particles are composed of a core of genetic material, either DNA or RNA, surrounded by a coat of protein. The function of the coat is to protect the viral genes from inactivation by adverse environmental factors, such as tissue nuclease enzymes which would otherwise digest a naked viral chromosome during its passage from cell to cell within a host. In a number of viruses the coat also plays an important part in the attachment of the virus to receptors on susceptible cells, and in many bacterial viruses the coat is further modified to facilitate the insertion of the viral genome through the tough structural barrier of the bacterial cell wall. The morphology of a variety of viruses is illustrated in Fig. 5.1.

The viral protein coat, or *capsid*, is composed of a large number of subunits, the *capsomeres*. This subunit structure is a fundamental property and is important from a number of aspects.

1 It leads to considerable economy of genetic information. This can be illustrated by considering some of the smaller viruses, which might, for example, have as a genome a single strand of RNA composed of about 3000 nucleotides and a protein coat with an overall composition of some 20 000 amino acid units. Assuming that one amino acid is coded for by a triplet of nucleotides, such a coat in the form of a single large protein would require a gene some 60 000 nucleotides in length. If, however, the viral coat comprised repeating units each composed of about 100 amino acids, only a section of about 300 nucleotides long would be required to specify the capsid protein, leaving genetic capacity for other essential functions.

2 Such a subunit structure permits the construction of the virus particles by a process in which the subunits self-assemble into structures held together by non-covalent intermolecular forces as occurs in the process of crystallization. This eliminates the need for a sequence of enzyme-catalysed reactions for coat synthesis. It also provides an automatic quality control system, as subunits which may have major structural defects fail to become incorporated into complete particles.

3 The subunit composition is such that the intracellular release of the viral genome from its coat involves only the dissociation of non-covalently bonded subunits, rather than the degradation of an integral protein sheath.

In addition to the protein coat, many animal virus particles are surrounded by a lipoprotein envelope which has generally been derived from the cytoplasmic membrane of their last host cell.

The geometry of the capsomeres results in their assembly into particles exhibiting one of two different architectural styles—helical or icosahedral symmetry (Fig. 5.2).

There is a third structural group comprising the poxviruses and many bacterial viruses, in which a number of major structural components can be identified and the overall geometry of the particles is complex.

3.1 Helical symmetry

Some virus particles have their protein subunits symmetrically packed in a helical array, forming hollow cylinders. The tobacco mosaic virus (TMV) is the classic example. X-ray diffraction data and electron micrographs have revealed that 16 subunits per turn of the helix project from a central axial hole that runs the length of the particle. The nucleic acid does not lie in this hole, but is

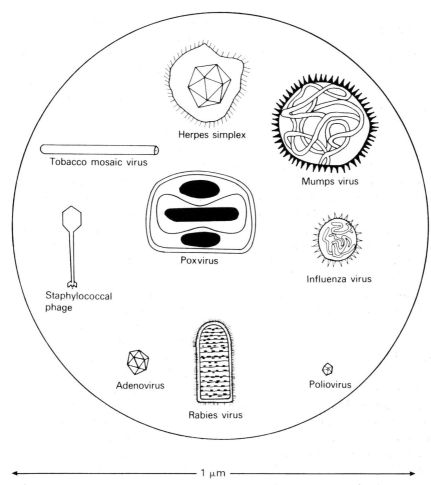

Fig. 5.1 The morphology of a variety of virus particles. The large circle indicates the relative size of a staphylococcus cell.

embedded into ridges on the inside of each subunit and describes its own helix from one end of the particle to the other.

Helical symmetry was thought at one time to exist only in plant viruses. It is now known, however, to occur in a number of animal virus particles. The influenza and mumps viruses, for example, which were first seen in early electron micrographs as roughly spherical particles, have now been observed as enveloped particles; within the envelope, the capsids themselves are helically symmetrical and appear similar to the rods of TMV, except that they are more flexible and are wound like coils of rope in the centre of the particle.

3.2 Icosahedral symmetry

The viruses in this architectural group have their capsomeres arranged in the form of regular icosahedra, i.e. polygons having 12 vertices, 20 faces and 30 sides. At each of the 12 vertices or corners of these icosahedral particles is a capsomere, called a *penton*, which is surrounded by five neighbouring units. Each of the 20 triangular faces contains an identical number of capsomeres which are surrounded by six neighbours and called *hexons*. In plant and bacterial viruses exhibiting this type of symmetry, the hexons and pentons are composed of the same polypeptide chains; in animal viruses, however, they may be distinct proteins. The number of hexons per capsid varies considerably in different viruses. Adenovirus, for example, is constructed from 240 hexons and 12 pentons, while the much smaller poliovirus is composed of 20 hexons and 12 pentons.

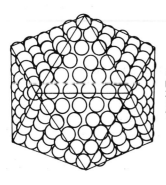

An icosahedral virus particle composed of 252 capsomeres 240 being hexons and 12 being pentons

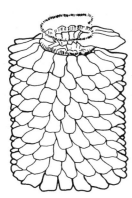

A helical virus partially disrupted to show the helical coil of viral nucleic acid embedded in the capsomeres

Fig. 5.2 Icosahedral and helical symmetry in viruses.

4 The effect of chemical and physical agents on viruses

Viruses generally exhibit greater sensitivity to chemical agents (biocides) than that shown by spore-forming organisms, but they may be more resistant than many species of bacteria, fungi and protozoa that do not form spores or cysts. Viruses can be divided into two major groups depending upon their sensitivity to biocides: the enveloped and the non-enveloped (naked) viruses. Enveloped viruses are generally large, and the presence of the lipid-containing envelope derived from the host cell enhances their susceptibility to chemical agents. Among naked viruses, the small ones such as picornaviruses (e.g. poliovirus) are among the most resistant to disinfection. Not all biocides have virucidal activity and the activity they do exhibit is subject to the environmental influences described in Chapter 11.

Biocides probably have multiple target sites on viral particles and the overall damage caused results in loss of viral infectivity (Table 5.1). When compared to bacterial cells, however, viruses present only a few structural targets to biocides: the envelope (when present), the glycoproteins, the capsid and the nucleic acid. The activity of biocides against the viral envelope has not been well documented but it can be expected that membrane-active agents such as phenolics and the cationic biocides (e.g. chlorhexidine and quaternary ammonium compounds — QACs) will act against the viral envelope, which is a typical unit membrane. The capsid is

Table 5.1 Possible virus–biocide interactions

Interaction	Consequence
Non-target sites attacked	Virus inactivation
Reversible adsorption of biocides to anti-receptors	Virus inactivation via loss of infectivity
	Reversible with the removal of the selective pressure (e.g. use of neutralizers)
Non-reversible adsorption to anti-receptors	Virus inactivation via loss of infectivity
Reversible conformational change of virus	Virus inactivation via loss of infectivity
	Reversible with the removal of the selective pressure
Destruction of the capsid	Inactivation of the virus
	Release of possible intact and infectious viral nucleic acid
Destruction of the nucleic acid within an intact capsid	Virus inactivation
Destruction of the capsid and the viral nucleic acid	Complete virus inactivation

probably the most important target site and any agents reacting strongly with protein amino groups (e.g. glutaraldehyde, ethylene oxide) or thiol groups (e.g. hypochlorite, iodine, ethylene oxide and hydrogen peroxide) may show virucidal activity. The release of an intact viral genome from a damaged capsid might be a cause for concern. The nucleic acid is the infectious part of the virus and its alteration/destruction by a biocide will result in viral inactivation. The size and nature of the genome and its interaction with the capsid (e.g. helical symmetry) certainly play a role in the sensitivity of the virus to biocides, and an increase in biocide concentration might result in an increase in the overall damage caused to a viral particle. In general, highly reactive biocides such as alkylating (e.g. glutaraldehyde) and oxidizing agents (e.g. peracetic acid) (Chapter 17) have good virucidal activity. However, other agents such as cationic biocides, phenolics and alcohols might have activity against enveloped viruses but a more limited effect on non-enveloped ones.

Physical agents such as heat and irradiation can inactivate viruses, and these processes, together with good hygiene and active immunization (Chapters 8, 9 and 23), are of vital importance in the control of human viral diseases. Most viruses are readily inactivated following exposure at 60°C for 30 minutes and thermal processes are used for eliminating viruses (e.g. HIV) from blood products. However, some species are more resistant, and hepatitis B for example can survive long periods of exposure to higher temperatures, probably because of the number of viral particles present at one time. Viruses can withstand low temperatures and are routinely stored at −40°C to −70°C. The enveloped viruses are extremely sensitive to drying on surfaces, whereas much longer survival times are seen with non-enveloped viruses.

UV irradiation can be used to eliminate viruses, especially airborne particles, by damaging viral nucleic acid, although again, small non-enveloped particles might be more resistant. Virus destruction can also be achieved by exposure to ionizing radiation (e.g. γ-rays, accelerated electrons), which is used in terminal sterilization processes applied to pharmaceutical and medical products (Chapter 20).

Because of their small size many species of virus can enter the pores of filter membranes used for sterilization of liquids, but particle entrapment by the membrane is often achieved as a result of adsorption processes. As a consequence, substantial reductions in viral concentration can result from filtration through membranes of appropriate characteristics, and adequate assurance of sterility may be achieved provided that the pre-sterilization bioburden is carefully controlled (Chapter 20).

5 Virus–host cell interactions

The precise sequence of events resulting from the infection of a cell by a virus will vary with different virus–host systems, but they will be variations of four basic themes.

1 Multiplication of the virus and destruction of the host cell.

2 Elimination of the virus from the cell and the infection aborted without a recognizable effect on the cells occurring.

3 Survival of the infected cell unchanged, except that it now carries the virus in a latent state.

4 Survival of the infected cell in a dramatically altered or transformed state, e.g. transformation of a normal cell to one having the properties of a cancerous cell.

6 Bacteriophages

Bacteriophages, or as they are more simply termed, phages, are viruses that have bacteria as their host cells. The name was first given by D'Herelle to an agent which he found could produce lysis of the dysentery bacillus *Shigella shiga*. D'Herelle was convinced that he had stumbled across an agent with tremendous medical potential. His phage could destroy *Sh. shiga* in broth culture so why not in the dysenteric gut of humans? Similar agents were found before long which were active against the bacteria of many other diseases, including anthrax, scarlet fever, cholera and diphtheria, and attempts were made to use them to treat these diseases. It was a great disappointment, however, that phages so virulent in their antibacterial activity

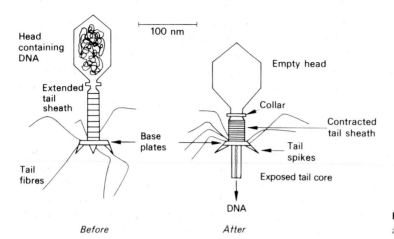

Head
containing
DNA

100 nm

Empty head

Extended
tail
sheath

Collar

Contracted
tail sheath

Base
plates

Tail
spikes

Tail
fibres

Exposed tail core

DNA

Before

After

Fig. 5.3 T-even phage structure before and after tail contraction.

in vitro proved impotent *in vivo*. A possible exception was cholera, where some success seems to have been achieved, and cholera phages were apparently used by the medical corps of the German and Japanese armies during World War II to treat this disease. Since the development of antibiotics, however, phage therapy has been abandoned.

Interest in bacterial viruses did not cease with the demise of phage therapy. They proved to be very much easier to handle in the laboratory than other viruses and had conveniently rapid multiplication cycles. They have, therefore, been used extensively as the experimental models for elucidating the biochemical mechanisms of viral replication. A vast amount of information has been collected about them and many of the important advances in molecular biology, such as the discovery of messenger RNA (mRNA), the understanding of the genetic code and the way in which genes are controlled, have come from work on phage–bacterium systems.

It is probable that all species of bacteria are susceptible to phages. Any particular phage will exhibit a marked specificity in selecting host cells, attacking only organisms belonging to a single species. A *Staphylococcus aureus* phage, for example, will not infect *Staph. epidermidis* cells. In most cases, phages are in fact strain-specific, only being active on certain characteristic strains of a given species.

Most phages are tadpole-shaped structures with heads which function as containers for the nucleic acid and tails which are used to attach the virus to its host cell. There are, however, some simple icosahedral phages and others that are helically symmetrical cylinders. The dimensions of the phage heads vary from the large T-even group (Fig. 5.3) of *Escherichia coli* phages (60 × 90 nm) to the much smaller ones (30 × 30 nm) of certain *Bacillus* phages. The tails vary in length from 15 to 200 nm and can be quite complex structures (Fig. 5.3). While the majority of phages have double-stranded DNA as their genetic material, some of the very small icosahedral and the helical phages have single-stranded DNA or RNA.

On the basis of the response they produce in their host cells, phages can be classified as *virulent* or *temperate*. Infection of a sensitive bacterium with a virulent phage results in the replication of the virus, lysis of the cell and release of new infectious progeny phage particles. Temperate phages can produce this lytic response, but they are also capable of a symbiotic response in which the invading viral genome does not take over the direction of cellular activity, the cell survives the infection and the viral nucleic acid becomes incorporated into the bacterial chromosome, where it is termed *prophage*. Cells carrying viral genes in this way are referred to as *lysogenic*.

6.1 The lytic growth cycle

The replication of virulent phage was initially studied using the T-even-numbered (T_2, T_4, and T_6)

phages of *E. coli*. These phages adsorb, by their long tail fibres, on to specific receptors on the surface of the bacterial cell wall. The base plate of the tail sheath and its pins then lock the phage into position on the outside of the cell. At this stage, the tail sheath contracts towards the head, while the base plate remains in contact with the cell wall and, as a result, the hollow tail core is exposed and driven through to the cytoplasmic membrane (Fig. 5.3). Simultaneously, the DNA passes from the head, through the hollow tail core and is deposited on the outer surface of the cytoplasmic membrane, from where it finds its own way into the cytoplasm. The phage protein coat remains on the outside of the cell and plays no further part in the replication cycle.

Within the first few minutes after infection, transcription of part of the viral genome produces 'early' mRNA molecules, which are translated into a set of 'early' proteins. These serve to switch off host cell macromolecular synthesis, degrade the host DNA and start to make components for viral DNA. Many of the early proteins duplicate enzymes already present in the host, concerned in the manufacture of nucleotides for cell DNA. However, the requirement for the production of 5-hydroxymethylcytosine-containing nucleotides, which replace the normal cytosine derivatives in T-even phage DNA, means that some of the early enzymes are entirely new to the cell. With the build-up of its components, the viral DNA replicates and also starts to produce a batch of 'late' mRNA molecules, transcribed from genes which specify the proteins of the phage coat. These late messages are translated into the subunits of the capsid structures, which condense to form phage heads, tails and tail fibres, and then together with viral DNA are assembled into complete infectious particles. The enzyme digesting the cell wall, lysozyme, is also produced in the cell at this stage and it eventually brings about the lysis of the cell and liberation of about 100 progeny viruses, some 25 minutes after infection.

As other phage systems have been studied, it has become clear that the T-even model of virulent phage replication is atypical in a number of respects. The large T-even genomes, with their coding capacity for about 200 proteins, give these phages a relatively high degree of independence from their hosts. Although relying on the host energy and protein-synthesizing systems they are capable of specifying a battery of their own enzymes. Most other phages have considerably smaller genomes. They tend to disturb the host cell metabolism to a much lesser extent than the T-even viruses, and also rely to a greater degree on pre-existing cell enzymes to produce components for their nucleic acid.

The lytic activity of the virulent phages can be demonstrated by mixing phage with about 10^7 sensitive indicator bacteria in 5 ml of molten nutrient agar. The mixture is then poured over the surface of a solid nutrient agar plate. On incubation, the phage particles will infect bacteria in their immediate neighbourhood, lysing them and producing a burst of progeny viruses. These particles then infect bacteria in the vicinity, producing a second generation of progeny and this sequence is repeated many times. In the meantime the uninfected bacteria produce a thick carpet or lawn of growth over the agar. As the lawn develops, clear holes or 'plaques' become obvious in it at each site of virus multiplication (Fig. 5.4). As each of these plaques is initiated by a single phage particle, they provide a means for titrating phage preparations.

6.2 Lysogeny

When a temperate phage is mixed with sensitive indicator bacteria and plated as described above, the

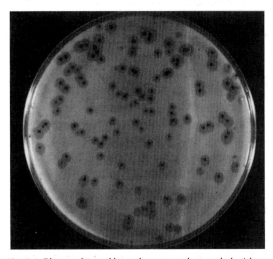

Fig. 5.4 Plaques formed by a phage on a plate seeded with *Bacillus subtilis*.

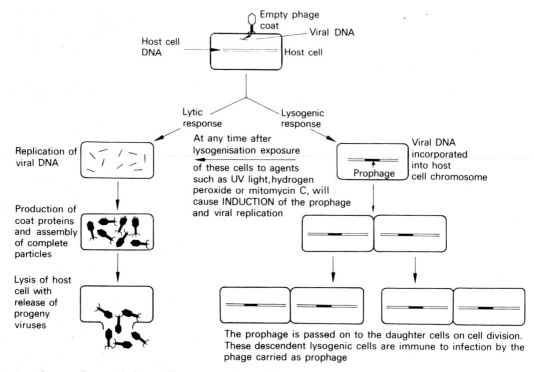

Fig. 5.5 Scheme to illustrate the lytic and lysogenic responses of bacteriophages.

reaction at each focus of infection is generally a combination of lytic and lysogenic responses. Some bacteria will be lysed and produce phage, others will survive as lysogenic cells, and the plaque becomes visible as a partial area of clearing in the bacterial lawn. It is possible to pick off cells from the central areas of these plaques and demonstrate that they carry prophage.

The phage lambda (λ) of *E. coli* is the temperate phage that has been most extensively studied. When any particular strain of *E. coli*, say K12, is infected with λ, the cells surviving the infection are designated *E. coli* K12(λ) to indicate that they are carrying the λ-prophage.

The essential features of lysogenic cells and the phenomenon of lysogeny are listed below and summarized in Fig. 5.5.

1 Integration of the prophage into the bacterial chromosome ensures that, on cell division, each daughter cell will acquire the set of viral genes.

2 In a normally growing culture of lysogenic bacteria, the majority of bacteria manage to keep their prophages in a dormant state. In a very small minority of cells, however, the prophage genes express themselves. This results in the multiplication of the virus, lysis of the cells and liberation of infectious particles into the medium.

3 Exposure of lysogenic cultures to certain chemical and physical agents, e.g. hydrogen peroxide, mitomycin C and ultraviolet light, results in mass lysis and the production of high titres of phage. This process is called *induction*.

4 When a lysogenic cell is infected by the same type of phage as it carries as prophage, the infection is aborted, the activity of the invading viral genes being repressed by the same mechanism that normally keeps the prophage in a dormant state.

5 Lysogeny is generally a very stable state, but occasionally a cell will lose its prophage and these 'cured' cells are once more susceptible to infection by that particular phage type.

Lysogeny is an extremely common phenomenon and it seems that most natural isolates of bacteria carry one or more prophages: some strains of *Staph.*

aureus have been shown to carry four or five different prophages.

The induction of a lysogenic culture to produce infectious phages, followed by lysogenization of a second strain of the bacterial species by these phages, results in the transmission of a prophage from the chromosome of one type of cell to that of another. On this migration, temperate bacteriophages can occasionally act as vectors for the transfer of bacterial genes between cells. This process is called *transduction* and it can be responsible for the transfer of such genetic factors as those that determine resistance to antibiotics (Chapter 13). In addition, certain phages have the innate ability to change the properties of their host cell. The classic example is the case of the β-phage of *Corynebacterium diphtheriae*. The acquisition of the β-prophage by non-toxin-producing strains of this species results in their conversion to diphtheria toxin-producers.

6.3 Epidemiological uses

Different strains of a number of bacterial species can be distinguished by their sensitivity to a collection of phages. Bacteria which can be typed in this way include *Staph. aureus* and *Salmonella typhi*. The particular strain of, say, *Staph. aureus* responsible for an outbreak of infection is characterized by the pattern of its sensitivity to a standard set of phages and then possible sources of infection are examined for the presence of that same phage type of *Staph. aureus*.

More recently, the fact that many of the chemical agents which cause the induction of prophage are carcinogenic has led to the use of lysogenic bacteria in screening tests for detecting potential carcinogens.

7 Human viruses

Viruses are, of course, important and common causes of disease in humans, particularly in children. Fortunately, most infections are not serious and, like the rhinovirus infections responsible for the common cold syndrome, are followed by the complete recovery of the patient. Many viral infections are in fact so mild that they are termed 'silent', to indicate that the virus replicates in the body without producing symptoms of disease. Occasionally, however, some of the viruses that are normally responsible for mild infections can produce serious disease. This pattern of pathogenicity is exemplified by the enterovirus group. Most enterovirus infections merely result in the symptomless replication of the virus in the cells lining the alimentary tract. Only in a small percentage of infections does the virus spread from this site via the bloodstream and the lymphatic system to other organs, producing a fever and possibly a skin rash in the host. On rare occasions enteroviruses like poliovirus can progress to the central nervous system where they may produce an aseptic meningitis or paralysis. There are a few virus diseases, such as rabies, which are invariably severe and have very high mortality rates.

Human viruses will cause disease in other animals. Some are capable of infecting only a few closely related primate species, others will infect a wide range of mammals. Under the conditions of natural infection viruses generally exhibit a considerable degree of tissue specificity. The influenza virus, for example, replicates only in the cells lining the upper respiratory tract.

Table 5.2 presents a summary of the properties of some of the more important human viruses.

7.1 Cultivation of human viruses

The cultivation of viruses from material taken from lesions is an important step in the diagnosis of many viral diseases. Studies of the basic biology and multiplication processes of human viruses also require that they are grown in the laboratory under experimental conditions. Human pathogenic viruses can be propagated in three types of cell systems.

7.1.1 Cell culture

Cells from human or other primate sources are obtained from an intact tissue, e.g. human embryo kidney or monkey kidney. The cells are dispersed by digestion with trypsin and the resulting suspension of single cells is generally allowed to settle in a vessel containing a nutrient medium. The cells will metabolize and grow and after a few days of incubation at

Table 5.2 Important human viruses and their properties

Group	Virus	Characteristics	Clinical importance
DNA viruses Poxviruses	Variola Vaccinia	Large particles 200–250 nm: complex symmetry	Variola is the smallpox virus, it produces a systemic infection with a characteristic vesicular rash affecting the face, arms and legs, and has a high mortality rate. Vaccinia has been derived from the cowpox virus and is used to immunize against smallpox
Adenoviruses	Adenovirus	Icosahedral particles 80 nm in diameter	Commonly cause upper respiratory tract infections; tend to produce latent infections in tonsils and adenoids; will produce tumours on injection into hamsters, rats or mice
Herpesviruses	Herpes simplex virus (HSV1 and HSV2)	Enveloped, icosahedral particles 150 nm in diameter	HSV1 infects oral membranes in children, >80% are infected by adolescence. Following the primary infection the individual retains the HSV1 DNA in the trigeminal nerve ganglion for life and has a 50% chance of developing 'cold sores'. HSV2 is responsible for recurrent genital herpes
	Varicella-zoster virus (VZV)	Enveloped, isocahedral particles 150 nm in diameter	Causes chickenpox in children; virus remains dormant in any dorsal root ganglion of the CNS; release of immune control in the elderly stimulates reactivation resulting in shingles
	Cytomegalovirus (CMV)	Enveloped, icosahedral particles 150 nm in diameter	CMV is generally acquired in childhood as a subclinical infection. About 50% of adults carry the virus in a dormant state in white blood cells. The virus can cause severe disease (pneumonia, hepatitis, encephalitis) in immunocompromised patients. Primary infections during pregnancy can induce serious congenital abnormalities in the fetus
	Epstein–Barr virus (EBV)	Enveloped, icosahedral particles 150 nm in diameter	Infections occur by salivary exchange. In young children they are commonly asymptomatic but the virus persists in a latent form in lymphocytes. Infection delayed until adolescence often results in glandular fever. In tropical Africa, a severe EBV infection early in life predisposes the child to malignant facial tumours (Burkitt's lymphoma)
Hepatitis viruses	Hepatitis B virus (HBV)	Spherical enveloped particle 42 nm in diameter enclosing an inner icosahedral 27-nm nucleocapsid	In areas such as South-East Asia and Africa, most children are infected by perinatal transmission. In the Western world the virus is spread through contact with contaminated blood or by sexual intercourse. There is strong evidence that chronic infections with HBV can progress to liver cancer
Papovaviruses	Papilloma virus	Naked icosahedra 50 nm in diameter	Multiply only in epithelial cells of skin and mucous membranes causing warts. There is evidence that some types are associated with cervical carcinoma
RNA viruses Myxoviruses	Influenza virus	Enveloped particles, 100 nm in diameter with a helically symmetric	These viruses are capable of extensive antigenic variation, producing new types against which the human population does not have effective immunity. These new antigenic

Table 5.2 *Continued*

Group	Virus	Characteristics	Clinical importance
		capsid; haemagglutinin and neuraminidase spikes project from the envelope	types can cause pandemics of influenza. In natural infections the virus only multiplies in the cells lining the upper respiratory tract. The constitutional symptoms of influenza are probably brought about by absorption of toxic breakdown products from the dying cells on the respiratory epithelium
Paramyxoviruses	Mumps virus	Enveloped particles variable in size, 110–170 nm in diameter, with helical capsids	Infection in children produces characteristic swelling of parotid and submaxillary salivary glands. The disease can have neurological complications, e.g. meningitis, especially in adults
	Measles virus	Enveloped particles variable in size, 120–250 nm in diameter, helical capsids	Very common childhood fever, immunity is life-long and second attacks are very rare
Rhabdoviruses	Rabies virus	Bullet-shaped particles, 75–180 nm, enveloped, helical capsids	The virus has a very wide host range, infecting all mammals so far tested; dogs, cats and cattle are particularly susceptible. The incubation period of rabies is extremely varied, ranging from 6 days up to 1 year. The virus remains localized at the wound site of entry for a while before passing along nerve fibres to central nervous system, where it invariably produces a fatal encephalitis
Reoviruses	Rotavirus	An inner core is surrounded by two concentric icosahedral shells producing particles 70 nm in diameter	A very common cause of gastroenteritis in infants. It is spread through poor water supplies and when standards of general hygiene are low. In developing countries it is responsible for about a million deaths each year
Picornaviruses	Poliovirus	Naked icosahedral particles 28 nm in diameter	One of a group of enteroviruses common in the gut of humans. The primary site of multiplication is the lymphoid tissue of the alimentary tract. Only rarely do they cause systemic infections or serious neurological conditions like encephalitis or poliomyelitis
	Rhinoviruses	Naked icosahedra 30 nm in diameter	The common cold viruses; there are over 100 antigenically distinct types, hence the difficulty in preparing effective vaccines. The virus is shed copiously in watery nasal secretions
	Hepatitis A virus (HAV)	Naked icosahedra 27 nm in diameter	Responsible for 'infectious hepatitis' spread by the oro-faecal route especially in children. Also associated with sewage contamination of food or water supplies
Togaviruses	Rubella	Spherical particles 70 nm in diameter, a tightly adherent envelope surrounds an icosahedral capsid	Causes German measles in children. An infection contracted in the early stages of pregnancy can induce severe multiple congenital abnormalities, e.g. deafness, blindness, heart disease and mental retardation

Table 5.2 *Continued*

Group	Virus	Characteristics	Clinical importance
Flaviviruses	Yellow fever virus	Spherical particles 40 nm in diameter with an inner core surrounded by an adherent lipid envelope	The virus is spread to humans by mosquito bites; the liver is the main target; necrosis of hepatocytes leads to jaundice and fever
	Hepatitis C virus (HCV)	Spherical particles 40 nm in diameter consisting of an inner core surrounded by an adherent lipid envelope	The virus is spread through blood transfusions and blood products. Induces a hepatitis which is usually milder than that caused by HBV
Filoviruses	Ebola virus	Long filamentous rods composed of a lipid envelope surrounding a helical nucleocapsid 1000 nm long, 80 nm in diameter	The virus is widespread amongst populations of monkeys. It can be spread to humans by contact with body fluids from the primates. The resulting haemorrhagic fever has a 90% case fatality rate
Retroviruses	Human T-cell leukaemia virus (HTLV-1)	Spherical enveloped virus 100 nm in diameter, icosahedral cores contain two copies of linear RNA molecules and reverse transcriptase	HTLV is spread inside infected lymphocytes in blood, semen or breast milk. Most infections remain asymptomatic but after an incubation period of 10–40 years in about 2% of cases, adult T-cell leukaemia can result
	Human immunodeficiency virus (HIV)	Differs from other retroviruses in that the core is cone-shaped rather than icosahedral	HIV is transmitted from person to person via blood or genital secretions. The principal target for the virus is the CD4+ T-lymphocyte cells. Depletion of these cells induces immunodeficiency
Hepatitis viruses	Hepatitis D virus (HDV)	An RNA-containing virus that can only replicate in cells co-infected with HBV. The spherical coat of HDV is composed of HBV capsid protein	The presence of the satellite HDV exacerbates the pathogenic effects of HBV producing severe hepatitis

37°C will form a continuous film or monolayer one cell thick. These cells are then capable of supporting viral replication. Cell cultures may be divided into three types according to their history.

1 Primary cell cultures, which are prepared directly from tissues.

2 Secondary cell cultures, which can be prepared by taking cells from some types of primary culture, usually those derived from embryonic tissue, dispersing them by treatment with trypsin and inoculating some into a fresh batch of medium. A limited number of subcultures can be performed with these sorts of cells, up to a maximum of about 50 before the cells degenerate.

3 There are now available a number of lines of cells, mainly originating from malignant tissue, which can be serially subcultured apparently indefinitely. These established cell lines are particularly convenient as they eliminate the requirement for fresh animal tissue for such sets or series of cultures. An example of these continuous cell lines are the famous HeLa cells, which were originally isolated

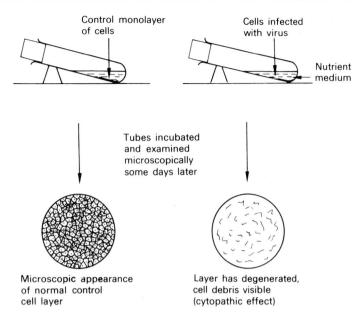

Fig. 5.6 The cytopathic effect of a virus on a tissue culture cell monolayer.

Microscopic appearance of normal control cell layer

Layer has degenerated, cell debris visible (cytopathic effect)

from a cervical carcinoma of a woman called Henrietta Lacks, long since dead but whose cells have been used in laboratories all over the world to grow viruses.

Inoculation of cell cultures with virus-containing material produces characteristic changes in the cells. The replication of many types of viruses produces the cytopathic effect (CPE) in which cells degenerate. This effect is seen as the shrinkage or sometimes ballooning of cells and the disruption of the monolayer by death and detachment of the cells (Fig. 5.6). The replicating virus can then be identified by inoculating a series of cell cultures with mixtures of the virus and different known viral antisera. If the virus is the same as one of the types used to prepare the various antisera, then its activity will be neutralized by that particular antiserum and CPE will not be apparent in that tube. Alternatively viral antisera labelled with a fluorescent dye can be used to identify the virus in the cell culture.

7.1.2 *The chick embryo*

Fertile chicken eggs, 10–12 days old, have been used as a convenient cell system in which to grow a number of human pathogenic viruses. Figure 5.7 shows that viruses generally have preferences for particular tissues within the embryo. Influenza viruses, for example, can be grown in the cells of the membrane bounding the amniotic cavity, while smallpox virus will grow in the chorioallantoic membrane. The growth of smallpox virus in the embryo is recognized by the formation of characteristic pock marks on the membrane. Influenza virus replication is detected by exploiting the ability of these particles to cause erythrocytes to clump together. Fluid from the amniotic cavity of the infected embryo is titrated for its haemagglutinating activity.

7.1.3 *Animal inoculation*

Experimental animals such as mice and ferrets have to be used for the cultivation of some viruses. Growth of the virus is indicated by signs of disease or death of the inoculated animal.

8 Multiplication of human viruses

The objective of viral replication is to ensure the multiplication of the virus by formation of virions (virus progeny) identical to the parent strain. Because of the structure of a virus, the multiplication cycle focuses mainly on the replication of viral DNA or RNA.

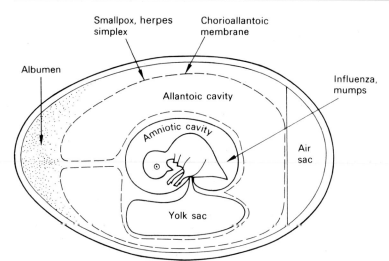

Fig. 5.7 A chick embryo showing the inoculation routes for virus cultivation.

The progress made in cell culture techniques has provided a better understanding of viral replication cycles. Human viruses generally have a slow multiplication cycle requiring from 4 to more than 40 hours (in some herpesviruses) for completion; this contrasts with bacterial viruses (bacteriophages) with a replication cycle as fast as 30 minutes. Certain viruses exhibit low infectivity; for example, picornavirus infectivity can be as low as 0.1% and rotavirus about 0.2%, and this makes the study of viral replication difficult.

In general, viral replication cycles, whatever the differences in detail, comprise events that can be separated into six discrete stages (Fig. 5.8):
• Attachment to the host cell
• Penetration of the host cell membrane
• Uncoating of the virus to release its core components
• Replication of the viral nucleic acids and translation of the genome
• Maturation or re-assembly of virions (i.e. progeny virus particles)
• Release of virions into the surrounding environment.

8.1 Attachment to the host cell

All viruses contain (glyco)protein materials on their surface, whether as an integral part of the capsid structure or in the form of spikes embedded in the viral envelope. These structures act as antireceptors that bind to a surface receptor on the target cells and hence they play an important role in the host–virus specificity, although some viruses may share common cell receptors. The virus–cell recognition event is similar to any protein–protein interaction in that it occurs through a stereospecific network of hydrogen bonds and lipophilic associations.

Viral attachment to the cell surface can be divided into three phases: (i) an initial contact mainly dependent on Brownian motion, (ii) a reversible phase during which electrostatic repulsion is reduced and (iii) irreversible changes in antireceptor–receptor configuration that initiates viral penetration through the cell membrane. A classic example of this process is the haemagglutinin antireceptor of influenza virus. It binds the terminal glycoside residues of gangliosides (cell surface glycolipids); this leads directly to the virus particle adhering to the cell. A similar interaction occurs during the attachment of HIV virus particles to T lymphocytes (see later).

8.2 Penetration of the viral particle

Once irreversibly attached to the cell surface, configuration changes of the complex anti-receptor–receptor initiate the penetration of the viral particle through the cell membrane. This energy-dependent

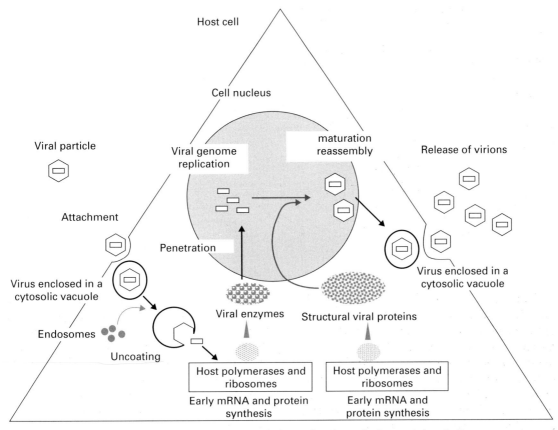

Fig. 5.8 Diagrammatic representation of the production and release of viral particles from an infected cell.

step occurs rapidly and operates by two mechanisms: endocytosis and fusion.

• During endocytosis, the association between receptor and anti-receptor draws the cell membrane to engulf the virus particle forming a cytosolic vacuole, similar to the process by which cells ingest other materials. Probably all non-enveloped viruses penetrate the cell in this manner, but some enveloped viruses such as orthomyxoviruses (e.g. influenza) also use this process.

• Fusion of the viral envelope and the cell membrane results in the direct release of the capsid into the cell cytoplasm. Herpesviruses and HIV penetrate their host cells in this manner. The precise biophysical details of the fusion process remain unknown.

8.3 Uncoating of the viral particle

Uncoating refers to the events after penetration which allow the virus to express its genome. For viruses that penetrate the cell via endocytosis, conformational changes in the virus coat and release of viral nucleocapsid into the cytoplasm result from acidification of the virus-containing cytosolic vacuoles following endosome fusion. Other viruses require only partial uncoating (e.g. reovirus) before transcription of their nucleic acid can begin, but in most cases the viral capsid completely disintegrates before viral functions start to be expressed. In some cases the nucleocapsid passes to the cell nucleus before uncoating occurs.

The uncoating process is increasingly studied because of its potential for antiviral chemotherapy. For example, amantadine and rimantadine (Fig. 5.9) are anti-influenza drugs, which function in part by inhibiting the envelope viral protein M2, resulting in the remaining association of the viral nucleocapsid with matrix proteins and preventing its transfer to the nucleus.

8.4 Replication of viral nucleic acids and translation of the genome

This stage of the viral replication cycle mainly involves three basic biochemical processes: the synthesis of new viral proteins (translation of the genome), RNA synthesis (transcription) and viral genome replication. There is a tremendous diversity in the structure, size and nature of the nucleic acid of mammalian viruses. There is no single pattern of replication, but all viruses make proteins with function to (i) alter the host cell metabolism in favour of virion production, (ii) ensure the replication of the viral genome and (iii) package the genome into virus particles. Viral protein synthesis can be divided into early and late protein synthesis. Early synthesis is concerned with the production of proteins involved in the replication of the viral genome such as polymerases, while late synthesis is more concerned with the production of structural components of the new virions. The mRNA molecules are, of course, translated on the cytoplasmic ribosomes.

The way in which the viral genome is replicated depends entirely on the nature of the nucleic acid carried by the virus. Positive strand RNA viruses (e.g. poliovirus) can use the parent RNA directly as mRNA, after the acquisition from the host cell of a terminal sequence enabling immediate translation. With negative strand RNA viruses (e.g. influenza virus), a positive RNA strand complementary in base sequence to the parent RNA has to be transcribed using an RNA-dependent RNA polymerase carried by the virus, as eukaryotic cells do not possess such enzymes.

Retroviruses (e.g. HIV) produce a proviral DNA from their positive strand RNA using the chemotherapeutically important reverse transcriptase enzyme. This is a unique enzyme acting both as RNA- and DNA-directed DNA polymerase, and as an associated RNAse activity. Its function is to produce a double-stranded proviral DNA, which is transported to the nucleus and integrated in the host genome under the control of a viral integrase. With the DNA-containing viruses, e.g. adenovirus, the nucleic acid passes to the nucleus where a host cell DNA-dependent RNA polymerase is used to transcribe part of the viral genome. The poxvirus, vaccinia, uses its own DNA-dependent RNA polymerase which is released during uncoating. For this virus the whole replication takes place in the cell cytoplasm, while for other DNA viruses, proteins synthesized in the cytoplasm are transported back to the nucleus where the virion assembly process takes place.

Although the replication of the viral genome is mainly under the control of polymerases, some complex viruses code for regulatory factors which suppress or accelerate cellular processes according to the need of the virus (e.g. *tat* gene in HIV).

The involvement of host cell enzymes in the replication of the viral proteins and genome severely limits the design of new antiviral drugs. However, unlike host mRNAs, which code directly for functional proteins, most viral genomes are polycistronic, which means that all the information is, or becomes, encoded in one piece of mRNA. As a result, the polyprotein produced by translation needs to be cleaved at appropriate positions for the different proteins to be functional. This post-translational protein processing offers targets for antiviral chemotherapy. Viruses that possess a polycistronic genome encode for a virus-specific protease, which is capable of performing cleavages at the correct place. Many of these viral proteases have been identified and characterized and have led to the discovery of several inhibitors, such as indinavir, sequinavir and ritonavir used for HIV chemotherapy.

8.5 Maturation or assembly of virions

As large amounts of viral materials accumulate within the cell, the role of structural proteins becomes evident. The structural proteins of small non-enveloped viruses (e.g. poliovirus) self-assemble once they are synthesized. Initially individual units form capsomeres, which then associate into capsids. The viral genome and associated proteins necessary for viral replication become engulfed in this new structure. Most non-enveloped viruses accumulate within the cytoplasm or nucleus and are only released when the cell lyses.

All enveloped human viruses acquire their phospholipid coating by budding through cellular membranes. For example, with the influenza virus, the capsid protein subunits are transported from the ribosomes to the nucleus, where they combine with new viral RNA molecules and are assembled into the helical capsids. The haemagglutinin and neuraminidase proteins that project from the envelope of the normal particles migrate to the cytoplasmic membrane where they displace the normal cell membrane proteins. The assembled nucleocapsids finally pass out from the nucleus, and as they impinge on the altered cytoplasmic membrane they cause it to bulge and bud off completed enveloped particles from the cell.

Other enveloped viruses, such as herpesviruses, assemble within the nucleus and acquire their envelope as they pass through the inner nuclear membrane. From here they pass into a vesicle that protects the virions from the cytoplasm and migrates to the cell surface.

The assembly of virions is not fully understood. It is thought that cellular factors such as chaperone proteins and the interactions between the viral nucleic acid and structural proteins might play an important role during the maturation process.

8.6 Release of virions into the surrounding environment

The release of virions ends the replication cycle of a virus. Two main release routes can be distinguished: budding and lysis. Most non-enveloped viruses accumulate within the cytoplasm or the nucleus and are only released when the cell lyses. The cell often self-disintegrates because normal cell housekeeping function is not maintained during viral replication. It has also been suggested that some viral proteases trigger the cell cytoplasmic membrane disintegration. Enveloped viruses usually exit the cell by budding. Virus particles are released in this way over a period of hours before the cell eventually dies. In the case of influenza virus, neuraminidase catalyses the cleavage of terminal neuraminic acid residues from cell surface gangliosides, which frees the virus particle from its interaction with the cell.

9 The problems of viral chemotherapy

Vaccination programmes have been very effective in the control of some viral diseases. Protection against smallpox was first demonstrated in 1796 by Jenner by inoculation with cowpox. Smallpox was later successfully eradicated. Poliovirus is also being eliminated thanks to a controlled intensive worldwide vaccination programme initiated by the World Health Organization. Such preventative methods are the most effective and economic way of controlling viral infections.

There are several possible biochemical target sites within the replication cycle of a virus (Table 5.3). The virus–receptor interaction, which is specific for the host cells (e.g. CD4–gp120 interaction between T lymphocytes and HIV), can potentially be blocked, although this approach would have a preventative rather than therapeutic role. There is greater potential for blocking the penetration and especially the uncoating processes. Some molecules (polypeptides) that bind to the viral coat are already being tested for their efficacy to block this viral replication step. However, the better prospects and most of the effective antiviral drugs available focus on the replication of viral core components, translation of the genome, and nucleic acid transcription and replication (e.g. DNA polymerase). Finally, it is possible that, to some extent, the maturation, assembly and release phase of virus particles could be blocked, although this process would be virus-dependent. For example, two very potent and highly selective neuraminidase inhibitors, zanamivir and ozaltamivir have been approved for clinical use against the influenza virus. These inhibitors prevent the shedding of virions and the transmission of infection.

With the increase in understanding of viral replication and in particular viral protein and nucleic acid synthesis, and the development of reliable and sophisticated antiviral assays, the young science of antiviral chemotherapy has progressed tremendously over the last 50 years. Acyclovir (Fig. 5.9) was probably the first truly effective and selective

Table 5.3 Possible target sites for chemotherapeutic agents

Target sites	Examples
Attachment, penetration and uncoating	Inhibition of HIV-1 attachment. Competition for CD4 receptors using a pentapeptide identical in sequence to the terminal amino acids of gp120*
	Inhibition of herpesvirus attachment. Inhibition of ribonucleotide reductase using a polypeptide*
	Inhibition of influenza virus attachment. Competition for cell receptor using a hexapeptide fusion sequence at the N-terminus of the haemagglutinin antireceptor*
Gene transcription and genome replication	Inhibition of viral coded reverse transcriptase using nucleoside analogues (e.g. ddI, 3TC, d4T, AZT)
	Inhibition of viral coded reverse transcriptase using non-nucleoside analogues (e.g. foscarnet)
	Inhibition of intracellular processing of viral proteins (e.g. alteration of glycosylation)†
	Inhibition of viral DNA replication using nucleoside analogues (e.g. idoxuridine against herpesvirus)
Inhibition of viral mRNA function	Use of oligonucleotides therapy (e.g. antisense nucleotides)†
Inhibition of viral DNA replication via the inhibition of specific polymerases	Use of nucleoside analogues such as acyclovir
	Foscarnet against herpesviruses
Inhibition of low molecular weight polypeptide gene products	Protease inhibitors such as indinavir, saquinavir (for HIV chemotherapy)

* Currently being studied and developed.
† Target site being considered for antiviral design and development.

antiviral agent. Viral polymerases have recently been the most widely studied target for antiviral chemotherapy, given that the replication of a virus is blocked by selectively blocking the production of viral nucleic acids. Nucleoside analogues such as acyclovir inhibit viral nucleic acid polymerases; this is probably the single most important chemotherapeutic interaction to date. For HIV chemotherapy, the inhibition of the viral encoded reverse transcriptase constitutes a major target site. Several nucleoside analogues such as didanosine (ddI), lamivudine (3TC), stavudine (d4T) and zidovudine (ZDV, formerly azidothymidine — AZT; Fig 5.9) are widely available. Nucleoside analogues are also used to inhibit the replication of viral DNA. For example, idoxiuridine (trifuridine) is incorporated into viral and cellular DNA instead of thymidine and is used for the treatment of herpes simplex virus and cytomegalovirus infections. Other non-nucleoside analogues such as nevirapine and foscarnet (a phosphate analogue; Fig. 5.9) are also employed in therapy, and oligonucleotides (nucleic acid oligomers) with base sequence complimentary to conserved regions of pro-viral DNA have been successful in the prevention of viral mRNA function. Oligonucleotide therapies can be divided into four separate approaches:

• Antisense nucleotides: production of an RNA sequence complementary to single-stranded viral RNA, which triggers the formation of double-stranded duplex, inhibiting viral RNA replication.
• Antigen methods: formation of triple helix of DNA preventing transcription.
• Decoy methods: production of synthetic decoys corresponding to a specific nucleic acid sequence which binds virally encoded regulatory proteins and affects transcription.
• Ribozymes: production of RNA molecules (oligo(ribo)nucleotides) inducing cleavage of other RNA sequences at specific sites.

Finally, there is an increased use of protease inhibitors (e.g. indinavir sulphate) that inhibit viral low molecular weight polypeptide gene products.

Despite the tremendous increase in antiviral

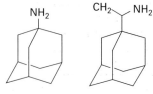

Acyclovir (nucleoside analogue
of guanosine)

Foscarnet (phosphate analogue;
trisodium salt of phosphonoformic acid)

AZT (nucleoside analogue
of thymidine)

d4T (nucleoside analogue of thymidine)

ddI (nucleoside analogue
of guanosine)

Amantadine

Rimantadine

Fig. 5.9 Examples of antiviral drugs.

drugs, there are several problems inherent in antiviral chemotherapy:
• Delay in treatment: many viral diseases only become apparent after extensive viral multiplication and tissue damage have occurred.
• Drug toxicity (e.g. nucleoside analogues): viral replication has considerable dependence on host cell enzyme systems that produce energy and synthesize proteins or other biopolymers. Furthermore, such compounds can also interfere with host regulatory genes, triggering cell apoptosis.
• Degradation and penetration of the antiviral drugs: the use of pro-drugs might improve drug absorption and other pharmacokinetics properties. For example, valacyclovir, a valyl ester of acyclovir is better absorbed into the gastrointestinal tract than the parent drug, and is cleaved by host enzymes into valine (a natural amino acid) and acyclovir.
• Finally, some viruses have developed resistance to antiviral drugs. HIV chemotherapy now involves

the use of at least two anti-HIV agents having different mechanisms of action (for example, zidovudine (AZT) + lamivudine (3TC) + indinavir (a protease inhibitor) or stavudine (d4T) + didanosine (ddI) ± indinavir), in order to minimize the development of HIV resistance to individual antiviral drugs, prolong the antiviral effect and improve outcome.

10 Tumour viruses

Experimental infection of animals has shown that certain viruses can induce cancer. This *oncogenic* activity can also be demonstrated *in vitro* in cell cultures. Cells surviving viral infection can change dramatically, acquiring the characteristics of tumour cells. These transformed cells exhibit frequent mitosis. They also lose the property of cell contact inhibition, so they tend to pile up on top of each other rather than remaining as organized monolayers.

Viral DNA can be recovered from cells transformed by DNA-containing viruses and in some cases these viral DNA sequences have been shown to be integrated into the host cell DNA. The oncogenic RNA-containing viruses possess the enzyme reverse transcriptase, which makes DNA copies of the viral RNA genome, and cells transformed by these retroviruses contain these DNA transcripts integrated into host cell DNA. It appears that the acquisition of DNA from oncogenic viruses can disturb the systems that normally regulate cell growth and division.

There is a now a substantial body of evidence that viruses are a major cause of cancer in humans, being involved in the genesis of some 20% of human cancers worldwide. It has also become clear, however, that less than 1% of individuals infected with these oncogenic viruses will develop cancer and that there may be intervals of many years before the cancer becomes apparent. There seems to be no single mechanism by which viruses induce tumours. Virus infection is one step in a multi-stage, multifactorial process. The acquisition of viral genes must be followed by other events such as environmental or dietary exposure to chemical carcinogens, or infection by other microorganisms if progression to cancer is to occur. The host genotype may also be a co-factor.

The Epstein–Barr virus (EBV) is a herpesvirus that is associated with the formation of lymphomas and nasopharyngeal carcinomas. It infects most humans but infections in childhood are generally asymptomatic. In young adults it can cause glandular fever, a chronic condition in which there is proliferation of white blood cells. After infection the virus becomes latent in B lymphocytes for the lifetime of the individual. *In vitro* the infection of B lymphocytes by EBV results in their transformation and proliferation. Normally *in vivo*, this EBV-induced proliferation of B cells is kept under control by the action of T-killer lymphocytes. In some African children infection with EBV induces Burkitt's lymphoma, a particularly malignant tumour of the jaw. The characteristic occurrence of this condition in hot humid regions of Africa where mosquitoes flourish has led to the hypothesis that infection with EBV has to be followed by malaria before the lymphomas will develop. Suppression of

T-cell activity is known to occur in malaria and it is thought that in this situation infection with the malarial parasite provides the co-factor that triggers tumour formation. Nasopharyngeal carcinoma is rare in the general human population. However, in certain parts of south China and in Cantonese populations that have emigrated to other parts of the world it is the most common form of cancer. Infection with EBV occurring at any age is the primary stage in the process. It then seems that the consumption of large amounts of smoked fish (a cultural characteristic of this group) exposes them to carcinogenic nitrosamines, which act as the co-factors to trigger cell proliferation.

The hepatitis B virus (HBV) is strongly associated with liver cancer. Studies have shown that people who are carrying this virus have a 200-fold increased risk of developing primary hepatocellular carcinoma. The typical pattern is that individuals infected with HBV in childhood develop chronic hepatitis, with the integration of part of the HBV genome into host cell chromosomes. Cirrhosis of the liver follows and eventually liver cancer develops some 20–50 years after the primary infection. The evidence suggests that the integration of viral DNA causes mutations in the host genes that regulate cell growth. This makes the liver cells more susceptible to exogenous carcinogens such as the fungal toxin aflatoxin and those generated by smoking tobacco. High alcohol consumption can be another co-factor.

The other viruses that are strongly implicated in human cancers include hepatitis C virus with liver cancer; certain of the human papilloma viruses that cause warts on epithelial surfaces and cervical, penile and anal carcinomas; human T-cell lymphotrophic virus type 1 with adult T-cell leukaemia/lymphoma syndrome and HIV with Kaposi's sarcoma.

11 The human immunodeficiency virus (HIV)

HIV is an enveloped RNA-containing virus. It has a cone-shaped nucleocapsid containing two copies of a positive-sense single-stranded RNA molecule and the enzyme reverse transcriptase. Some 70 glycoprotein spikes project from the envelope. These contain the binding site for the CD4 protein present on the surface of T4-helper lymphocytes and ensure that the virus attaches to these cells. The main way in which people become infected is by the transmission of free virus or infected CD4+ T lymphocytes during heterosexual and male homosexual activity. Infection can also result from infected blood, particularly between drug abusers who share hypodermic needles. Health professionals whose work might bring them into contact with infected blood are also at risk. In the days before the screening of blood donors for HIV, clotting factor VIII prepared from infected blood also infected people with haemophilia. Vertical transmission also occurs, about 20% of babies born to HIV-positive mothers are infected. In the 20 years since the first reports, acquired immune deficiency syndrome (AIDS) has developed into one of the most devastating diseases to afflict the human population. The World Health Organization estimated that by December 2001 more than 60 million people had become infected with HIV and that over 20 million had died of the disease. The problem is critical in sub-Saharan Africa where 2.3 million people died of AIDS in 2001.

After the primary infection, the virus is transported to lymph nodes where it replicates extensively in CD4+ lymphocytes. The number of these white cells declines and high titres of virus are found in the blood. Most patients experience a brief glandular fever-like illness at this stage, with characteristically persistent swollen lymph nodes. The number of the virus-specific CD8+ cytotoxic T lymphocytes then increases and this is associated with a reduction in the viral load in the blood to a low constant level; the population of CD4+ cells also recovers. There then follows an asymptomatic phase, which can last anything from 1 to 15 years. During this phase, most of the infected cells are located in lymph nodes where the virus is replicating actively. Enormous numbers of viral particles (10^{10}) are produced per day, but the CD8+ cytotoxic lymphocytes destroy virus-infected cells and more CD4+ cells replace those killed. In this way the concentration of virus in the bloodstream is maintained at relatively low levels, although patients are infectious. As the years go by, it becomes increasing difficult to replace the CD4+ helper lymphocytes. It also seems that HIV mutates, producing virions that become progressively more variable and difficult for the immune system to control. As a result, the number of virus particles in the blood increases and the population of CD4+ cells gradually declines. When the count of these cells falls below 200 per µl of blood, the immune system becomes seriously compromised and the individual becomes susceptible to infection by a range of opportunist pathogens including fungi, protozoa, bacteria and other viruses. Infections with *Candida albicans*, *Pneumocystis carinii*, *Mycobacterium tuberculosis*, cytomegalovirus and EBV are particularly common and will eventually kill the patient. While the CD4+ cells are the primary target, the virus also attacks muscle tissue and cells in the peripheral and central nervous system, resulting in the final stages of the disease, in major weight loss, myopathy, dementia and collapse of brain function.

The replication cycle of HIV has been investigated in great detail in the hope that it will reveal ways of inhibiting the production of progeny viruses. The process starts when the glycoprotein spikes (gp120) in the virus envelope recognize and bind to the CD4+ receptors in the cytoplasmic membranes of the T4 helper lymphocytes. The fusion of the viral envelope and the cell membrane then leads to the entry of the HIV core into the cell. The core is uncoated, releasing the two RNA molecules and the reverse transcriptase into the cytoplasm. The RNA is copied by reverse transcriptase into a single strand of DNA, which is then duplicated to form a double-stranded DNA copy of the original viral RNA genome. This DNA moves into the host cell nucleus where it is integrated as proviruses into a host cell chromosome. These integrated proviruses can lie dormant in the cell or can be expressed, producing viral mRNA and proteins. The viral genome codes for envelope proteins (env), capsid proteins (gag) and enzymes involved in viral multiplication (pol). An important feature of HIV replication is that the polyprotein products of these genes have to be cleaved by a viral protease enzyme to produce the functional proteins. The viral proteins and new copies of the viral RNA are then assembled into new virions that bud off from the infected cell and can repeat the HIV replication cycle in other CD4+ cells.

Enormous efforts have been made to develop chemotherapeutic agents for HIV. While there is no prospect of drugs that will eliminate the provirus from the populations of host lymphocytes, considerable progress has been made in the development of agents that preserve the stock of CD4+ cells in infected individuals and prevent the progression of the infection to AIDS. A major advance in this field was the discovery of the protease inhibitors such as saquinavir, ritonavir and indinavir. These compounds inhibit HIV replication by blocking the action of the protease that cleaves the viral polyproteins to produce the functional proteins. Currently a protease inhibitor is administered along with two reverse transcriptase inhibitors such as AZT, d4T or ddI. This triple therapy has been termed highly active anti-retroviral therapy (HAART). It reduces the numbers of HIV particles in the blood, restores lost immune functions and slows the progression to AIDS. Unfortunately, it has no effect on latently infected CD4+ so it does not clear the HIV infection. Patients who stop using the drugs experience a rapid rebound in levels of the virus in the blood and progression of the disease. The requirement for this life-long suppressive therapy makes the treatment extremely expensive. In the areas of the world where the disease is rampant, lack of funds makes the cost of treatment prohibitive.

Despite huge investments of human and financial resources it has not yet proved possible to develop a vaccine that would protect against HIV infection. Research into HIV vaccines presents several particularly difficult problems. The imprecise operation of the viral reverse transcriptase enzyme ensures that antigenic variants are produced at high frequencies. The fact that HIV targets cells involved in the immune response brings special difficulties. For example, it might be thought that a virus-specific antibody that prevented the virus binding to its target host cell might produce a protective response. However, the binding of antibodies onto virus particles results in ingestion of the viruses by phagocytes and therefore infection of these cells. The current aim is to stimulate both virus-specific antibody and T-cell responses and to ensure that the vaccine produces the local mucosal immunity necessary to protect the genital and rectal epithelia.

Lack of an animal model and ethical considerations in the conduct of clinical trials have compounded the problem and slowed progress in vaccine development.

The AIDS pandemic is out of control in parts of the world (sub-Saharan Africa and southern and south-east Asia) and the lack of access to effective chemotherapy means that the prognosis is bleak for the millions of people who are HIV-positive. Sexual intercourse is now the main mode of infection and if the pandemic is to be contained, sexually active individuals have to be persuaded to reduce the number of their partners and to practise safe sex using condoms.

12 Prions

The causative agents of the neurodegenerative diseases bovine spongiform encephalopathy (BSE), scrapie in sheep and Creutzfeldt–Jakob disease (CJD) in humans used to be referred to as slow viruses. However, it is now clear that they are caused by a distinct class of infectious agents termed *prions* that have unique and disturbing properties. They can be recovered from the brains of infected individuals as rod-like structures which are oligomers of a 30-kDa glycoprotein. They are devoid of nucleic acid and are extremely resistant to heating and ultraviolet irradiation. They also fail to produce an immune response in the host. Just how such proteins can replicate and be infectious has only recently been understood. It seems that a glycoprotein (designated PrPc) with the same amino acid sequence as the prion (PrPsc) but with a different tertiary structure, is present in the membranes of normal neurons of the host. The evidence suggests that the prion form of the protein combines with the normal form and alters its configuration to that of the prion. The newly formed prion can then in turn modify the folding of other PrPc molecules. In this way the prion protein is capable of autocatalytic replication. As the prions slowly accumulate in the brain, the neurons progressively vacuolate. Holes eventually appear in the grey matter and the brain takes on a sponge-like appearance. The clinical symptoms take a long time to develop, up to 20 years in humans, but the disease has an inevitable progression to paralysis, dementia and death.

It is now clear that the large-scale outbreak of BSE that began in the UK during the 1980s resulted from feeding cattle with supplements prepared from sheep and cattle offal. The recognition of this fact led to changes in animal feed policies and eventually to the imposition of a ban on the human consumption of bovine brain, spinal cord and lymphoid tissues that were considered to be potentially infectious. Unfortunately people had been consuming potentially contaminated meat for a number of years. Concerns that the agent had already been disseminated to humans in the food chain were realized in 1996 with the advent of a novel human disease that was called *variant* or vCJD. This condition was unusual as it attacked young adults with an average age of 30 rather than 60-year-olds that typically succumb to classical sporadic CJD. Studies on the experimental transmission of prions to mice provided evidence that vCJD represents infection by the BSE agent. The pathology in the mouse brain induced by the vCJD agent and the incubation time of the disease are different from that of classical CJD and very similar to that of BSE. Gel electrophoresis of the polypeptides from the brains of infected mice revealed that the different transmissible spongiform encephalitis agents have characteristic molecular signatures. These signatures are based on the lengths of protease-resistant fragments and the glycosylation patterns on the prion molecules. The patterns from vCJD agent were very different patterns from those of the classical CJD but remarkably similar to those formed by BSE.

Since 1996 there has been a slow but gradual increase in the numbers of confirmed cases of vCJD. By March 2002 the number of deaths in the UK from vCJD had reached 109. As the average incubation time for vCJD is not yet known, it is difficult to estimate how many more cases will develop. The measures taken to protect the public will hopefully have prevented any further human infections but sadly there is no effective treatment available for those who have already contracted the disease.

13 Further reading

Balfour, H. H. (1999) Antiviral drugs. *N Engl J Med*, **340**, 1255–1268.

Belay, E. (1999) Transmissible spongiform encephalopathies in humans. *Annu Rev Microbiol*, **53**, 283–314.

Collinge, J., Sidle, K. C., Meads, J., Ironside, J. & Hill, A. F. (1996) Molecular analysis of prion strain variation and the aetiology of 'new variant' CJD. *Nature*, **383**, 685–690.

Dalgleish, A. G. (1991) Viruses and cancer. *Br Med Bull*, **47**, 21–46.

Dimmock, N. J., Easton, A. J. & Leppard, K. N. (2001) *Introduction to Modern Virology*, 5th edn. Blackwell Science, Oxford.

Hanke, T. (2001) Prospect for a prophylactic vaccine for HIV. *Br Med Bull*, **58**, 205–218.

Levy, J. A. (1998) *HIV and the Pathogenesis of AIDS*, 2nd edn. ASM Press, Herndon, VA.

McCance, D. J. (1998) *Human Tumour Viruses*. ASM Press, Washington, DC.

Maillard, J-Y. (2001) Virus susceptibility to biocides: an understanding. *Rev Med Microbiol*, **12**, 63–74.

Morrison, L. (2001) The global epidemiology of HIV/AIDS. *Br Med Bull*, **58**, 7–18.

Oxford, J. S., Coates, A. R. M., Sia, D. Y., Brown, K. & Asad, S. Potential target sites for antiviral inhibitors of human immunodeficiency virus (HIV). *J Antimicrob Chemother*, **23**, S9–S27.

Pattison, J. (1998) The emergence of bovine spongiform encephalopathy. *Emerg Infect Dis*, **4**, 390–394.

Prusiner, S. B. (1996) Molecular biology and pathogenesis of prion diseases *Trends Biochem Sci*, **21**, 482–487.

Weber, J. (2001) The pathogenesis of HIV-I infection. *Br Med Bull*, **58**, 61–72.

Chapter 6
Protozoa

Tim Paget

1 Introduction

1.1 Parasitism

Parasitism is a specific type of interaction between two organisms that has many features in common with other infectious processes, but host–parasite interactions often operate over a longer timescale than those seen with other pathogens. This extended process results in significant host–parasite interaction at the cellular and organismal level. It is known, for example, that some parasites alter the behaviour of the host, while others, such as *Giardia lamblia*, induce biochemical change in the host cells at the site of infection (the duodenal epithelium). Most parasites have a life cycle that often involves several hosts; this means that survival and transmission between different hosts requires the parasite to exhibit more than one physiologically distinct form.

1.2 Habitats

Parasites inhabit a wide range of habitats within their hosts. Some parasites will inhabit only one site throughout their life cycle, but many move to various sites within the body. Such movement may require the formation of motile cellular forms, and it will produce a significant change in the physiology and morphology of the parasite as a result of environmental change. Parasites moving from the gut to other tissues, for example, will encounter higher levels of oxygen, changes in pH and significant exposure to the host immune response. When life cycles involve more than one host organism these changes are greater. The reasons for such movement include evasion of host immune attack and to aid transmission.

1.3 Physiology of parasitic protozoa

Parasitic protozoa, like their free-living counterparts, are single-celled eukaryotic organisms that utilize flagella, cilia or amoeboid movement for motility. The complexity of some parasite life cycles means that some species may exhibit, at different times, more than one form of motility. All pathogenic protozoa are heterotrophs, using carbohydrates or amino acids as their major source of carbon and energy. Some parasitic protozoa utilize oxygen to generate energy through oxidative phosphorylation, but many protozoan parasites lack mitochondria, or have mitochondria that do not function like those in mammalian cells. As a result of this adaptation many parasites exhibit a fermentative metabolism that functions even in the presence of oxygen. The reason for the utilization of less efficient fermentative pathways is not clear, but it is presumably due in part to the fact that such parasites survive in environments where oxygen is only present occasionally or at low levels. For some parasites oxygen is toxic, and they appear to utilize it possibly in an effort to remove it and thus maintain an anaerobic metabolism.

The metabolism of parasites is highly adapted, with many possessing unique organelles such as kienetoplasts and hydrogenosomes. Many synthetic pathways that are found in other eukaryotes are absent because many metabolic intermediates or precursors such as lipids, amino acids and nucleotides are actively scavenged from their environment. This minimizes energy expenditure, which is finely balanced in parasites and means that the membrane of parasitic protozoa is rich in transporters. Secretion of haemolysins, cytolysins, proteolytic enzymes, toxins, antigenic and immunomodulatory molecules that reduce host immune response also occurs in pathogenic protozoa.

Survival of parasites is partly due to their high rate of reproduction, which may be either sexual or asexual; some organisms such as *Plasmodium* exhibit both forms of reproduction in their life cycle. Simple fission is characteristic of many amoeba, but some species also undergo nuclear division in the cystic state (cysts are forms required for survival outside the host) with each nucleus giving rise to new trophozoites (the growing, motile and pathogenic form).

2 Blood and tissue parasites

This section considers the life cycles, disease and pathology of some blood and tissue parasites; this is not an exhaustive list but covers some of the most important species. These diseases are commonly associated with travel to tropical and subtropical countries, but diseases such as leishmaniasis are frequently seen in southern Spain and France. It should also be noted that climate change is altering the geographical distribution of many parasitic diseases.

2.1 Malaria

Malaria has been a major disease of humankind for thousands of years. Despite the availability of drugs for treatment, malaria is still one of the most important infectious diseases of humans, with approximately 200–500 million new cases and 1–2.5 million deaths each year. Protozoa of the genus *Plasmodium* cause malaria and four species are responsible for the disease in humans: *P. falciparum*, *P. vivax*, *P. ovale* and *P. malariae*. *P. falciparum* and *P. vivax* account for the vast majority of cases, although *P. falciparum* causes the most severe disease. Other species of plasmodia infect reptiles, birds and other mammals. Malaria is spread to humans by the bite of female mosquitoes of the genus *Anopheles* but transmission by inoculation of infected blood and through congenital routes is also seen. These mosquitoes feed at night and their breeding sites are primarily in rural areas.

2.1.1 Disease

The most common symptom of malaria is fever, although chills, headache, myalgia and nausea are frequently seen and other symptoms such as vomiting, diarrhoea, abdominal pain and cough occasionally appear. In all types of malaria, the periodic febrile response (fever) is caused by rupture of mature schizonts (one of the cell forms arising as part of the life cycle). In *P. vivax* and *P. ovale* malaria fever occurs every 48 hours, whereas in *P. malariae*, maturation occurs every 72 hours. In falciparum malaria fever may occur every 48 hours, but is usually irregular, showing no distinct periodicity. Apart

83

from anaemia, most physical findings in malaria are often non-specific and offer little aid in diagnosis, although enlargement of some organs may be seen after prolonged infection. If the diagnosis of malaria is missed or delayed, especially with *P. falciparum* infection, potentially fatal complicated malaria may develop. The most frequent and serious complications of malaria are cerebral malaria and severe anaemia.

2.1.2 Life cycle

Plasmodia have a complex life cycle (Fig. 6.1) involving a number of life cycle stages and two hosts. The human infective stage comprises the sporozoites (approximately $1 \times 7\,\mu m$), which are produced by sexual reproduction in the midgut of the anopheline mosquito (vector) and migrate to its salivary gland. When an infected *Anopheles* mosquito bites a human, sporozoites are injected into the bloodstream and are thought to enter liver parenchymal cells within 30 minutes of inoculation. In these cells the parasite differentiates into a spherical, multinucleate schizont which may contain 2000–40 000 uninucleate merozoites. This process of growth and development is termed exo-erythrocytic schizogony. This exo-erythrocytic phase usually takes between 5 and 21 days, depending on the species of *Plasmodium*; however, in *P. vivax* and *P. ovale* the maturation of schizonts may be delayed for up to 1–2 years. These 'quiescent' parasites are called hypnozoites. Clinical illness is caused by the erythrocytic stage of the parasite life cycle; no disease is associated with sporozoites, the developing liver stage of the parasite, the merozoites released from the liver, or gametocytes.

The common symptoms of malaria are due to the rupture of erythrocytes when erythrocytic schizonts mature (Fig. 6.2a). This release of parasite material triggers a host immune response, which in turn induces the formation of inflammatory cytokines, reactive oxygen intermediates and other cellular products. These pro-inflammatory molecules play a prominent role in pathogenesis, and are probably responsible for the fever, chills, sweats, weakness and other systemic symptoms associated with malaria. In *P. falciparum* malaria, infected erythrocytes adhere to the endothelium of capillaries and postcapillary venules, leading to obstruction of the microcirculation and localized anoxia. The pathogenesis of anaemia appears to involve haemolysis or phagocytosis of parasitized erythrocytes and ineffective erythropoiesis.

2.2 Trypanosomatids

The family Trypanosomatidae consists of two genera, *Trypanosoma* and *Leishmania*. These are important pathogens of humans and domestic animals and the diseases they cause constitute serious medical and economic problems. Because these protozoans have a requirement for haematin obtained from blood, they are called haemoflagellates. The life cycles of both genera involve insect and vertebrate hosts and have up to eight life cycle stages, which differ in the placement and origin of the flagellum. Trypanosomatids have a unique organelle called the kinetoplast. This appears to be a special part of the mitochondrion and is rich in DNA. Two types of DNA molecules, *maxicircles* that encode mainly certain important mitochondrial enzymes, and *minicircles*, which serve a function in the process of RNA editing, have been found in the kinetoplast. Replication of trypanosomatids occurs by single or multiple fission, involving first the kinetoplast, then the nucleus, and finally the cytoplasm. There are four major diseases associated with this group: Chagas disease is caused by *Trypanosoma cruzi*; sleeping sickness (African trypanosomiasis) is associated with *Trypanosoma brucei*; cutaneous and mucocutaneous leishmaniasis are caused by a range of species including *Leishmania tropica*, *Leishmania major*, *Leishmania mexicana*, *Leishmania amazonensis* and *Leishmania braziliensis*; and visceral leishmaniasis, which is also known as kala-azar, is typically caused by *Leishmania donovani*.

2.2.1 American trypanosomiasis (Chagas disease)

Chagas disease begins as a localized infection that is followed by parasitaemia and colonization of internal organs and tissues. Infection may first be evidenced by a small tumour (chagoma) on the skin. Symptoms of the disease include fever, oedema and

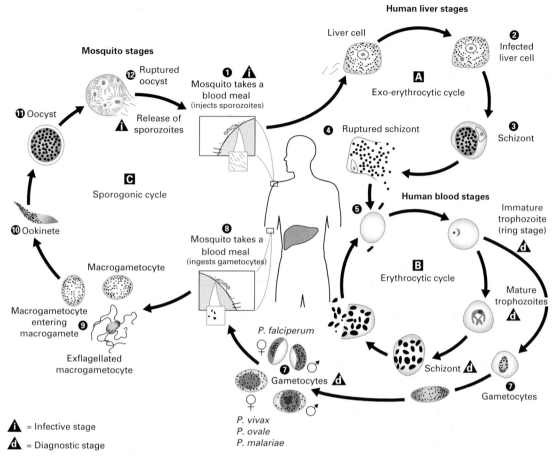

Fig. 6.1 The malaria parasite life cycle involves two hosts. During a blood meal, a malaria-infected female *Anopheles* mosquito inoculates sporozoites into the human host (**1**). Sporozoites infect liver cells (**2**) and mature into schizonts (**3**), which rupture and release merozoites (**4**). (Of note, in *P. vivax* and *P. ovale* a dormant stage (hypnozoites) can persist in the liver and cause relapses by invading the bloodstream weeks, or even years later.) After this initial replication in the liver (exo-erythrocytic schizogony, **A**), the parasites undergo asexual multiplication in the erythrocytes (erythrocytic schizogony, **B**). Merozoites infect red blood cells (**5**). The ring stage trophozoites mature into schizonts, which rupture releasing merozoites (**6**). Some parasites differentiate into sexual erythrocytic stages (gametocytes) (**7**). Blood stage parasites are responsible for the clinical manifestations of the disease. The gametocytes, male (microgametocytes) and female (macrogametocytes), are ingested by an *Anopheles* mosquito during a blood meal (**8**). The parasite's multiplication in the mosquito is known as the sporogonic cycle (**C**). While in the mosquito's stomach, the microgametes penetrate the macrogametes, generating zygotes (**9**). The zygotes in turn become motile and elongated (ookinetes) (**10**), which invade the midgut wall of the mosquito where they develop into oocysts (**11**). The oocysts grow, rupture and release sporozoites (**12**), which make their way to the mosquito's salivary glands. Inoculation of the sporozoites into a new human host perpetuates the malaria life cycle (**1**).

myocarditis (infection of the heart muscle) with or without heart enlargement, and meningo-encephalitis in children. The acute disease is frequently subclinical and patients may become asymptomatic carriers; this chronic phase may result, after 10–20 years, in cardiopathy. Chagas disease is transmitted by cone-nosed triatomine bugs of several genera (*Triatoma, Rhodnius* and *Panstrongylus*) and in nature the disease exists among wild mammals and their associated triatomines. Human trypanosomiasis is seen in almost all countries of the Americas, including the

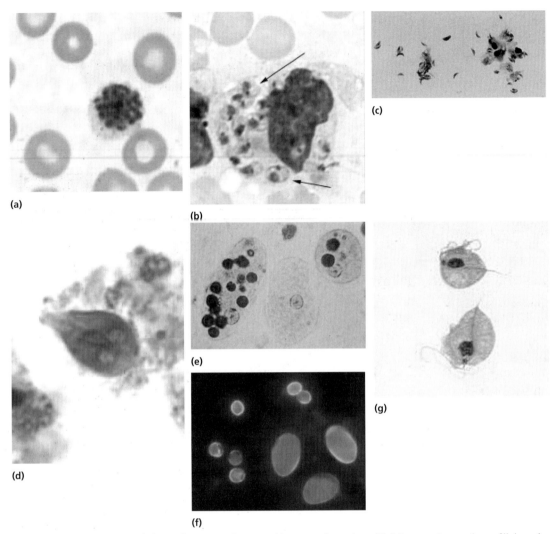

Fig. 6.2 (a) Mature schizonts of *Plasmodium vivax*. *P. vivax* schizonts are large, have 12–24 merozoites, and may fill the red blood cell (RBC). RBCs are enlarged 1.5–2 times and may be distorted. Under optimal conditions Schüffner's dots may be seen. (b) *Leishmania tropica* amastigotes within an intact macrophage. (c) *Toxoplasma gondii* trophozoites in the bronchial secretions from an HIV-infected patient. (d) Trophozoites of *Giardia intestinalis*. Each cell has two nuclei and is 10–20 μm in length. (e) Trophozoites of *Entamoeba histolytica* with ingested erythrocytes, which appear as dark inclusions. (f) Oocysts of *Cryptosporidium parvum* (upper left) and cysts of *Giardia intestinalis* (lower right) labelled with immunofluorescent antibodies. (g) Trophozoites of *Trichomonas vaginalis*.

southern United States, but the main foci are in poor rural areas of Latin America.

T. cruzi exhibits two cell types in vertebrate hosts, a blood form termed a trypomastigote, and in the tissues (mainly heart, skeletal and smooth muscle, and reticulo-endothelial cells) the parasite occurs as an amastigote (Fig. 6.3). Trypomastigotes ingested when the insect takes a blood meal from an infected host transform into epimastigotes in the intestine. Active reproduction occurs and in 8–10 days, metacyclic trypomastigote forms appear which are flushed out of the gut with the faeces of the insect. These organisms are able to penetrate the vertebrate host only through the mucosa or

Triatomine bug stages   **Human stages**

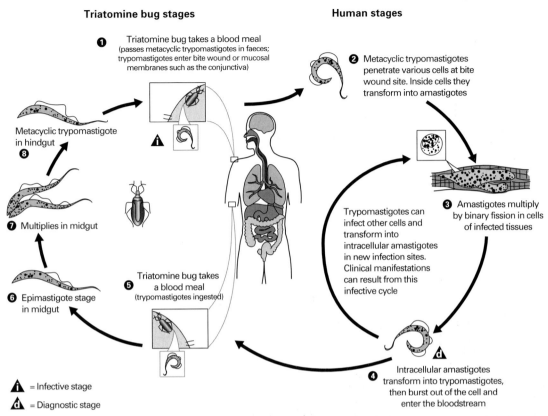

Fig. 6.3 An infected triatomine insect vector (or 'kissing' bug) takes a blood meal and releases trypomastigotes in its faeces near the site of the bite wound. Trypomastigotes enter the host through the wound or through intact mucosal membranes, such as the conjunctiva (1). Common triatomine vector species for trypanosomiasis belong to the genera *Triatoma*, *Rhodinius* and *Panstrongylus*. Inside the host, the trypomastigotes invade cells, where they differentiate into intracellular amastigotes (2). The amastigotes multiply by binary fission (3) and differentiate into trypomastigotes, and then are released into the circulation as bloodstream trypomastigotes (4). Trypomastigotes infect cells from a variety of tissues and transform into intracellular amastigotes in new infection sites. Clinical manifestations can result from this infective cycle. The bloodstream trypomastigotes do not replicate (different from the African trypanosomes). Replication resumes only when the parasites enter another cell or are ingested by another vector. The 'kissing' bug becomes infected by feeding on human or animal blood that contains circulating parasites (5). The ingested trypomastigotes transform into epimastigotes in the vector's midgut (6). The parasites multiply and differentiate in the midgut (7) and differentiate into infective metacyclic trypomastigotes in the hindgut (8). *Trypanosoma cruzi* can also be transmitted through blood transfusions, organ transplantation, transplacentally, and in laboratory accidents.

abrasions of the skin; hence, transmission does not necessarily occur at every blood meal. Within the vertebrate the trypomastigotes transform into amastigotes, which, after a period of intracellular multiplication at the portal of entry, are released into the blood as trypanosomes; these invade other cells or tissues, becoming amastigotes again.

The pathology of the infection is associated with inflammatory reactions in infected tissues. These can lead to acute myocarditis and destruction-specific ganglia. Parasite enzymes may also cause cell and tissue damage. In the absence of parasites, an autoimmune pathological process seems to be mediated by T lymphocytes (CD4+) (see Chapter 8) and by the production of certain cytokines; these induce a polyclonal activation of B lymphocytes and the secretion of large quantities of autoantibodies.

2.2.2 African trypanosomiasis (sleeping sickness)

Sleeping sickness (African trypanosomiasis) is caused by *Trypanosoma brucei*, of which there are two morphologically indistinguishable subspecies: *T. brucei rhodesiense* and *T. brucei gambiense*. After infection the parasite undergoes a period of local multiplication then enters the general circulation via the lymphatics. Recurrent fever, headache, lymphadenopathy and splenomegaly may occur. Later, signs of meningo encephalitis appear, followed by somnolence (sleeping sickness), coma and death.

T. brucei, unlike *T. cruzi*, multiplies in the blood or cerebrospinal fluid. Trypanosomes ingested by a feeding fly must reach the salivary glands within a few days, where they reproduce actively as epimastigotes attached to the microvilli of the salivary gland until they transform into metacyclic trypomastigotes, which are found free in the lumen. Around 15–35 days after infection the fly becomes infective through its bite.

The pathology of the infection is due to inflammatory changes associated with an induced autoimmune demyelination of nerve cells. Interestingly, the immunosuppressive action of components of the parasite's membrane are probably responsible for frequent secondary infections such as pneumonia. Liberation of common surface antigens (the mechanism involved in immune evasion) in every trypanolytic crisis (episode of trypanosome lysis) leads to antibody and cell-mediated hypersensitivity reactions. It is believed that some cytotoxic and pathological processes are the result of biochemical and immune mechanisms.

2.2.3 Cutaneous and mucocutaneous leishmaniasis

Leishmaniasis is the term used for diseases caused by species of the genus *Leishmania* that are transmitted by the bite of infected sandflies. The lesions of cutaneous and mucocutaneous leishmaniasis are localized to the skin and mucous membranes. Visceral leishmaniasis is a much more severe disease, which involves the entire reticulo-endothelial system, and is discussed in section 2.2.4 of this chapter. Cutaneous leishmaniasis appears 2–3 weeks after the bite of an infected sandfly as a small cutaneous papule; this slowly develops and often becomes ulcerated and develops secondary infections. Secondary or diffuse lesions may develop. The disease is usually chronic but may occasionally be self-limiting. Leishmaniasis from a primary skin lesion may involve the oral and nasopharyngeal mucosa. *Leishmania* species that infect man are all morphologically similar and only exhibit one form, the intracellular amastigotes (3–6 μm long and 1.5–3 μm in diameter). Promastigotes (Fig. 6.2b) are found in the sandfly.

In mammalian hosts amastigotes are phagocytosed by macrophages, but resist digestion and divide actively in the phagolysosome (Fig. 6.4). The female sandfly ingests parasites in the blood meal from an infected person or animal and these pass into the stomach where they transform into promastigotes, and multiply actively. The parasites attach to the walls of the oesophagus, midgut and hindgut of the fly, and some eventually reach the proboscis and are inoculated into a new host.

The obvious symptoms of this infection are caused by the uptake of parasites by local macrophages. Host response to infection produces tubercle-like structures designed to limit the spread of infected cells. Some lesions may resolve spontaneously after a few months but other types of lesion may become chronic, sometimes with lymphatic and bloodstream dissemination. In infections due to *L. braziliensis* there is a highly destructive spread of infected macrophages to the oral or nasal mucosa. In *L. mexicana*, *L. amazonensis* and *L. aethiopica* infections the disease becomes more disseminated. The immunological response of the host plays an important factor in determining the precise pathology of the disease and this is apparent by the more severe type of infection seen in individuals with HIV. In Europe and Africa several rodents may act as reservoirs of the disease, but in countries such as India, transmission can occur in a man–sandfly–man cycle without rodent intervention. In rural semi-arid zones of Latin

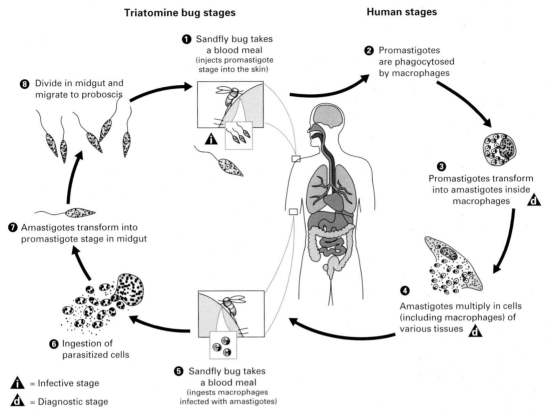

Triatomine bug stages

Human stages

❶ Sandfly bug takes a blood meal (injects promastigote stage into the skin)

❷ Promastigotes are phagocytosed by macrophages

❽ Divide in midgut and migrate to proboscis

❸ Promastigotes transform into amastigotes inside macrophages

❼ Amastigotes transform into promastigote stage in midgut

❹ Amastigotes multiply in cells (including macrophages) of various tissues

❻ Ingestion of parasitized cells

❺ Sandfly bug takes a blood meal (ingests macrophages infected with amastigotes)

▲ = Infective stage

△ = Diagnostic stage

Fig. 6.4 Leishmaniasis is transmitted by the bite of female phlebotomine sandflies. The sandflies inject the infective stage, promastigotes, during blood meals (**1**). Promastigotes that reach the puncture wound are phagocytosed by macrophages (**2**) and transform into amastigotes (**3**). Amastigotes multiply in infected cells and affect different tissues, depending in part on the *Leishmania* species (**4**). This originates the clinical manifestations of leishmaniasis. Sandflies become infected during blood meals on an infected host when they ingest macrophages infected with amastigotes (**5, 6**). In the sandfly's midgut, the parasites differentiate into promastigotes (**7**), which multiply and migrate to the proboscis (**8**).

America, both wild and domestic dogs enter the epidemiological chain and the vector is a common sandfly, *Lutzomyia longipalpis*, abundant in and around houses. The disease is more common in children in both Latin America and the Mediterranean area.

2.2.4 Visceral leishmaniasis (kala-azar)

Like cutaneous leishmaniasis, visceral leishmaniasis begins with a nodule at the site of inoculation but this lesion rarely ulcerates and usually disappears in a few weeks. However, symptoms and signs of systemic disease such as undulating fever, malaise, diarrhoea, organ enlargement and anaemia subsequently develop. In more serious cases of visceral leishmaniasis the parasites, which can resist the internal body temperature, invade internal organs (liver, spleen, bone marrow and lymph nodes), where they occupy the reticulo-endothelial cells. The pathogenic mechanisms of the disease are not fully understood, but enlargement occurs in those organs that exhibit marked cellular alteration such as hyperplasia. Parasitized macrophages replace tissue in the bone marrow. Patients with advanced disease are prone to superinfection with other organisms.

2.3 *Toxoplasma gondii*

The term coccidia describes a group of protozoa that contains the organism *Cryptosporidium* (see intestinal parasites) as well as a number of important veterinary parasites. *Toxoplasma gondii* is an intestinal coccidian but the major pathology of infection is associated with other tissues and organs. *T. gondii* infects members of the cat family as definitive hosts and has a wide range of intermediate hosts. Infection is common in many warm-blooded animals, including humans. In most cases infection is asymptomatic, but devastating disease can occur congenitally in children as a result of infection during pregnancy. *T. gondii* infection in humans is a worldwide problem, although the rates of human infection vary from country to country. The reasons for these variations are thought to be environmental factors, cultural habits and the presence of domestic and native animal species. The frequency of postnatal toxoplasmosis acquired by eating raw meat and by ingesting food contaminated by oocysts from cat faeces (oocyst formation is greatest in the domestic cat) is unknown but it likely to be high. Widespread natural infection is possible because infected animals may excrete millions of resistant oocysts, which can survive in the environment for prolonged periods (months–years). Mature oocysts are approximately 12 μm in diameter and contain eight infective sporozoites.

T. gondii infection in most animals including humans is asymptomatic. However, severe disease in humans is observed only in congenitally infected children and in immunosuppressed individuals. The most common symptom associated with postnatal infection in humans is lymphadenitis which may be accompanied by fever, malaise, fatigue, muscle pains, sore throat and headache (flu-like symptoms). Typically infection resolves spontaneously in weeks or months, but in immunosuppressed individuals, a fatal encephalitis may occur producing symptoms such as headache, disorientation, drowsiness, hemiparesis, reflex changes and convulsions. Prenatal *T. gondii* infections often target the brain and retina and can cause a wide spectrum of clinical disease. Mild disease may consist of impaired vision, whereas severely diseased children may exhibit a 'classic tetrad' of signs: retinochoroiditis, hydrocephalus, convulsions and intracerebral calcifications. Hydrocephalus is the least common but most dramatic lesion of congenital toxoplasmosis.

The life cycle of *T. gondii* was only fully described in the early 1970s when felines including domestic cats were identified as the definitive host. Various warm-blooded animals can serve as intermediate hosts. *T. gondii* is transmitted by three mechanisms: congenitally, through the consumption of uncooked infected meat and via faecal matter contamination. Figure 6.5 shows the life cycle of *T. gondii*. Cats acquire toxoplasma by ingesting any of three infectious stages of the organism: the rapidly multiplying forms, tachyzoites, the dormant bradyzoites (cysts) in infected tissue and the oocysts shed in faeces. The probability of infection and the time between infection and the shedding of oocysts varies with the stage of *T. gondii* ingested. Fewer than 50% of cats shed oocysts after ingesting tachyzoites or oocysts, whereas nearly all cats shed oocysts after ingesting bradyzoites. When a cat ingests tissue cysts, the cyst wall is dissolved by intestinal and gut proteolytic enzymes, which causes the release of bradyzoites. These enter the epithelial cells of the small intestine and initiate the formation of numerous asexual generations before the sexual cycle begins. At the same time that some bradyzoites invade the surface epithelia, other bradyzoites penetrate the lamina propria and begin to multiply as tachyzoites (trophozoites) (Fig. 6.2c). Within a few hours, tachyzoites may disseminate to other tissues through the lymph and blood. Tachyzoites can enter almost any type of host cell and multiply until it is filled with parasites; the cell then lyses and releases more tachyzoites to enter new host cells. The host usually controls this phase of infection, and as a result the parasite enters the 'resting' stage in which bradyzoites are isolated in tissue cysts. Tissue cysts are formed most commonly in the brain, liver and muscles. These cysts usually cause no host reaction and may remain dormant for the life of the host. In intermediate hosts, such as humans, the extra-intestinal cycle of *T. gondii* is similar to the cycle in cats except that there is no sexual stage.

Most cases of toxoplasmosis in humans are probably acquired by the ingestion of either tissue cysts in infected meat or oocysts in food contaminated

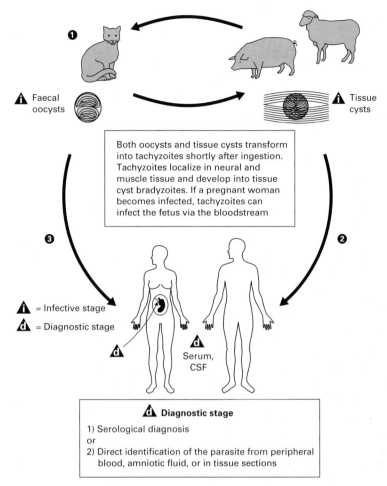

Both oocysts and tissue cysts transform into tachyzoites shortly after ingestion. Tachyzoites localize in neural and muscle tissue and develop into tissue cyst bradyzoites. If a pregnant woman becomes infected, tachyzoites can infect the fetus via the bloodstream

① Faecal oocysts

① Tissue cysts

③

②

① = Infective stage

ⓓ = Diagnostic stage

ⓓ

ⓓ Serum, CSF

ⓓ Diagnostic stage

1) Serological diagnosis
or
2) Direct identification of the parasite from peripheral blood, amniotic fluid, or in tissue sections

Fig. 6.5 Members of the cat family (Felidae) are the only known definitive hosts for the sexual stages of *Toxoplasma gondii* and thus are the main reservoirs of infection. Cats become infected with *T. gondii* by carnivorism (**1**). After tissue cysts or oocysts are ingested by the cat, viable organisms are released and invade epithelial cells of the small intestine where they undergo an asexual cycle followed by a sexual cycle and then form oocysts, which are then excreted. The unsporulated oocyst takes 1–5 days after excretion to sporulate (become infective). Although cats shed oocysts for only 1–2 weeks, large numbers may be shed. Oocysts can survive in the environment for several months and are remarkably resistant to disinfectants, freezing and drying, but are killed by heating to 70°C for 10 minutes. Human infection may be acquired in several ways: (A) ingestion of undercooked infected meat containing *Toxoplasma* cysts (**2**); (B) ingestion of the oocyst from faecally contaminated hands or food (**3**); (C) organ transplantation or blood transfusion; (D) transplacental transmission; (E) accidental inoculation of tachyzoites. The parasites form tissue cysts, most commonly in skeletal muscle, myocardium and brain; these cysts may remain throughout the life of the host.

with cat faeces. Bradyzoites from the tissue cysts or sporozoites released from oocysts invade intestinal epithelia and multiply. *T. gondii* may spread both locally to mesenteric lymph nodes and to distant organs by invading the lymphatic and blood systems. Focal areas of necrosis (caused by localized cell lysis) may develop in many organs. The extent of the disease is usually determined by the extent of injury to infected organs, especially to vital and vulnerable organs such as the eye, heart and adrenals.

Opportunist toxoplasmosis in immune suppressed patients usually represents reactivation of chronic infection. The predominant lesion of toxo-plasmosis—encephalitis in these patients—is necrosis, which often results in multiple abscesses, some as large as a tennis ball.

3 Intestinal parasites

Gut protozoan parasites include *Entamoeba histolytica*, *Giardia lamblia*, *Dientamoeba fragilis*, *Balantidium* sp., *Isospora* sp. and *Cryptosporidium parvum*. All these organisms are transmitted by the faecal–oral route and most of them are cosmopolitan in their distribution. A good example of this is *Giardia*, which is found in nearly all countries of the world. In many developed countries, including the UK and USA, it is one of the most commonly identified waterborne infectious organisms. *Cryptosporidium*, like *Toxoplasma*, has a complex life cycle utilizing both sexual and asexual reproduction. In contrast, *Giardia* and *Entamoeba* have simple life cycles utilizing only asexual reproduction. These latter organisms are members of a small group of eukaryotes that do not have mitochondria. It had long been assumed that they never had mitochondria, but recent studies showing the presence of mitochondrial-like enzymes and structural proteins suggest that it is more likely that this organelle was lost as a result of metabolic/physiological adaptation.

3.1 *Giardia lamblia* (syn. *intestinalis*, *duodenalis*)

Giardia lamblia is the causative agent of giardiasis—a severe diarrhoeal disease. The incidence of *Giardia* infection worldwide ranges from 1.5% to 20% but is probably significantly higher in countries where standards of hygiene are poor. The most common route of spread is via the faecal–oral route, although spread can also occur through ingestion of contaminated water and these modes of transmission are particularly prevalent in institutions, nurseries and day-care centres. Recent outbreaks and epidemics in the UK, USA and Eastern Europe have been caused by drinking contaminated water from community water supplies or directly from rivers and streams. Many animals harbour

Giardia species that are indistinguishable from *G. lamblia*, and this has raised the question of the existence of animal reservoirs of *Giardia*. Recent findings of *Giardia*-infected animals in watersheds from which humans acquired giardiasis, and the successful interspecies transfer of these organisms suggests that giardiasis is a zoonotic infection. More recently, it has been recognized that *Giardia* infection may be transmitted by sexual activity, particularly among homosexual men.

This organism exhibits only two life cycle forms: the vegetative bi-nucleate trophozoite (10–20 µm long by 2–3 µm wide) (Fig. 6.2d) and the transmissible quadra-nucleate cyst (10–12 µm long by 1–3 µm wide). Trophozoites have four pairs of flagella and an adhesive disc, which is thought to help adhesion to the intestinal epithelium. Division in trophozoites is by longitudinal fission.

It was long believed that *Giardia* was a non-pathogenic commensal. However, we now know that *Giardia* can produce disease ranging from a self-limiting diarrhoea to a severe chronic syndrome. Immune-competent individuals with giardiasis may exhibit some or all of the following signs and symptoms: diarrhoea or loose, foul-smelling stools; steatorrhoea (fatty diarrhoea); malaise; abdominal cramps; excessive flatulence; fatigue and weight loss. Infected individuals with an immune deficiency or protein-calorie malnutrition may develop a more severe disease and will exhibit symptoms such as interference with the absorption of fat and fat-soluble vitamins, retarded growth, weight loss, or a coeliac disease-like syndrome.

Giardia infection is initiated by ingestion of viable cysts (Fig. 6.6); the infective dose of which can be a low as one cyst, although infection initiated by 10–100 viable cysts is more likely. As the cysts pass through the stomach the low pH and elevated CO_2 induce excystation (cyst–trophozoite transformation). From each cyst two complete trophozoites emerge and these rapidly undergo division then attach to the duodenal and jejunal epithelium. Once attached, they will undergo division, and 4–7 days later they will detach and begin to round up and form cysts (encystment). This process is thought to be induced in response to bile. The first cysts are found in faeces after 7–10 days.

The underlying pathology of giardiasis is not

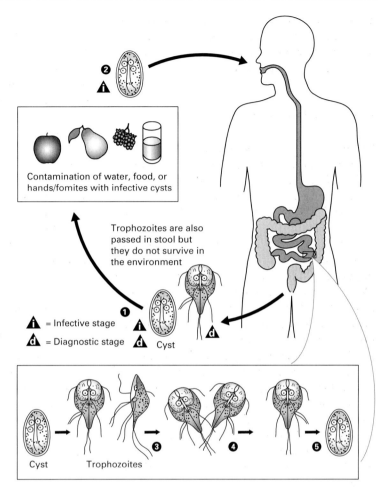

Fig. 6.6 Cysts are resistant forms and are responsible for transmission of giardiasis. Both cysts and trophozoites can be found in the faeces (diagnostic stages) (**1**). The cysts are hardy, and can survive several months in cold water. Infection occurs by the ingestion of cysts in contaminated water, food or by the faecal–oral route (hands or fomites) (**2**). In the small intestine, excystation releases trophozoites (each cyst produces two trophozoites) (**3**). Trophozoites multiply by longitudinal binary fission, remaining in the lumen of the proximal small bowel where they can be free or attached to the mucosa by a ventral sucking disc (**4**). Encystation occurs as the parasites transit toward the colon. The cyst is the stage found most commonly in non-diarrhoeal faeces (**5**). Because the cysts are infectious when passed in the stool or shortly afterwards, person-to-person transmission is possible. While animals are infected with *Giardia*, their importance as a reservoir is unclear.

Contamination of water, food, or hands/fomites with infective cysts

Trophozoites are also passed in stool but they do not survive in the environment

⚠ = Infective stage ⚠

🛡 = Diagnostic stage 🛡 Cyst

① Cyst Trophozoites ③ ④ ⑤

fully understood. The trophozoites do not invade the mucosa, and although their presence may have some physical effects on the surface it is more likely that some of the pathology is caused by inflammation of the mucosal cells of the small intestine causing an increased turnover rate of intestinal mucosal epithelium. The immature replacement cells have less functional surface area and less digestive and absorptive ability. This would account for the microscopic changes seen in infected epithelia. It has been suggested that other mechanisms may exist, e.g. toxin production, but to date no such molecule has been observed.

3.2 *Entamoeba histolytica*

Entamoeba histolytica is the causative agent of amoebic dysentery; another infection transmitted via the faecal–oral route. The severity of this and related pathologies caused by this organism can vary from diarrhoea associated with the intestinal infection to extra-intestinal amoebiasis producing hepatic and often lung infection. The prevalence of amoebiasis in developing countries reflects the lack of adequate sanitary systems. It had long been known that most infections associated with *E. histolytica* are asymptomatic, but in the late 1980s a separate, but morphologically and biochemically similar species, *E. dispar*, was identified. This was shown to be non-pathogenic but commonly misidentified as *E. histolytica* and thus the cause of 'asymptomatic *Entamoeba* infection'.

E. histolytica has a relatively simple life cycle and, like *Giardia*, exhibits only two morphological forms: the trophozoite and cyst stages. Trophozoites (Fig. 6.2e) vary in size from 10 to 60 µm and are actively motile. The cyst is spherical, 10–20 µm in diameter, with a thin transparent wall. Fully mature cysts contain four nuclei.

Symptoms of amoebic dysentery are associated with mucosal invasion and ulceration. Mucosal erosion causes diarrhoea, the severity of which increases with the level of invasion and colonization. Symptoms can also be affected by the site of the infection. Peritonitis as a result of perforation has been reported in connection with severe amoebic infection. Extra-intestinal amoebiasis is usually associated with liver infection, causing abscesses and/or enlargement. The abscess appears as a slowly enlarging liver mass and will cause noticeable pain. Jaundice may also occur due to blockage of the bile. Pleural, pulmonary, and pericardial infection results from metastatic spread from the liver, but can also manifest in other parts of the viscera or give rise to a brain abscess. However, these complications are uncommon.

The life cycle of *E. histolytica* (Fig. 6.7) is simple, but the ability of trophozoites to infect sites other than the intestine make it more complex than that of *Giardia*. Infection is initiated by ingestion of mature cysts, and again, excystation occurs during transit through the gut. After this, trophozoites rapidly divide by simple fission to produce four amoebic cells, which undergo a second division; thus each cyst yields eight trophozoites. Survival outside the host depends on the resistant cyst form.

The pathology of the disease is only partially understood. The process of tissue invasion has been well studied and involves binding and killing of the host cells by specific adhesin molecules and the action of a pore-forming protein, amoebapore. The initial superficial ulcer may deepen into the submucosa and become chronic. Spread may occur by direct extension, by undermining of the surrounding mucosa until it sloughs, or by penetration that can lead to perforation. If the trophozoites gain access to the vascular or lymphatic circulation, metastases may occur first to the liver and then by direct extension or further metastasis to other organs, including the brain.

3.3 *Cryptosporidium parvum*

Cryptosporidium parvum is a ubiquitous coccidian parasite that causes cryptosporidiosis in man; however, other species are known to cause infection in immunocompromised patients. The life cycle of the parasite is complex but is completed in a single host. Infection follows the ingestion of oocysts associated with contaminated water or food. According to the World Health Organization (WHO) the health significance of *C. parvum* is high due to the persistence of the organism in the environment. Cattle represent the most important reservoir of *C. parvum* but other mammals, domestic and wild, can be infected and act as carriers of the disease, even if asymptomatic. It is now known that a number of genetically distinct subspecies exist that can be divided into two groups. Group I comprises organisms that are human infective only (soon to be reclassified as *C. hominis*). Group II comprises organisms that infect a wider range of hosts. There have been several large outbreaks of this infection in the UK and USA, in which water was identified as the initial vehicle for transmission. Members of this genus are intracellular parasites infecting the intestinal mucosal epithelium. The two major life cycle forms are the oval oocyst and the sporozoite.

C. parvum infections are often asymptomatic, but symptoms such as profuse watery diarrhoea, stomach cramps, nausea, vomiting and fever are typical. The symptoms can last from several days to a few weeks in immunocompetent individuals, but in immunocompromised patients infection can become chronic, lasting months or even years. The mean infective dose for immunocompetent people is dependent on the strain of *C. parvum* but it is considered to be approximately 100 cells, and infants are more vulnerable to infection. Diarrhoea is a major cause of childhood mortality and morbidity as well as malnutrition in developing countries. *Cryptosporidium* is the third most common cause of infective diarrhoea in children in such countries, and consequently it plays a role in the incidence of childhood malnutrition.

Cryptosporidium infection has a higher nutritional impact in boys than girls, due to an increased need for micronutrients in boys to build up larger muscle mass. However, breast-feeding does offer

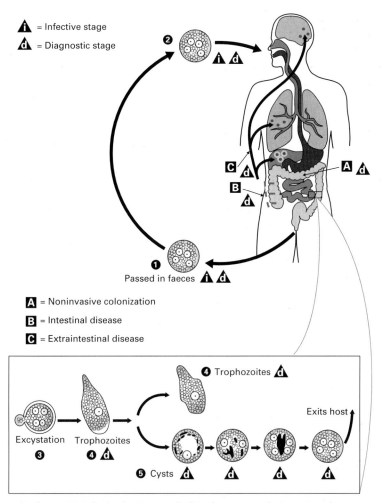

Fig. 6.7 Cysts are passed in faeces (**1**). Infection by *Entamoeba histolytica* occurs by ingestion of mature cysts (**2**) in faecally contaminated food, water or hands. Excystation (**3**) occurs in the small intestine and trophozoites (**4**) are released, which migrate to the large intestine. The trophozoites multiply by binary fission and produce cysts (**5**), which are passed in the faeces (**1**). Because of the protection conferred by their walls, the cysts can survive days to weeks in the external environment and are responsible for transmission. (Trophozoites can also be passed in diarrhoeal stools, but are rapidly destroyed once outside the body, and if ingested would not survive exposure to the gastric environment.) In many cases, the trophozoites remain confined to the intestinal lumen (**A**, non-invasive infection) of individuals who are asymptomatic carriers, passing cysts in their stool. In some patients the trophozoites invade the intestinal mucosa (**B**, intestinal disease), or through the bloodstream, extra-intestinal sites such as the liver, brain and lungs (**C**, extra-intestinal disease), with resultant pathological manifestations. It has been established that the invasive and non-invasive forms represent two separate species, respectively, *E. histolytica* and *E. dispar*. However, not all persons infected with *E. histolytica* will have invasive disease. These two species are morphologically indistinguishable. Transmission can also occur through faecal exposure during sexual contact (in which case not only cysts, but also trophozoites could prove infective).

some protection against infection. In immunocompromised individuals *Cryptosporidium* infection causes a severe gastroenteritis, and often the parasites infect other epithelial tissues causing pneumonia; the mortality rate due to *C. parvum* in AIDS patients is between 50% and 70%. Infection occurs when oocysts (Fig. 6.2f) excyst following environmental stimuli (typical intestinal conditions) and

parasitize the epithelial cells which line the intestine wall (Fig. 6.8). After several further stages of the cycle, two forms of oocyst are produced; soft-walled oocysts re-initiate infection of neighbouring enterocytes while hard-walled cysts are expelled in the faeces.

Little is known about the mechanism by which these organisms cause disease. They are known to invade cells but this process is atypical in that the parasites form a vacuole just below the epithelial cell membrane. During infection a variety of changes are seen such as partial villous atrophy, crypt lengthening and inflammation; these responses are probably due in part to cell damage that occurs during the growth of the intracellular forms. It has also been proposed that parasite enzymes and/or immune-mediated mechanisms may also be involved. It should be remembered, however, that cryptosporidiosis is resolved by the immune system in healthy patients normally within 3 weeks.

4 Trichomonas and free-living amoebas

4.1 *Trichomonas vaginalis*

Trichomonas vaginalis is a common sexually transmitted parasite. Infection rates vary from 10% to 50% with the highest reported rates found in the USA. Infections are usually asymptomatic or mild although symptomatic infection is most common in women. Trichomonads are all anaerobes and contain hydrogenosomes. This organelle is found in very few other anaerobic eukaryotes and is often termed the 'anaerobic mitochondrion'. A number of functions have been assigned to it, and it has been shown to function in the generation of ATP. This organism does not exhibit a life cycle as only the motile (flagellate/amoeboid) trophozoite (Fig. 6.2g) has been seen and division is by binary fission. Trichomonads have a pear-shaped body 7–15 μm long, a single nucleus, three to five forward-directed flagella, and a single posterior flagellum that forms the outer border of an undulating membrane.

Trichomoniasis in women is frequently chronic and is characterized by vaginal discharge and dysuria. The inflammation of the vagina is usually diffuse and is characterized by reddening of the vaginal wall and migration of polymorphonuclear leucocytes into the vaginal lumen (these form part of the vaginal discharge).

Because there is no resistant cyst, transmission from host to host must be direct. The inflammatory response in trichomoniasis is the major pathology associated with this organism; however, the mechanisms of induction are not known. It is likely that mechanical irritation resulting from contact between the parasite and vaginal epithelium is a major cause of this response but the organism produces high concentrations of acidic end-products and polyamines, both of which would also irritate local tissues.

4.2 Free-living opportunist amoebas

The free-living opportunist amoebas are an often forgotten group of protozoans. The two major

Fig. 6.8 Life cycle of *Cryptosporidium*. Sporulated oocysts, containing four sporozoites, are excreted by the infected host through faeces and possibly other routes such as respiratory secretions (**1**). Transmission of *Cryptosporidium parvum* occurs mainly through contact with contaminated water (e.g. drinking or recreational water). Occasionally food sources, such as chicken salad, may serve as vehicles for transmission. Many outbreaks in the USA have occurred in water parks, community swimming pools and day-care centres. Zoonotic transmission of C. *parvum* occurs through exposure to infected animals or exposure to water contaminated by faeces of infected animals (**2**). Following ingestion (and possibly inhalation) by a suitable host (**3**), excystation (**a**) occurs. The sporozoites are released and parasitize epithelial cells (**b, c**) of the gastrointestinal tract or other tissues such as the respiratory tract. In these cells, the parasites undergo asexual multiplication (schizogony or merogony) (**d, e, f**) and then sexual multiplication (gametogony) producing microgamonts (male, **g**) and macrogamonts (female, **h**). Upon fertilization of the macrogamonts by the microgametes (**i**), oocysts (**j, k**) develop that sporulate in the infected host. Two different types of oocysts are produced, the thick-walled oocyst, which is commonly excreted from the host (**j**) and the thin-walled oocyst (**k**), which is primarily involved in autoinfection. Oocysts are infective upon excretion, thus permitting direct and immediate faecal–oral transmission. (From: Juranek DD. Cryptosporidiosis. In: *Hunter's Tropical Medicine*, 8th edn. Edited by GT Strickland.)

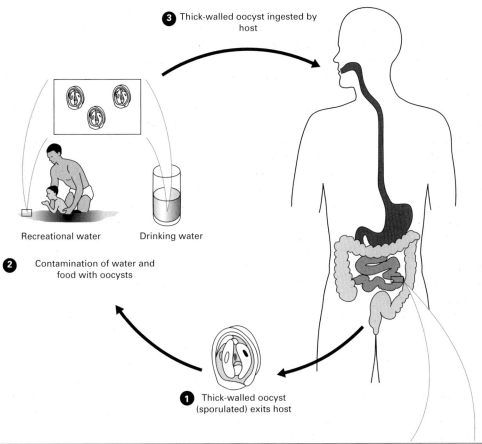

3 Thick-walled oocyst ingested by host

Recreational water

Drinking water

2 Contamination of water and food with oocysts

1 Thick-walled oocyst (sporulated) exits host

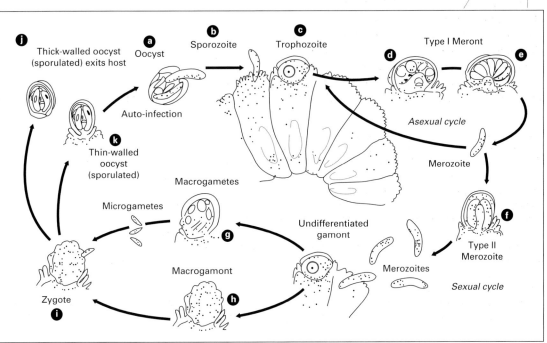

j Thick-walled oocyst (sporulated) exits host

a Oocyst

b Sporozoite

c Trophozoite

Type I Meront

d

e

Auto-infection

k Thin-walled oocyst (sporulated)

Asexual cycle

Merozoite

Macrogametes

Microgametes

Undifferentiated gamont

f Type II Merozoite

g

Merozoites

Sexual cycle

Macrogamont

h

Zygote

i

groups, *Naegleria* and *Acanthamoeba*, infect humans and both can cause fatal encephalitis. Both types of infections are rare, with less than 200 cases of *Naegleria fowleri* infection recorded worldwide and approximately 100–200 cases of *Acanthamoeba* ulcerative keratitis per year. This disease is commonly associated with contact lens use and it is thought that infection is caused by a combination of corneal trauma and dirty contact lenses. Both types of amoeba produce resistant cysts and *Naegleria* also exhibits a flagellate form. Both *Acanthamoeba* and *Naegleria* are free-living inhabitants of fresh water and soil, but *Naegleria fowleri* (the human pathogen) reproduces faster in warm waters up to 46°C. Treatment of water by chlorination or ozonolysis does not entirely eliminate cysts and both amoebae have been isolated from air-conditioning units.

Naegleria fowleri is the causative agent of primary amoebic meningo-encephalitis, a rapidly fatal disease that usually affects children and young adults. In all cases, contact with amoebae occurs as a result of swimming in infected fresh water. The organisms enter the brain via the olfactory tract after amoebae are inhaled or splashed into the olfactory epithelium. The incubation period ranges from 2 to 15 days and depends both on the size of the inoculum and the virulence of the strain. The disease appears with the sudden onset of severe frontal headache, fever, nausea, vomiting and stiff neck. Symptoms develop rapidly to lethargy, confusion and coma and in all cases to date the patient died within 48–72 hours.

Acanthamoeba castellanii, *A. culbertsoni* and other pathogenic *Acanthamoeba* species can cause opportunist lung and skin infections in immunocompromised individuals. Where amoebae spread from such lesions to the brain, they can cause a slowly progressive and usually fatal encephalitis. In addition, *Acanthamoeba* can cause an ulcerating keratitis in healthy individuals, usually in association with improperly sterilized contact lenses. The presence of cysts and trophozoites in alveoli or in multiple nodules or ulcerations of the skin characterizes acanthamoebic pneumonitis and dermatitis. Spread of amoebae to the brain produces an encephalitis, characterized by neurological changes, drowsiness, personality changes and seizures in the early stages of infection, which progress to altered mental status, lethargy and cerebellar ataxia, finally ending in coma and death. *Acanthamoeba* keratitis is characterized by painful corneal ulcerations that fail to respond to the usual anti-infective treatments. The infected and damaged corneal tissue may show a characteristic annular infiltrate and congested conjunctivae. If not successfully treated, the disease progresses to corneal perforation and loss of the eye or to a vascularized scar over thinned cornea, with impaired vision.

5 Host response to infection

Mechanisms to control parasitic protozoa are similar to those utilized for other infectious agents; they can be divided into non-specific mechanism(s) and specific mechanism(s) involving the immune system. The best studied non-specific mechanisms include those that affect the entry of parasites into the red blood cell. The sickle cell haemoglobin trait and lack of the Duffy factor on the erythrocyte surface make the red cell more resistant to invasion by *Plasmodium*. These traits are commonly found in populations from malaria-endemic regions. A second example of a non-specific factor is the presence of trypanolytic factors in the serum of humans which confer resistance to *T. brucei*, Although non-specific factors can play a key role in resistance, usually they work in conjunction with the host's immune system.

5.1 Immune response

Unlike most other types of infection, protozoan diseases are often chronic, lasting for months to years. When associated with a strong host immune response, this type of long-term infection is apt to result in a high incidence of immunopathology. Until recently the importance of host immune response in controlling many parasite infections was not fully appreciated, but the impact of HIV infection on many parasitic diseases has highlighted this relationship.

Different parasites elicit different humoral and/or cellular immune responses. In malaria and trypanosome infections, antibody appears to play a major role in immunity, although it would seem that for many organisms both humoral and cellular immunity are required for killing of parasites. Cellular immunity is believed to be the most important mechanism in the killing of *Leishmania* and *Toxoplasma*. Cytokines are involved in the control of both the immune response and also the pathology of many parasitic diseases. Helper (h) and cytotoxic (c) T cells play major roles in the induction/control of the response. The various subsets of these produce different profiles of cytokines. For example, the Th1 subset produces gamma interferon (IFN-γ) and interleukin-2 (IL-2) and is involved in cell-mediated immunity. In contrast, the Th2 subset produces IL-4 and IL-6, and is responsible for antibody-mediated immunity. The induction of the correct T-cell response is key to recovery. The Th1 subset and increased IFN-γ are important for the control of *Leishmania*, *T. cruzi* and *Toxoplasma* infections, whereas the Th2 response is more important in parasitic infections in which antibody is a major factor. It is important to recognize that the cytokines produced by one T-cell subset can up- or down-regulate the response of other T-cell subsets; IL-4 will down-regulate Th1 cells for example. The cytokines produced by T and other cell types do not act directly on the parasites but induce changes in the metabolism of glucose, fatty acid and protein in other host cells. Cytokines can also stimulate cell division and, therefore, clonal expansion of T- and B-cell subsets. This can lead to increased antibody production and/or cytotoxic T-cell numbers. The list of cytokines and their functions is growing rapidly, and it would appear that these chemical messages influence all phases of the immune response. They are also clearly involved in the multitude of physiological responses (fever, decreased food intake, etc.) observed in an animal's response to a pathogen, and in the pathology that results.

5.2 Immune pathology

The protozoa can elicit humoral responses in which antigen–antibody complexes are formed and these can trigger coagulation and complement systems. Immune complexes have been found circulating in serum and deposited in the kidneys where they may contribute to conditions such as glomerulonephri-

tis. In other tissues these complexes can also induce localized hypersensitivities. It is thought that this type of immediate hypersensitivity is responsible for various clinical syndromes including blood hyperviscosity, oedema and hypotension.

Another important form of antibody-mediated pathology is autoimmunity. Autoantibodies to a number of different host antigens (e.g. red blood cells, laminin, collagen and DNA) have been demonstrated. These autoantibodies may play a role in the pathology of parasitic diseases by exerting a direct cytotoxic effect on the host cells, e.g. autoantibodies that coat red blood cells produce haemolytic anaemia; they may also cause damage through a build up of antigen–antibody complexes.

Many parasites can elicit the symptoms of disease through the action of their surface molecules such as the pore-forming proteins of *E. histolytica* that induce contact-dependent cell lysis, and trypanosome glycoproteins that can fix and activate complement resulting in the production of biologically active and toxic complement fragments. A range of parasite-derived enzymes such as proteases and phospholipases can cause cell destruction, inflammatory responses and gross tissue pathology.

5.3 Immune evasion

Parasites exhibit a number of mechanisms that allow them to evade host immune response. Two such mechanisms are displayed by trypanosomes, which are able to exhibit both antigenic masking and antigenic variation. Masking means the parasite becomes coated with host components and therefore is not recognized as foreign, and antigenic variation results in surface antigens being changed during the course of an infection, so again the immune response is evaded. Parasites can also suppress the host's immune response either to the parasite specifically or to foreign antigens in general. This, however, can cause a number of problems, as general immune suppression may make the individual more susceptible to secondary infection.

6 Control of protozoan parasites

It is now clear that the best approach for the suc-

Table 6.1 Common anti-protozoal drugs and their modes of action

Drug	Mode of action (if known)	Mechanism of selectivity	Target organism(s)
Dapsone	Co-factor synthesis	Unique target	*Plasmodium* spp.
Proguanil	Co-factor synthesis	Differences in the target	*Plasmodium* spp.
Pyrimethamine	Co-factor synthesis	Differences in the target	*Plasmodium* spp.
Sulphonamides	Co-factor synthesis	Differences in the target	*Plasmodium* spp.
Benznidazole	Nucleic acid synthesis	Activation in the parasite	*Trypanosoma* spp.
Chloroquine	Nucleic acid synthesis	Differential uptake	*Plasmodium* spp.
Mefloquine	Nucleic acid synthesis	Differential uptake	*Plasmodium* spp.
Metronidazole	Nucleic acid synthesis	Activation in the parasite	*Giardia, Trichomonas, Entamoeba*
Pentamidine	Nucleic acid synthesis	Differential uptake	*Leishmania* spp.
Quinine	Nucleic acid synthesis	Differential uptake	*Plasmodium* spp.
Eflornithine	Protein function	Differences in the target	*T. brucei gambiense*
Tetracycline	Protein function	Differential uptake	*Plasmodium* spp.
Benzimadazoles	Microtubule function	Differences in the target	*Giardia, Trichomonas*
Amphotericin B	Membrane function	Differences in the target	*Leishmania* spp.
Atovaquone	Energy metabolism	Differences in the target	*Plasmodium* spp.
Melarasaprol	Energy metabolism	Target pathway more important in the parasite	*T. brucei gambiense*
Primaquine	Energy metabolism	Differences in the target	*Trypanosoma* spp.

cessful control of parasites requires the integration of a number of methods, which draw upon our increasing understanding of the parasites' life cycle, epidemiology and host response to infection.

6.1 Chemotherapy

The origins of chemotherapy are closely linked to the development of anti-parasitic agents, but there has been slow progress in the development of new and novel anti-protozoal agents over the past 30 years. Recently, with the support of the WHO and government-sponsored research, new anti-parasitic drugs are slowly coming into the market. Interestingly there are still a number of protozoan parasite infections such as cryptosporidiosis for which there is no effective treatment.

6.1.1 Mechanisms of action and selective toxicity

For many of the commonly used anti-protozoal drugs the modes of action and mechanisms of selective toxicity are well understood, although for some the precise mechanism remains unclear. The most

common anti-protozoal drugs and their modes of action are shown in Table 6.1.

Considering the drugs in relation to modes of action, dapsone and the sulphonamides block the biosynthesis of tetrahydrofolate by inhibiting dihydropteroate synthetase, while the 2,4-diaminopyrimidines (proguanil and pyrimethamine) block the same pathway but at a later step catalysed by dihydrofolate reductase.

The drugs that interfere with nucleic acid synthesis include those that bind to the DNA and intercalate with it such as chloroquine, mefloquine and quinine, and pentamidine that is unable to intercalate but probably interacts ionically. Other compounds such as benznidazole and metronidazole may alkylate DNA through activation of nitro groups via a one electron reduction step. Several of these compounds, however, including chloroquine, mefloquine, quinine and metronidazole have more than one potential mode of action. Chloroquine, for example, inhibits the enzyme haem polymerase, which functions to detoxify the cytotoxic molecule haem that is generated during the degradation of haemoglobin. Metronidazole is reduced in the parasite cell and forms a number of cytotoxic intermediates, which can cause damage not only to DNA but also to membranes and proteins.

Tetracycline targets protein synthesis in *Plasmodium* via a similar mechanism to that seen in bacteria: inhibition of chain elongation and peptide bond formation. Eflornithine interferes with the metabolism of the amino acid ornithine in *T. brucei gambiense* by acting as a suicide substrate for the enzyme ornithine decarboxylase.

Albendazole has recently been shown to have significant anti-giardial activity, although its mode of action is unclear. In leishmania, amphotericin B binds to the membrane sterol ergosterol making the plasma membrane leaky to ions and small molecules (e.g. amino acids), while the anti-protozoal drugs atovaquone and primaquine bind to the cytochrome bc_1 complex and inhibit electron flow. The anti-trypanosomal drug melarsaprol is most likely to act by blocking glycolytic kinases, especially the cytoplasmic pyruvate kinase, although they may also disrupt the reduction of trypanothione.

6.1.2 Drug resistance

As with bacteria, drug resistance in some parasites such as *Plasmodium* is a major problem and tends to appear where chemotherapy has been used extensively. This problem is exacerbated by the fact there are so few drugs available for the control of some parasites. Parasites utilize the same five basic resistance mechanisms that are displayed by bacteria: 1) metabolic inactivation of the drug; 2) use of efflux pumps; 3) use of alternative metabolic pathways; 4) alteration of the target; 5) elevation of the amount of target enzyme.

6.2 Other approaches to control

The early success in malaria control can be attributed to the use of professional spray teams who treated the inside of huts with DDT, without any direct involvement of the infected population. However, the problem with pesticides like DDT is that they lack specificity, and as application is not always well directed there is often destruction of a wide range of insects, which may have undesirable side-effects. Further problems include the accumu-

lation of pesticide residues in the food chain and pesticide resistance in the target organism. Window screens and bed nets do prevent mosquito bites, however, and there has been a lot of interest in using bed nets impregnated with insecticide. Environmental control was a major form of control used before the development of modern insecticides. A good example of this is mosquito control through the removal of breeding sites by drainage, land reclamation projects, removal of vegetation overhanging water, speeding up water flow in canals and periodic drainage and drying out of canals. Life cycle forms that enter the water system, such as cysts and oocysts of *Giardia* and *Cryptosporidium*, can present a major public health problem. These forms are often resistant to common disinfection methods and require physical removal from waters. Cysts and oocysts can be destroyed by use of proper sewage treatments like anaerobic digestion, but these systems require regular maintenance in order to remain effective.

6.2.1 Biological control

Biological control is an active but developing area. Genetic control of insect vectors, particularly the use of irradiated sterile males, has been widely publicized, and the release of chemically sterile males has been attempted to control anopheline mosquitoes. Other similar methods include the release of closely related species within the environment in order to produce sterile hybrids. Genetically modified mosquitoes are currently being developed that are resistant to *Plasmodium* infection, and larvivorous fish have also been employed for mosquito control; other organisms considered for the same purpose include bacteria, fungi, nematodes and predatory insects. One of the best studied agents is the bacterium *Bacillus thuringiensis*; the spore or the isolated toxin from this species can be used as a very effective and specific insecticide.

6.2.2 Vaccination

Where exposure to infection is likely to occur, killing the parasite as it enters the host is a sensible approach to control. There are two options available, chemoprophylaxis or vaccination. Unfortunately long-term chemotherapy can have adverse side-effects, and in the absence of symptoms members of the 'at risk' population may fail to take the treatment. Vaccination would seem to be the ideal method of parasite control, as life-long resistance may result from just a single treatment. Despite a huge amount of effort, the only successful parasite vaccines are those for the control of veterinary parasites. However, there has been some success with the development of recombinant vaccines for the control of malaria. The recent development of DNA vaccines may be of use in the control of parasites. In this method the DNA encoding an important parasite protein is injected into host cells and the foreign 'vaccinating' protein is synthesized in or on the surface of the cell. This intracellular foreign protein enters the cell's major histocompatibility complex (MHC) class 1 pathway resulting in a cell-mediated immune response. In contrast, a protein that is extracellular enters the MHC class 2 pathway, which results primarily in an antibody or humoral response.

7 Acknowledgement

The figures for this chapter originate in the copyright-free DPDx website maintained by the United States Centre for Disease Control Division of Parasitic Diseases; this source is gratefully acknowledged.

Chapter 7

Principles of microbial pathogenicity and epidemiology

Peter Gilbert and David Allison

1 Introduction

Microorganisms are ubiquitous, and the majority of them are free-living and derive their nutrition from inert organic and inorganic materials. The association of humans with such microorganisms is generally harmonious, as the majority of those encountered are benign and, indeed, are often vital to commerce, health and a balanced ecosystem. Each of us unwittingly carries a population of bacterial cells on our skin and in our gut that outnumbers cells carrying our own genome by ten to one. In spite of this the tissues of healthy animals and plants are essentially microbe-free. This is achieved through provision of a number of non-specific defences to those tissues, and specific defences such as antibodies (see Chapters 8 and 23) that may be acquired after exposure to particular agents. Breach of these defences by microorganisms, through the expression of virulence factors and adaptation to a pathogenic mode of life, or following disease, accidental trauma, catheterization or implantation of medical devices may lead to the establishment of microbial infections.

The ability of bacteria and fungi to establish infections of plants, animals and man varies considerably. Some are rarely, if ever, isolated from infected tissues, while opportunist pathogens (e.g. *Pseudomonas aeruginosa*) can establish themselves only in compromised individuals. Only a few species of bacteria may be regarded as obligate pathogens, for which animals or plants are the only reservoirs for their existence (e.g. *Neisseria gonorrhoeae*). Viruses (Chapter 5) on the other hand must parasitize host cells in order to replicate and are therefore inevitably associated with disease. Even among the viruses and obligate bacterial pathogens the degree of virulence varies, in that some are able to co-exist with the host without causing overt disease (e.g. staphylococci), while others will always cause some detriment to the host organism. Organisms such as these invariably produce their effects, directly or indirectly, by actively growing on or in the host tissues.

Other groups of microorganisms may cause disease through ingestion, by the victim, of substances (toxins) produced during microbial growth on foods (e.g. *Clostridium botulinum*, botulism; *Bacillus cereus*, vomiting). The organisms themselves do not have to survive and grow in the victim for the effects of the toxin to be felt. Whether such organisms should be regarded as pathogenic is debatable, but they must be considered in any account of microbial pathogenicity.

Animals and plants constantly interact with bacteria present within their environment. For an infection to develop, such microorganisms must remain associated with the host and increase their numbers more rapidly than they can either be eliminated or killed. This balance relates to the ability of the bacterium to mobilize nutrients and multiply in the face of innate defences and a developing immune response by the now compromised host.

The greater the number of bacterial cells associated with the initial challenge to the host, the greater will be the chance of a successful colonization. If the pathogen does not arrive at its 'portal of entry' to the body or directly at its target tissues in sufficient number, then an infection will not ensue. The minimum number of viable microorganisms that is required to cause infection and thereby disease is called the 'minimum infective number' (MIN). The MIN varies markedly between the various pathogens and is also affected by the general health and immune status of the individual host. The course of an infection can be considered as a sequence of separate events that includes initial contact with the pathogen, its consolidation and spread between and within organs and its eventual elimination (Fig. 7.1). Growth and consolidation of the microorganisms at the portal of entry commonly involves the formation of a microcolony (biofilm, see Chapter 3). Biofilms and microcolonies are collections of microorganisms that are attached to surfaces and enveloped within exopolymer matrices (glycocalyx) composed of polysaccharides, glycoproteins and/or proteins. Growth within the matrix not only protects the pathogens against opsonization and phagocytosis by the host but also modulates their micro-environment and reduces the effectiveness of many antibiotics. The localized high cell densities present within the biofilm com-

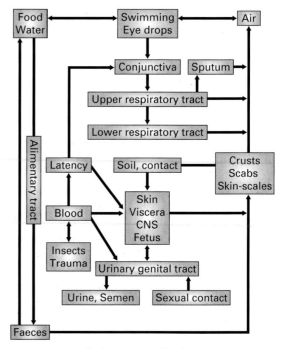

Fig. 7.1 Routes of infection, spread and transmission of disease.

munities also initiate production, by the colonizing organism, of extracellular virulence factors such as toxins, proteases and siderophores (low molecular weight ligands responsible for the solubilization and transport of iron (III) in microbial cells). These help combat the host's innate defences and also promote the acquisition of nutrients by the pathogen.

Viruses are incapable of growing extracellularly and must therefore rapidly gain entry to cells, generally epithelial in nature, at their initial site of entry. Once internalized, in the non-immune host, they are to a large extent protected against the non-specific host defences. Following these initial consolidation events, the organisms may expand into surrounding tissues and/or disperse, via the blood, plasma, lymph or nerves, to distant tissues in order to establish secondary sites of infection or to consolidate further. While in some instances the microorganism is able to colonize the host indefinitely and remain viable for many years (e.g. chicken pox, cold sores) more generally it succumbs to the heightened defences of the host, and in order to survive must either infect other individuals or survive in the general environment.

2 Portals of entry

2.1 Skin

The part of the body that is most widely exposed to microorganisms is the skin. Intact skin is usually impervious to microorganisms and its surface is of acid pH and contains relatively few nutrients that are favourable for microbial growth. The vast majority of organisms falling onto the skin surface will die, while the survivors must compete with the commensal microflora for nutrients in order to grow. These commensals, which include coryneform bacteria, staphylococci and yeasts, derive nutrients from compounds like urea, hormones (e.g. testosterone) and fatty acids found in the apocrine and epocrine secretions. Such organisms are highly adapted to growth in this environment and will normally prevent the establishment of chance contaminants of the skin. Infections of the skin itself, such as ringworm (*Trichophyton mentagrophytes*) and warts, rarely, if ever, involve penetration of the epidermis. Infection can, however, occur through the skin following trauma such as burns, cuts and abrasions and, in some instances, through insect or animal bites or the injection of contaminated medicines. In recent years extensive use of intravascular and extravascular medical devices and implants has led to an increase in the occurrence of hospital-acquired infection. Commonly these infections involve the growth of skin commensals such as *Staphylococcus epidermidis* when associated with devices that penetrate the skin barrier. The organism grows as an adhesive biofilm upon the surfaces of the device, and infection arises either from contamination of the device during its implantation or by growth along it of the organism from the skin. In such instances the biofilm sheds bacterial cells to the body and may give rise to a bacteraemia (the presence of bacteria in the blood).

The weak spots, or Achilles heels, of the body occur where the skin ends and mucous epithelial tissues begin (mouth, anus, eyes, ears, nose and urinogenital tract). These mucous membranes present a much more favourable environment for microbial growth than the skin, in that they are warm, moist and rich in nutrients. Such membranes, nevertheless, possess certain characteristics that allow them to resist infection. The majority, for example, possess their own highly adapted commensal microflora that must be displaced by any invading organisms. The resident flora varies greatly between different sites of the body, but is usually common to particular host species. Each site can be additionally protected by physicochemical barriers such as extreme acid pH in the stomach, the presence of freely circulating non-specific antibodies and/or opsonins, and/or by macrophages and phagocytes (see Chapter 8). All infections start from contact between these tissues and the potential pathogen. Contact may be direct, from an infected individual to a healthy one; or indirect, and may involve inanimate vectors such as soil, food, drink, air and airborne particles. These may directly contact the body or be ingested or inhaled or enter wounds via infected bed linen and clothing. Indirect contact may also involve animal vector intermediates (carriers).

2.2 Respiratory tract

Air contains a large amount of suspended organic matter and, in enclosed occupied spaces, may hold up to 1000 microorganisms/m^3. Almost all of these airborne organisms are non-pathogenic bacteria and fungi, of which the average person would inhale approximately 10 000 per day. The respiratory tract is protected against this assault by a mucociliary blanket that envelops the upper respiratory tract and nasal cavity. Both present a tortuous path down which microbial particles travel and inevitably impact upon these surfaces to become trapped within an enveloping blanket of mucus. Beating cilia move the mucus coating to the back of the throat where it, together with adherent particles, is swallowed. The alveolar regions of the lower respiratory tract have additional protection in the form of alveolar macrophages. To be successful, a pathogen must avoid being trapped in the mucus and swallowed, and if deposited in the alveolar sacs must avoid engulfment by macrophages or resist subsequent digestion by them. The possession of surface adhesins, specific for epithelial receptors, aids attachment of the invading microorganism and avoidance of removal by the mucociliary blanket. Other strategies include the export of ciliostatic toxins (i.e. *Corynebacterium diphtheriae*) that paralyse the cilial bed. As the primary defence of the respiratory tract is the mucociliary blanket, it is easy to envisage how infection with respiratory viruses (i.e. influenza virus kills respiratory epithelia) or the chronic inhalation of tobacco smoke (increases mucin production and decreases the proportion of ciliated epithelial cells) increases the susceptibility of individuals to infection.

2.3 Intestinal tract

The intestinal tract must contend with whatever it is given in terms of food and drink. The extreme acidity and presence of digestive enzymes in the stomach will kill many of the bacteria challenging it, and the gastrointestinal tract carries its own commensal flora of yeast and lactobacilli that afford protection by, for example, competing with potential pathogens like *Helicobacter pylori*. Bile salts are mixed with the semi-digested solids exiting from the stomach into the small intestine. These salts not only neutralize the stomach acids but also contain surfactants that are able to solubilize the outer membrane of many Gram-negative bacteria. As a consequence, the small intestine is generally free from microorganisms and can be readily colonized by suitably adapted pathogens. The lower gut on the other hand is highly populated by commensal microorganisms (10^{11} g^{-1} gut tissue) that are often associated with the intestinal wall, either embedded in layers of protective mucus or attached directly to the epithelial cells. The pathogenicity of incoming bacteria and viruses depends upon their ability to survive passage through the stomach and duodenum and upon their capacity for attachment to, or penetration of, the gut wall, despite competition from the commensal flora and the presence of secretory antibodies (Chapter 8).

2.4 Urinogenital tract

In healthy individuals, the bladder, ureters and urethra are sterile, and sterile urine constantly flushes the urinary tract. Organisms invading the urinary tract must avoid being detached from the epithelial surfaces and washed out during urination. In the male, as the urethra is long (c. 20 cm), bacteria must be introduced directly into the bladder, possibly through catheterization. In the female, the urethra is much shorter (c. 5 cm) and is more readily traversed by microorganisms that are normally resident within the vaginal vault. Bladder infections are therefore much more common in the female. Spread of the infection from the bladder to the kidneys can easily occur through reflux of urine into the ureter. As for the implantation of devices across the skin barrier (above), long-term catheterization of the bladder will promote the occurrence of bacteriuria (the presence of bacteria in the urine) with all of the associated complications.

Lactic acid in the vagina gives it an acidic pH (5.0); this, together with other products of metabolism inhibits colonization by most bacteria, except some lactobacilli that constitute the commensal flora. Other types of bacteria are unable to establish themselves in the vagina unless they have become extremely specialized. These species of microorganism tend to be associated with sexually transmitted infections.

2.5 Conjunctiva

The conjunctiva is usually free of microorganisms and protected by the continuous flow of secretions from lachrymal and other glands, and by frequent mechanical cleansing of its surface by the eyelid periphery during blinking. Lachrymal fluids contain a number of inhibitory compounds, together with lysozyme, that can enzymically degrade the peptidoglycan of Gram-positive bacteria such as staphylococci. Damage to the conjunctiva, caused through mechanical abrasion or reductions in tear flow, will increase microbial adhesion and allow colonization by opportunist pathogens. The likelihood of infection is thus promoted by the use of soft and hard contact lenses, physical damage, exposure to chemicals, or damage and infection of the eyelid border (blepharitis).

3 Consolidation

To be successful, a pathogen must be able to survive at its initial portal of entry, frequently in competition with the commensal flora and generally subject to the attention of macrophages and wandering white blood cells. Such survival invariably requires the organism to attach itself firmly to the epithelial surface. This attachment must be highly specific in order to displace the commensal microflora, and subsequently governs the course of an infection. Attachment can be mediated through provision, on the bacterial surface, of adhesive substances such as mucopeptide and mucopolysaccharide slime layers, fimbriae (Chapter 3), pili (Chapter 3) and agglutinins (Chapter 8). These are often highly specific in their binding characteristics, differentiating, for example, between the tips and bases of villi in the large bowel and the epithelial cells of the upper, mid and lower gut. Secretory antibodies, which are directed against such adhesions, block the initial attachment of the organism and thereby confer resistance to infection.

The outcome of the encounter between the tissues and potential pathogens is governed by the ability of the microorganism to multiply at a faster rate than it is removed from those tissues. Factors that influence this are the organism's rate of growth, the initial number arriving at the site and their ability to resist the efforts of the host tissues at removing/starving/killing them. The definition of *virulence* for pathogenic microorganisms must therefore relate to the minimum number of cells required to initiate an infection (MIN). This will vary between individuals, but will invariably be lower in compromised hosts such as those who are catheterized, diabetics, smokers and cystic fibrotics, and those suffering trauma such as malnutrition, chronic infection or physical damage. A number of the individual factors that contribute towards virulence are discussed below.

3.1 Resistance to host defences

Most bacterial infections confine themselves to the surface of epithelial tissue (e.g. *Bordetella pertussis*, *Corynebacterium diphtheriae*, *Vibrio cholerae*). This is, to a large extent, a reflection of their inability to combat that host's deeper defences. Survival at these sites is largely due to firm attachment to the epithelial cells. Such organisms manifest disease through the production and release of toxins (see below).

Other groups of organisms regularly establish systemic infections after traversing the epithelial surfaces (e.g. *Brucella abortus*, *Salmonella typhi*, *Streptococcus pyogenes*). This property is associated with their ability either to gain entry into susceptible cells and thereby enjoy protection from the body's defences, or to be phagocytosed by macrophages or polymorphs yet resist their lethal action and multiply within them. Other organisms are able to multiply and grow freely in the body's extracellular fluids. Microorganisms have evolved a number of different strategies that allow them to suppress the host's normal defences and thereby survive in the tissues.

3.1.1 Modulation of the inflammatory response

Growth of microorganisms releases cellular products into their surrounding medium, many of which cause non-specific inflammation associated with dilatation of blood vessels. This increases capillary flow and access of phagocytes to the infected site. Increased lymphatic flow from the inflamed tissues carries the organisms to lymph nodes where further antimicrobial and immune forces come into play (Chapter 8). Many of the substances that are released by microorganisms in this fashion are chemotactic towards polymorphs that tend, therefore, to become concentrated at the site of infection: this is in addition to the inflammation and white blood cell accumulation that is associated with antibody binding and complement fixation (Chapter 8). Many organisms have adapted mechanisms that allow them to overcome these initial defences. Thus, virulent strains of *Staphylococcus aureus* produce a mucopeptide (peptidoglycan), which suppresses early inflammatory oedema, and related factors that suppress the chemotaxis of polymorphs.

3.1.2 Avoidance of phagocytosis

Resistance to phagocytosis is sometimes associated

with specific components of the cell wall and/or with the presence of capsules surrounding the cell wall. Classic examples of these are the M-proteins of the streptococci and the polysaccharide capsules of the pneumococci. The acidic polysaccharide K-antigens of *Escherichia coli* and *Salmonella typhi* behave similarly, in that (i) they can mediate attachment to the intestinal epithelial cells, and (ii) they render phagocytosis more difficult. Generally, possession of an extracellular capsule will reduce the likelihood of phagocytosis.

Microorganisms are more readily phagocytosed when coated with antibody (opsonized). This is due to the presence on the white blood cells of receptors for the Fc fragment of IgM and IgG (discussed in Chapter 8). Avoidance of opsonization will clearly enhance the chances of survival of a particular pathogen. A substance called protein A is released from actively growing strains of *Staph. aureus*, which acts by non-specific binding to IgG at the Fc region (see also Chapter 8), at sites both close to, and remote from, the bacterial surface. This blocks the Fc region of bound antibody masking it from phagocytes. Protein A–IgG complexes remote from the infection site will also bind complement, thereby depleting it from the plasma and negating its actions near to the infection site.

3.1.3 Survival following phagocytosis

Death of microorganisms following phagocytosis can be avoided if the microorganisms are not exposed to the killing and digestion processes within the phagocyte. This is possible if fusion of the lysosomes with phagocytic vacuoles can be prevented. Such a strategy is employed by virulent *Mycobacterium tuberculosis*, although the precise mechanism is unknown. Other bacteria seem able to grow within the vacuoles despite lysosomal fusion (*Listeria monocytogenes*, *Sal. typhi*). This can be attributed to cell wall components that prevent access of the lysosomal substances to the bacterial membranes (e.g. *Brucella abortus*, mycobacteria) or to the production of extracellular catalase which neutralizes the hydrogen peroxide liberated in the vacuole (e.g. staphylococci).

If microorganisms are able to survive and grow within phagocytes, they will escape many of the other body defences such as the lymph nodes, and be distributed around the body. As the lifespan of phagocytes is relatively short then such bacteria will eventually be delivered to the liver and gastrointestinal tract where they are 're-cycled'.

3.1.4 Killing of phagocytes

An alternative strategy is for the microorganism to kill the phagocyte. This can be achieved by the production of leucocidins (e.g. staphylococci, streptococci) which promote the discharge of lysosomal substances into the cytoplasm of the phagocyte rather than into the vacuole, thus directing the phagocyte's lethal activity towards itself.

4 Manifestation of disease

Once established, the course of a bacterial infection can proceed in a number of ways. These can be related to the relative ability of the organism to penetrate and invade surrounding tissues and organs. The vast majority of pathogens, being unable to combat the defences of the deeper tissues, consolidate further on the epithelial surface. Others, which include the majority of viruses, penetrate the epithelial layers, but no further, and can be regarded as partially invasive. A small group of pathogens are fully invasive. These permeate the subepithelial tissues and are circulated around the body to initiate secondary sites of infection remote from the initial portal of entry (Fig. 7.1).

Other groups of organisms may cause disease through ingestion by the victim of substances produced during microbial growth on foods. Such diseases may be regarded as intoxications rather than as infections and are considered later (section 5.1.1). Treatment in these cases is usually an alleviation of the harmful effects of the toxin rather than elimination of the pathogen from the body.

4.1 Non-invasive pathogens

Bordetella pertussis (the aetiological agent of whooping cough) is probably the best described of these pathogens. This organism is inhaled and rapidly localizes on the mucociliary blanket of the lower respiratory tract. This localization is very selective and is thought to involve agglutinins on the organism's surface. Toxins produced by the organism inhibit ciliary movement of the epithelial surface and thereby prevent removal of the bacterial cells to the gut. A high molecular weight exotoxin is also produced during the growth of the organism which, being of limited diffusibility, pervades the subepithelial tissues to produce inflammation and necrosis. *C. diphtheriae* (the causal organism of diphtheria) behaves similarly, attaching itself to the epithelial cells of the respiratory tract. This organism produces a low molecular weight, diffusible toxin that enters the blood circulation and brings about a generalized toxaemia.

In the gut, many pathogens adhere to the gut wall and produce their effect via toxins that pervade the surrounding gut wall or enter the systemic circulation. *Vibrio cholerae* and some enteropathic *E. coli* strains localize on the gut wall and produce toxins that increase vascular permeability. The end result is a hypersecretion of isotonic fluids into the gut lumen, acute diarrhoea and, as a consequence, dehydration that may be fatal in juveniles and the elderly. In all these instances, binding to epithelial cells is not essential but increases permeation of the toxin and prolongs the presence of the pathogen.

4.2 Partially invasive pathogens

Some bacteria, and the majority of viruses, are able to attach to the mucosal epithelia and then penetrate rapidly into the epithelial cells. These organisms multiply within the protective environment of the host cell, eventually killing it and inducing disease through erosion and ulceration of the mucosal epithelium. Typically, members of the genera *Shigella* and *Salmonella* utilize such mechanisms in infections of the gastrointestinal tract. These bacteria attach to the epithelial cells of the large and small intestines, respectively, and, following their entry into these cells by induced pinocytosis, multiply rapidly and penetrate laterally into adjacent epithelial cells. The mechanisms for such attachment and movement are unknown but involve a transition from a non-motile to motile phenotype. Some species of salmonellae produce, in addition, exotoxins that induce diarrhoea (section 4.1). There

are innumerable serotypes of *Salmonella*, which are primarily parasites of animals but are important to humans in that they colonize farm animals such as pigs and poultry and ultimately infect foods derived from them. *Salmonella* food poisoning (salmonellosis), therefore, is commonly associated with inadequately cooked meats, eggs and also with cold meat products that have been incorrectly stored following contact with the uncooked product. Dependent upon the severity of the lesions induced in the gut wall by these pathogens, red blood cells and phagocytes pass into the gut lumen, along with plasma, and cause the classic 'bloody flux' of bacillary dysentery. Similar erosive lesions are produced by some enteropathic strains of *E. coli*.

Viral infections such as influenza and the 'common cold' (in reality 300–400 different strains of rhinovirus) infect epithelial cells of the respiratory tract and nasopharynx, respectively. Release of the virus, after lysis of the host cells, is to the void rather than to subepithelial tissues. The residual uninfected epithelial cells are rapidly infected resulting in general degeneration of the tracts. Such damage not only predisposes the respiratory tract to infection with opportunist pathogens such as *Neisseria meningitidis* and *Haemophilus influenzae* but it also causes the associated fever.

4.3 Invasive pathogens

Invasive pathogens either aggressively invade the tissues surrounding the primary site of infection (active spread) or are passively transported around the body in the blood, lymph, cerebrospinal, axonal or pleural fluids (passive spread). Some, especially aggressive organisms, move both passively and actively, setting up multiple, expansive secondary sites of infection in various organs.

4.3.1 Active spread

Active spread of microorganisms through normal subepithelial tissues is difficult in that the gel-like nature of the intercellular materials physically inhibits bacterial movement. Induced death and lysis of the tissue cells produces, in addition, a highly viscous fluid, partly due to undenatured DNA. Physical damage, such as wounds, rapidly seal with fibrin clots, thereby reducing the effective routes for spread of opportunist pathogens. Organisms such as *Strep. pyogenes*, *Cl. perfringens* and, to some extent, the staphylococci, are able to establish themselves in tissues by virtue of their ability to produce a wide range of extracellular enzyme toxins. These are associated with killing of tissue cells, degradation of intracellular materials and mobilization of nutrients. A selection of such toxins will be considered briefly.

1 *Haemolysins* are produced by most of the pathogenic staphylococci and streptococci. They have a lytic effect on red blood cells, releasing iron-containing nutrients.

2 *Fibrinolysins* are produced by both staphylococci (staphylokinase) and streptococci (streptokinase). These toxins indirectly activate plasminogen and so dissolve fibrin clots that the host forms around wounds and lesions to seal them. The production of fibrinolysins therefore increases the likelihood of the infection spreading. Streptokinase may be employed clinically in conjunction with streptodornase (Chapter 25) in the treatment of thrombosis.

3 *Collagenases* and *hyaluronidases* are produced by most of the aggressive invaders of tissues. These are able to dissolve collagen fibres and the hyaluronic acids that function as intercellular cements; this causes the tissues to break up and produce oedematous lesions.

4 *Phospholipases* are produced by organisms such as *Cl. perfringens* (alpha-toxin). These toxins kill tissue cells by hydrolysing the phospholipids that are present in cell membranes.

5 *Amylases*, *peptidases* and *deoxyribonuclease* mobilize many nutrients that are released from lysed cells. They also decrease the viscosity of fluids present at the lesion by depolymerization of their biopolymer substrates.

Organisms possessing the above toxins, particularly those also possessing *leucocidins*, are likely to cause expanding oedematous lesions at the primary site of infection. In the case of *Cl. perfringens*, a soil microorganism that has become adapted to a saprophytic mode of life, infection arises from an accidental contamination of deep wounds when a process similar to that seen during the decomposition of a carcass ensues (gangrene). This organism is most likely to spread through tissues when blood circulation, and therefore oxygen tension, in the affected areas is minimal.

Abscesses formed by streptococci and staphylococci can be deep-seated in soft tissues or associated with infected wounds or skin lesions; they become localized through the deposition of fibrin capsules around the infection site. Fibrin deposition is partly a response of the host tissues, but is also partly a function of enzyme toxins such as *coagulase*. Phagocytic white blood cells can migrate into these abscesses in large numbers to produce significant quantities of pus. Such pus, often carrying the infective pathogen, might be digested by other phagocytes in the late stages of the infection or discharged to the exterior or to the capillary and lymphatic network. In the latter case, blocked capillaries might serve as sites for secondary lesions. Toxins liberated from the microorganisms during their growth in such abscesses can freely diffuse to the rest of the body to set up a generalized toxaemia.

Sal. typhi, *Sal. paratyphi* and *Sal. typhimurium* are serotypes of *Salmonella* (section 4.2) that are not only able to penetrate into intestinal epithelial cells and produce exotoxins, but are also able to penetrate beyond into subepithelial tissues. These organisms therefore produce a characteristic systemic disease (typhoid and enteric fever), in addition to the usual symptoms of salmonellosis. Following recovery from such infection the organism is commonly found associated with the gall bladder. In this state, the recovered person will excrete the organism and become a reservoir for the infection of others.

4.3.2 Passive spread

When invading microorganisms have crossed the epithelial barriers they will almost certainly be taken up with lymph in the lymphatic ducts and be delivered to filtration and immune systems at the local lymph nodes. Sometimes this serves to spread infections further around the body. Eventually, spread may occur from local to regional lymph nodes and thence to the bloodstream. Direct entry to the bloodstream from the primary portal of entry is rare and will only occur when the organism damages the blood vessels or if it is injected directly into them. This might be the case following an insect bite or surgery. Bacteraemia such as this will often lead to secondary infections remote from the original portal of entry.

5 Damage to tissues

Damage caused to the host organism through infection can be direct and related to the destructive presence of microorganisms (or to their production of toxins) in particular target organs; or it can be indirect and related to interactions of the antigenic components of the pathogen with the host's immune system. Effects can therefore be closely related to, or remote from, the infected organ.

Symptoms of the infection can in some instances be highly specific, relating to a single, precise pharmacological response to a particular toxin; or they might be non-specific and relate to the usual response of the body to particular types of trauma. Damage induced by infection will therefore be considered in these categories.

5.1 Direct damage

5.1.1 *Specific effects*

For the host, the consequences of infection depend to a large extent upon the tissue or organ involved. Soft tissue infections of skeletal muscle are likely to be less damaging than, for instance, infections of the heart muscle and central nervous system. Infections associated with the epithelial cells that make up small blood vessels can block or rupture them to produce anoxia or necrosis in the tissues that they supply. Cell and tissue damage is generally the result of a direct local action by the microorganisms, usually concerning action at the cytoplasmic membranes. The target cells are usually phagocytes and are generally killed (e.g. by *Brucella, Listeria, Mycobacterium*). Interference with membrane function through the action of enzymes such as phospholipase causes the affected cells to leak. When lysosomal membranes are affected, the lysosomal enzymes disperse into the cells and tissues causing them, in turn, to autolyse. This is mediated through the vast battery of enzyme toxins available to these organisms (section 4). If these toxins are

produced in sufficient concentration they may enter the circulatory systems to produce a generalized toxaemia. During their growth, other pathogens liberate toxins that possess very precise, singular pharmacological actions. Diseases mediated in this manner include diphtheria, tetanus and scarlet fever.

In diphtheria, the organism C. *diphtheriae* confines itself to epithelial surfaces of the nose and throat and produces a powerful toxin which affects an elongation factor involved in eukaryotic protein biosynthesis. The heart and peripheral nerves are particularly affected, resulting in myocarditis (inflammation of the myocardium) and neuritis (inflammation of a nerve). Little damage is produced at the infection site.

Tetanus occurs when Cl. *tetani*, ubiquitous in the soil and the faeces of herbivores, contaminates wounds, especially deep puncture-type lesions. These might be the result of a minor trauma such as a splinter, or a major one such as a motor vehicle accident. At these sites, tissue necrosis, and possibly also microbial growth, reduce the oxygen tension to allow this anaerobe to multiply. Its growth is accompanied by the production of a highly potent toxin that passes up peripheral nerves and diffuses locally within the central nervous system. The toxin has a strychnine-like action and affects normal function at the synapses. As the motor nerves of the brainstem are the shortest, the cranial nerves are the first affected, with twitches of the eyes and spasms of the jaw (lockjaw).

A related organism, Cl. *botulinum*, produces a similar toxin that may contaminate food if the organism has grown in it and if conditions are favourable for anaerobic growth. Meat pastes and pâtés are likely sources. This toxin interferes with acetylcholine release at cholinergic synapses and also acts at neuromuscular junctions. Death from this toxin eventually results from respiratory failure.

Many other organisms are capable of producing intoxication following their growth on foods. Most common among these are the staphylococci and strains of *Bacillus cereus*. Some strains of *Staph. aureus* produce an enterotoxin which acts upon the vomiting centres of the brain. Nausea and vomiting therefore follow ingestion of contaminated foods

111

and the delay between eating and vomiting varies between 1 and 6 hours depending on the amount of toxin ingested. *Bacillus cereus* also produces an emetic toxin but its actions are delayed and vomiting can follow up to 20 hours after ingestion. The latter organism is often associated with rice products and will propagate when the rice is cooked (spore activation) and subsequently reheated after a period of storage.

Scarlet fever is produced following infection with certain strains of *Strep. pyogenes*. These organisms produce a potent toxin that causes an erythrogenic skin rash that then accompanies the more usual effects of a streptococcal infection.

5.1.2 Non-specific effects

If the infective agent damages an organ and affects its functioning, this can manifest itself as a series of secondary disease features that reflect the loss of that function to the host. Thus, diabetes may result from an infection of the islets of Langerhans, paralysis or coma from infections of the central nervous system, and kidney malfunction from loss of tissue fluids and its associated hyperglycaemia. In this respect virus infections almost inevitably result in the death and lysis of the host cells. This will result in some loss of function by the target organ. Similarly, exotoxins and endotoxins can also be implicated in non-specific symptoms, even when they have well-defined pharmacological actions. Thus, a number of intestinal pathogens (e.g. *V. cholerae*, *E. coli*) produce potent exotoxins that affect vascular permeability. These generally act through adenylate cyclase, raising the intracellular levels of cyclic AMP (adenosine monophosphate). As a result of this the cells lose water and electrolytes to the surrounding medium, the gut lumen. A common consequence of these related, yet distinct, toxins is acute diarrhoea and haemo-concentration. Kidney malfunction might well follow and in severe cases lead to death. Symptomologically there is little difference between these conditions and the food poisoning induced by ingestion of staphylococcal enterotoxin. The latter toxin is formed by the organisms during their growth on infected food substances and is absorbed actively from the gut. It acts, not at the epithelial cells of the gut, but at the vomiting centre of the central nervous system causing nausea, vomiting and diarrhoea within 6 hours (above).

5.2 Indirect damage

Inflammatory materials are released not only from necrotic cells but also directly from the infective agent. Endotoxins are derived from the parts that form the bacterial cell rather than being deliberately exported cellular products. Thus, during the growth and autolysis of Gram-negative bacteria components of their cell envelopes, such as lipopolysaccharide (see Chapter 3) are shed to the environment. Endotoxins tend to be less toxic than exotoxins and have much less precise pharmacological actions. Indeed, it is not always clear to what extent these can be related to actions by the host or by the pathogen. Reactions include local inflammation, elevations in body temperature, aching joints, and head and kidney pain. Inflammation causes swelling, pain and reddening of the tissues, and sometimes loss of function of the organs affected. These reactions may sometimes be the major sign and symptom of the disease.

While various toxic effects have been attributed to these endotoxins, their role in the establishment of the infection, if any, remains unclear. The most notable effect of these materials is their ability to induce a high body temperature (pyrogenicity) (Chapters 3 and 19). The pyrogenic effect of lipopolysaccharide relates to the action of the lipid-A component directly upon the hypothalamus and also to its direct action on macrophages and phagocytes. Elevation of body temperature follows within 1–2 hours. In infections such as meningitis the administration of antibiotics may cause such a release of pyrogen that the resultant inflammation and fever is fatal. In such instances antibiotics are co-administered with steroids to counter this effect. The pyrogenic effects of lipid-A are unaffected by moist heat treatment (autoclave). Growth of Gram-negative organisms such as *Pseudomonas aeruginosa* in stored water destined for use in terminally sterilized products will cause the final product to be pyrogenic. Processes for the destruction of pyrogen associated with glassware, and tests for the absence of pyrogen in water and product therefore form an important part of parenteral drug manufacture (Chapter 19).

Many microorganisms minimize the effects of the host's defence system against them by mimicking the antigenic structure of the host tissue. The eventual immunological response of the host to infection then leads to the autoimmune destruction of itself. Thus, infections with *Mycoplasma pneumoniae* can lead to production of antibody against normal group O erythrocytes with concomitant haemolytic anaemia.

If antigen released from the infective agent is soluble, antigen–antibody complexes are produced. When antibody is present at a concentration equal to or greater than the antigen, such as in the case of an immune host, these complexes precipitate and are removed by macrophages present in the lymph nodes. When antigen is present in excess, the complexes, being small, continue to circulate in the blood and are eventually filtered off by the kidneys, becoming lodged in kidney glomeruli and in the joints. Localized inflammatory responses in the kidneys are sometimes then initiated by the complement system (Chapter 8). Eventually the filtering function of the kidneys becomes impaired, producing symptoms of chronic glomerulonephritis.

6 Recovery from infection: exit of microorganisms

The primary requirement for recovery is that multiplication of the infective agent is brought under control, that it ceases to spread around the body and that the damaging consequences of its presence are arrested and repaired. Such control is brought about by the combined function of the phagocytic, immune and complement systems. A successful pathogen will not seriously debilitate its host; rather, the continued existence of the host must be ensured in order to maximize the dissemination of the pathogen within the host population. From the microorganism's perspective the ideal situation is where it can persist permanently within the host and be constantly released to the environment. While this is the case for a number of virus infections (chickenpox, herpes) and for some bacterial ones, it is not common. Generally, recovery from

infection is accompanied by complete destruction of the organism and restoration of a sterile tissue. Alternatively, the organism might return to a commensal relationship with the host on the epithelial and skin surface.

Where the infective agent is an obligate pathogen, a means must exist for it to infect other individuals before its eradication from the host organism. The route of exit is commonly related to the original portal of entry (Fig. 7.1). Thus, pathogens of the intestinal tract are liberated in the faeces and might easily contaminate food and drinking water. Infective agents of the respiratory tract might be exhaled during coughing, sneezing or talking, survive in the associated water droplets and infect, through inhalation, nearby individuals. Infective agents transmitted by insect and animal vectors may be spread through those same vectors, the insects/animals having been themselves infected by the diseased host. For some 'fragile' organisms (e.g. *N. gonorrhoeae*, *Treponema pallidum*), direct contact transmission is the only means of spread between individual hosts. In these cases, intimate contact between epithelial membranes, such as occurs during sexual contact, is required for transfer to occur. For opportunist pathogens, such as those associated with wound infections, transfer is less important because the pathogenic role is minor. Rather, the natural habitat of the organism serves as a constant reservoir for infection.

7 Epidemiology of infectious disease

Spread of a microbial disease through a population of individuals can be considered as vertical (transferred from one generation to another) or horizontal (transfer occurring within genetically unrelated groups). The latter can be divided into common source outbreaks, relating to infection of a number of susceptible individuals from a single reservoir of the infective agent (i.e. infected foods), or propagated source outbreaks, where each individual provides a new source for the infection of others.

Common source outbreaks are characterized by a sharp onset of reported cases over the course of a single incubation period and relate to a common experience of the infected individuals. The number of cases will persist until the source of the infection is removed. If the source of the infection remains (i.e. a reservoir of insect vectors) then the disease becomes endemic to the exposed population with a constant rate of infection. Propagated source outbreaks, on the other hand, show a gradual increase in reported cases over a number of incubation periods and eventually decline when the majority of susceptible individuals in the population have been affected. Factors that contribute to propagated outbreaks of infectious disease are the infectivity of the agent (I), the population density (P) and the numbers of susceptible individuals in it (F). The likelihood of an epidemic occurring is given by the product of these three factors (i.e. FIP). Increases in any one of them might initiate an outbreak of the disease in epidemic proportions. Thus, reported cases of particular diseases show periodicity, with outbreaks of epidemic proportion occurring only when FIP exceeds certain critical threshold values, related to the infectivity of the agent. Outbreaks of measles and chickenpox therefore tend to occur annually in the late summer among children attending school for the first time. This has the effect of concentrating all susceptible individuals in one, often confined, space at the same time. The proportion of susceptible individuals can be reduced through rigorous vaccination programmes (Chapter 9). Provided that the susceptible population does not exceed the threshold FIP value, then herd immunity against epidemic spread of the disease will be maintained.

Certain types of infectious agent (e.g. influenza virus) are able to combat herd immunity such as this through undergoing major antigenic changes. These render the majority of the population susceptible, and their occurrence is often accompanied by spread of the disease across the entire globe (pandemics).

8 Further reading

Salyers, A. A. & Drew, D. D. (2001) *Microbiology: Diversity, Disease and the Environment*. Fitzgerald Science Press, Bethesda, MD.

Smith, H. (1990) Pathogenicity and the microbe *in vivo*. *J Gen Microbiol*, **136**, 377–393.

Wilson, M., McNab, R. & Henderson, B. (2002) *Bacterial Disease Mechanisms*. Cambridge University Press, Cambridge.

Part 2

Antimicrobial Agents

Chapter 8

Basic aspects of the structure and functioning of the immune system

Mark Gumbleton and James Furr

1 Introduction

1.1 Historical perspective and scope of immunology

Progress in immunological science has been driven by the need to understand and exploit the generation of immune states exemplified now by the use of modern vaccines. From almost the first recorded observations, it was recognized that persons who had contracted and recovered from certain infectious diseases were not susceptible (i.e. were immune) to the effects of the same disease when re-exposed to the infection. Thucydides, over 2500 years ago, described in detail an epidemic in Athens (which could have been typhus or plague) and noted that sufferers were 'touched by the pitying care of those who had recovered because they were themselves free of apprehension, for no-one was ever attacked a second time or with a fatal result'.

Since that time many attempts have been made to induce this immune state. In ancient times the process of variolation (the inoculation of live organisms of smallpox obtained from the diseased pustules of patients who were recovering from the disease) was practised extensively in India and China. The success rate was very variable and often depended on the skill of the variolator. In the late 18th century Edward Jenner, an English country doctor, observed the similarity between the pustules of smallpox and those of cowpox, a disease that affected the udders of cows. He also observed that milkmaids who had contracted cowpox by the handling of diseased udders were immune to smallpox. Jenner deliberately inoculated a young boy with cowpox, and after the boy's recovery, inoculated him again with the contents of a pustule taken from a patient suffering from smallpox; the boy did not succumb to infection from this first, or any subsequent challenges, with the smallpox virus. Even though the mechanisms by which this protection against smallpox were not understood, Jenner's work had shown proof of principle that the harmless stimulation of our adaptive immune system (see below) was capable of generating an immune state against a specific disease, and thereby provided the basis for the process we now understand as vaccination. The cowpox virus is otherwise known as the vaccinia virus and the term vaccine was introduced by Pasteur to commemorate Jenner's work.

In 1801 Jenner prophesied the eradication of smallpox by the practice of vaccination. In 1967 smallpox infected 10 million people worldwide. The World Health Organization (WHO) initiated a programme of confinement and vaccination with the aim of eradicating the disease. In Somalia in 1977 the last case of naturally acquired smallpox occurred, and in 1979 the WHO announced the total eradication of smallpox, thus fulfilling Jenner's prophecy. Many vaccine products are now available designed to provide protection against a range of infectious diseases. Their value has been proven in national vaccine programmes leading to dramatic reductions in morbidity and mortality of such diseases as diphtheria, pertussis, mumps, measles, rubella, hepatitis A and B.

Further progress in the understanding of the complex nature and functioning of the immune system has been gained through the recognition that many varied forms of pathology, beyond that of infectious disease *per se*, have an underlying immunological basis, including such diseases as asthma, diabetes, rheumatoid arthritis and many forms of cancer. A basic knowledge of how the immune system functions is essential for health professionals involved in understanding the nature of disease and rationalizing therapeutic strategies. This chapter aims to provide a sound overview of the structure and functioning of the immune system and impart the reader with knowledge which will serve as a platform for the study of more complex specialized texts if and when required.

1.2 Definitions and outline structure of the immune system

The primary function of the immune system is to defend against and eliminate 'foreign' material, and to minimize any damage that may be caused as a result of the presence of such material. The term 'foreign' includes not only potentially pathogenic microorganisms but also cells recognized as 'non-self' and therefore foreign such as the human body's own virally infected or otherwise transformed (e.g. cancerous) host cells. Foreign material would also include allogeneic (within species) or xenogeneic (between species) transplant tissue and therapeutic proteins administered as medicines if they arose from a different species or were of human origin but had undergone inappropriate post-translational modifications during manufacture or contained impurities. It is also possible that small organic-based drugs may form adducts with endogenous proteins leading to the generation of an immunogen. A good example of such adduct formation is that between the serum protein albumin and the glucuronide metabolite of some non-steroidal anti-inflammatory drugs. This adduct is proposed as the basis of some hypersensitivity reactions.

For clarity there are a number of terms that should be defined at this point. An organism which has the ability to cause disease is termed a *pathogen*. The term *virulence* is used to indicate the degree of *pathogenicity* of a given strain of microorganism. Reduction in the virulence of a pathogen is termed *attenuation*; this can eventually result in an organism losing its virulence completely and it is then termed *avirulent*.

An *antigen* is a component of the 'foreign' material that gives rise to the primary interaction with the body's immune system. If the antigen elicits an immune response it may then be termed an *immunogen*. Within a given antigen, e.g. a protein, there will be *antigenic determinants* or *epitopes*, which actually represent the antigen recognition sites for our *adaptive immune system* (see below). For example, within a protein antigen, an epitope for an antibody response will comprise 5–20 amino acids that arise either as part of a linear chain or as a cluster of amino acids brought together conformationally by the folding of the protein. Antibodies (otherwise known as immunoglobulins — Ig) are produced and secreted into biological fluids by our adaptive immune system, are widely used in *in vitro* diagnosis and have been investigated in therapeutics as a means of targeting drugs to specific sites in the body. A *monoclonal antibody* refers to an antibody nominally recognizing only a single antigen (e.g. a single protein) and within which only a single common epitope (e.g. clusters comprising a common single specific amino acid sequence or pattern) is recognized. In contrast, a *polyclonal antibody* refers to an antibody nominally recognizing only a single antigen but within which a number of different epitopes (e.g. clusters comprising different amino acid sequences or patterns) are recognized.

The immune system is broadly considered to exhibit two forms of response:

1 The *innate immune response*, which is non-specific, displays no time lag in responsiveness, and is not intrinsically affected by prior contact with infectious agent.

2 The *adaptive immune response*, which displays a time lag in response, involves highly specific recognition of antigen and affords the generation of immunological memory. An example of immunological memory is that provided by the generation of specific lymphocyte memory cell populations following vaccination with an antigen (e.g. diphtheria toxoid). These memory cells reside over a long term in our lymphoid tissue and permit a more rapid and pronounced protective immunological response upon future exposure to the same antigen.

The adaptive immune system is further subdivided into:

(a) *Humoral immunity* within which the effector cells are *B lymphocytes* and where antigen recognition occurs through interactions with antibodies.

(b) *Cell-mediated immunity* within which the effector cells are *T lymphocytes* and where antigen recognition occurs through interactions of peptide antigen (presented on the surface of other cell types) with *T-cell receptors (TCR)* on the plasma membrane of T lymphocytes. In cell-mediated immunity the peptide antigen must be presented to T lymphocytes by other cell types in association with a class of plasma membrane molecules termed *major histocompatibility complex (MHC) proteins*.

1.3 Cells of the immune system

A schematic overview of the cells involved in both the innate and adaptive components of the immune response is shown in Fig. 8.1. The majority of cells involved in the immune system arise from progenitor cell populations within the bone marrow. The differentiation of these progenitor cells is under the control of a variety of growth factors, e.g. granulocyte- or macrophage-colony stimulating factors (G-CSF and M-CSF, respectively) released by monocyte and macrophage cells as well as by fibroblasts and activated endothelial cells. These growth factors promote the growth and maturation of monocyte and granulocyte populations within the bone marrow before their release into the lymphoid and blood circulations.

The key cells of the innate immune system include the following. (A) *Mononuclear phagocytic* cells which comprise the short-lived (< 8 h) monocytes in the blood circulation and which migrate into tissues and undergo further differentiation to give rise to the long-lived and key effector cell — the macrophage. (B) The *granulocyte cell* populations which include the neutrophil, basophil and eosinophil. (C) The *mast cell* which is a tissue-resident cell that is triggered by tissue damage or infection to release numerous initiating factors leading to an inflammatory response. Such factors include histamine, leukotrienes B4, C4, D4, pro-inflammatory cytokines (signal proteins released by leucocytes — white blood cells), e.g. TNF-α, and chemotactic substances such as interleukin-8 (IL-8). The sudden degranulation of the contents of mast cells is also responsible for the acute anaphylactic reactions to bee stings, penicillins, nuts etc. (D) The *natural killer* (NK) cell which has a phenotype similar to that of lymphocytes but lacks their specific recognition receptors. The NK cell exploits non-specific recognition to elicit cytotoxic actions against host cells infected with virus and those host cells that have acquired tumour cell characteristics.

The lymphocyte populations also arise from bone marrow progenitor cells. The B lymphocytes mature or differentiate in the bone marrow before leaving to circulate in the blood and lymph, while T lymphocytes undergo maturation in the thymus. Antibodies mediating the effector functions of the

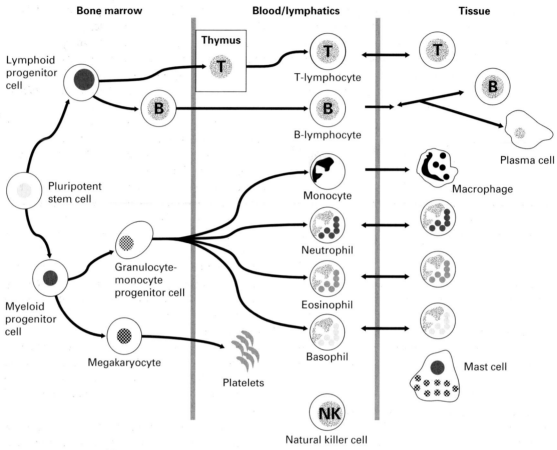

Fig. 8.1 An overview of the cells involved in the immune response: both innate and adaptive components. The cells arise from a pluripotent progenitor cell within the bone marrow, with their growth and differentiation controlled by numerous growth factors. The T lymphocytes differentiate in the thymus gland.

humoral immune system are produced and secreted from a differentiated B lymphocyte cell population termed plasma cells.

2 The innate immune system

2.1 Innate barriers at epidermal and mucosal surfaces

Innate defence against the passage of potentially pathogenic microorganisms across epidermal and mucosal barriers involves a range of non-specific mechanisms. Commensal microorganisms upon

mucosal surfaces and upon membranes such as skin and conjunctiva constitute one such mechanism. These commensals are, under normal circumstances, non-pathogenic, and help prevent colonization by pathogenic strains. There are also a number of physical and chemical barriers against microbial entry, including the flow of fluid secretions from tear ducts, the urogenital tract and the skin. Many of these secretions possess bacteristatic or bactericidal activity due to their low pH or the presence of hydrolytic enzymes such as lysozyme (a peptidoglycan hydrolase). Similarly, the mucus barrier, covering mucosal surfaces such as the epithelium of the lung, serves as a false binding platform for microorganisms, preventing them interacting with the underlying host cells. In the normal state the hydrated mucus barrier is efficiently cleared under the driving force of beating cilia. The serious lung infections manifest in cystic fibrosis arise because of the inability of patients to clear the bacteria-laden dehydrated mucus effectively.

2.2 Innate defence once epidermal or mucosal barriers have been compromised

The function of the innate defence system against microorganisms that have penetrated into interstitial tissues and the vascular compartment relies largely upon the processes of phagocytosis (see section 2.2.3) and of activation of the alternative complement pathway (see section 2.2.4). However, the functions of the innate system when exposed to microbial infection are also critical to the recruitment and activation of cells of the adaptive immune response (see later).

The main cells mediating phagocytosis are the mononuclear phagocytic cells and granulocyte cell populations; of the latter neutrophils are particularly important. For such cells to function, they must possess receptors to sense signals from their environment. In executing their effector functions they need to secrete a range of molecules that will recruit or activate other immune cells to a site of infection.

Before consideration of the process of phagocytosis, an overview of the mononuclear phagocytic cell and granulocyte cell populations will be given.

2.2.1 *Mononuclear phagocytic cells*

The mononuclear phagocytic cells include monocytes and macrophages. The monocyte comprises approximately 5% of the circulating blood leucocyte population and is a short-lived cell (circulating in blood ≤8 h), but which migrates into tissue to give rise to the tissue macrophage. The macrophage constitutes a long-lived, widely distributed heterogeneous population of cell types which bear different names within different tissues, such as the migrating Kupffer cell within the liver or the fixed mesangial cell within the kidney glomerulus.

The mononuclear phagocytic cells secrete a wide range of molecules too numerous to list in full here. However, these secretions include:

1 Molecules which can break down or permeabilize microbial membranes and thereby mediate extracellular killing of microorganisms, e.g. enzymes (lysozyme or cathepsin G), bactericidal reactive oxygen species and cationic proteins.

2 Cytokines which can provide innate protective antiviral (e.g. interferon-α or -β) and anti-tumour (e.g. tumour necrosis factor — TNF-α) activity against other host cells. A group of cytokines termed chemokines can also serve to chemoattract other leucocytes into an area of ongoing infection or inflammation, for example IL-8 which attracts neutrophils. Yet another group of cytokines has pro-inflammatory actions (e.g. IL-1 and TNF-α) which, among other outcomes, will lead to activation of endothelial and leucocyte cells promoting increased leucocyte extravasation into tissues and in the case of IL-1 activate T-lymphocyte populations.

3 Bioactive lipids (e.g. thromboxanes, prostaglandins and leukotrienes), which further promote the inflammatory response through actions to increase capillary vasodilation and permeability.

The mononuclear phagocytic cells also possess numerous receptors that interact with their environment. These cells possess, among others:

• Receptors for chemotaxis toward microorganisms, e.g. receptors for secreted bacterial peptides such as formylmethionyl peptide.

• Receptors for complement proteins that serve as leucocyte activators (e.g. C3a and C5a; see section 2.2.4) or complement proteins that serve to coat (to opsonize) microorganisms (e.g. C3b). An opsonized microbial surface more readily adheres to a phagocyte membrane, with the opsonin triggering enhanced activity of the phagocyte itself.

• Receptors for promoting adherence such as lectin receptors interacting with carbohydrate moieties on the surface of the microorganism, or receptors for Fc domains (non-antigen-recognition domains) of antibodies which opsonize microorganisms (e.g. the receptor for the Fc domain of IgG is Fcγ), or integrin receptors for cell–cell adhesion (e.g. promoting interaction between a macrophage and T lymphocyte).

121

• Receptors for cytokines including those involved in macrophage activation (e.g. interferon-γ — IFN-γ) or limiting macrophage mobility (e.g. macrophage inhibitory factor — MIF) and hence increasing cell retention at a site of infection.

2.2.2 Granulocyte cell populations

The granulocyte cell populations include the neutrophils, basophils and eosinophils. The short-lived (~2–3 days) neutrophil is the most abundant granulocyte (comprising >90% of all circulating blood granulocytes) and is the most important in terms of phagocytosis; indeed this is the main function of the neutrophil. The receptors and secretions of the neutrophil are similar to those of the macrophage, although notably the neutrophil does not present antigen via MHC class II proteins (see later). The neutrophil is recruited to sites of tissue infection or inflammation by a neutrophil-specific chemotactic factor (IL-8) and is also chemoattracted and activated by some of the same factors described for mononuclear phagocytic cells, including complement protein C3a, bacterial formylmethionyl peptides and leukotrienes. Like macrophages, neutrophils undergo a respiratory burst and are

very effective generators of reactive oxygen species.

Eosinophils are poor phagocytic cells and have a specialized role in the extracellular killing of parasites such as helminths, which cannot be physically phagocytosed. Basophils are non-phagocytic cells.

2.2.3 Phagocytosis

Macrophages and neutrophils in particular demonstrate a high capacity for the physical engulfment of particles such as microorganisms or microbial fragments from their immediate extracellular environment. This process (Fig. 8.2) comprises a number of steps.
• Chemotaxis of the phagocyte toward the microorganism through signals arising from the microorganism itself (e.g. formylmethionyl peptide), signals arising from complement proteins (e.g. C3a and C5a) generated as part of the activation of the alternative complement pathway (see below), or signals due to release of inflammatory factors (e.g. leukotrienes) secreted by other leucocyte cells situated at the site of an infection.
• Adherence of the microorganism to the surface of the phagocyte (step A in Fig. 8.2), involving:

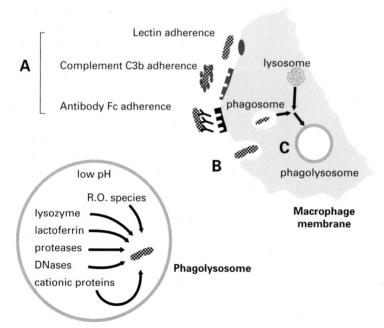

Fig. 8.2 Schematic of phagocytosis showing: (step A) adherence of the microorganism to the surface of the phagocyte; (step B) membrane activation of the phagocyte; (step C) enclosure of phagocytosed material within the phagosome and subsequently the phagolysosome. The mediators of the phagolysosome degradation of the microorganism are shown in the enlarged phagolysosome insert.

adhesion through lectin receptors present on the surface of the phagocyte which interact with carbohydrate moieties on the surface of the microorganism; adhesion through complement C3b receptors present on the surface of the phagocyte interacting with C3b molecules that have opsonized the surface of the microorganism; adhesion through Fc receptors which interact with the Fc domain of antibodies that have opsonized the surface of a microorganism.

• Membrane activation of the phagocyte actin–myosin contractile network to extend pseudopodia around the attached microorganism (step B in Fig. 8.2). Membrane activation will also lead to the generation of a 'respiratory burst' by the phagocyte which involves an increase in the activity of the phagocyte membrane NADPH oxidase which converts molecular oxygen into bactericidal reactive oxygen species such as superoxide anion ($\bullet O_2^-$), hydrogen peroxide (H_2O_2), and in particular hydroxyl radicals ($\bullet OH$) and halogenated oxygen metabolites ($HOCl^-$).

• The enclosure of phagocytosed material, initially within a membranous vesicle termed a phagosome. Here, cationic proteins such as defensins and reactive oxygen species begin microbial membrane degradation. This is followed within minutes by fusion of the phagosome with a lysosome to form a phagolysosome, whose contents are at an acidic pH of ~5 which is optimal for the continued active breakdown of microbial structural components (step C in Fig. 8.2).

2.2.4 Alternative complement pathway

The alternative complement pathway fulfils a critical role in innate immune defence. The complement system comprises at least 20 different serum proteins, many are known by the letter C and a number, e.g. C3. Many of the complement proteins are zymogens, i.e. pro-enzymes requiring proteolytic cleavage to be enzymatically active themselves; some are regulatory in function. The cleavage products of complement proteins are distinguished from their precursor by the suffix 'a' or 'b', e.g. C3a and C3b, with the suffix 'b' generally denoting the larger fragment that stays associated with a microbial membrane, and the suffix 'a' generally denoting the

smaller fragment that diffuses away. The activation of the complement pathway occurs in a cascade sequence with amplification occurring at each stage, such that each individual enzyme molecule activated at one stage generates multiple activated molecules at the next. In the 'resting' state, in the absence of infection, the complement proteins are inactive or have only a low level of spontaneous activation. The cascade is tightly regulated by both soluble and membrane-bound associated proteins. The regulation of the complement pathway prevents inappropriate activation of the cascade (i.e. when there is no infection present) and also minimizes damage to host cells during an appropriate complement response to a microbial infection. Complement activation is normally localized to the site(s) of infection.

There are three main biological functions of the alternative complement pathway.

• Opsonization of microbial membranes. This involves the covalent binding of complement proteins to the surface of microbial membranes. This opsonization or coating by complement proteins promotes adherence of the opsonized microbial component(s) to the cell membranes of phagocytic cells. The complement protein C3b is a potent opsonin.

• Activation of leucocytes. This involves complement proteins acting upon leucocytes, either at the site of infection or at some distance away, with the result of raising the level of functioning of the leucocytes in immune defence. For example, C3a is a potent leucocyte chemoattractant and also an activator of the respiratory burst.

• Lysis of the target cell membrane. This involves a collection of complement proteins associating upon the surface of a microbial membrane to form a membrane attack complex (MAC), which leads to the formation of membrane pores and, ultimately, microbial cell lysis.

Figure 8.3 shows a highly schematized view of the activation cascade for the alternative complement pathway upon a microbial membrane surface. The activation steps in the alternative pathway are also shown in Fig. 8.7, which contrasts with the activation steps in the classical complement pathway involving antibody.

The pivotal protein in the alternative pathway is

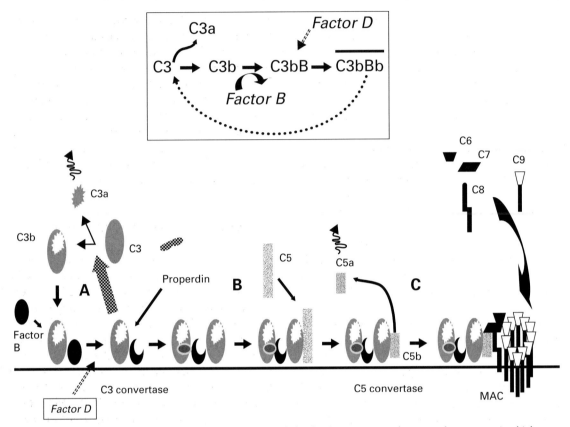

Fig. 8.3 A highly schematized overview of the activation cascade for the alternative complement pathway on a microbial membrane surface. In the presence of a microbial membrane the C3b formed by C3 tickover deposits on the microbial membrane (step A). C3a diffuses away leading to leucocyte activation. The deposited C3b leads to the generation of a stabilized C3 convertase (step B) which, through a positive feedback loop, leads to the amplified cleavage of more C3. Some C3b associates with the C3 convertase to generate a C5 convertase (step C) which will eventually lead to the generation of an MAC.

C3 (195 kDa). Under normal circumstances (in the absence of infection) C3 is cleaved very slowly through reaction with water or trace amounts of proteolytic enzyme to give C3b and C3a. The C3b formed is susceptible to nucleophilic attack by water and is rapidly inactivated to give iC3b. The C3a is not generated in sufficient amounts to lead to leucocyte activation and is rapidly inactivated. This normal low-level cleavage of the C3 molecule is termed 'C3 tickover' and it provides low levels of starting material, i.e. C3b, which will be required for full activation of the alternative complement pathway in the case of a microbial infection.

In the presence of a microbial membrane the C3b formed by C3 tickover will be susceptible to nucleophilic attack by hydroxyl or amine groups on the membrane surface, leading to the covalent attachment of C3b to the membrane (step A in Fig. 8.3). Once C3b has attached the membrane, factor B can bind to form a molecule termed C3bB. This complex is stabilized by a soluble protein called properdin. Factor D then enzymatically cleaves the bound factor B to generate a molecule termed C3bBb which is the C3 convertase of the alternative pathway (Fig. 8.3 inset).

This newly generated stable C3 convertase enzymatically cleaves C3 to generate further C3b and C3a molecules, leading to leucocyte activation (by

C3a) and greater deposition of C3b on the microbial membrane and hence further generation of C3 convertase molecules. In effect the microbial membrane has activated a positive feedback loop with cleavage of C3 to generate high amounts of C3b and C3a molecules.

The deposited C3b not only leads to the formation of the C3 convertase but also coats the microbial membrane as an opsonin and so promotes binding to phagocyte cell membranes. Some of the deposited C3b associates with the newly formed C3 convertase to generate a complex termed C3bBb3b, which is the C5 convertase of the alternative pathway (step B in Fig. 8.3). This C5 convertase binds the complement protein C5 and cleaves it into C5a (a leucocyte activator) and C5b (an opsonin). The C5b remains associated with the membrane and acts as a platform for the sequential binding of complement proteins C6, C7, C8 (step C in Fig. 8.3). The α-chain of the C8 molecule penetrates into the microbial membrane and mediates conformational changes in the incoming C9 molecules such that C9 becomes amphipathic (simultaneously containing hydrophilic and hydrophobic groups). In this form it is capable of insertion through the microbial membrane where it mediates a polymerization process that gives the MAC. The MAC generates transmembrane channels within the microbial membrane with the osmotic pressure of the cell leading to influx of water and eventual microbial cell lysis.

Differences between host cell membranes and microbial cell membranes mean that the cascade is only activated in the presence of microorganisms, so C3 tickover cannot give rise to full activation of the alternative pathway in the absence of microbial membrane. Stable deposition of a functional C3 convertase only occurs on the microbial cell surface. The differences that exist include, for example:

• lipopolysaccharide or peptidoglycan on microbial membranes that promote the binding of C3b;
• the high sialic acid content of host cell membranes that promotes the dissociation of any C3 convertase formed on host surfaces;
• the presence of specific host cell membrane proteins that also serve a key regulatory function.

Decay activating factor (DAF) or complement receptor type I (CR1) are host cell membrane proteins that serve to competitively block the binding of factor B with C3b and hence inhibit formation of a C3 convertase; they also promote disassembly of any C3 convertase formed. Membrane cofactor protein (MCP) and CR1 are further host cell membrane proteins that promote the displacement of factor B from its binding with C3b. Host cell membranes also possess a protein, CD59, which prevents the unfolding of C9 — a required step for membrane insertion to form an effective MAC.

3 The humoral adaptive immune system

The humoral immune response is mediated through antibody–antigen interactions. B lymphocytes in their naïve state, unstimulated by antigen, possess antibody molecules on their cell membrane, which serve a surveillance function to recognize any invading antigen. A B lymphocyte that has bound antigen is capable of differentiating into a plasma cell which, under the influence of signals from helper T cells, produces a fuller repertoire of antibody molecules (i.e. a fuller range of antibody classes), which are then secreted from the plasma cell into the extracellular environment to bring about a range of humoral effector functions.

3.1 B-lymphocyte antigens

As briefly discussed in section 1.2, a B-cell antigen is a substance or molecule specifically interacting with an antibody, and which may lead to the further production of antibody and an immunological response. Typically B-lymphocyte antigens are proteins within which the epitopes each comprise clusters of 5–20 amino acid residues in size. B-lymphocyte epitopes arise most commonly from the three-dimensional folding of proteins (i.e. conformational epitopes), although they may also comprise a sequential linear sequence of amino acids within the polypeptide chain (linear epitopes). As a general rule, there is a gradient of increasing immunogenicity with increasing molecular weight of protein. Further, the higher the structural complexity of the protein or polypeptide antigen then the higher the level of immunogenicity it is likely to exhibit. Thus, a polypeptide comprising a single amino acid such as polylysine may be expected to be a weaker immunogen than a protein of equivalent molecular weight but comprising a diverse range of amino acids.

Polysaccharides tend not to be good immunogens for B lymphocytes. When a polysaccharide serves as the sole immunogen, the humoral response obtained is termed 'T-cell-independent' because the polysaccharide does not elicit helper T-lymphocyte co-operation (see section 4). The consequences of a T-cell-independent humoral response include the lack of production of memory B-cell populations and the lack of synthesis by the plasma cell of the full range of antibody subclasses, i.e. T-cell-independent humoral responses mainly involve the production of IgM antibody. For improved immunogenicity carbohydrate antigens are conjugated to proteins which allow a more effective 'T-cell dependent' humoral response, i.e. one that affords the generation of memory B-cell populations and of the synthesis of the full range of antibody subclasses. This strategy is used in a number of current vaccine products, e.g. meningococcal group C conjugate vaccine comprises the capsular polysaccharide antigen of *Neisseria meningitidis* group C conjugated to *Corynebacterium diphtheriae* protein. Pure nucleic acid and lipid serve as very poor antigens.

3.2 Basic structure of antibody molecule

Figure 8.4 shows an antibody monomer comprising a four-polypeptide subunit structure, where the subunits are linked through disulphide bonding. The basic monomer structure can be considered the same for all the different classes of antibody (see below) even though some may form higher order structures, e.g. IgM is a pentamer comprising five antibody monomer units.

The subunits of the antibody monomer comprise two identical 'heavy' polypeptide chains and two identical 'light' polypeptide chains, with each of these containing a 'constant' region and a 'variable' region. The light chain variable regions (V_L) and the heavy chain variable regions (V_H) are the parts of the antibody molecule involved in antigen recognition. Specifically, antibodies produced by different B lymphocytes or plasma cells will have variable regions possessing different amino acid sequences leading to differences in antibody variable region surface conformation. At the extreme tips of the variable regions are hypervariable domains that serve the specific antigen recognition function discriminating between, for example, diphtheria toxin and tetanus toxin. The structural differences in the variable and hypervariable domains enable different antibodies to recognize different structural epitopes; this meets the needs of the immune system to combat a large and diverse range of antigens.

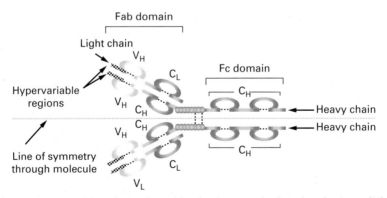

Fig. 8.4 An antibody monomer comprising a four-polypeptide subunit structure, where the subunits are linked through disulphide bonding. The Fab fragment is concerned with antigen recognition, while the Fc region determines the various effector functions of antibodies. A horizontal line of symmetry can be drawn through the antibody structure bisecting the molecule into a single heavy chain and a single light chain and clearly showing the bivalency in antigen recognition.

A horizontal line of symmetry can be drawn through the antibody structure in Fig 8.4, bisecting the molecule into two equivalent halves each containing a single heavy chain and a single light chain and clearly showing the antibody monomer to possess bivalency in its ability to interact with antigen, i.e. each antibody monomer can bind two epitopes, although the epitopes bound by a single antibody must be identical. The antigen recognition domain of an antibody monomer is termed the Fab domain. The structure of the constant region of the heavy chain (C_H) does not influence the antigen recognition function of the molecule but defines the different classes of antibody that are produced and hence the effector functions arising from antigen–antibody interaction; this heavy chain constant region is termed the Fc domain.

An analogy that may assist visualization of the function of an antibody molecule is one that views it as a hand (Fab domain) attached to the arm (Fc domain) (Fig. 8.4). The palm of the hand (variable region) can take up different shapes to allow the fingertips (hypervariable regions) to gain a very precise interaction with an object (antigen). At the wrist (hinge region) the hand is highly flexible relative to the arm (Fc domain) to allow the hand and fingertips (Fab domain) maximum flexibility to orientate an interaction with objects (antigen). The structure of the arm (Fc domain) does not influence interaction with an object (antigen). Once the object (antigen) has interacted with the fingertips (hypervariable regions) of the hand then the arm (Fc domain) can mediate a variety of effector functions.

A B lymphocyte and plasma cell can produce different classes of antibody depending on the stage of immune activation and on the intercellular signals that the B lymphocyte and plasma cell receive from other effector cells within the immune system. As stated above, the class of antibody is determined by the structure of the Fc domain and the different classes of antibodies possess different effector functions. The basic classes of antibodies are: IgM (heavy chain constant region defined as μ); IgA (heavy chain constant region defined as α); IgD (heavy chain constant region defined as δ); IgG (heavy chain constant region defined as γ) and IgE (heavy chain constant region defined as ε). The different classes of antibody can be remembered using the acronym MADGE. In addition to the heavy chain constant region classes, there are two light chain constant region classes, κ and λ; however, these do not mediate different antibody effector functions.

Each B lymphocyte and the plasma cell that derives from it is capable of producing all the different antibody classes. However, all the antibody classes produced by a single B lymphocyte and its derived plasma cell will recognize only a single epitope, i.e. recognize only a single specific set of chemical features within a sequence or pattern of amino acid residues. In other words, all antibodies produced by a single B lymphocyte, and its derived plasma cell, possess the same Fab domain recognizing the same antigenic determinant but clearly may possess different Fc domains capable of mediating different effector functions. Thus the same epitope can stimulate various different forms mediated via the IgM, IgA, IgD, IgG, IgE classes of humoral immune attack.

Within the antibody pool it is estimated that there are approximately 10^9 different epitope recognition specificities, sufficient to cover the range of pathogens likely to be encountered in life. This enormous diversity in antigen recognition is due to the amino acid sequence diversity in the variable and hypervariable domains of the antibody molecule. However, this large diversity cannot result from the presence of an equivalent number of separate protein coding genes; the human genome project has estimated there to be only approximately 30 000 protein coding genes. Rather, the clonal diversity in antigen recognition is due in the main to a process termed gene rearrangement, which occurs in each B lymphocyte during maturation in the bone marrow. For example, the DNA coding for a single heavy chain molecule will result from the splicing together of genes from four separate regions termed a <u>V</u>ariable region gene, a <u>D</u>iversity region gene, a <u>J</u>oining region gene and a <u>C</u>onstant region gene. There are approximately 100 V genes, 25 D genes and 50 J genes. Gene rearrangement will allow combinatorial freedom for any V, D and J genes to splice together providing a large number of VDJ combined gene product permutations and hence diversity in antigen recognition. Inaccurate splicing together of the regional genes at the V–D and D–J junctions further increases diversity, as does the process of random nucleotide insertion. The <u>C</u>onstant region genes will dictate the different classes of antibody and not the antigen recognition specificity. An additional process which occurs in a B-lymphocyte memory cell population while it resides within the lymphoid tissue is that of somatic mutation, in which only very slight changes in antibody Fab domains occur through single base mutations. Sometimes these mutations prove advantageous by increasing the affinity of an antibody to the same original epitope. Under these circumstances the antibody clone with the highest binding affinity to the original target epitope will proliferate and dominate. The light chain gene also comprises <u>V</u>, <u>J</u> and <u>C</u> regions and the V and J genes undergo a similar rearrangement to that described for the heavy chain, and hence further add to diversity. The heavy chain and light chain polypeptides are joined together via disulphide bond formation following protein synthesis of the individual heavy and light chains. In summary, all antibodies produced by a single B lymphocyte and its derived plasma cell are 'programmed' to recognize only a single antigen recognition feature determined by the recombination pattern of the <u>V</u>, <u>D</u> and <u>J</u> genes (heavy chain) and the <u>V</u> and <u>J</u> genes (light chain). The class of antibody is determined by further excisions within the DNA to allow the same VDJ gene combination to lie next to a different <u>C</u> gene, which codes for the structure of the antibody constant region and therefore determines antibody class. The five <u>C</u> gene classes are μ, α, δ, γ and ε, although various subclasses also exist. Antibody class switching is not a random process but one that is regulated by helper T-lymphocyte cytokine secretions.

3.3 Clonal selection and expansion

Within the body there may exist at any one time only a handful of naïve B lymphocytes capable of recognizing the same epitope. The meeting of an antigen and a naïve B lymphocyte capable of recognizing an epitope within the antigen occurs through the delivery of antigen to lymphoid tissues of the spleen, lymph nodes and local lymphoid tissue within mucosal surfaces (mucosal associated lymphoid tissue, MALT) and skin (SALT). This lymphoid tissue is rich in lymphocytes. Further, a proportion of B lymphocytes will always be recirculating from the lymphoid tissue through the lymph and blood circulations and so able to encounter circulating antigen.

Antigen will be specifically recognized by IgM molecules present on the surface of the naïve B lymphocyte. Following this antigen-driven selection of a specific B-lymphocyte clone, the clone will undergo repeated cell divisions. Some of the daughter cells will differentiate into short-lived (2–3 days) plasma cells able to secrete antibody of different classes to combat the initial primary antigen exposure. Other clonal daughter cells will become long-lived B-lymphocyte memory cells populating the lymphoid tissue and spreading around the body through the lymph and blood circulations. These cells will provide 'immunological memory' able to generate a more rapid and pronounced secondary response upon subsequent exposure to the original antigen (Fig. 8.5).

This process of clonal selection and expansion to form memory cell populations is the basis of vaccination. The initial introduction of antigen gives rise to a primary response (Fig. 8.6) in which there is a significant latent period before increased serum antibody levels are observed; the main antibody response is IgM production, although some IgG is

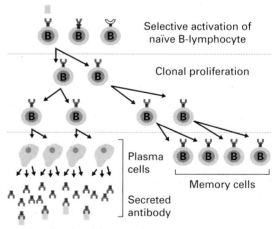

Fig. 8.5 Clonal proliferation of B lymphocytes. Following antigen-driven selection of a specific B-lymphocyte clone, it will undergo repeated cell divisions to give effector cell populations and memory cell populations.

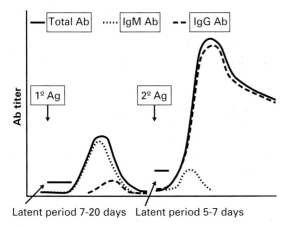

Fig. 8.6 Primary and secondary responses to antigen. A primary response of the humoral system involves a significant latent period before elevated serum antibody levels are seen; the major serum antibody generated is IgM. Memory cell populations provide the basis of the secondary response, which displays a significant reduction in the latency period to achieve elevated serum antibody. The antibody serum levels are greater than in the primary response and involve mainly IgG.

also synthesized and secreted. Upon re-exposure to the same antigen a secondary response is elicited. The features of the secondary response include: a reduced latent period between antigen challenge and increases in serum antibody (e.g. latent period of 5–7 days for the secondary response versus 7–20 days for the primary response); an antibody response dominated by IgG which is more pronounced with higher serum levels achieved. In the absence of helper T lymphocyte involvement (T-cell-independent humoral responses, e.g. where antigen is carbohydrate alone) B-lymphocyte memory cell populations are not produced, and antibody class switching is restricted. Hence, under these circumstances, the primary and secondary antibody responses to antigen challenge are essentially indistinguishable and exhibit a prolonged latent period, relatively low levels of serum antibody produced, and IgM as the main serum antibody.

3.4 Humoral immune effector functions

The humoral immune response is mediated by the initial antibody–antigen interaction, but with the different antibody classes offering a range of effector functions. The effector functions of antibodies include those described below.

3.4.1 Cognitive function on B-lymphocyte cell surface

Antibody on the surface of naïve or memory B lymphocytes serves to recognize and bind specific antigen; IgM serves this main cognitive function. It exists as a pentamer of five monomer units with an antigen valency of 10 and is extremely efficient at binding antigen. IgD appears to function mainly on the surface of B lymphocytes and may also contribute to cognition in some way.

3.4.2 Neutralization of antigen by secreted antibody

Secreted antibody, in particular IgG, IgA and IgM, can bind antigen and sterically hinder the interaction of toxins, viruses, bacteria, etc. with host cell surfaces. In the circulatory and interstitial fluids IgG (which exists as a monomer with an antigen valency of 2) is the main antibody that fulfils this role in the secondary response, while IgM is the main antibody produced in the primary response. IgA has specific roles in mucosal immunity.

3.4.3 Opsonization of antigen

Secreted antibody, in particular IgG, opsonizes antigenic material and in doing so promotes association (e.g. through Fcγ receptors) of the antigenic material with phagocyte membranes. Occupancy of the Fc receptor by the antibody also serves to activate a phagocyte's killing mechanisms.

3.4.4 Mucosal immunity

Mucosal immunity involves the interaction of antibody with antigen at mucosal surfaces such as those of the gastrointestinal tract, lung or urogenital tract. The major antibody of the mucosal lining fluid is IgA, which exists as a dimer of two monomer units (antigen valency of 4). IgA is actively secreted across mucosal epithelium into the lining fluid; it will neutralize antigen and may also serve as an op-sonin. IgA is also present in secretions such as tears, saliva, etc. but it has a limited role in systemic immunity.

3.4.5 Antibody-dependent cell cytotoxicity (ADCC)

Through specific binding to antigen upon the surface of membranes perceived as 'foreign', e.g. microbial cells or host cells virally infected or otherwise transformed, antibody can direct (through its Fc domains) the close association of 'killing' cells, such as neutrophils, eosinophils, NK cells and even cytotoxic T lymphocytes, with the 'foreign' membrane. This close association depends upon the antibody's Fc domain binding to the respective Fc receptor present on the surface membrane of the 'killing' cell. The release of cytotoxic molecules into the extracellular environment in close proximity to the 'foreign' cell enables the efficient and targeted release of cytotoxic molecules. IgG is the main antibody of systemic body fluids and is an important mediator of ADCC, although IgE and IgA may undertake this role in certain circumstances, e.g. against certain parasites IgE directs ADCC mediated by eosinophils.

3.4.6 Immediate hypersensitivity

Mast cells express high affinity receptors (Fcε) that bind the Fc domain of IgE antibodies. In the absence of antigen these receptors are occupied by the IgE monomer (antigen valency of 2) secreted previously from plasma cells. In this circumstance the IgE molecules are serving a cognitive function which, upon appropriate antigen binding, results in aggregation of the membrane-bound IgE and causes immediate mast cell degranulation and release of inflammatory mediators. Mast cells possess in their membranes IgE monomers able to recognize different antigenic epitopes. This contrasts with each single B lymphocyte, which possesses IgM antibody on its surface membrane that performs a cognitive function but is capable of recognizing only a single epitope specificity.

3.4.7 Neonatal immunity

The neonate lacks the ability to mount a full immunological response, accordingly maternal IgG is transported across the placenta late in pregnancy and is also absorbed across the gastrointestinal tract from breast milk. Maternal IgA secreted into breast milk will also provide mucosal protection for the neonate.

3.4.8 Activation of the classical complement pathway

A complement cascade similar to that of the alternative pathway can be activated through specific antibody–antigen interactions. The antibodies that activate the classical complement pathway are IgM and IgG.

Key steps in the activation of the classical pathway are shown in Fig. 8.7, where a contrast is also drawn to the alternative pathway. In the classical pathway the initiating step is the specific binding of IgG or IgM to antigen. Once this occurs, a complement protein termed C1 (which comprises a single C1q subunit, two C1r subunits and two C1s subunits) binds to adjacent Fc domains in the antibody–antigen complex. This binding of C1 activates the catalytic activity of the C1r subunits, and in turn the C1s subunits. The activated C1s subunits cleave C4 into C4b and C4a; the latter can diffuse away and serve as a leucocyte activator. The C4b covalently associates with the antibody –antigen complex on the surface of a microbial membrane and can serve as an opsonin. A further complement protein, C2, binds to this membrane complex to give C4b2. The C1s subunit then enzymically cleaves the bound C2a to generate on the membrane a new complex termed C4b2b, which is the C3 convertase of the classical pathway. (In some texts the C2a is referred to as the larger subunit remaining with the membrane while C2b is the smaller subunit that diffuses away.)

This C3 convertase molecule is distinct from that within the alternative pathway, but it is from this point onwards that parallels can be drawn between the two cascades.

The host proteins that serve key regulatory functions within the alternative pathway (DAF, CR1

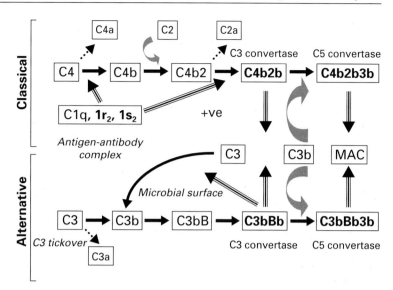

Fig. 8.7 The classical and alternative complement pathways.

factor I, CD59) also serve similar functions within the classical pathway. However, in contrast to the alternative pathway the activation step in the classical pathway requires specific antibody–antigen interactions. In this context the C1 protein can only become catalytically active when it is bound to at least two adjacent Fc domains. In the case of the IgG and IgM molecules the Fc domains will only align adjacent to each other when the corresponding Fab domains bind antigen. Further, when C1 is free in the circulation it is bound to a protein termed C1 inhibitor (C1-INH) which prevents any possible activation of C1 in the absence of antibody. Once C1 binds to adjacent Fc domains within an antibody–antigen complex C1-INH is displaced.

The functions of the classical complement pathway are similar to those described for the alternative pathway, i.e. opsonization, leucocyte activation and membrane lysis of target cells. The classical pathway can additionally lead to complement protein deposition upon insoluble antibody–antigen immune complexes circulating within blood, and in doing so promote the clearance of such potentially harmful complexes by Kupffer cells of the liver. The presence of two complement pathways provides for rapid (alternative) and specific (classical) activation of a key defence mechanism, and offers greater protection

against the development of microbial resistance mechanisms.

4 Cell-mediated adaptive immune system

Cell-mediated adaptive immune responses are mediated by T lymphocytes which arise from bone marrow progenitor cells and undergo maturation in the thymus before release into the systemic blood and lymph circulations (Fig. 8.1). There are a number of parallels that can be drawn between the B-lymphocyte-mediated immune response and the T-lymphocyte-mediated response. First, membrane-bound antibodies serve the cognitive function for B lymphocytes, while the cognitive function for T lymphocytes is served by T-cell receptors (TCR) present on the cell's plasma membrane surface. Second, in response to antigen T lymphocytes, like B lymphocytes, will undergo clonal proliferation and form a population clone of memory T cells specific for a single epitope. Third, each single B lymphocyte and plasma cell that derives from it is capable of producing antibodies that will only recognize a single epitope. In the same manner each single T cell is programmed to make T-cell receptors of only a single specificity able to recognize only a single specific set of chemical features within a T-cell epitope. This is achieved for the TCR in a similar manner to that for antibodies in that different gene segments termed V-D-J are brought together by the process of gene rearrangement into single RNA products. The recombined RNA will code for the polypeptide chains that make up the TCR. When all the possible recombinations are considered, the number of different TCR molecules that an individual can make is in excess of 10^9, a number similar to the primary antigen recognition repertoire of T cells.

There are two general classes of T lymphocytes: helper T lymphocytes and cytotoxic T lymphocytes. The latter function to kill host cells that have undergone a transformation such as a viral infection or cancer and they recognize specific antigens on the surface of host cells that have arisen as a result of such cell transformation. Through this specific antigen recognition, the cytotoxic T cell becomes closely apposed to the target host cell and is activated to synthesize and release cytotoxic secretory products (e.g. pore-forming molecules such as perforins) leading to lysis of the affected host cell. In contrast, the helper T cell can be viewed as the co-ordinator of the adaptive immune system, providing appropriate activation signals, in the form of secreted cytokines, to promote the functioning of both the cytotoxic T-cell populations and that of the antibody-producing B-lymphocyte and plasma cell populations. The actions of the helper T-cell populations also promote the function of the innate immune system, for example IFN-γ released by helper T cells increases the phagocytic activity of macrophages. The helper T cells are further divided into Th1 and Th2 subpopulations depending upon the nature of cytokines they secrete and, as a consequence, the arms of the immune system they predominantly influence. The Th1 helper T cells mainly regulate cell-mediated immunity through expression of cytokines such as IL-2, IL-12 and IFN-γ, which modulate cytotoxic T-cell and NK cell function. The Th2 helper T cells regulate humoral immunity through expression of cytokines such as IL-2, IL-4, IL-5, IL-6 and IL-10.

4.1 T-lymphocyte antigen recognition and MHC proteins

Epitopes for T lymphocytes comprise exclusively linear peptide sequences. T lymphocytes are unable to respond to carbohydrate, lipid or nucleic acid material and they only respond to peptide antigen when it is presented to the T lymphocyte by surface proteins on the plasma membrane of host cells. These surface proteins are termed major histocompatibility complex (MHC) proteins and can be subdivided into two main classes. MHC class I proteins are expressed on the surface of all nucleated host cell membranes and present peptide antigen to cytotoxic T lymphocytes. MHC class II proteins are expressed only on a more specialized group of cells termed antigen-presenting cells (APCs), and present peptide antigen to helper T lymphocytes.

Such a distinct cellular distribution of MHC proteins and restriction in presentation to discrete T-lymphocyte subpopulations may be remembered by considering the different T-lymphocyte functions. That is, all cells of the body have the potential to become infected with virus and undergo a cancerous change and hence all cells must have the capacity to be destroyed by the actions of cytotoxic T cells. As such, all cells of the body must possess MHC I molecules to afford antigen presentation to cytotoxic T cells. In contrast, as a co-ordinator cell of the immune system, the helper T cell must be able to respond to its environment in order to give appropriate signals or 'help' to other immune cells. Specialized APCs with the capacity to phagocytose interstitial proteinaceous material therefore undertake the function of 'environmental sampling'. MHC class II proteins expressed on the surface of APCs will present peptide antigen to helper T lymphocytes.

APCs include the macrophage tissue cell population, specialized APCs such as dendritic cells within the lymphatic system or Langerhans cells within the skin. B lymphocytes also serve the function of an APC because they interact with protein antigen through high affinity surface IgM molecules. Subsequently, they internalize the protein antigen for processing to generate peptides that will be presented by MHC II molecules expressed on the B-

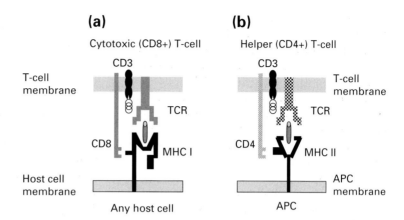

Fig. 8.8 The process of MHC presentation of peptide and interaction with T-lymphocyte receptor (TCR). Cytotoxic T lymphocytes (CD8+) interact with MHC I (a), while helper T lymphocytes (CD4+) interact with MHC II (b).

lymphocyte cell surface. Another cell type that can serve the function of an APC is the endothelial cell, which can be induced to express MHC II molecules by the action of the cytokine IFN-γ. It should not be overlooked that the APC can itself become infected with virus and undergo cancerous transformation, and therefore the APC, in addition to MHC II molecules, will also express the full complement of MHC I molecules on its surface.

This process of MHC presentation of peptide and interaction with T-lymphocyte receptor is shown in Fig. 8.8. A foreign peptide presented by a MHC molecule will be recognized by a TCR expressed on the surface of an appropriate T lymphocyte. Once a particular TCR recognizes a peptide sequence as foreign, intracellular signals to activate the T cell are sent via the CD3 complex present within the T-cell membrane. The recognition of peptide as foreign will lead to an immune response. Beyond antigen presentation, the interaction between MHC molecule and T lymphocyte also serves to identify that the T lymphocyte and host cell membrane arise from the same embryonic tissue. Tremendous inter-individual differences or more specifically polymorphisms exist in the MHC proteins within a population. The T lymphocyte undertakes this MHC surveillance through the possession of accessory molecules. Cytotoxic T lymphocytes possess CD8+ molecules which interact with MHC I (Fig. 8.8a), while helper T lymphocytes possess CD4+ molecules which interact with MHC II (Fig. 8.8b); hence the use of the terms

CD8+ lymphocytes to refer to cytotoxic T cells and CD4+ lymphocytes to refer to helper T cells.

4.2 Processing of proteins to allow peptide presentation by MHC molecules

Peptide epitope presented by MHC I is derived from the processing of proteins (e.g. a viral protein) synthesized within the actual cell that eventually will present the peptide to cytotoxic T lymphocytes. The MHC I molecule is composed of two polypeptide chains, an α-chain which has α1, α2 and α3 domains, and a second polypeptide termed β_2-microglobulin. The α1 and β2 domains form a peptide-binding cleft which can accommodate peptides up to 11 amino acids in length. Figure 8.9a shows the processing of a protein into peptide fragments for presentation by MHC I. The synthesized protein (indicated by an asterisk) is present in the cytoplasm of the cell and is degraded by a subcellular organelle termed a proteasome. The derived peptide fragments are actively transported, via a TAP peptide transporter, into the lumen of the endoplasmic reticulum (ER) where they fit within the binding clefts of MHC I molecules. From the ER the MHC I with bound peptide is transported to the trans-Golgi network (TGN), from which it is transported via endosomes to the plasma membrane where the MHC I molecule with bound peptide is accessible to surveillance by cytotoxic CD8+ T lymphocytes.

Peptide epitopes presented by MHC II are derived from proteins present within the extracellular

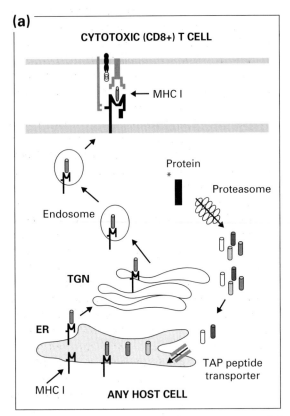

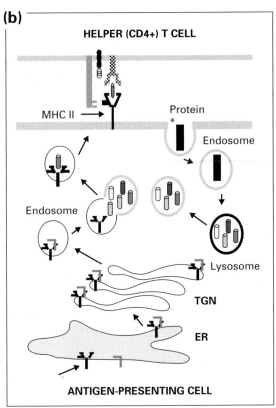

Fig. 8.9 Schematic of the processing of a protein into peptide fragments for presentation by MHC. (a) The synthesized protein (*) is present in the cytoplasm of the cell and is degraded into peptide by the proteasome. The derived peptide fragments are presented by MHC I to cytotoxic CD8+ T lymphocytes. (b) Protein (*) is endocytosed by an APC (antigen-presenting cell) and processed into peptide within lysosomes. The derived peptide fragments are presented by MHC II to helper CD4+ T lymphocytes.

fluid and are presented to helper T lymphocytes by APCs. The MHC II molecule is composed of two polypeptide chains, an α-chain which has α1 and α2 domains, and a β-chain which has β1 and β2 domains. The α1 and β1 domains form a peptide-binding cleft that can accommodate peptides up to 20 amino acids in length. Figure 8.9b shows the processing of a protein into peptide fragments for presentation by MHC II. In this case the protein (indicated by an asterisk) is internalized from the extracellular fluid by the APC and restricted to an endosomal compartment without access to the APC's cytoplasm. The endosome delivers the protein to a lysosome compartment which degrades the protein into peptide fragments, after which the peptide fragments are returned to an endosome compartment. In the lumen of the ER the MHC II molecule becomes associated with another protein termed an invariant chain which blocks access of peptides to the binding cleft of the MHC II molecule; The MHC II–invariant chain complex is transferred to the TGN and then to an endosomal compartment. At this point the endosomes that contain the processed peptide and the MHC II molecules merge, and the invariant chain disintegrates, allowing peptides access to the MHC II-binding cleft. The MHC II molecules with bound peptide are transported to the plasma membrane where they are accessible to surveillance by helper CD4+ T lymphocytes.

5 Some clinical perspectives

This section is intended to provide a brief overview of some clinical issues that exemplify the basic aspects of immune system functioning discussed previously.

5.1 Transplantation rejection

Transplantation is the process of transferring cells, tissues or organs — termed a graft — from one location to another. An autologous graft refers to a transplant between two sites within the same individual, e.g. skin graft from the thigh to the hand. An allogeneic graft refers to a transplant between two genetically different individuals of the same species, e.g. kidney transplant from a donor to a recipient individual. A xenogenic graft refers to a transplant across different species, e.g. pig to human.

The tempo of clinical rejection, in for example kidney transplantation, is often categorized by the following stages:

• Hyperacute rejection occurs within minutes to hours following revascularization of a graft. The cause is due to the presence of preformed circulating antibody (IgG) that reacts with the blood cell antigens (the ABO system), or MHC I molecules or other poorly defined antigens. This should now be a rare event clinically as recipients are tested (cross-matched) before transplantation for the presence of antibodies reactive with cells of the donor.

• Acute rejection occurs within weeks to months following transplantation and involves humoral (antibody) and cell-mediated induced cytotoxicity. Damage may be reversed with early diagnosis and more aggressive immunosuppressive therapy.

• Chronic rejection occurs many months to even years following transplantation. The pathology is characterized by fibrosis and may require differential diagnosis to distinguish between a chronic rejection event and the recurrence of the original disease that necessitated transplantation in the first place.

The major alloantigens (i.e. antigens responsible for rejection of allogeneic grafts) are the MHC proteins. Although there are two distinct classes of MHC protein (described in section 4.1) the MHC molecules actually comprise a number of subclasses which vary further in the general nature of peptides that they will accept within their binding clefts. The MHC I molecules are composed of three subclasses, MHC IA, MHC IB and MHC IC, on each nucleated cell of the body; all three subclasses are simultaneously expressed. The MHC II molecules are also composed of three subclasses, MHC II DR, MHC II DP and MHC II DQ, and again on each APC all three subclasses of MHC II molecule are simultaneously expressed. APCs, like other cells in the body, will also express MHC I molecules on their surface in addition to MHC II.

As indicated previously, the major cause of allogeneic tissue transplantation rejection is the polymorphic nature of the MHC phenotype between individuals. Polymorphism in MHC arises within the population because the genes for each of the MHC subclasses can exist in multiple different forms or alleles. For example, in humans there are at least 52 different forms of the MHC IB gene and at least 24 different forms of the MHC IA gene. It follows that individuals in a population can possess any one of the 52 different forms of MHC IB gene and any one of the 24 different forms of MHC 1A gene, so the number of different combinations for the six classes of MHC proteins is many millions. The situation is further complicated by the fact that each individual inherits and co-expresses a set of MHC I and II genes from each parent. This means that on each nucleated cell of the body there will be co-expressed paternally derived and maternally derived versions of the MHC IA, MHC IB and MHC IC molecules. The same principle will apply for co-expression upon APCs of paternal and maternal MHC II protein subclasses.

This tremendous polymorphism is important in immune defence because it allows the broadest possible scope of peptide antigen presentation, and thus the best chance of survival of a population as a whole, but it also confers the very high probability of MHC mismatch during allogeneic transplantation. As a result of the mode of MHC inheritance, the highest probability of a MHC tissue match between individuals that are not genetically identical twins will be that obtained between siblings, where there is a 1 in 4 chance of a sibling possessing an exact match for all the MHC I and MHC II subclasses. The MHC proteins are also termed human leucocyte antigens (HLA), and HLA tissue typing is undertaken routinely before transplantation to gain improved matches between donor and recipient. In kidney transplantation it has been found that matching the MHC IA, IB and IIDR genes in particular appears to improve short- and long-term graft survival.

The main target for the modern immunosuppressants such as cyclosporin and tacrolimus is inhibition of cytokine gene transcription in a highly selective manner in the helper T-lymphocyte populations. The consequence of this is to inhibit helper T-cell auto-activation and helper T-cell co-activation of cytotoxic T lymphocytes and of B lymphocytes, and thus considerably 'damp down' cell-mediated and humoral immune responses to the graft.

5.2 Hypersensitivity

Hypersensitivity can be defined as an exaggerated response of the immune system leading to host tissue damage. However, some of the immune responses described in the hypersensitivity classification below are, in some circumstances, appropriate responses to invading antigen. For example, a component in what is an appropriate immune response to tissue transplant rejection can be defined as a type II hypersensitivity reaction.

On the basis of the highly influential Gell and Coombs' classification scheme, there are four categories of hypersensitivity.

• *Type I — immediate hypersensitivity*. This is also called anaphylactic or acute hypersensitivity. It involves IgE antibody and is mediated via degranulation of mast cells leading to release of preformed factors which promote an influx of immune cells to the site of mast cell activation and initiation of a rapid inflammatory reaction. In the extreme case the inflammatory response extends beyond the localized site of initiation and affects systemic tissues leading to life-threatening anaphylactic reactions such as those documented to penicillin, to peanut antigen, or to bee sting antigen. Examples of localized type I hypersensitivity would include hay fever. The term 'allergy' has become synonymous with type I hypersensitivity.

• *Type II hypersensitivity — antibody-mediated*

cytotoxicity. This is caused by antibodies that are directed against cell surface antigens. IgG and IgM are the key antibodies involved that direct cytotoxic events against the cell surface with which they interact. The cytotoxic events would include activation of the classical complement pathway leading to the formation of a MAC, and the attraction and activation of killing cells such as NK cells or phagocytes which can bind to the antigen–antibody complex via receptors for antibody Fc domains or complement C3b. Type II hypersensitivity disorders include blood transfusion reactions arising from mismatch of the blood ABO antigens between donor and recipient, or haemolytic disease of the newborn. Autoimmune disorders such as myasthenia gravis, Goodpasture's syndrome and autoimmune haemolytic anaemias are initiated by autoantibodies reacting against 'self' tissue.

• *Type III hypersensitivity — complex-mediated*. This involves the formation of large antigen–antibody complexes that circulate in the blood, are usually coated by complement proteins and removed by phagocytosis. If this process is compromised for any reason then the antigen–antibody complexes will be deposited in tissue capillary beds, with kidney deposition being clinically the most important site. This deposition of high molecular weight antigen–antibody complexes in the glomerular capillaries of the kidney can lead to a condition termed glomerulonephritis which involves disruption of the glomerular basement membrane, destruction of glomeruli and ultimately renal failure which may necessitate organ transplantation. Systemic lupus erythematosus is a condition where autoantibodies are directed against the host's DNA and RNA with subsequent complement-coated immune complexes deposited throughout systemic tissues such as in the kidney, skin, joints and brain.

• *Type IV hypersensitivity — cell-mediated*. This results from inappropriate accumulation of macrophages at a localized site, and may or may not involve the presence of antigen. Under conditions of ongoing localized infection or inflammation, macrophages release proteases, which destroy infected or otherwise damaged tissue. However, with the inappropriate recruitment and/or activation of excessive numbers of macrophages, continuing damage to normal tissue may result, leading to chronic inflammation. The recruitment and activation of macrophages in type IV hypersensitivity is augmented by the activity of helper T lymphocytes (specifically the Th1 subpopulation). Examples of type IV hypersensitivity include granuloma formation and contact dermatitis. Granulomas are initiated and maintained by the recruitment of macrophages into the site of a persistent source of antigen or toxic material. A granuloma is a fibrotic core of tissue composed of tissue cells and macrophages surrounded by lymphocytes and then further surrounded by layers of calcified collagenous material. The disease sarcoidosis is a granulomatous disease of unknown cause but characterized by granuloma nodule formation in the lung and skin, among other sites.

6 Summary

The immune system is a complex body system whose various functions display a high level of inter-regulation. As such, any attempt to describe the functioning of the immune system within a single chapter will inevitably represent an oversimplification. However, the authors consider this chapter to be a comprehensive, but nevertheless basic, overview of the immune system that will serve as a sound foundation for further reading on the clinical immunological basis of disease or for the consultation of more specialized texts on immunological function.

The discussion in this chapter is structured by delineating the immune system into innate and adaptive responses. The innate system, responding immediately but non-specifically to antigen, is complimentary to the adaptive immune system which reacts in a highly specific manner to antigen but which displays a delay in its response. It should not be forgotten, however, that the functionings of the two systems are intimately related, showing dependency upon each other for the optimal maintenance of health.

7 Further reading

Abbas, A. K., Lichtman, A. H. & Pober, J. S. (2000) *Cellular and Molecular Immunology*. WB Saunders, Philadelphia and London. [Strong on experimental observations that form the basis for the science of immunology at the molecular, cellular, and whole-organism levels, and the resulting conclusions.]

Clancy, J. & Morgan, J. (2001) *Basic Concepts in Immunology: A Student's Survival Guide*. McGraw-Hill, New York and London. [Foundation text.]

Janeway, C., Travers, P., Capra, J. D. & Walport, M. J. (2001) *Immunobiology: The Immune System in Health and Disease*. Garland Press, New York. [Medical and basic immunology with emphasis on concepts.]

Parkin, J. & Cohen, B. (2001) An overview of the immune system. *Lancet*, **357**, 1777–1789.

Playfair, J. H. L. (2000) *Immunology at a Glance*. Blackwell Science, Oxford. [Pictorial based primer for immunological novices.]

Roitt, R. & Delves, P. J. (2001) *Roitt's Essential Immunology*, 10th edn. Blackwell Science, Oxford. [Classic introductory text.]

Roitt, I. & Rabson, A. (2000) *Really Essential Medical Immunology*. Blackwell Science, Oxford. [Contains essential immunological information for medical students and other health professionals.]

Chapter 9

Vaccination and immunization

Peter Gilbert and David Allison

1 Introduction

People rarely suffer from the same infectious disease twice. When such re-infections occur it is with an antigenically modified strain (common cold, influenza), the patient is immunocompromised (immunosuppressive drugs, immunological disorders) or a long time has elapsed since the first infection. Alternatively the patient may have failed to eliminate the primary infection that has then remained latent and emerges in a modified or similar form (herpes simplex, cold sores; herpes zoster, chickenpox). Immunity against re-infection was recognized long before the discovery of the causal agents of infectious disease.

Efforts were therefore made towards developing treatment strategies that might generate immunity to infection. An early development was the attempted control of smallpox (variola major) through the deliberate introduction, under the skin of healthy individuals, of material taken from active smallpox lesions. Such treatments produced single localized lesions and commonly, but not always, protected the recipient from contracting full-blown smallpox. The process became known as variolation and, unknown to its practitioners, attenuated the disease through changing the route of infection of the causal organism from respiratory transmission to cutaneous. Unfortunately, occasional cases of smallpox resulted from such treatment. Further developments recognized that immunity developed towards one disease often brings with it cross-immunity towards another related condition. Cowpox is a disease of cattle that can be transmitted to man. Symptoms are similar but less severe than those of smallpox. Material taken from active cowpox (vaccinia) lesions was therefore substituted into the variolation procedures. This conferred much of the protection against smallpox that had become associated with variolation but without the associated risks. This discovery, by Edward Jenner, made over two centuries ago, became known as

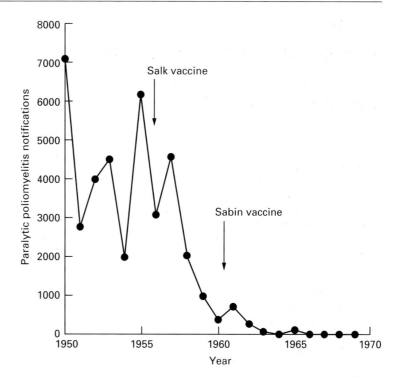

Fig. 9.1 Reported incidence of paralytic poliomyelitis in England and Wales during the 1950s and 1960s. After the introduction of vaccination programmes the incidence of this disease dropped from an endemic incidence of c. 5000 cases per year to fewer than 10.

vaccination and heralded a new era in disease control. The term vaccination is now widely used to describe prophylactic measures that use living microorganisms or their products to induce immunity. The more general term immunization describes procedures that induce immunity in the recipient but which do not necessarily involve the use of microorganisms. Nowadays vaccination and immunization procedures are used not only to protect the individual against infection but also to protect communities against epidemic disease. Such public health measures have met with spectacular success, as illustrated in Fig. 9.1 for the incidence of paralytic poliomyelitis. In those instances where there is no reservoir of the pathogen other than in infected individuals, and survival outside the host is limited (i.e. smallpox, poliomyelitis and measles) then such programmes, worldwide, have the potential to eradicate the disease permanently.

2 Spread of infection

Infectious diseases may either be spread from a common reservoir of the infectious agent that is distinct from the diseased individuals (common source) or they might transfer directly from a diseased individual to a healthy one (propagated source).

2.1 Common source infections

In common source infections, the reservoir of infection might be animate (e.g. insect vectors of malaria and yellow fever) or they might be inanimate (infected drinking water, cooling towers, contaminated food supply). In the simplest of cases the source of the infection is transient (i.e. food sourced to a single retail outlet, or to an isolated event such as a wedding reception). In such instances the onset of new cases is rapid, phased over 1–1.5 incubation periods, and the decline in new cases closely follows the elimination of the source (Fig. 9.2). This leads to an acute outbreak of infection limited socially and geographically to those linked with the source. Such an incident was epitomized by the outbreak of *Escherichia coli* O157 infections in Lanarkshire in the winter of 1996 that was linked to a single retail

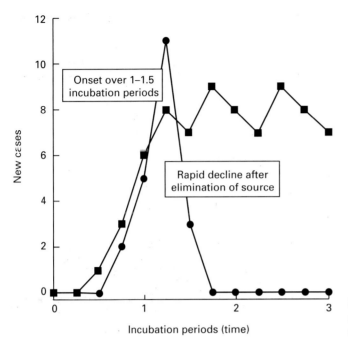

Fig. 9.2 Incidence pattern for common source outbreaks of infection where the source persists (■) and where it is short-lived (●).

outlet. If the source of the infection persists beyond the onset, then the incidence of new cases is maintained at a level that is commensurate with the infectivity of the pathogen and the frequency of exposure of individuals. In this manner, if cases of the variant Creutzfeldt–Jakob disease (vCJD), first recognized in the mid-1990s, relate to human exposure to bovine spongiform encephalopathy (BSE)-infected beef in the early 1980s, then the incidence of vCJD will increase over 1–1.5 incubation periods (i.e. 10–15 years) and be sustained for as long as such meat had remained on sale. In such a scenario vCJD related to a single common source outbreak, could persist for another 20–30 years.

For those infectious diseases that are transmitted to humans via insect vectors then onset and decline phases of epidemics are rarely observed other than as reflections of the seasonal variation in the prevalence of the insect. Rather, the disease is endemic within the population group and has a steady incidence of new cases. Diseases such as these are generally controlled by public health measures and environmental control of the vector with vaccination and immunization being deployed to protect individuals (e.g. yellow fever vaccination).

2.2 Propagated source infections

Propagated outbreaks of infection relate to the direct transmission of an infective agent from a diseased individual to a healthy, susceptible one. Mechanisms of such transmission were described in Chapter 7 and include inhalation of infective aerosols (measles, mumps, diphtheria), direct physical contact (syphilis, herpes virus) and, where sanitation standards are poor, through the introduction of infected faecal material into drinking water (cholera, typhoid) or onto food (*Salmonella, Campylobacter*). The ease of transmission, and hence the rate of onset of an epidemic (Fig. 9.3) relates not only to the susceptibility status and general state of health of the individuals concerned but also to the virulence properties of the organism, the route of transmission, the duration of the infective period associated with the disease, behavioural patterns, age of the population group and the population density (i.e. urban versus rural).

Each infective individual will be capable of transmitting the disease to the susceptible individuals that they encounter during their infective period. The number of persons to which a single infective

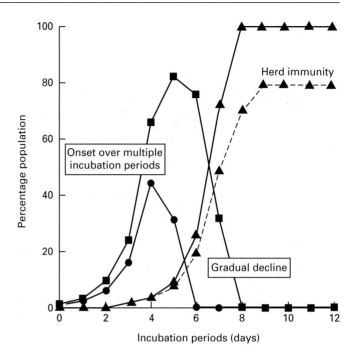

Fig. 9.3 Propagated outbreaks of infection showing the incidence of new cases (●), diseased individuals (■) and recovered immune (▲). The dotted line indicates the incidence pattern for an incompletely mixed population group.

individual might transmit the disease, and hence the rate of occurrence of the infection within the population, will depend upon the population density with respect to susceptible and infective individuals, the degree and nature of their social interaction, and the duration and timing of the infective period. Clearly if infectivity precedes the manifestation of disease, then spread of the infection will be greater than if these were concurrent. As each infected individual will, in turn, become a source of infection then this leads to a near exponential increase in the incidence of disease. Figure 9.3 shows the incidence of disease within a theoretical population group. This hypothetical group is perfectly mixed, and all individuals are susceptible to the infection. The model infection has an incubation period of 1 day and an infective period of 2 days commencing at the onset of symptoms with recovery occurring 1 day later. For the sake of this illustration it has been assumed that each infective individual will infect two others per day until all of the population group have contracted the disease (solid lines). In practice, however, the rate of transmission will decrease as the epidemic progresses, as the recovered individuals will become immune to further infection, reducing

the population density of susceptible individuals, and thereby the likelihood of onward transmission. Epidemics therefore often cease before all members of the community have been infected (Fig. 9.3, dotted line). If the proportion of immune individuals within a population group can be maintained above this threshold level then the likelihood of an epidemic arising from a single isolated infection incident is small (herd immunity). The threshold level itself is a function of the infectivity of the agent and the population density. Outbreaks of measles and chickenpox therefore tend to occur annually in the late summer among children attending school for the first time. This has the effect of concentrating all susceptible individuals in one, often confined, space and thereby reducing the proportion of immune subjects to below the threshold for propagated transmission.

An effective vaccination programme is therefore one that can maintain the proportion of individuals who are immune to a given infectious disease above the critical threshold level. Such a programme will not prevent isolated cases of infection but will prevent these from becoming epidemic.

3 Objectives of a vaccine/immunization programme

There is the potential to develop a protective vaccine/immunization programme for each and every infectious disease. Whether or not such vaccines are developed and deployed is related to the severity and economic impact of the disease upon the community as well as the effects upon the individual. Various factors governing the likelihood of an immunization programme being adopted are discussed below, while the principles of immunity, and of the production and quality control of immunological products are discussed in Chapters 8 and 23, respectively.

3.1 Severity of the disease

The severity of the disease, not only in terms of its morbidity and mortality and the probability of permanent injury to its survivors, but also in the likelihood of infection must be sufficient to warrant the development and routine deployment of a vaccine and its subsequent use. Thus, whilst influenza vaccines are constantly reviewed and stocks maintained, the control of influenza epidemics through vaccination is not recommended. Rather, those groups of individuals, such as the elderly, who are at special risk from the infection are protected.

Vaccines to be included within a national immunization and vaccination programme are chosen to reflect the infection risks within that country. Additional immunization, appropriate for persons travelling abroad, is intended not only to protect the at-risk individual, but also to prevent importing the disease into an unprotected home community.

3.2 Effectiveness of the vaccine/immunogen

Vaccination and immunization programmes seldom confer 100% protection against the target disease. More commonly the degree of protection is c. 60–95%. In such instances, while individuals receiving treatment will have a high probability of becoming immune, virtually all members of a community must be treated in order to reduce the actual proportion of susceptible individuals to below the threshold for epidemic spread of the dis-

ease. Anti-diphtheria and anti-tetanus prophylaxis, which utilize toxoids, are among the most efficient immunization programmes, whereas the performance of BCG is highly variable, and cholera vaccine (killed) gives little personal protection and is virtually useless in combating epidemics,

3.3 Safety

No medical or therapeutic procedure comes without some risk to the patient. All possible steps are taken to ensure safety, quality and efficacy of vaccines and immunological products (Chapter 23). The risks associated with immunization procedures must be constantly reviewed and balanced against the risks of, and associated with, contracting the disease. In this respect, smallpox vaccination in the UK was abandoned in the mid-1970s as the risks associated with vaccination then exceeded the predicted number of deaths that would follow importation of the disease. Shortly after this, in May 1980, the World Health Assembly pronounced the world to be free of smallpox. Similarly, the incidence of paralytic poliomyelitis in the USA and UK in the late 1990s was low with the majority of cases being related to vaccine use. As the worldwide elimination of poliomyelitis approaches, there is much debate as to the value of the live (Sabin) vaccine outside of an endemic area.

Public confidence in the safety of vaccines and immunization procedures is essential if compliance is to match the needs the community. In this respect public concern and anxiety, in the mid-1970s, over the perceived safety of pertussis vaccine led to a reduction in coverage of the target group from c. 80% to c. 30%. Major epidemics of whooping cough, with over 100 000 notified cases, followed in 1977–1979 and 1981–1983. By 1992, public confidence had returned, coverage had increased to 92% and there were only 4091 reported cases. Similarly, links have been claimed between the incidence of autism in children and the change in the UK from single measles and German measles vaccines to the combined MMR vaccine. Such claims are unfounded but have nevertheless decreased the uptake of the MMR vaccine and, thereby, increased the likelihood and magnitude of future measles epidemics.

3.4 Cost

Cheap effective vaccines are an essential component of the global battle against infectious disease. It was estimated that the 1996 costs of the USA childhood vaccination programme, directed against polio, diphtheria, pertussis, tetanus, measles and tuberculosis, was $1 for the vaccines and $14 for the programme costs. The newer vaccines, particularly those that have been genetically engineered, are considerably more expensive, putting the costs beyond the budgets of many developing countries.

3.5 Longevity of the immunity

The ideal of any vaccine is to provide lifelong protection of the individual against disease. Immunological memory (Chapter 8) depends on the survival of cloned populations of small B and T lymphocytes (memory cells). These small lymphocytes have a lifespan in the body of c. 15–20 years. Thus, if the immune system is not boosted, either by natural exposure to the organism or by re-immunization, then immunity gained in childhood will be attenuated or lost completely by the age of 30. Those vaccines that provide only poor protection against disease have proportionately reduced time-spans of effectiveness. Equally many of the immunization protocols are less effective, and have less duration, when administered to immunologically naïve individuals (neonates) rather than adults. Yellow fever vaccination, which is highly effective, must therefore be repeated at 10-year intervals, while typhoid vaccines are only effective for 1–3 years. Whether or not immunization in childhood is boosted at adolescence or in adult life depends on the relative risks associated with the infection as a function of age.

4 Classes of immunity

The theoretical background that underlies immunity to infection has been discussed in detail in Chapter 8. Immunity to infection may be passively acquired through the receipt of preformed, protective antibodies or it may be actively acquired through an immune response following deliberate or accidental exposure to microorganisms or their component parts. Active acquired immunity might involve either or both of the humoral and cell-mediated responses.

4.1 Passive acquired immunity

Humoral antibodies of the IgG class are able to cross the placenta from mother to fetus. These antibodies will provide passive protection of the newborn against those diseases which involve humoral immunity and to which the mother is immune. In this fashion, newborn infants in the UK have passive protection against tetanus, but not against tuberculosis. The latter requires cell-mediated immunity. Secreted antibodies are also passed to the gut of newborn together with the first deliveries of breast milk (colostrum). Such antibodies provide some passive protection against infections of the gastrointestinal tract.

Maternally acquired antibodies will react not only with antigen associated with a threatening infection but also with antigens introduced to the body as part of an immunization programme. Premature immunization, i.e. before degradation and elimination of the maternal antibodies, will therefore reduce the potency of an administered vaccine. This aspect of the timing of a course of vaccinations is discussed later.

Administration of preformed antibodies, taken from animals, from pooled human serum, or from human cell lines is often used to treat an existing infection (e.g. tetanus, diphtheria) or condition (venomous snake bite). Pooled human serum may also be administered prophylactically, within a slow-release vehicle, for those persons entering parts of the world where diseases such as hepatitis A are endemic. Such administrations confer no long-term immunity and will interfere with concurrent vaccination procedures.

4.2 Active acquired immunity

Active acquired immunity (Chapter 8) relates to exposure of the immune system to antigenic materials. Such exposure might be related to a naturally occurring or vaccine-associated infection, or it might be associated with the direct introduction of non-viable antigenic material into the body. The latter might occur through insect or animal bites and stings, inhalation, ingestion or deliberate injection. The route of exposure to antigen will influence the nature of the subsequent immune response. Thus, injection of antigen will lead primarily to humoral (IgG, IgM) production, while exposure of epithelial tissues (gut, respiratory tract) will lead not only to the production of secretory antibodies (IgA, IgE) but also, through the common immune response, to a stimulation of humoral antibody.

The magnitude and specificity of an immune response depends not only upon the duration of the exposure to antigen but also upon its time-concentration profile. During a naturally occurring infection the levels of antigen in the host are very small at onset and localized to the portal of entry to the host. As the amounts of antigen are small they will react only with a small, highly defined subgroup of small lymphocytes. These will undergo transformation to produce various antibody classes specific to the antigen and undergo a clonal expansion of their number. These immune responses and the progress of the infection will progress simultaneously. With time microorganisms will release greater amounts of antigenic materials that will, in turn, react with an increasing number of cloned lymphocytes, to produce yet more antibody. Eventually the antibody levels will be sufficient to bring about the elimination, from the host, of the infecting organism. Antibody levels will then decline with the net result of this encounter being the clonal expansion of particular small lymphocytes relating to a highly specific 'immunological memory' of the encounter.

This situation should be contrasted with the injection of a non-replicating immunogen. Often the amount of antigen introduced is large when compared with the levels present during the initial stages of an infection. In a non-immune animal the antigens will react not only with those lymphocytes that are capable of producing antibody of high specificity but also with those of a lower specificity. Antibody (high and low specificity) produced will react with and remove the residual antigen. The immune response will cease after this initial (primary) challenge. On a subsequent (secondary) challenge the antigen will react with residual preformed antibody relating to the first challenge together with a more specific subgroup of the original cloned lymphocytes. As the number of challenges is increased then the proportion of stimulated lymphocytes that are specific to the antigen becomes increased. After a sufficient number of consecutive challenges the magnitude and specificity of the immune response matches that which would occur during a natural infection with an organism bearing the antigen. This pattern of exposure brings with it certain problems. Firstly, as the introduced immunogen will react preferentially with preformed antibody rather than lymphocytes then sufficient time must elapse between exposures so as to allow the natural loss of antibody to occur. Secondly, immunity to infection will only be complete after the final challenge with immunogen. Thirdly, low specificity antibody produced during the early exposures to antigen might be capable of cross-reaction with host tissues to produce an adverse response to the vaccine.

5 Classes of vaccine

Vaccines may be considered as representing live microorganisms, killed microorganisms or purified bacterial and viral components (component vaccines). Recent innovations have included the introduction of DNA vaccines that encode for the transcription of antigen when introduced directly into host tissues or that might be delivered by virus vectors (i.e. adenovirus). Some aspects of these vaccine classes are discussed below.

5.1 Live vaccines

Vaccines may be live, infective microorganisms, attenuated with respect to their pathogenicity but retaining their ability to infect, or they might be genetically engineered such that one mildly infective organism has been modified so that it causes the expression of antigens from an unrelated pathogen.

Two major advantages stem from the use of live vaccines. Firstly, the immunization mimics the course of a natural infection such that only a single exposure is required to render an individual immune. Secondly, the exposure may be mediated through the natural route of infection (e.g. oral) thereby stimulating an immune response that is appropriate to a particular disease (e.g. secretory antibody as a primary defence against poliomyelitis virus in the gut).

Disadvantages associated with the use of live vaccines are also apparent. Live attenuated vaccines, administered through the natural route of infection, will be replicated in the patient and could be transmitted to others. If attenuation is lost during this replicative process then infections might result (see poliomyelitis, below). A second, major disadvantage, of live vaccines is that the course of their action, and possible side-effects, might be affected by the infection and immunological status of the patient.

5.2 Killed and component vaccines

As these vaccines are unable to evoke a natural infection profile with respect to the release of antigen then they must be administered on a number of occasions. Immunity is not complete until the course of immunization is complete and, with the exception of toxin-dominated diseases (diphtheria, tetanus) where the immunogen is a toxoid, will never match the performance of live vaccine delivery. Specificity of the immune response generated in the patient is initially low. This is particularly the case when the vaccine is composed of a relatively crude cocktail of killed cells where the immune response is directed only partly towards antigenic components of the cells that are associated with the infection process. This increases the possibility of adverse reactions in the patient. Release profiles of these immunogens can be improved through their formulation with adjuvants (Chapters 8 and 23), and the immunogenicity of certain purified bacterial components such as polysaccharides can be improved by their conjugation to a carrier.

5.3 DNA vaccines

A recent development, associated with research into gene therapy, has been the use of DNA encoding specific virulence factors of defined pathogens to evoke an immune response. The DNA is introduced directly into tissue cells by means of a transdermal gene-gun and is transcribed by the recipient cells. Accordingly the host responds to the antigenic material produced as though it were an infection. The course of release of the antigen reflects that of a natural infection and, therefore, a highly specific response is invoked. Eventually the introduced DNA is lost from the recipient cells and antigen release ceases. To date the approach has been used with some success in veterinary medicine but has not yet been employed for humans.

6 Routine immunization against infectious disease

6.1 Poliomyelitis vaccination

Poliovirus, a picornavirus, has three immunologically distinct types (I, II and III). The first phase of poliomyelitis infection is an acute infection of lymphoid tissues associated with the gastrointestinal tract (Peyer's patches), during which time the virus can be found in the throat and in faeces. The second phase is characterized by an invasion of the bloodstream, and in the third phase the virus migrates from the bloodstream into the meninges. Infections range in severity from clinically inapparent (>90%) to paralytic. Paralytic poliomyelitis is a major illness, but only occurs in 0.1–2% of infected individuals. It is characterized by the destruction of large nerve cells in the anterior horn of the brain resulting in varying degrees of paralysis. Unvaccinated adults are at greater risk from paralytic infection than children. The infection is transmitted by the faecal–oral route.

Polio is the only disease, at present, for which both live and killed vaccines compete. Since the introduction of the killed virus (Salk) in 1956 and the live attenuated virus (Sabin) in 1962 there has been a remarkable decline in the incidence of poliomyelitis (Fig. 9.1). The inactivated polio vaccine (IPV) contains formalin-killed poliovirus of all three serotypes. On injection, the vaccine stimulates the production of antibodies of the IgM and IgG class that neutralize the virus in the second stage of infection. A course of three injections at monthly intervals produces long-lasting immunity to all three poliovirus types.

The live, oral polio vaccine (OPV) is widely used

in many countries, including the UK and USA. Its main advantages over the IPV vaccine are its lower cost and easier administration. OPV contains attenuated poliovirus of each of the three types and is administered, as a liquid, onto the tongue. The vaccine strains infect the gastrointestinal mucosa and oropharynx, promoting the common immune response, and involving both humoral and secretory antibodies. IgA, secreted within the gut epithelium, provides local resistance to the first stages of poliomyelitis infection. OPV therefore provides protection at an earlier stage of the infection than does IPV. Infection of epithelial cells with one strain of enterovirus, however, often inhibits simultaneous infection by related strains. At least three administrations of OPV are therefore required, with each dosing conferring immunity to one of the vaccine serotypes. These doses must be separated by a period of at least 1 month in order to allow the previous infection to lapse. Booster vaccinations are also provided to cover the eventuality that some other enterovirus infection, present at the time of vaccination, had reduced the response to the vaccine strains.

Faecal excretion of vaccine virus will occur and may last for up to 6 weeks post-treatment. Such released virus will spread to close contacts and infect/(re-)immunize them. Vaccine-associated poliomyelitis may occur through reversion of the attenuated strains to the virulent wild-type, particularly with types II and III and is estimated to occur once per 4 million doses. As the wild-type virus can be isolated in faeces, infection may occur in unimmunized contacts as well as vaccine recipients. Since the introduction of OPV, notifications of paralytic poliomyelitis in the UK have dropped spectacularly. However, from 1985 to 1995, 19 of the 28 notified cases of paralytic poliomyelitis were associated with revertant vaccine strains (14 recipients, 5 contacts). As the risk of natural infections with poliomyelitis within developed countries has now diminished markedly, the greater risk resides with the live vaccine strains. Proposals are therefore now being considered that in the developed world OPV should be replaced with IPV.

6.2 Measles, mumps and rubella vaccination (MMR)

Measles, mumps and rubella (German measles) are infectious diseases, with respiratory routes of transmission and infection, caused by members of the paramyxovirus group. Each virus is immunologically distinct and has only one serotype. Whilst the primary multiplication sites of these viruses are within the respiratory tract, the diseases are associated with viral multiplication elsewhere in the host.

6.2.1 Measles

Measles is a severe, highly contagious, acute infection that frequently occurs in epidemic form. After multiplication within the respiratory tract the virus is transported throughout the body, particularly to the skin where a characteristic maculopapular rash develops. Complications of the disease can occur, particularly in malnourished children, the most serious being measles encephalitis that can cause permanent neurological injury and death.

A live vaccine strain of measles was introduced in the USA in 1962 and to the UK in 1968. A single injection produces high-level immunity in over 95% of recipients. Moreover, as the vaccine induces immunity more rapidly than the natural infection, it may be used to control the impact of measles outbreaks. The measles virus cannot survive outside of an infected host. Widespread use of the vaccine therefore has the potential, as with smallpox, of eliminating the disease worldwide. Mass immunization has reduced the incidence of measles to almost nil, although a 15-fold increase in the incidence was noted in the USA between 1989 and 1991 because of poor compliance with the vaccine.

6.2.2 Mumps

Mumps virus infects the parotid glands to cause swelling and a general viraemia. Complications include pancreatitis, meningitis and orchitis, the latter occasionally leading to male sterility. Infections can also cause permanent unilateral deafness at any age. In the absence of vaccination, infection occurs in >90% of individuals by age 15 years. A live attenuated mumps vaccine has been available since 1967 and has been part of the juvenile vaccination programme in the UK since 1988 when it was included as part of the MMR triple vaccine (see below).

6.2.3 *Rubella*

Rubella is a mild, often subclinical infection that is common among children aged between 4 and 9 years. Infection during the first trimester of pregnancy brings with it a major risk of abortion or congenital deformity in the fetus (congenital rubella syndrome, CRS).

Rubella immunization was introduced to the UK in 1970 for prepubertal girls and non-immune women intending to start families. The vaccine utilizes a live, cold-adapted Wistar RA2713 vaccine strain of the virus. The major disadvantage of the vaccine is that, as with the wild-type, the fetus can be infected. While there have been no reports of CRS associated with use of the vaccine, the possible risk makes it imperative that women do not become pregnant within 1 month of vaccination. Prepubertal girls were immunized to extend the period of immunity through the child-bearing years. Until 1988 boys were not routinely protected against rubella. Their susceptibility to the virus was thought to maintain the natural prevalence of the disease in the community and thereby reinforce the vaccine-induced immunity in vaccinated, adult females. This proved to be not the case. Rather cases of CRS could be related to incidence of the disease in younger children within the family. Rubella vaccine is now given to both sexes at the age of 12–15 months as part of the MMR programme (below).

6.2.4 *MMR vaccine*

MMR vaccine was introduced to the UK in 1988 for young children of both sexes, replacing single antigen measles vaccine. It consists of a single dose of a lyophilized preparation of live attenuated strains of the measles, mumps and rubella viruses. MMR had previously been deployed in the USA and Scandinavia for a significant number of years without any indication of increased adverse reaction or of decreased sero-conversion over separate administration of the component parts. Immunization results in sero-conversion to all three viruses in >95% of re-cipients. For maximum effect MMR vaccine is recommended for children of both sexes aged 12–15 months but can also be given to non-immune adults. From October 1996 a second dose of MMR was recommended for children aged 4 years in order to prevent the re-accumulation of sufficient susceptible children to sustain future epidemics. Single antigen rubella vaccine continues to be given to girls aged 10–14 years, if they have not previously received MMR vaccine.

In recent years several research papers have attributed an increase in autism to the introduction of the triple vaccine. This has led to a decreased public confidence in the vaccine. Detailed examination of the literature, and also the results of several clinical studies, have now indicated that there is no association between use of the triple vaccine and autism. This is backed up by over 20 years of successful deployment of the vaccine outside of the UK. Currently much effort is being made to restore confidence in the vaccine in order to avoid the lack of compliance leading to the occurrence of measles epidemics.

6.3 Tuberculosis

Tuberculosis (TB) is a major cause of death and morbidity worldwide, particularly where poverty, malnutrition and poor housing prevail. Human infection is acquired by inhalation of *Mycobacterium tuberculosis* and *M. bovis*. Tuberculosis is primarily a disease of the lungs, causing chronic infection of the lower respiratory tract, but may spread to other sites or proceed to a generalized infection (miliary tuberculosis). Active disease can result either from a primary infection or from a subsequent reactivation of a quiescent infection. Following inhalation, the mycobacteria are taken up by alveolar macrophages where they survive and multiply. Circulating macrophages and lymphocytes, attracted to the site, carry the organism to local lymph nodes where a cell-mediated immune response is triggered. The host, unable to eliminate the pathogen, contains them within small granulomas or tubercles. If high numbers of mycobacteria are present then the cellular responses can result in tissue necrosis. The tubercles contain viable pathogens that may persist for the remaining life of the host. Reactivation of the healed primary lesions is thought to account for over two-thirds of all newly reported cases of the disease.

The incidence of TB in the UK declined 10-fold between 1948 and 1987, since when just over 5000 new cases have been notified each year. Those most at risk include pubescent children, health service staff and individuals intending to stay for more than 1 month in countries where TB is endemic.

A live vaccine is required to elicit protection against TB, as both antibody and cell-mediated immunity are required for protective immunity. Vaccination with BCG (bacille Calmette-Guérin), derived from an attenuated *M. bovis* strain, is commonly used in countries where TB is endemic. The vaccine was introduced in the UK in 1953 and was administered intradermally to children aged 13–14 years and to unprotected adults. Efficacy in the UK has been shown to be > 70% with protection lasting at least 15 years. In other countries, where the general state of health and well-being of the population is less than in the developed world, the efficacy of the vaccine has been shown to be significantly less than this.

Because of the risks of adverse reaction to the vaccine by persons who have already been exposed to the disease a sensitivity test must be carried out before immunization with BCG. A Mantoux skin test assesses an individual's sensitivity to a purified protein derivative (PPD) prepared from heat-treated antigens (tuberculin) extracted from *M. tuberculosis*. A positive test implies past infection or past, successful immunization. Those with strongly positive tests may have active disease and should be referred to a chest clinic. However, many people with active TB, especially disseminated TB, sero-convert from a positive to a negative skin test. Results of the skin test must therefore be interpreted with care.

Much debate surrounds the use of BCG vaccine, a matter of some importance, considering that TB kills c. 3 million people annually and that drug-resistant strains have emerged. While the vaccine has demonstrated some efficacy in preventing juvenile TB, it has little prophylactic effect against post-primary TB in those already infected. One solution is to bring forward the BCG immunization to include neonates. Immunization at 2–4 weeks of age will ensure that immunization precedes infection,

and also negates the requirement for a skin test. Passive acquired maternal antibody to TB is unlikely to interfere with the effectiveness of the immunization as immunity relates to a cell-mediated response. Alternative strategies involve improvement of the vaccine possibly through the introduction, into the BCG strain, of genes that encode protective antigens of *M. tuberculosis*.

6.4 Diphtheria, tetanus and pertussis (DTP) immunization

Immunization against these unrelated diseases is considered together because the vaccines are non-living and are often co-administered as a triple vaccine as part of the juvenile vaccination programme.

6.4.1 Diphtheria

This is an acute, non-invasive infectious disease associated with the upper respiratory tract (Chapter 7). The incubation period is from 2 to 5 days although the disease remains communicable for up to 4 weeks. A low molecular weight toxin is produced which affects myocardium, nervous and adrenal tissues. Death results in 3–5% of infected children. Diphtheria immunization protects by stimulating the production of an antitoxin. This antitoxin will protect against the disease but not against infection of the respiratory tract. The immunogen is a toxoid, prepared by formaldehyde treatment of the purified toxin (Chapter 23) and administered while adsorbed to an adjuvant, usually aluminium phosphate or aluminium hydroxide. The primary course of diphtheria prophylaxis consists of three doses starting at 2 months of age and separated by an interval of at least 1 month. The immune status of adults may be determined by administration of Schick test toxin, which is essentially a diluted form of the vaccine.

6.4.2 Tetanus

Tetanus is not an infectious disease but relates to the production of a toxin by germinating spores and vegetative cells of *Clostridium tetani* that might infect a deep puncture wound. The organism, which may be introduced into the wound from the soil, grows anaerobically at such sites. The toxin is adsorbed into nerve cells and acts like strychnine on nerve synapses (Chapter 7). Tetanus immunization employs a toxoid and protects by stimulating the production of antitoxin. This antitoxin will neutralize the toxin as the organisms release it and before it can be adsorbed into nerves. As the toxin is produced only slowly after infection then the vaccine, which acts rapidly, may be used prophylactically in those non-immunized persons who have recently suffered a candidate injury. The toxoid, as with diphtheria toxoid, is formed by reaction with formaldehyde and is adsorbed onto an inorganic adjuvant. The primary course of tetanus prophylaxis consists of three doses starting at 2 months of age and is separated by an interval of at least 1 month.

6.4.3 Pertussis (whooping cough)

Caused by the non-invasive respiratory pathogen *Bordetella pertussis*, whooping cough (Chapter 7) may be complicated by bronchopneumonia, repeated post-tussis vomiting leading to weight loss, and to cerebral hypoxia associated with a risk of brain damage. Until the mid-1970s the mortality from whooping cough was about one per 1000 notified cases with a higher rate for infants under 1 year of age. A full course of vaccine, which consists of a suspension of killed *Bord. pertussis* organisms (Chapter 23), gives complete protection in > 80% of recipients. The primary course of pertussis prophylaxis consists of three doses starting at 2 months of age and separated by an interval of at least 1 month.

6.4.4 DTP vaccine combinations and administration

The primary course of DTP protection consists of three doses of a combined vaccine, each dose separated by at least 1 month and commencing not earlier than 2 months of age. In such combinations the pertussis component of the vaccine acts as an additional adjuvant for the toxoid elements. Monovalent pertussis and tetanus vaccines, and combined vaccines lacking the pertussis component (DT) are available. If pertussis vaccination is contraindicated or refused then DT vaccine alone should be offered. The primary course of pertussis vaccination is considered sufficient to confer lifelong protection, especially as the mortality associated with disease declines markedly after infancy. The risks associated with tetanus and diphtheria infection persist throughout life. DT vaccination is therefore repeated before school entry, at 4–5 years of age, and once again at puberty.

6.5 *Haemophilus influenzae* type b (Hib) immunization

Seven different capsular serotypes of *Haemophilus influenzae* type b (Hib) are associated with respiratory infection in young children. The most common presentation of these infections is as meningitis, frequently associated with bacteraemia. The sequelae, following Hib infection, include deafness, convulsions and intellectual impairment. The fatality rate is c. 4–5% with 8–11% of survivors having permanent neurological disorders. The disease, which is rare in children under 3 months, peaks both in its incidence and severity at 12 months of age. Infection is uncommon after 4 years of age. Before the introduction of Hib vaccination the incidence of the disease in the UK was estimated at 34 per 100 000. The vaccine utilizes purified preparations of the polysaccharide capsule of the major serotypes. Polysaccharides are poorly immunogenic and must be conjugated onto a protein carrier to enhance their efficacy. Hib vaccines are variously conjugated onto diphtheria and tetanus toxoids (above), group B meningococcal outer-membrane protein and a nontoxic derivative of diphtheria toxin (CRM197) and can now be mixed and co-administered with the DTP vaccine. Three doses of the vaccine are recommended, separated by 1 month. No reinforcement is recommended at 4 years of age as the risks from infection are negligible at this time. To avoid possible interactions, Hib vaccine was required, at its introduction, to be administered at a different body site to DTP. Sufficient evidence has now been gathered as to render this recommendation unnecessary.

6.6 Meningococcal immunization

Meningococcal meningitis and septicaemia are systemic infections caused by strains of *Neisseria meningitidis*. There are at least 13 serotypes of which groups B and C are most common. In the UK type B accounts for approximately two-thirds of reported cases with type C accounting for the remaining third. Type C meningitis is not usually found in this country but is epidemic, particularly in the summer months, in other parts of the world. The most recent increases in meningococcal disease have been associated with group C infections in young adolescents. Group C meningitis is most common in the under 1-year-old group but its mortality is greatest in adolescents. Overall mortality from meningococcal disease is around 10%. The commonest manifestation is meningitis but in around 15–20% of cases septicaemia predominates. Mortality rates are much greater in septicaemic cases. At present there is no available vaccine for group B meningococcus but vaccines are available for groups A and C. As with the Hib vaccine the preparations are intended to invoke an immune responsiveness towards the polysaccharide component of the pathogens. Early vaccines were of a purified polysaccharide worked in adults and were of little efficacy in the most at-risk group of infants. The new MenC conjugate vaccine uses a similar technology to Hib and conjugates the polysaccharide components to a carrier protein (usually diphtheria toxin or tetanus toxoid). The resultant vaccine is effective in the very young and is suitable for infants. The vaccine is administered along with DTP and Hib at 2, 3 and 4 months. A single dose is sufficient to immunize individuals over 12 months of age and has been used to provide cover for teenagers, adolescents and young adults.

Group C vaccine is available for those travelling to areas of the world where the infections are epidemic (e.g. Kenya).

7 Juvenile immunization schedule

The timing of the various components of the juvenile vaccination programme is subject to continual review. In the 1960s, the primary course of DTP vaccination consisted of three doses given at 3, 6 and 12 months of age, together with OPV. This separation gave adequate time for the levels of induced

Table 9.1 Children's immunization schedule for UK (1996)

Vaccine	Age	Notes
BCG	Neonatal (1st month)	If not, at 13–14 years
DTP, Hib, MenC Poliomyelitis	1st dose 2 months 2nd dose 3 months 3rd dose 4 months	Primary course
MMR	12–15 months	Any time over 12 months
Booster DT	3–5 years	3 years after primary course
Poliomyelitis	3–5 years	
MMR booster	3–5 years	
BCG	10–14 years	If not in infancy
Booster DT	13–18 years	

antibody to decline between successive doses of the vaccines. Current recommendations (Table 9.1) accelerate the vaccination programme with no reductions in its efficacy. Thus, MMR vaccination has replaced separate measles and rubella prophylaxis and BCG vaccination may now be given at birth. DTP vaccination occurs at 2, 3 and 4 months to coincide with administration of Hib and MenC. It is imperative that as many individuals as possible benefit from the vaccination programme. Fewer visits to the doctor's surgery translate into improved patient compliance and less likelihood of epidemic spread of the diseases in question. The current recommendations minimize the number of separate visits to the clinic while maximizing the protection generated.

8 Immunization of special risk groups

While not recommended for routine administration, vaccines additional to those represented in the juvenile programme are available for individuals in special risk categories. These categories relate to occupational risks or risks associated with travel abroad. Such immunization protocols include those directed against cholera, typhoid, meningitis (type A), anthrax, hepatitis A and B, influenza, Japanese encephalitis, rabies, tick-borne encephalitis and yellow fever.

9 Further reading

Mims, C. A., Nash, A. & Stephen, J. (2001) *Mims' Pathogenesis of Infectious Disease*, 5th edn. Academic Press, London.

Salisbury, D. M. & Begg, N. T. (1996) *Immunisation Against Infectious Disease.* HMSO, London (updated every 4–5 years).

Salyers, A. A. & Whitt, D. D. (1994) *Bacterial Pathogenesis: A Molecular Approach.* American Society for Microbiology Press, Washington.

Chapter 10
Types of antibiotics and synthetic antimicrobial agents

A Denver Russell

1 Antibiotics

1.1 Definition

An antibiotic was originally defined as a substance, produced by one microorganism, which inhibited the growth of other microorganisms. The advent of synthetic methods has, however, resulted in a modification of this definition and an antibiotic now refers to a substance produced by a microorganism, or to a similar substance (produced wholly or partly by chemical synthesis), which in low concentrations inhibits the growth of other microorganisms. Chloramphenicol was an early example.

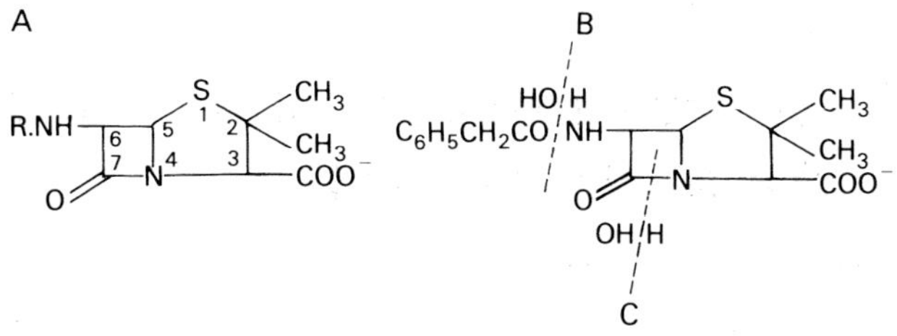

Fig. 10.1 A, General structure of penicillins; B, removal of side chain from benzylpenicillin; C, site of action of β-lactamases.

Antimicrobial agents such as sulphonamides (section 13.1) and the 4-quinolones (section 13.7), produced solely by synthetic means, are often referred to as antibiotics.

1.2 Sources

There are three major sources from which antibiotics are obtained.

1 Microorganisms. For example, bacitracin and polymyxin are obtained from some *Bacillus* species; streptomycin, tetracyclines, etc. from *Streptomyces* species; gentamicin from *Micromonospora purpurea*; griseofulvin and some penicillins and cephalosporins from certain genera (*Penicillium, Acremonium*) of the family Aspergillaceae; and monobactams from *Pseudomonas acidophila* and *Gluconobacter* species. Most antibiotics in current use have been produced from *Streptomyces* spp.

2 Synthesis. Chloramphenicol is now usually produced by a synthetic process.

3 Semisynthesis. This means that part of the molecule is produced by a fermentation process using the appropriate microorganism and the product is then further modified by a chemical process. Many penicillins and cephalosporins (section 2) are produced in this way.

In addition, it has been suggested that (a) some bacteriophages (Chapter 5) might have an important role to play in the chemotherapy of bacterial infections, and (b) plant products might prove to be a potentially fruitful source of new antimicrobial agents.

2 β-Lactam antibiotics

There are several different types of β-lactam anti-biotics that are valuable, or potentially important, antibacterial compounds. These will be considered briefly.

2.1 Penicillins and mecillinams

The penicillins (general structure, Fig. 10.1A) may be considered as being of the following types.

1 Naturally occurring. For example, those produced by fermentation of moulds such as *Penicillium notatum* and *P. chrysogenum*. The most important examples are benzylpenicillin (penicillin G) and phenoxymethylpenicillin (penicillin V).

2 Semisynthetic. In 1959, scientists at Beecham Research Laboratories succeeded in isolating the penicillin 'nucleus', 6-aminopenicillanic acid (6-APA; Fig. 10.1A: R represents H). During the commercial production of benzylpenicillin, phenylacetic (phenylethanoic) acid ($C_6H_5.CH_2.COOH$) is added to the medium in which the *Penicillium* mould is growing (see Chapter 22). This substance is a precursor of the side-chain (R; see Fig. 10.2) in benzylpenicillin. Growth of the organism in the absence of phenylacetic acid led to the isolation of 6-APA; this has a different R_F value from benzylpenicillin, which allowed it to be detected chromatographically.

A second method of producing 6-APA came with the discovery that certain microorganisms produce enzymes, penicillin amidases (acylases), which catalyse the removal of the side-chain from benzylpenicillin (Fig. 10.1B).

Acylation of 6-APA with appropriate substances results in new penicillins being produced that differ only in the nature of the side-chain (Table 10.1; Fig. 10.2). Some of these penicillins have considerable activity against Gram-negative as well as Gram-positive bacteria, and are thus broad-spectrum

Drug	R	Drug	R	Drug	R

1 — $C_6H_5CH_2CO-$

2 — $C_6H_5OCH_2CO-$

3 — (structure with OCH₃, CO, OCH₃)

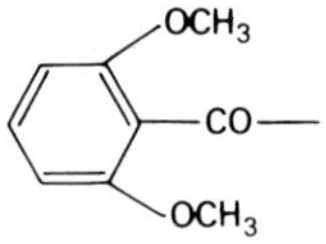

4 — (phenyl isoxazole with CH₃)

5 — (2-Cl phenyl isoxazole with CH₃)

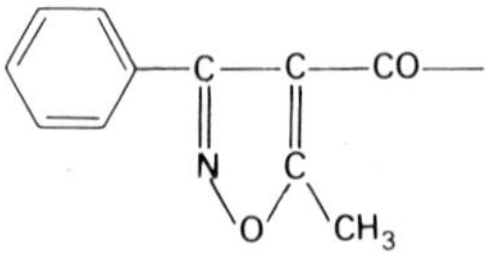

6 — (Cl, F phenyl isoxazole with CH₃)

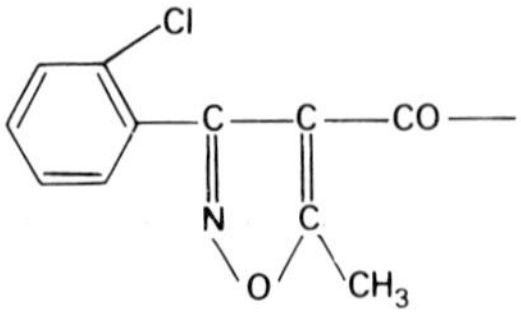

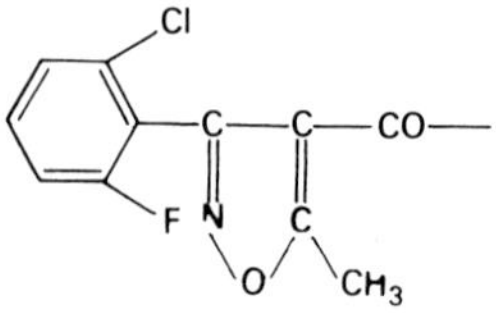

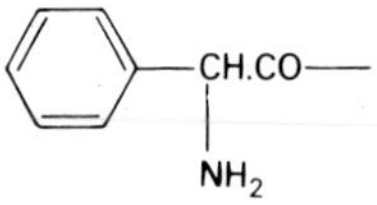

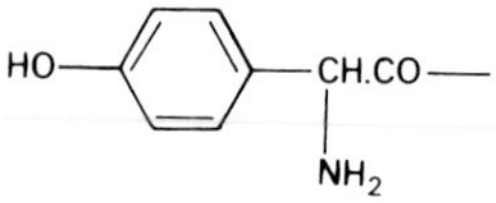

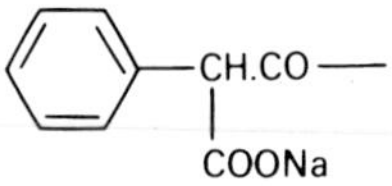

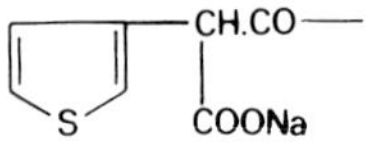

7 — CH.CO— with NH₂

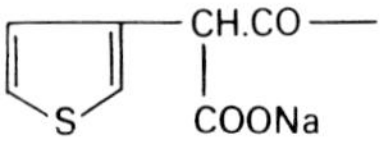

8 — HO— CH.CO— with NH₂

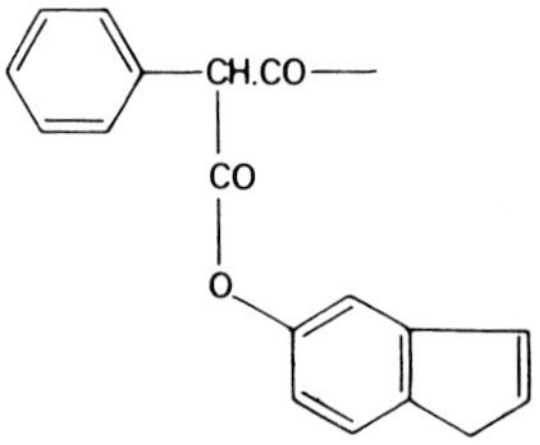

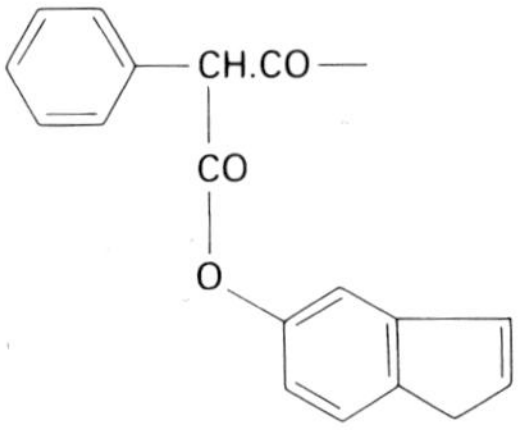

9 — CH.CO— with COONa

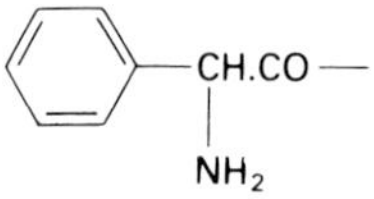

10 — (thiophene) CH.CO— with COONa

11 — (thiophene) CH.CO— with COONa

12 — CH.CO— CO—O—(indene)

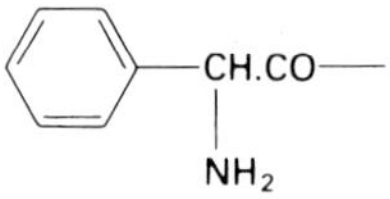

13 — CH.CO— CO—O—(indene)

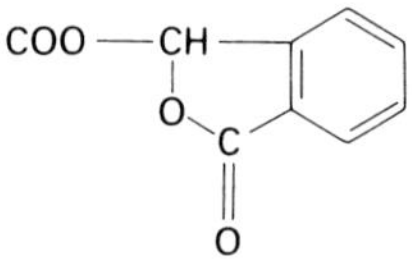

14 — CH.CO— NH₂ — At 3: $COOCH_2O.C.C(CH_3)_3$, O

15 — CH.CO— NH₂ — At 3: $COO-CH$ (phthalide)

16 — CH.CO— NH₂ — At 3: $COOCH_2CH_2O.COOC_2H_5$ / $COOCH(CH_3)_3O.COOC_2H_5$

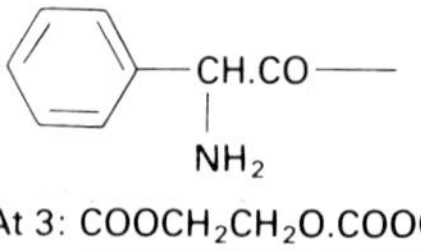

17 — CH.CO— NH—CO—(piperazinedione)

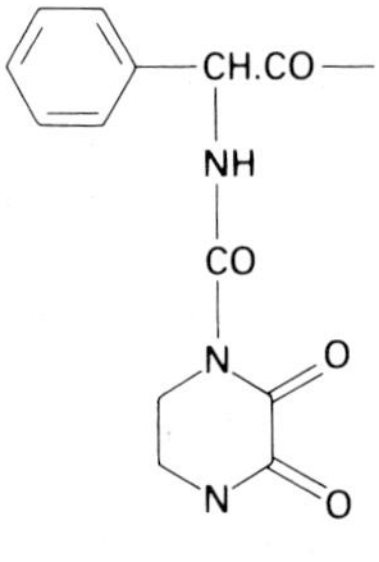

18 — CH.CO— NH—CO—(pyrazolidinone)

19 — CH.CO— NH—CO—(imidazolidinone)—N—$SO_2.CH_3$

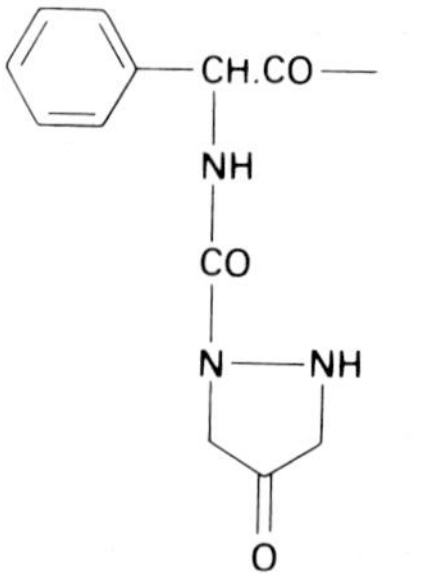

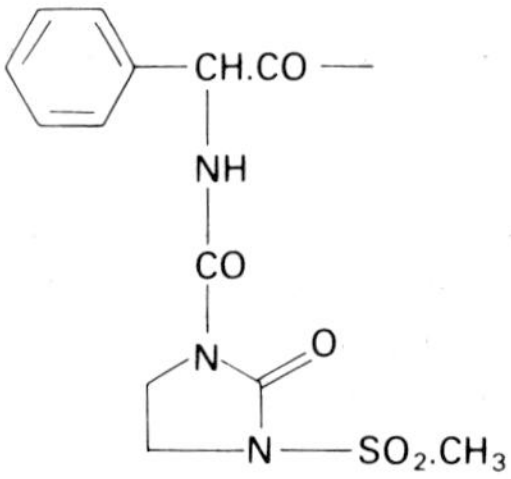

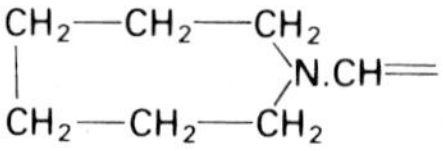

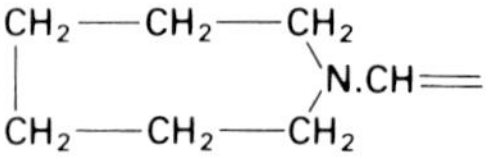

20 — $CH_2-CH_2-CH_2$ / $CH_2-CH_2-CH_2$ N.CH=

21 — $CH_2-CH_2-CH_2$ / $CH_2-CH_2-CH_2$ N.CH= — At 3: $COOCH_2O.C.C(CH_3)_3$, O

antibiotics. Pharmacokinetic properties may also be altered.

The sodium and potassium salts are very soluble in water but they are hydrolysed in solution, at a temperature-dependent rate, to the corresponding penicilloic acid (Fig. 10.3A), which is not antibacterial. Penicilloic acid is produced at alkaline pH or (via penicillenic acid; Fig. 10.3B) at neutral pH, but

Table 10.1 The penicillins and mecillinams

Penicillin	Orally effective	Stability to β-lactamases from		Activity versus			Ester	Hydrolysed after absorption
		Staph. aureus	Gram -ve	Gram -ve*	Ps. aeruginosa			
1 Benzylpenicillin	–	–	–	–	–		–	–
2 Phenoxymethylpenicillin	+	–	–	–	–		–	–
3 Methicillin	–	+	+	–	–		–	–
4 Oxacillin	+	+	+	–	–		–	–
5 Cloxacillin	+	+	+	–	–		–	–
6 Flucloxacillin	+	+	+	–	–		–	–
7 Ampicillin	+	–	–	+	–		–	–
8 Amoxycillin	+	–	–	+	–		–	–
9 Carbenicillin	–	–	+	+	+		–	–
10 Ticarcillin	–	–	+	+	+		–	–
11 Temocillin	+	+	+	+	+		–	–
12 Carfecillin } Carbenicillin esters	+	–	+	+	+		+	+
13 Indanyl carbenicillin (carindacillin) }	+	–	+	+	+		+	+
14 Pivampicillin } Ampicillin esters	+	–	–	+	–		+	+
15 Talampicillin }	+	–	–	+	–		+	+
16 Bacampicillin }	+	–	–	+	–		+	+
17 Piperacillin } Substituted ampicillins	–	–	–	+	+		–	–
18 Azlocillin }	–	–	–	+	+		–	–
19 Mezlocillin }	–	–	–	+	+		–	–
20 Mecillinam } 6-β-amidino- penicillins	–	NR	V	+	–		–	–
21 Pivmecillinam }	+	NR	V	+	–		+	+

* Except *Ps. aeruginosa*. All penicillins show some degree of activity against Gram-negative cocci.

+, applicable. –, inapplicable. NR, not relevant: mecillinam and pivmecillinam have no effect on Gram-positive bacteria: V, variable.

Note: **1** Esters give high urinary levels. **2** Hydrolysis of these esters by enzyme action after absorption from the gut mucosa gives rapid and high blood levels. **3** For additional information on resistance to β-lactamase inactivation, see Chapter 13. **4** In general, all penicillins are active against Gram-positive bacteria, although this may depend on the resistance of the drug to β-lactamase (see column 3): thus, benzylpenicillin is highly active against strains of *Staphylococcus aureus* which do not produce β-lactamase, but is destroyed by β-lactamase-producing strains. **5** Temocillin number (11) is less active against Gram-positive bacteria than ampicillin or the ureidopenicillins (substituted ampicillins). **6** Not all of the antibiotics listed above are currently available, but are included to illustrate the stages in development of the penicillins.

◀

Fig. 10.2 Examples of the side-chain R in various penicillins and mecillinams (the numbers 1–21 correspond to those in Table 10.1). Numbers 20 (mecillinam) and 21 (pivmecillinam) are 6-β-amidinopenicillanic acids (mecillinams). Number 11 (temocillin) has a methoxy (—OCH$_3$) group at position 6α; this confers high β-lactamase stability on the molecule.

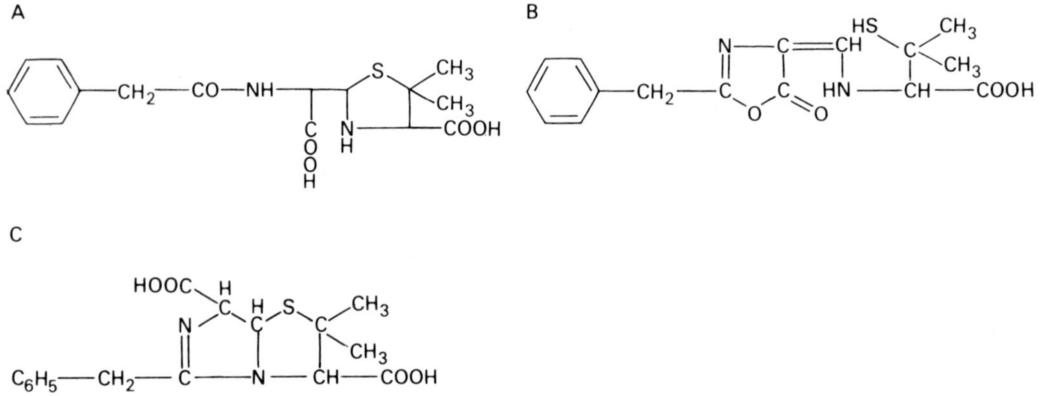

Fig. 10.3 Degradation products of benzylpenicillin in solution: A, penicilloic acid; B, penicillenic acid; C, penillic acid.

at acid pH a molecular re-arrangement occurs, giving penillic acid (Fig. 10.3C). Instability in acid medium logically precludes oral administration, as the antibiotic may be destroyed in the stomach; for example at pH 1.3 and 35°C methicillin has a half-life of only 2–3 minutes and is therefore not administered orally, whereas ampicillin, with a half-life of 600 minutes, is obviously suitable for oral use.

Benzylpenicillin is rapidly absorbed and rapidly excreted. However, certain sparingly soluble salts of benzylpenicillin (benzathine, benethamine and procaine) slowly release penicillin into the circulation over a period of time, thus giving a continuous high concentration in the blood.

Pro-drugs (e.g. carbenicillin esters, ampicillin esters; Fig. 10.2, Table 10.1) are hydrolysed by enzyme action after absorption from the gut mucosa to produce high blood levels of the active antibiotic, carbenicillin and ampicillin, respectively.

Several bacteria produce an enzyme, β-lactamase (penicillinase; see Chapter 13), which may inactivate a penicillin by opening the β-lactam ring, as in Fig. 10.1C. However, some penicillins (Table 10. l) are considerably more resistant to this enzyme than others, and consequently may be extremely valuable in the treatment of infections caused by β-lactamase-producing bacteria. In general, the penicillins are active against Gram-positive bacteria; some members (e.g. amoxycillin) are also effective against Gram-negative bacteria, although not *Pseudomonas aeruginosa*, whereas others (e.g. ticarcillin) are also active against this organism. In

particular, substituted ampicillins (piperacillin and the ureidopenicillins, azlocillin and mezlocillin) appear to combine the properties of ampicillin and carbenicillin. Temocillin is the first penicillin to be completely stable to hydrolysis by β-lactamases produced by Gram-negative bacteria.

The 6-β-amidinopenicillanic acids, mecillinam and its ester pivmecillinam, have unusual antibacterial properties, as they are active against Gram-negative but not Gram-positive organisms.

2.2 Cephalosporins

In the 1950s, a species of *Cephalosporium* (now known as *Acremonium*: see Chapter 22) isolated near a sewage outfall off the Sardinian coast was studied at Oxford and found to produce the following antibiotics.

1 An acidic antibiotic, cephalosporin P (subsequently found to have a steroid-like structure).
2 Another acidic antibiotic, cephalosporin N (later shown to be a penicillin, as its structure was based on 6-APA).
3 Cephalosporin C, obtained during the purification of cephalosporin N; this is a true cephalosporin, and from it has been obtained 7-aminocephalosporanic acid (7-ACA; Fig. 10.4), the starting point for new cephalosporins.

Cephalosporins consist of a six-membered dihydrothiazine ring fused to a β-lactam ring. Thus, the cephalosporins (Δ^3-cephalosporins) are structurally related to the penicillins (section 2.1). The

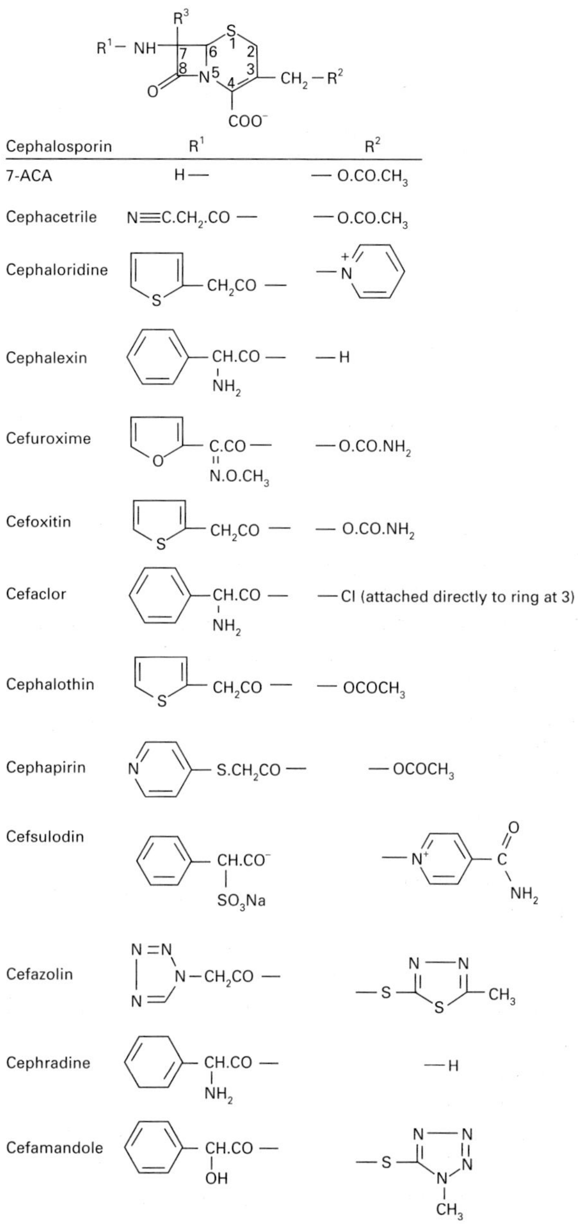

Fig. 10.4 (*above and overleaf*) General structure of cephalosporins and examples of side-chains R and R^2. (R^3 is $-OCH_3$ in cefoxitin and cefotetan and $-H$ in other members.) Cephalosporins containing an ester group at position 3 are liable to attack by esterases *in vivo*.

position of the double bond in Δ^3-cephalosporins is important, as Δ^2-cephalosporins (double bond between 2 and 3) are not antibacterial irrespective of the composition of the side-chains.

2.2.1 Structure-activity relationships

The activity of cephalosporins (and other β-lactams) against Gram-positive bacteria depends on antibiotic affinity for penicillin-sensitive

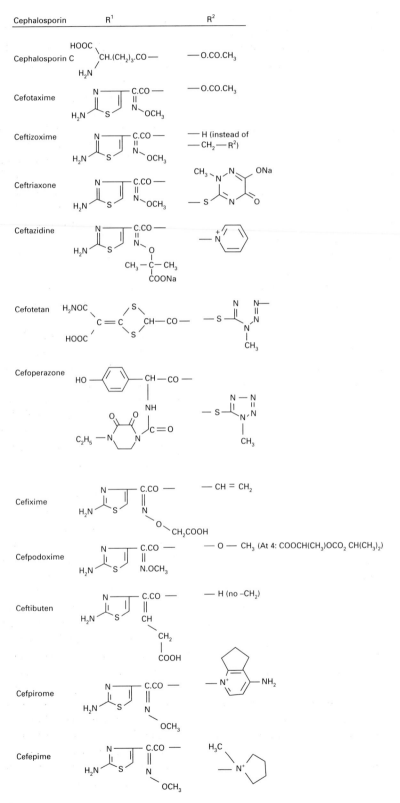

Fig. 10.4 *Continued*

enzymes (PSEs) detected in practice as penicillin-binding proteins (PBPs). Resistance results from altered PBPs or, more commonly, from β-lactamases. Activity against Gram-negative bacteria depends upon penetration of β-lactams through the outer membrane, resistance to β-lactamases found in the periplasmic space and binding to PBPs. (For further information on mechanisms of action and bacterial resistance, see Chapters 12 and 13). Modifications of the cephem nucleus (Fig. 10.4) at 7α, i.e. R^3, by addition of methoxy groups increase β-lactamase stability but decrease activity against Gram-positive bacteria because of reduced affinity for PBPs. Side-chains containing a 2-aminothiazolyl group at R^1, e.g. cefotaxime, ceftizoxime, ceftriaxone and ceftazidime, yield cephalosporins with enhanced affinity for PBPs of Gram-negative bacteria and streptococci. An iminomethoxy group ($-C=N.OCH_3$) in, for example, cefuroxime provides β-lactamase stability against common plasmid-mediated β-lactamases. A propylcarboxy group ($(CH_3)_2-C-COOH$) in, for example, ceftazidime increases β-lactamase resistance and also provides activity against *Ps. aeruginosa*, whilst at the same time reducing β-lactamase induction capabilities.

Further examples of the interplay of factors in antibacterial activity are demonstrated by the following findings.

1 7α-methoxy substitution of cefuroxime, cefamandole and cephapirin produces reduced activity against *E. coli* because of a lower affinity for PBPs;

2 similar substitution of cefoxitin produces enhanced activity against *E. coli* because of greater penetration through the outer membrane of the organism.

In cephalosporins susceptible to β-lactamases, opening of the β-lactam ring occurs with concomitant loss of the substituent at R^2 (except in cephalexin, where R^2 represents H; see Fig. 10.4). This is followed by fragmentation of the molecule. Provided that they are not inactivated by β-lactamases, the cephalosporins generally have a broad spectrum of activity, although there may be a wide variation. *Haemophilus influenzae*, for example, is particularly susceptible to cefuroxime; see also Table 10.2.

2.2.2 Pharmacokinetic properties

Pharmacokinetic properties of the cephalosporins depend to a considerable extent on their chemical nature, e.g. the substituent R^2. The 3-acetoxymethyl compounds such as cephalothin, cephapirin and cephacetrile are converted *in vivo* by esterases to the antibacterially less active 3-hydroxymethyl derivatives and are excreted partly as such. The rapid excretion means that such cephalosporins have a short half-life in the body. Replacement of the 3-acetoxymethyl group by a variety of groups has rendered other cephalosporins much less prone to esterase attack. For example, cephaloridine has an internally compensated betaine group at position 3 (R^2) and is metabolically stable.

Cephalosporins such as the 3-acetoxymethyl derivatives described above, cephaloridine and cefazolin are inactive when given orally. For good oral absorption, the 7-acyl group (R^1) must be based on phenylglycine and the amino group must remain unsubstituted. The R^2 substituent must be small, non-polar and stable; a methyl group is considered desirable but might decrease antibacterial activity. Earlier examples of oral cephalosporins are provided by cephalexin, cefaclor and cephradine (Table 10.2). Newer oral cephalosporins such as cefixime, cefpodoxime and ceftibuten show increased stability to β-lactamases produced by Gram-negative bacteria.

Like cefuroxime axetil (also given orally), cefpodoxime is an absorbable ester. During absorption, esterases remove the ester side-chain, liberating the active substance into the blood. Cefixime and ceftibuten are non-ester drugs characterized by activity against Gram-positive and Gram-negative bacteria, although *Ps. aeruginosa* is resistant.

Parenterally administered cephalosporins that are metabolically stable and that are resistant to many types of β-lactamases include cefuroxime, cefamandole, cefotaxime and cefoxitin, which has a 7β-methoxy group at R^2. Injectable cephalosporins with anti-pseudomonal activity include ceftazidime, cefsulodin and cefoperazone.

Side-chains of the various cephalosporins, including those most recently developed, are presented in Fig. 10.4 and a summary of the properties of these antibiotics in Table 10.2.

Table 10.2 The cephalosporins*

Group	Examples	Staphylococci†	Staphylococcal β-lactamase	Streptococci‡	Enterobacteria	Enterobacterial β-lactamases	Neisseria	Haemophilus	Ps. aeruginosa	Comment
Oral cephalosporins	Cephalexin, cephradine, cefaclor, cefadroxil	++	++	+	V	V	+	(+)	R	
	Cefixime, ceftibuten	+	++	++	V	V	++	++	R	Newer oral cephalosporins
	Cefuroxime axetil	++	++	++	V	V	++	++	R	Absorbable ester
	Cefpodoxime axetil	++	++	++	V	V	++	++	R	Absorbable ester
Injectable cephalosporins (β-lactamase susceptible)	Cephaloridine, cephalothin, cephacetrile, cefazolin	++	+	+	V	V	+	(+)	R	
Injectable cephalosporins (improved β-lactamase stability)	Cefuroxime, cefoxitin, cefamandole	++	++	++	++	++	++	++	R	Cefoxitin shows activity against *Bacteroides fragilis*
Injectable cephalosporins (still higher β-lactamase stability)	Cefotaxime, ceftazidime, ceftizoxime, ceftriaxone (also the oxacephem, latamoxef, section 2.4)	++	++	+++	+++	+++	+++	+++	R (ceftazidime +++)	Latamoxef has high activity against *B. fragilis*
Injectable cephalosporins (anti-pseudomonal activity)	Cefoperazone	++	++	+	V	V	++	++	++	
	Cefsulodin	(+)	++	(+)				R	+++	
Injectable cephalosporins (other)	Cefotetan	(+)			+++	+++			R	Inhibits *B. fragilis*

* Early cephalosporins were spelt with 'ph', more recently with 'f'.
† Methicillin-resistant *Staph. aureus* (MRSA) strains are resistant to cephalosporins.
‡ Enterococci are resistant to cephalosporins.
+++, excellent; ++, good; +, fair; (+), poor; R, resistant; V, variable.

2.3 Clavams

The clavams differ from penicillins (based on the penam structure) in two respects, namely the replacement of sulphur in the penicillin thiazolidine ring (Fig. 10.1) with oxygen in the clavam oxazolidine ring (Fig. 10.5A) and the absence of the side-chain at position 6. Clavulanic acid, a naturally occurring clavam isolated from *Streptomyces clavuligerus*, has poor antibacterial activity but is a

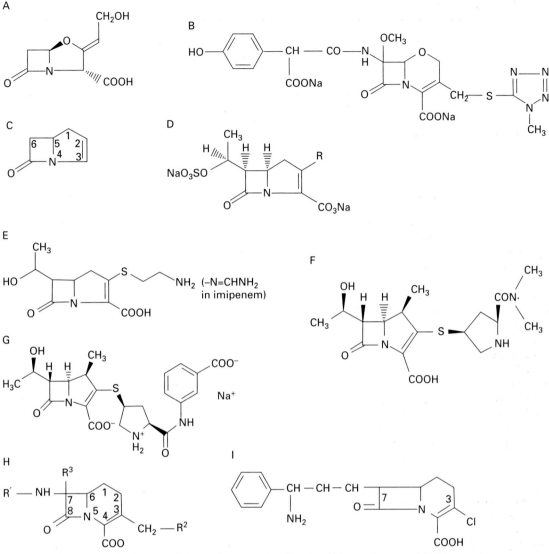

Fig. 10.5 A, clavulanic acid; B, latamoxef; C, 1-carbapenems; D, olivanic acid (general structure); E, thienamycin; F, meropenem; G, ertapenem; H, 1-carbacephems; I, loracarbef.

potent inhibitor of staphylococcal β-lactamase and of most types of β-lactamases produced by Gram-negative bacteria, especially those with a 'penicillinase' rather than a 'cephalosporinase' type of enzyme action.

A significant development in chemotherapy has been the introduction into clinical practice of a combination of clavulanic acid with a broad-spectrum, but β-lactamase-susceptible, penicillin,

amoxycillin. The spectrum of activity has been extended to include *Ps. aeruginosa* by combining clavulanic acid with the β-lactamase-susceptible penicillin, ticarcillin.

2.4 1-Oxacephems

In the 1-oxacephems, for example latamoxef (moxalactam, Fig. 10.5B), the sulphur atom in the dihydrothiazine cephalosporin ring system is replaced by oxygen. This would tend to make the molecule chemically less stable and more susceptible to inactivation by β-lactamases. The introduction of the 7-α-methoxy group (as in cefoxitin, Fig. 10.4), however, stabilizes the molecule. Latamoxef is a broad-spectrum antibiotic with a high degree of stability to most types of β-lactamases, and is highly active against the anaerobe *B. fragilis*.

2.5 1-Carbapenems

The 1-carbapenems (Fig. 10.5C) comprise a family of fused β-lactam antibiotics. They are analogues of penicillins or clavams, the sulphur (penicillins) or oxygen (clavams) atom being replaced by carbon. Examples are the olivanic acids (section 2.5.1) and thienamycin and imipenem (section 2.5.2).

2.5.1 Olivanic acids

The olivanic acids (general structure, Fig. 10.5D) are naturally occurring β-lactam antibiotics which have, with some difficulty, been isolated from culture fluids of *Strep. olivaceus*. They are broad-spectrum antibiotics and are potent inhibitors of various types of β-lactamases.

2.5.2 Thienamycin and imipenem

Thienamycin (Fig. 10.5E) is a broad-spectrum β-lactam antibiotic with high β-lactamase resistance. Unfortunately, it is chemically unstable, although the *N*-formimidoyl derivative, imipenem, overcomes this defect. Imipenem (Fig. 10.5E) is stable to most β-lactamases but is readily hydrolysed by kidney dehydropeptidase and is administered with a dehydropeptidase inhibitor, cilastatin. Meropenem, marketed more recently, is more stable than imipenem to this enzyme and may thus be administered without cilastatin. Its chemical structure is depicted in Fig. 10.5F. Ertapenem (Fig. 10.5G) has properties similar to those of meropenem but affords the additional advantage of once-daily dosing.

2.6 1-Carbacephems

In the 1-carbacephems (Fig. 10.5H), the sulphur in the six-membered dihydrothiazine ring of the cephalosporins (based on the cephem structure, see Fig. 10.4) is replaced by carbon. Loracarbef (Fig. 10.5I) is a newer oral carbacephem which is highly active against Gram-positive bacteria, including staphylococci.

2.7 Nocardicins

The nocardicins (A to G) have been isolated from a strain of *Nocardia* and comprise a novel group of β-lactam antibiotics (Fig. 10.6A). Nocardicin A is the most active member, and possesses significant activity against Gram-negative but not Gram-positive bacteria.

2.8 Monobactams

The monobactams are monocyclic β-lactam antibiotics produced by various strains of bacteria. A novel nucleus, 3-aminomonobactamic acid (3-AMA, Fig. 10.6B), has been produced from naturally occurring monobactams and from 6-APA. Several monobactams have been tested and one (aztreonam, Fig. 10.6C) has been shown to be highly active against most Gram-negative bacteria and to be stable to most types of β-lactamases. It is not destroyed by staphylococcal β-lactamases but is inactive against all strains of *Staph. aureus* tested. *Bacteroides fragilis*, a Gram-negative anaerobe, is resistant to aztreonam, probably by virtue of the β-lactamase it produces, and this conclusion is supported by the finding that a combination of the monobactam with clavulanic acid (section 2.3) is ineffective against this organism.

2.9 Penicillanic acid derivatives

Penicillanic acid derivatives are synthetically produced β-lactamase inhibitors. Penicillanic acid sulphone (Fig. 10.6D) protects ampicillin from hydrolysis by staphylococcal β-lactamase and some, but not all, of the β-lactamases produced by Gram-negative bacteria, but is less potent than

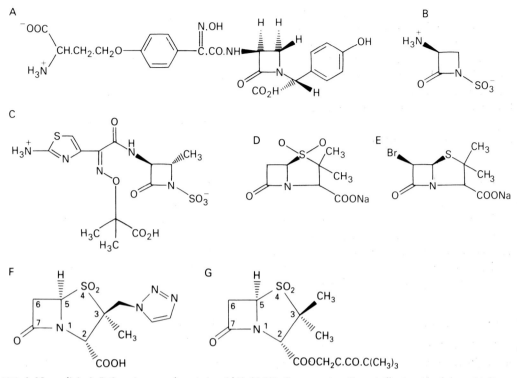

Fig. 10.6 A, Nocardicin A; B, 3-aminomonobactamic acid (3-AMA); C, aztreonam; D, penicillanic acid sulphone (sodium salt); E, β-bromopenicillanic acid (sodium salt); F, tazobactam; G, sulbactam.

clavulanic acid. β-Bromopenicillanic acid (Fig. 10.6E) inhibits some types of β-lactamases.

Tazobactam (Fig. 10.6F) is a penicillanic acid sulphone derivative marketed as a combination with piperacillin. Alone it has poor intrinsic antibacterial activity but is comparable to clavulanic acid in inhibiting β-lactamase activity.

Sulbactam (Fig. 10.6G) is a semisynthetic 6-desaminopenicillin sulphone structurally related to tazobactam. Not only is it an effective inhibitor of many β-lactamases but it is also active alone against certain Gram-negative bacteria. It is used clinically in combination with ampicillin.

2.10 Hypersensitivity

Some types of allergic reaction, for example immediate or delayed-type skin allergies, serum sickness-like reactions and anaphylactic reactions, may occur in a proportion of patients given penicillin treatment. There is some, but not complete, cross-allergy with cephalosporins.

Contaminants of high molecular weight (considered to have arisen from mycelial residues from the fermentation process) may be responsible for the induction of allergy to penicillins; their removal leads to a marked reduction in the antigenicity of the penicillin. It has also been found, however, that varying amounts of a non-protein polymer (of unknown source) may also be present in penicillin and that this also may be antigenic.

The interaction of a non-enzymatic degradation product, D-benzylpenicillenic acid (formed by cleavage of the thiazolidine ring of benzylpenicillin in solution; see Fig. 10.3B), with sulphydryl or amino groups in tissue proteins, to form hapten-protein conjugates, is also of importance. In particular, the reaction between D-benzylpenicillenic acid and the ε-amino group of lysine (α,ε-diamino-*n*-caproic acid, $NH_2(CH_2)_4.CH(NH_2).COOH$) residues

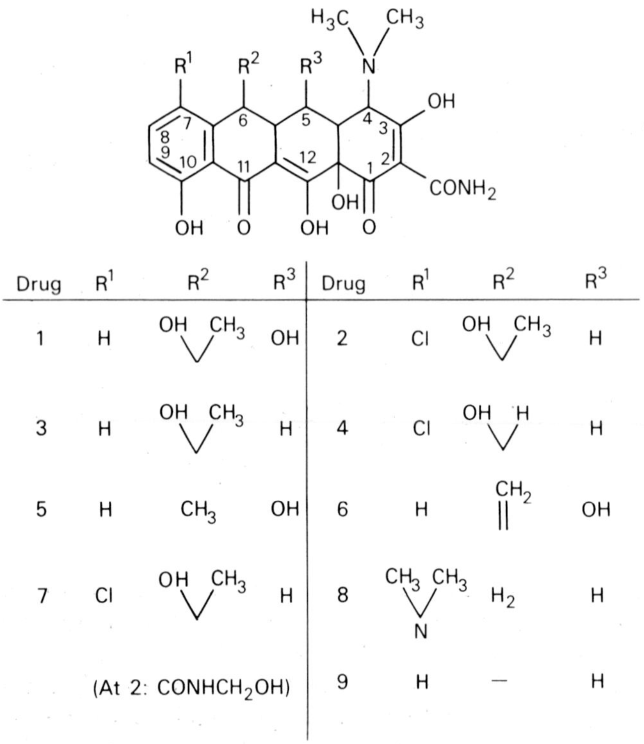

Drug	R^1	R^2	R^3	Drug	R^1	R^2	R^3
1	H	OH CH₃	OH	2	Cl	OH CH₃	H
3	H	OH CH₃	H	4	Cl	OH H	H
5	H	CH₃	OH	6	H	CH₂	OH
7	Cl	OH CH₃	H	8	CH₃ CH₃ N	H₂	H
	(At 2: CONHCH₂OH)			9	H	—	H

Fig. 10.7 Tetracycline antibiotics:
1, oxytetracycline; 2, chlortetracycline;
3, tetracycline; 4, demethylchlortetracycline;
5, doxycycline; 6, methacycline; 7, clomocycline;
8, minocycline; 9, thiacycline (a thiatetracycline
with a sulphur atom at 6).

is to be noted, because these D-benzylpenicilloyl derivatives of tissue proteins function as complete penicillin antigens.

3 Tetracycline group

3.1 Tetracyclines

There are several clinically important tetracyclines, characterized by four cyclic rings (Fig. 10.7). They consist of a group of antibiotics obtained as by-products from the metabolism of various species of *Streptomyces*, although some members may now be thought of as being semisynthetic. Thus, tetracycline (by catalytic hydrogenation) and clomocycline are obtained from chlortetracycline, which is itself produced from *Strep. aureofaciens*. Methacycline is obtained from oxytetracycline (produced from *Strep. rimosus*) and hydrogenation of methacycline gives doxycycline. Demethylchlortetracycline is produced by a mutant strain of *Strep.*

aureofaciens. Minocycline is a derivative of tetracycline.

The tetracyclines are broad-spectrum antibiotics, i.e. they have a wide range of activity against Gram-positive and Gram-negative bacteria. *Ps. aeruginosa* is less sensitive, but is generally susceptible to tetracycline concentrations obtainable in the bladder. Resistance to the tetracyclines (see also Chapter 13) develops relatively slowly, but there is cross-resistance, i.e. an organism resistant to one member is usually resistant to all other members of this group. However, tetracycline-resistant *Staph. aureus* strains may still be sensitive to minocycline. Suprainfection ('overgrowth') with naturally tetracycline-resistant organisms, for example *Candida albicans* and other yeasts, and filamentous fungi, affecting the mouth, upper respiratory tract or gastrointestinal tract, may occur as a result of the suppression of tetracycline-susceptible microorganisms.

Thiatetracyclines contain a sulphur atom at position 6 in the molecule. One derivative, thiacycline,

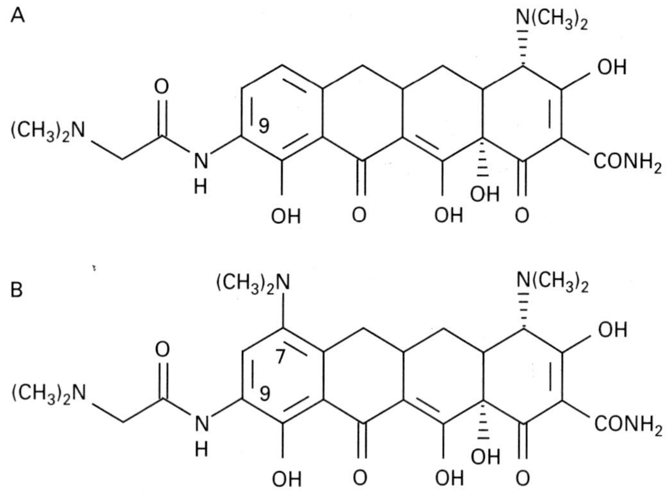

A

B

Fig. 10.8 Structures of two tetracycline analogues, which are members of the new glycylcycline group of antibiotics: A, *N,N*-dimethylglycylamido-6-demethyl-6-deoxytetracycline; B, *N,N*-dimethylglycylamidominocycline.

is more active than minocycline against tetracycline-resistant bacteria. Despite toxicity problems affecting its possible clinical use, thiacycline could be the starting point in the development of a new range of important tetracycline-type antibiotics.

The tetracyclines are no longer used clinically to the same extent as they were in the past because of the increase in bacterial resistance.

3.2 Glycylcyclines

The glycylcyclines (Fig. 10.8) represent a new group of tetracycline analogues. They are novel tetracyclines substituted at the C-9 position with a dimethylglycylamido side-chain. They possess activity against bacteria that express resistance to the older tetracyclines by an efflux mechanism (Chapter 13).

4 Rifamycins

Rifamycins A to E have been described. From rifamycin B are produced rifamide (rifamycin B diethylamide) and rifamycin SV, which is one of the most useful and least toxic of the rifamycins.

Rifampicin (Fig. 10.9), a bactericidal antibiotic, is active against Gram-positive bacteria (including *Mycobacterium tuberculosis*) and some Gram-

negative bacteria (but not Enterobacteriaceae or pseudomonads). It has been found to have a greater bactericidal effect against *M. tuberculosis* than other antitubercular drugs, is active orally, penetrates well into cerebrospinal fluid and is thus of use in the treatment of tuberculous meningitis (see also section 13.5).

Rifampicin possesses significant bactericidal activity at very low concentrations against staphylococci. Unfortunately, resistant mutants may arise very rapidly, both *in vitro* and *in vivo*. It has thus been recommended that rifampicin should be combined with another antibiotic, e.g. vancomycin, in the treatment of staphylococcal infections.

Rifabutin may be used in the prophylaxis of *M. avium* complex infections in immunocompromised patients and in the treatment, with other drugs, of pulmonary tuberculosis and non-tuberculous mycobacterial infections.

5 Aminoglycoside-aminocyclitol antibiotics

Aminoglycoside antibiotics contain amino sugars in their structure. Deoxystreptamine-containing members are neomycin, framycetin, gentamicin, kanamycin, tobramycin, amikacin, netilmicin and sisomicin. Both streptomycin and dihydrostreptomycin contain streptidine, whereas the aminocycli-

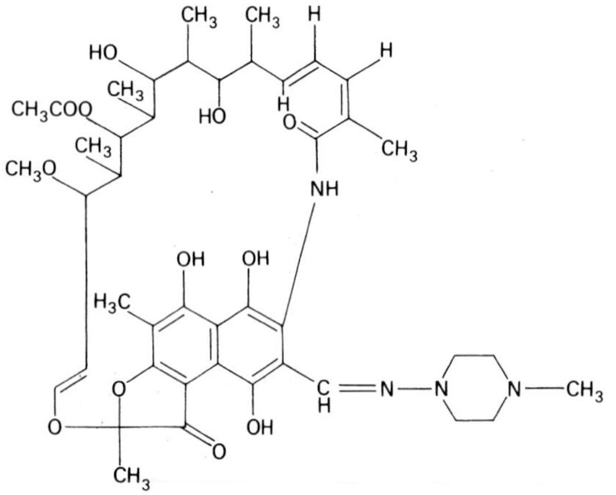

Fig. 10.9 Rifampicin.

tol spectinomycin has no amino sugar. Examples of chemical structures are provided in Fig. 10.10.

Streptomycin (Fig. 10.10A) was isolated by Waksman in 1944, and its activity against *M. tuberculosis* ensured its use as a primary drug in the treatment of tuberculosis. Unfortunately, its ototoxicity and the rapid development of resistance have tended to modify its usefulness, and although it still remains a useful drug against tuberculosis it is usually used in combination with other antibiotics. Streptomycin also shows activity against other types of bacteria, for example against various Gram-negative bacteria and some strains of staphylococci. Dihydrostreptomycin has a similar antibacterial action but is more toxic.

Kanamycin (a complex of three antibiotics, A, B and C; Fig. 10.10B) is active in low concentrations against various Gram-positive (including penicillin-resistant staphylococci) and Gram-negative bacteria. It is a recognized second-line drug in the treatment of tuberculosis.

Gentamicin (a mixture of three components, C_1, C_{1a} and C_2; Fig. 10.10C) is active against many strains of Gram-positive and Gram-negative bacteria, including some strains of *Ps. aeruginosa*. Its activity is greatly increased at pH values of about 8. It is often administered in conjunction with a β-lactam to delay the development of resistance. Gentamicin is the most important aminoglycoside antibiotic, is the aminoglycoside of choice in the UK and is widely used for treating serious infections. As with other members of this group, side-effects are dose-related, dosage must be given with care, plasma levels should be monitored and treatment should not normally exceed 7 days.

Paromomycin finds special use in the treatment of intestinal amoebiasis (it is amoebicidal against *Entamoeba histolytica*) and of acute bacillary dysentery.

Neomycin is poorly absorbed from the alimentary tract when given orally, and is usually used in the form of lotions and ointments for topical application against skin and eye infections. Framycetin consists of neomycin B with a small amount of neomycin C, and is usually employed locally.

A desirable property of newer aminoglycoside antibiotics is increased antibacterial activity against resistant strains, especially improved stability to aminoglycoside-modifying enzymes (Chapter 13). Alteration in the 3′-position of kanamycin B (Fig. 10.10B) to give 3′-deoxykanamycin B (tobramycin) changes the activity spectrum. Amikacin (Fig. 10.10D) has a substituted aminobutyryl in the amino group at position 1 in the 2-deoxystreptamine ring and this enhances its resistance to some, but not all, types of aminoglycoside-modifying enzymes, as it has fewer sites of modification. Netilmicin (*N*-ethylsisomicin) is a semisynthetic derivative of sisomicin but is less susceptible than sisomicin to some types of bacterial enzymes.

The most important of these antibiotics are amikacin, tobramycin, netilmicin and especially gentamicin.

6 Macrolides

6.1 Older members

The macrolide antibiotics are characterized by possessing molecular structures that contain large (12–16-membered) lactone rings linked through glycosidic bonds with amino sugars.

The most important members of this group are erythromycin (Fig. 10.11), oleandomycin, triacetyloleandomycin and spiramycin. Erythromycin is active against most Gram-positive bacteria, *Neisseria*, *H. influenzae* and *Legionella pneumophila*, but not against the Enterobacteriaceae; its activity is

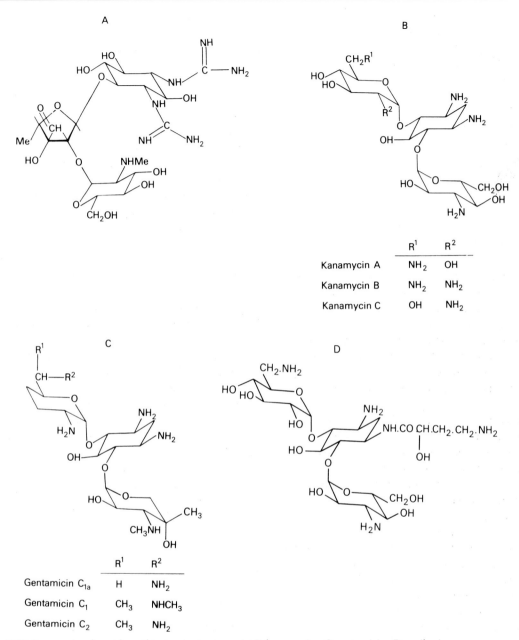

Fig. 10.10 Some aminoglycoside antibiotics: A, streptomycin; B, kanamycins; C, gentamicins; D, amikacin.

	R^1	R^2
Kanamycin A	NH_2	OH
Kanamycin B	NH_2	NH_2
Kanamycin C	OH	NH_2

	R^1	R^2
Gentamicin C_{1a}	H	NH_2
Gentamicin C_1	CH_3	$NHCH_3$
Gentamicin C_2	CH_3	NH_2

pH-dependent, increasing with pH up to about 8.5. Erythromycin estolate is more stable than the free base to the acid of gastric juice and is thus employed for oral use. The estolate produces higher and more prolonged blood levels and distributes into some tissues more efficiently than other dosage forms. *In vivo*, it hydrolyses to give the free base.

Staphylococcus aureus is less sensitive to erythromycin than are pneumococci or haemolytic streptococci, and there may be a rapid development

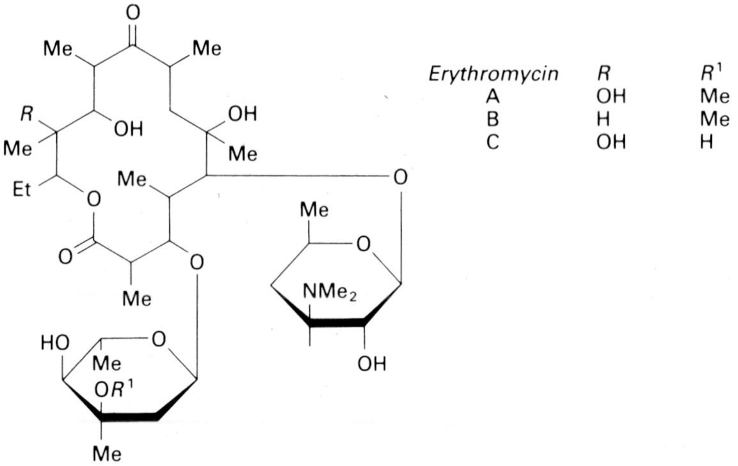

Fig. 10.11 Erythromycins: erythromycin is a mixture of macrolide antibiotics consisting largely of erythromycin A.

Erythromycin	R	R¹
A	OH	Me
B	H	Me
C	OH	H

of resistance, especially of staphylococci, *in vitro*. However, *in vivo* with successful short courses of treatment, resistance is not usually a serious clinical problem. On the other hand, resistance is likely to develop when the antibiotic is used for long periods.

Oleandomycin, its ester (triacetyloleandomycin) and spiramycin have a similar range of activity to erythromycin but are less potent. Resistance develops only slowly in clinical practice. However, cross-resistance may occur between all four members of this group.

6.2 Newer members

The new macrolides are semisynthetic molecules that differ from the original compounds in the substitution pattern of the lactone ring system (Table 10.3, Figs 10.12 and 10.13).

Roxithromycin has similar *in vitro* activity to erythromycin but enters leucocytes and macrophages more rapidly with higher concentrations in the lysosomal component of the phagocytic cells. It is likely to become an important drug against *Legionella pneumophila*. Clarithromycin and azithromycin are also of value.

7 Lincosamides

Lincomycin and clindamycin (Fig. 10.14A, B) are

Table 10.3 Newer macrolide derivatives of erythromycin

Lactone ring structure	Example	Derivative of erythromycin
14-membered	Erythromycin	—
	Roxithromycin	Methoxy-ethoxy-methyloxine
	Clarithromycin	Methyl
	Dirithromycin	Oxazine
15-membered	Azithromycin	Deoxo-aza-methyl-homo

active against Gram-positive cocci, except *Enterococcus faecalis*. Gram-negative cocci tend to be less sensitive and enterobacteria are resistant. Although not related structurally to the macrolides (section 6), the lincosamides have a similar mechanism of action. Cross-resistance may occur between lincosamides, streptogramins and macrolides, but some erythromycin-resistant organisms may be sensitive to lincosamides.

8 Streptogramins

Pristinamycin and virginiamycin are two streptogramins that have been long been known. Pristinamycin is a mixture of synergistic components, pristinamycins I and II, the former being a macrolide and the latter a depsipeptide.

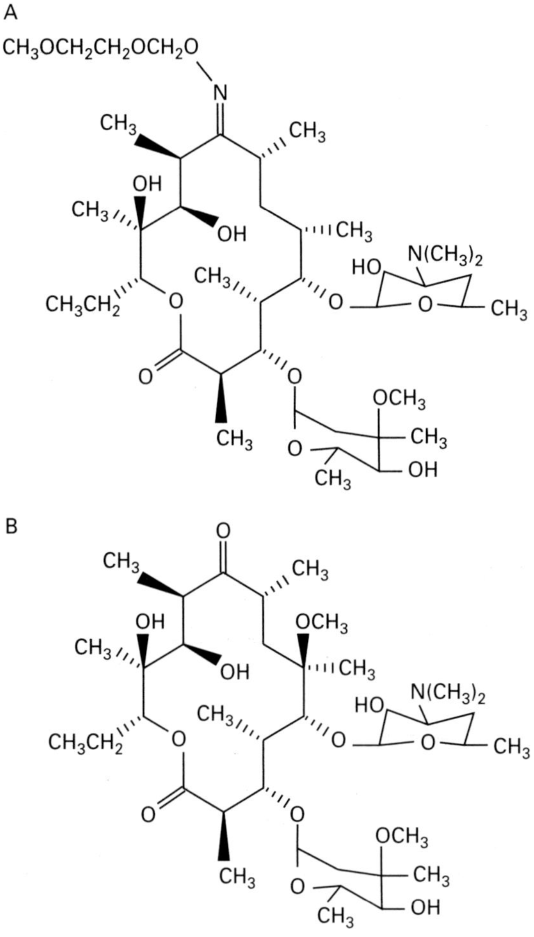

A

CH₃OCH₂CH₂OCH₂O

B

Fig. 10.12 Examples of newer 14-membered macrolides: A, roxithromycin; B, clarithromycin.

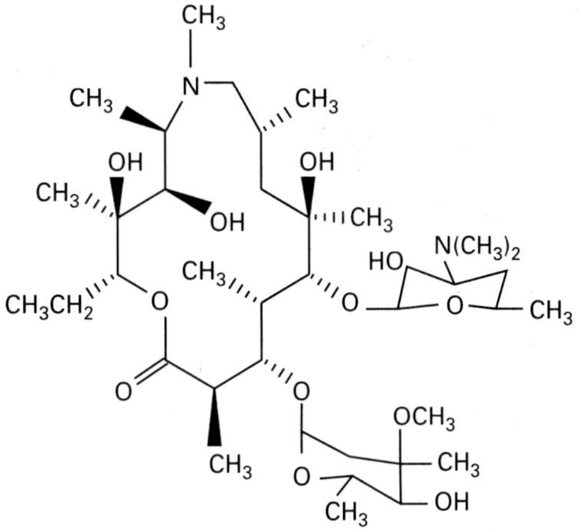

Fig. 10.13 Structure of azithromycin (15-membered macrolide).

The MLS (macrolides, lincosamides, streptogramins) group of antibiotics all inhibit protein synthesis by binding to the 50S ribosomal subunit. Resistance mechanisms specific to individual members occur but resistance to all may be conferred by a single mechanism that involves 23S rRNA. However, it is claimed that the quinupristin-dalfopristin combination does not demonstrate cross-resistance to other antibiotics within the MLS group or to other antibiotics.

9 Polypeptide antibiotics

The polypeptide antibiotics comprise a rather diverse group. They include:

1 Bacitracin, with activity against Gram-positive but not Gram-negative bacteria (except Gram-negative cocci);

2 Polymyxins, which are active against many types of Gram-negative bacteria (including *Ps. aeruginosa* but excluding cocci, *Serratia marcescens* and *Proteus* spp.) but not Gram-positive organisms; and

3 Antitubercular antibiotics, capreomycin and viomycin.

Because of its highly toxic nature when administered parenterally, bacitracin is normally restricted to external usage.

Two important new streptogramins are quinupristin (Fig. 10.15A) and dalfopristin (Fig. 10.15B), which are derivatives of pristinamycin I and IIA, respectively. Individually, the two components are bacteristatic but in combination they act synergistically to produce a bactericidal effect by inhibiting early (dalfopristin) and late (quinupristin) phases of bacterial protein synthesis. These two antibiotics are used intravenously in combination (ratio 30:70) for the treatment of serious or life-threatening infections associated with vancomycin-resistant *Enterococcus faecium* bacteraemia, although the effect against this organism is bacteristatic.

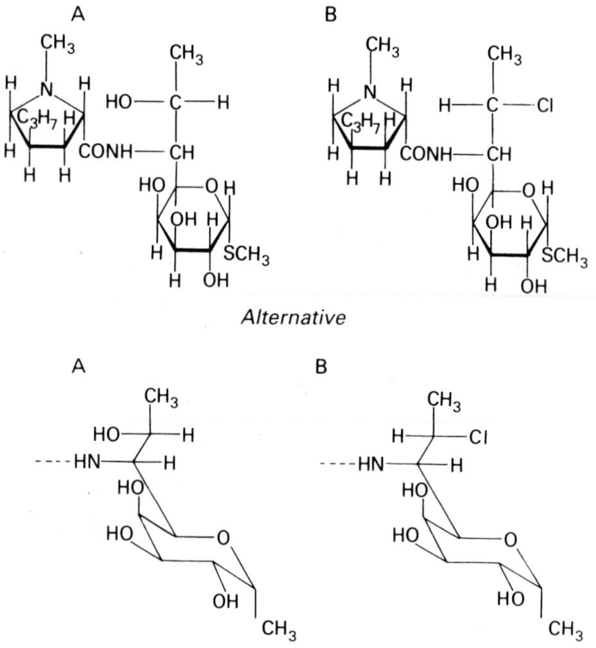

Fig. 10.14 Lincosamides: A, lincomycin; B, clindamycin.

The antibacterial activity of five members (A to E) of the polymyxin group is of a similar nature. However, they are all nephrotoxic, although this effect is much reduced with polymyxins B and E (colistin). Colistin sulphomethate sodium is the form of colistin used for parenteral administration. Sulphomyxin sodium, a mixture of sulphomethylated polymyxin B and sodium bisulphite, has the action and uses of polymyxin B sulphate, but is less toxic.

Capreomycin and viomycin show activity against *M. tuberculosis* and may be regarded as being second-line antitubercular drugs.

10 Glycopeptide antibiotics

Two important glycopeptide antibiotics are vancomycin and teicoplanin.

10.1 Vancomycin

Vancomycin is an antibiotic isolated from *Strep. orientalis* and has an empirical formula of $C_{66}H_{75}Cl_2N_9O_4$ (mol. wt 1448); it has a complex tricyclic glycopeptide structure. Modern chromatographically purified vancomycin gives rise to fewer side-effects than the antibiotic produced in the 1950s.

Vancomycin is active against most Gram-positive bacteria, including methicillin-resistant strains of *Staph. aureus* and *Staph. epidermidis*, *Enterococcus faecalis*, *Clostridium difficile* and certain Gram-negative cocci. Gram-negative bacilli, mycobacteria and fungi are not susceptible. Vancomycin-resistant enterococci are now posing a clinical problem in hospitals, however.

Vancomycin is bactericidal to most susceptible bacteria at concentrations near its minimum inhibitory concentration (MIC) and is an inhibitor of bacterial cell wall peptidoglycan synthesis, although at a site different from that of β-lactam antibiotics (Chapter 12).

Employed as the hydrochloride and administered by dilute intravenous injection, vancomycin is indicated in potentially life-threatening infections that cannot be treated with other effective, less toxic, antibiotics. Oral vancomycin is the drug of choice in the treatment of antibiotic-induced pseudomembranous colitis associated with the administration

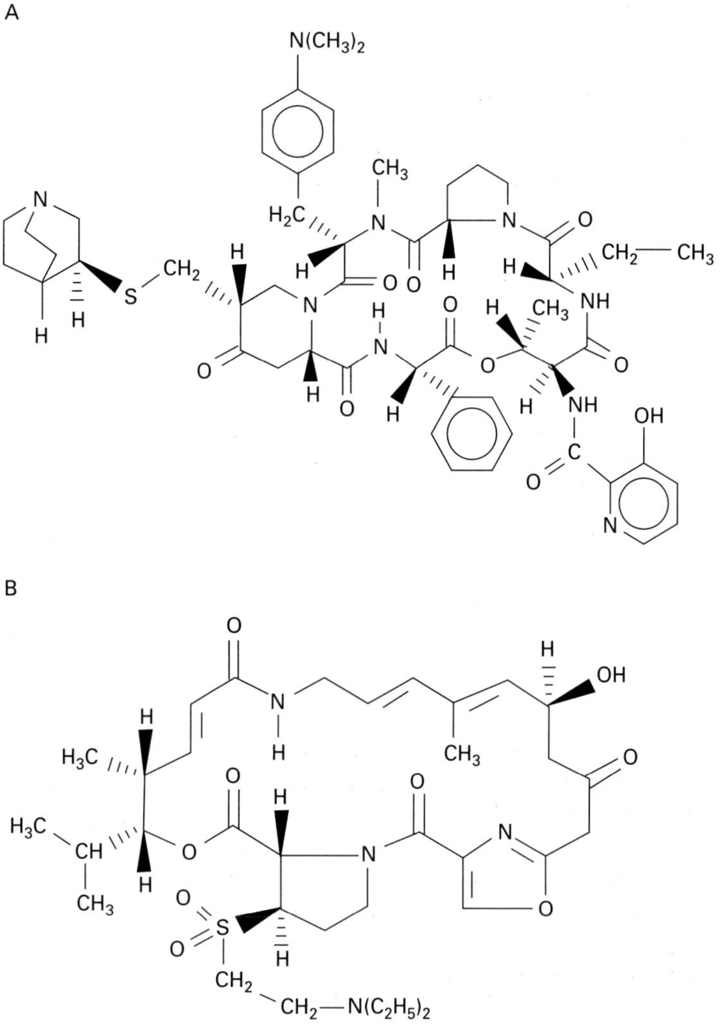

Fig. 10.15 Streptogramins: A, quinupristin; B, dalfopristin.

of antibiotics such as clindamycin and lincomycin (section 7).

10.2 Teicoplanin

Teicoplanin is a naturally occurring complex of five closely related tetracyclic molecules. Its mode of action and spectrum of activity are essentially similar to vancomycin, although it might be less active against some strains of coagulase-negative staphylococci. Teicoplanin can be administered by intramuscular injection.

11 Miscellaneous antibacterial antibiotics

Antibiotics described here (Fig. 10.16) are those which cannot logically be considered in any of the other groups above.

11.1 Chloramphenicol

Originally produced from a *Streptomyces*, chloramphenicol (Fig. 10.16A) has since been totally synthesized. It has a broad spectrum of activity, but exerts a bacteristatic effect. It has antirickettsial ac-

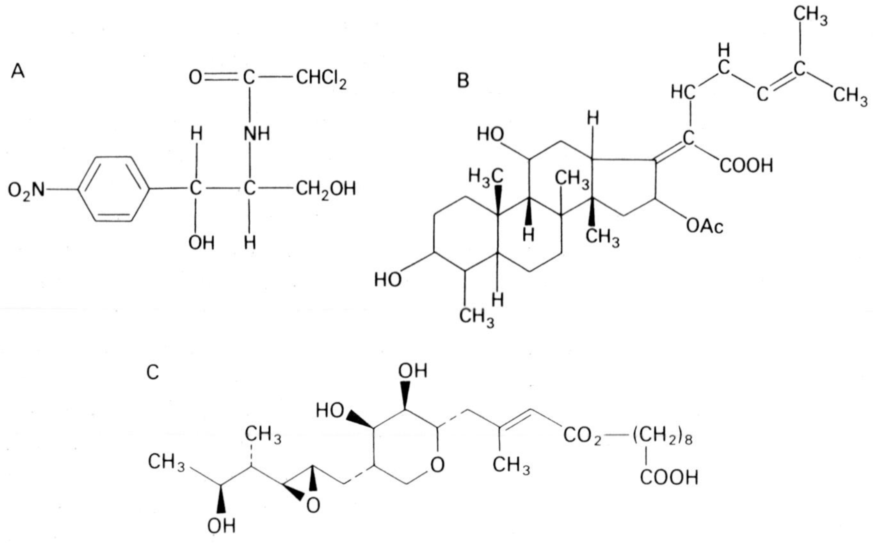

Fig. 10.16 Miscellaneous antibiotics: A, chloramphenicol; B, fusidic acid; C, mupirocin.

tivity and is inhibitory to the larger viruses. Unfortunately, aplastic anaemia, which is dose-related, may result from treatment in a proportion of patients. It should thus not be given for minor infections and its usage should be restricted to cases where no effective alternative exists, e.g. typhoid fever resistant to other antibiotics (see Chapter 14). Some bacteria (see Chapter 13) can produce an enzyme, chloramphenicol acetyltransferase, that acetylates the hydroxyl groups in the side-chain of the antibiotic to produce, initially, 3-acetoxychloramphenicol and, finally, 1,3-diacetoxychloramphenicol, which lacks antibacterial activity. The design of fluorinated derivatives of chloramphenicol that are not acetylated by this enzyme could be a significant finding, although toxicity may be a problem.

The antibiotic is administered orally as the palmitate, which is tasteless; this is hydrolysed to chloramphenicol in the gastrointestinal tract. The highly water-soluble chloramphenicol sodium succinate is used in the parenteral formulation, and thus acts as a pro-drug. A semisynthetic derivative of chloramphenicol, thiamphenicol, is claimed to be less toxic than chloramphenicol.

11.2 Fusidic acid

Employed as a sodium salt, fusidic acid (Fig. 10.16B) is active against many types of Gram-positive bacteria, especially staphylococci, although streptococci are relatively resistant. It is employed in the treatment of staphylococcal infections, including strains resistant to other antibiotics. However, bacterial resistance may occur *in vitro* and *in vivo*.

11.3 Mupirocin (pseudomonic acid A)

Mupirocin (Fig. 10.16C) is the main fermentation product obtained from *Ps. fluorescens*. Other pseudomonic acids (B, C and D) are also produced. Mupirocin is active predominantly against staphylococci and most streptococci, but *Enterococcus faecalis* and Gram-negative bacilli are resistant. There is also evidence of plasmid-mediated mupirocin resistance in some clinical isolates of *Staph. aureus*. Mupirocin is employed topically in eradicating nasal and skin carriage of staphylococci, including methicillin-resistant *Staph. aureus* (MRSA) colonization.

12 Antifungal antibiotics

In contrast to the wide range of antibacterial antibiotics, there are very few antifungal antibiotics that can be used systemically. Lack of toxicity is, as always, of paramount importance, but the differences in structure of, and some biosynthetic processes in, fungal cells (Chapter 4) mean that antibacterial antibiotics are usually inactive against fungi.

Fungal infections are normally less virulent in nature than are bacterial or viral infections but may, nevertheless, pose a problem in individuals with a depressed immune system, e.g. AIDS sufferers.

12.1 Griseofulvin

This is a metabolic by-product of *Penicillium griseofulvum*. Griseofulvin (Fig. 10.17A) was first isolated in 1939, but it was not until 1958 that its antifungal activity was discovered. It is active against the dermatophytic fungi, i.e. those such as *Trichophyton* causing ringworm. It is ineffective against *Candida albicans*, the causative agent of oral thrush and intestinal candidiasis, and against bacteria, and there is thus no disturbance of the normal bacterial flora of the gut.

Griseofulvin is administered orally in the form of tablets. It is not totally absorbed when given orally, and one method of increasing absorption is to reduce the particle size of the drug. Griseofulvin is deposited in the deeper layers of the skin and in hair keratin, and is therefore employed in chemotherapy of fungal infections of these areas caused by susceptible organisms.

12.2 Polyenes

Polyene antibiotics are characterized by possessing a large ring containing a lactone group and a hydrophobic region consisting of a sequence of four to seven conjugated double bonds. The most important polyenes are nystatin and amphotericin B (Fig. 10.17B and C, respectively).

Nystatin has a specific action on *C. albicans* and is of no value in the treatment of any other type of infection. It is poorly absorbed from the gastrointestinal tract; even after very large doses, the blood level is insignificant. It is administered orally in the treatment of oral thrush and intestinal candidiasis infections.

Amphotericin B is particularly effective against systemic infections caused by *C. albicans* and *Cryptococcus neoformans*. It is poorly absorbed from the gastrointestinal tract and is thus usually administered by intravenous injection under strict medical supervision. Amphotericin B methyl ester (Fig. 10.17C) is water-soluble, unlike amphotericin B itself, and can be administered intravenously as a solution. The two forms have equal antifungal activity but higher peak serum levels are obtained with the ester. Although the ester is claimed to be less toxic, neurological effects have been observed. An ascorbate salt has recently been described which is water-soluble, of similar activity and less toxic. Lipid-based and liposomal formulations of amphotericin are also available which exhibit lower toxicity than conventional aqueous formulations; they may therefore be given in higher doses.

13 Synthetic antimicrobial agents

13.1 Sulphonamides

Sulphonamides were introduced by Domagk in 1935. It had been shown that a red azo dye, prontosil (Fig. 10.18B), had a curative effect on mice infected with β-haemolytic streptococci; it was subsequently found that *in vivo*, prontosil was converted into sulphanilamide. Chemical modifications of the nucleus of sulphanilamide (see Fig. 10.18A) gave compounds with higher antibacterial activity, although this was often accompanied by greater toxicity. In general, it may be stated that the sulphonamides have a broadly similar antibacterial activity but differ widely in pharmacological actions.

Bacteria that are almost always sensitive to the sulphonamides include *Strep. pneumoniae*, β-haemolytic streptococci, *Escherichia coli* and *Proteus mirabilis*; those almost always resistant include *Enterococcus faecalis*, *Ps. aeruginosa*, indole-positive *Proteus* and *Klebsiella*; whereas bacteria showing a marked variation in response include *Staph. aureus*, gonococci, *H. influenzae* and hospital strains of *E. coli* and *Pr. mirabilis*.

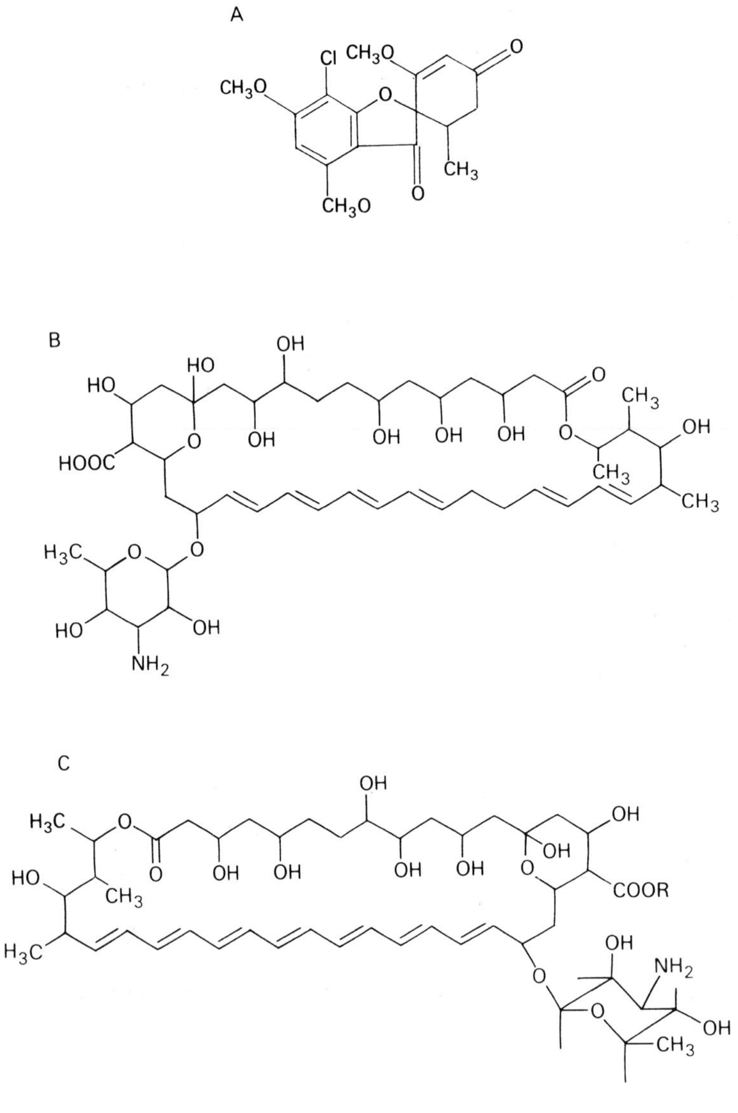

Fig. 10.17 Antifungal antibiotics: A, griseofulvin; B, nystatin; C, amphotericin (R = H) and its methyl ester (R = CH₃).

The sulphonamides show considerable variation in the extent of their absorption into the bloodstream. For example, sulphadimidine and sulphadiazine are rapidly absorbed, whereas succinylsulphathiazole and phthalylsulphathiazole are poorly absorbed and are excreted unchanged in the faeces.

From a clinical point of view, the sulphonamides were extremely useful for the treatment of uncomplicated urinary tract infections caused by *E. coli* in domiciliary practice, although their value has diminished in recent years due to resistance develop-ment. They have also been employed in treating meningococcal meningitis (again, the number of sulphonamide-resistant meningococcal strains is a current problem) and superficial eye infections.

13.2 Diaminopyrimidine derivatives

Small-molecule diaminopyrimidine derivatives were shown in 1948 to have an antifolate action. Subsequently, compounds were developed that were highly active against human cells (e.g. the use of methotrexate as an anticancer agent), protozoa

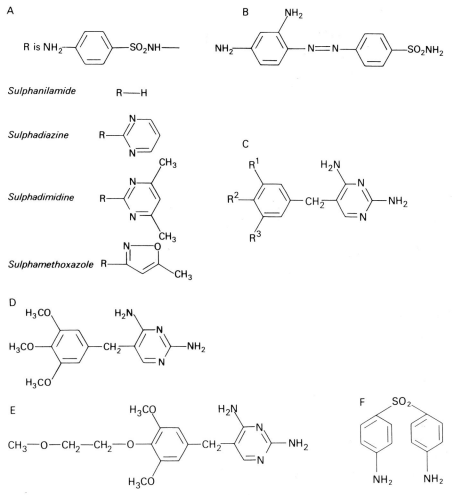

Fig. 10.18 A, Some sulphonamides; B, prontosil rubrum; C, unsubstituted diaminobenzylpyrimidines; D, trimethoprim; E, tetroxoprim; F, dapsone.

(e.g. the use of pyrimethamine in malaria) or bacteria (e.g. trimethoprim: Fig. 10.18D). Unsubstituted diaminobenzylpyrimidines (Fig. 10.18C) bind poorly to bacterial dihydrofolate reductase (DHFR). The introduction of one, two or especially three methoxy groups (as in trimethoprim) produces a highly selective antibacterial agent. A more recent antibacterial addition is tetroxoprim (2,4-diamino-5-(3′,5′-dimethoxy-4′-methoxyethoxybenzyl) pyrimidine; Fig. 10.18E) which retains methoxy groups at R^1 and R^3 and has a methoxyethoxy group at R^2. Trimethoprim and tetroxoprim have a broad spectrum of activity but

resistance can arise from a non-susceptible target site, i.e. an altered DHFR (see Chapter 13).

13.3 Co-trimoxazole

Co-trimoxazole is a mixture of sulphamethoxazole (five parts) and trimethoprim (one part). The reason for using this combination is based upon the *in vitro* finding that there is a 'sequential blockade' of folic acid synthesis, in which the sulphonamide is a competitive inhibitor of dihydropteroate synthetase and trimethoprim inhibits DHFR (see Chapter 12). The optimum ratio of the two components may not be achieved *in vivo* and arguments continue as to the clinical value of co-trimoxazole, with many advocating the use of trimethoprim alone. Co-trimoxazole is the agent of choice in treating pneumonias caused by *Pneumocystis carinii*, a yeast (although it had been classified as a proto-zoan). *Pneumocystis carinii* is a common cause of pneumonia in patients receiving immunosuppressive therapy and in those with AIDS.

13.4 Dapsone

Dapsone (diaminodiphenylsulphone; Fig. 10.18F) is used specifically in the treatment of leprosy. However, because resistance to dapsone is unfortunately now well known, it is recommended that dapsone be used in conjunction with rifampicin and clofazimine.

13.5 Antitubercular drugs

The three standard drugs used in the treatment of tuberculosis were streptomycin (considered above), *p*-aminosalicylic acid (PAS) and isoniazid (isonicotinylhydrazide, INH; synonym, isonico-tinic acid hydrazine, INAH). The tubercle bacillus rapidly becomes resistant to streptomycin, and the role of PAS was mainly that of preventing this development of resistance.

The current approach is to treat tuberculosis in two phases: an *initial* phase where a combination of three drugs is used to reduce the bacterial level as rapidly as possible, and a *continuation* phase in which a combination of two drugs is employed. Front-line drugs are isoniazid, rifampicin, strepto-mycin and ethambutol. Pyrazinamide, which has good meningeal penetration, and is thus particularly useful in tubercular meningitis, may be used in the initial phase to produce a highly bactericidal response.

Isoniazid has no significant effect against organisms other than mycobacteria. It is given orally. Cross-resistance between it, streptomycin and rifampicin has not been found to occur.

When bacterial resistance to these primary agents exists or develops, treatment with the sec-ondary antitubercular drugs has to be considered. The latter group comprises capreomycin, cycloser-ine, some of the newer macrolides (azithromycin, clarithromycin), 4-quinolones (e.g. ciprofloxacin, ofloxacin) and prothionamide (no longer marketed in the UK). Prothionamide, pyrazinamide and ethionamide are, like isoniazid, derivatives of isoni-cotinic acid. The *British National Formulary* no longer lists ethionamide as being a suitable antitu-bercular drug. Chemical structures of the above, and of thiacetazone (not used nowadays because of its side-effects) are presented in Fig. 10.19.

There has, unfortunately, been a global resur-gence of tuberculosis in recent years. Multiple drug-resistant *M. tuberculosis* (MDRTB) strains have been isolated in which resistance has been acquired to many drugs used in the treatment of this disease.

13.6 Nitrofuran compounds

The nitrofuran group of drugs (Fig. 10.20) is based on the finding over 40 years ago that a nitro group in the 5 position of 2-substituted furans endowed these compounds with antibacterial activity. Many hundreds of such compounds have been synthe-sized, but only a few are in current therapeutic use. In the most important nitrofurans, an azomethine group, —CH=N—, is attached at C-2 and a nitro group at C-5. Less important nitrofurans have a vinyl group, —CH=CH—, at C-2.

Biological activity is lost if:
1 the nitro ring is reduced;
2 the —CH=N— linkage undergoes hydrolytic de-composition; or
3 the —CH=CH— linkage is oxidized.

The nitrofurans show antibacterial activity against a wide spectrum of microorganisms, but fu-raltadone has now been withdrawn from use be-cause of its toxicity. Furazolidone has a very high activity against most members of the Enterobacteri-aceae, and has been used in the treatment of diar-rhoea and gastrointestinal disturbances of bacterial origin. Nitrofurantoin is used in the treatment of urinary tract infections; antibacterial levels are not reached in the blood and the drug is concentrated in the urine. It is most active at acid pH. Nitrofurazone is used mainly as a topical agent in the treatment of burns and wounds and also in certain types of ear infections. The nitrofurans are believed to be mutagenic.

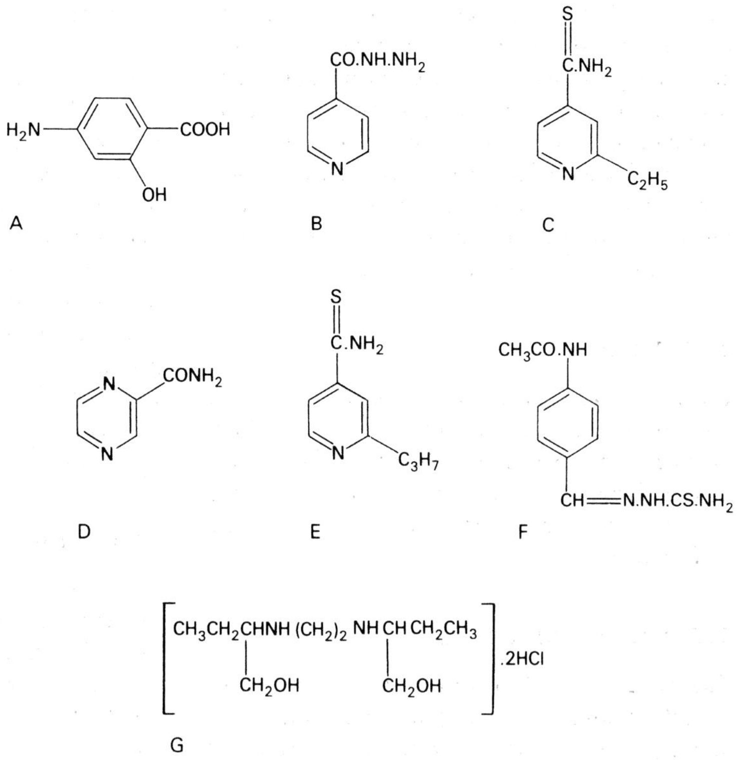

Fig. 10.19 Antitubercular compounds (see text also for details of antibiotics): A, PAS; B, isoniazid; c, ethionamide; D, pyrazinamide; E, prothionamide; F, thiacetazone; G, ethambutol.

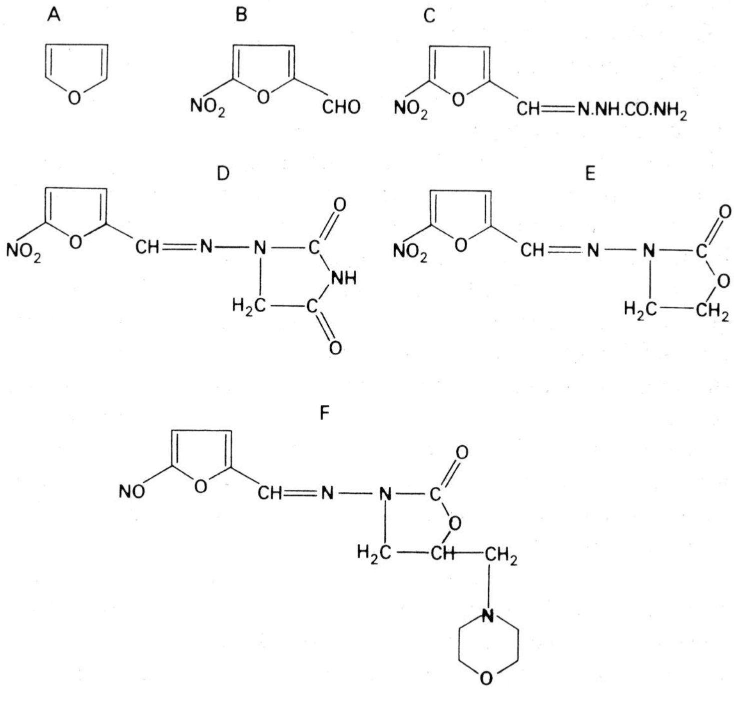

Fig. 10.20 A, Furan; B, 5-nitrofurfural; C–F, nitrofuran drugs: respectively C, nitrofurazone, D, nitrofurantoin, E, furazolidone and F, furaltadone.

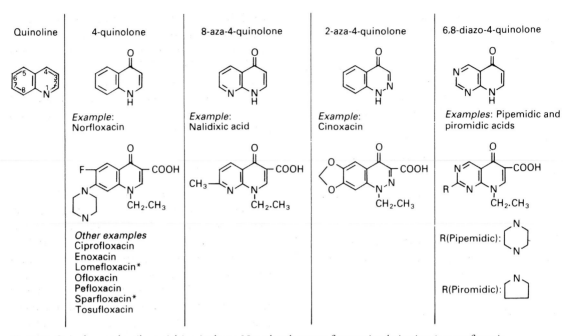

Fig. 10.21 Quinolone and antibacterial 4-quinolones. Note that the newer fluoroquine derivatives (e.g. norfloxacin, ciprofloxacin, ofloxacin) have a 6-fluoro and a 7-piperazino substituent. Drugs marked with an asterisk are difluorinated quinolones, with a second fluorine atom at C-8.

13.7 4-Quinolone antibacterials

Over 10 000 quinolone antibacterial agents have now been synthesized. Nalidixic acid is regarded as the progenitor of the new quinolones. It has been used for several years as a clinically important drug in the treatment of urinary tract infections. Since its clinical introduction, other 4-quinolone antibacterial agents have been synthesized, some of which show considerably greater antibacterial potency. Furthermore, this means that many types of bacteria not susceptible to nalidixic acid therapy may be sensitive to the newer derivatives. The most important development was the introduction of a fluorine substituent at C-6, which led to a considerable increase in potency and spectrum of activity compared with nalidixic acid. These second-generation quinolones are known as fluoroquinolones, examples of which are ciprofloxacin and norfloxacin (Fig. 10.21).

Nalidixic acid is unusual in that it is active against several different types of Gram-negative bacteria, whereas Gram-positive organisms are resistant.

However, the newer fluoroquinolone derivatives show superior activity against Enterobacteriaceae and *Ps. aeruginosa*, and their spectrum also includes staphylococci but not streptococci. Extensive studies with norfloxacin have demonstrated that its broad spectrum, high urine concentration and oral administration make it a useful drug in the treatment of urinary infections. Ciprofloxacin may be used in the treatment of organisms resistant to other antibiotics; it can also be used in conjunction with a β-lactam or aminoglycoside antibiotic, e.g. when severe neutropenia is present.

The third and most recently developed generation of quinolones has maintained many of the properties of the second generation; examples are lomefloxacin, sparfloxacin (both difluorinated derivatives) and temafloxacin (a trifluorinated derivative). Lomefloxacin has a sufficiently long half-life to allow once-daily dosing, but adverse photosensitivity reactions are now being recognized. Sparfloxacin retains high activity against Gram-negative bacteria but has enhanced activity against Gram-positive cocci and anaerobes. Temafloxacin

Table 10.4 Antimicrobial imidazoles

Antimicrobial or other activity	Examples
Antibacterial	Metronidazole, tinidazole: anaerobic bacteria only
Antiprotozoal	Metronidazole, tinidazole
Anthelmintic	Mebendazole
Antifungal	Clotrimazole, miconazole, econazole, ketoconazole
	Newer imidazoles: fluconazole, itraconazole

has, unfortunately, been withdrawn from clinical use because of unexpected severe haemolytic and nephrotoxic reactions.

13.8 Imidazole derivatives

The imidazoles comprise a large and diverse group of compounds with properties encompassing antibacterial (metronidazole), antiprotozoal (metronidazole), antifungal (clotrimazole, miconazole, ketoconazole, econazole) and anthelmintic (mebendazole) activity: see Table 10.4.

Metronidazole (Fig. 10.22A) inhibits the growth of pathogenic protozoa, very low concentrations being effective against the protozoa *Trichomonas vaginalis*, *Entamoeba histolytica* and *Giardia lamblia*. It is also used to treat bacterial vaginosis caused by *Gardnerella vaginalis*. Given orally, it cures 90–100% of sexually transmitted urogenital infections caused by *T. vaginalis*. It has also been found that metronidazole is effective against anaerobic bacteria, for example *B. fragilis*, and against facultative anaerobes grown under anaerobic, but not aerobic, conditions. Metronidazole is administered orally or in the form of suppositories.

Other imidazole derivatives include clotrimazole (Fig. 10.22B), miconazole (Fig. 10.22C) and econazole (Fig. 10.22D), all of which possess a broad antimycotic spectrum with some antibacterial activity and are used topically. Miconazole is used topically but can also be administered by intravenous or intrathecal injection in the treatment of severe systemic or meningeal fungal infections. Newer imidazoles are (a) ketoconazole (Fig. 10.22E),

which is used orally for the treatment of systemic fungal infections (but not when there is central nervous system involvement or where the infection is life-threatening), (b) fluconazole (Fig. 10.22F), which is given orally or by intravenous infusion in the treatment of candidiasis and cryptococcal meningitis. Itraconazole is well absorbed when given orally after food.

13.9 Flucytosine

Flucytosine (5-fluorocytosine; Fig. 10.22G) is a narrow-spectrum antifungal agent with greatest activity against yeasts such as *Candida*, *Cryptococcus* and *Torulopsis*. Evidence has been presented which shows that, once inside the fungal cell, flucytosine is deaminated to 5-fluorouracil (Fig. 10.22H). This is converted by the enzyme pyrophosphorylase to 5-fluorouridine monophosphate (FUMP), diphosphate (FUDP) and triphosphate (FUTP), which inhibits RNA synthesis; 5-fluorouracil itself has poor penetration into fungi. *Candida albicans* is known to convert FUMP to 5-fluorodeoxyuridine monophosphate (FdUMP), which inhibits DNA synthesis by virtue of its effect on thymidylate synthetase. Resistance can occur *in vivo* by reduced uptake into fungal cells of flucytosine or by decreased accumulation of FUTP and FdUMP.

13.10 Synthetic allylamines

Terbinafine (Fig. 10.22I), a member of the allylamine class of antimycotics, is an inhibitor of the enzyme squalene epoxidase in fungal ergosterol biosynthesis. Terbinafine is orally active, is fungicidal and is effective against a broad range of dermatophytes and yeasts. It can also be used topically as a cream.

13.11 Synthetic thiocarbamates

The synthetic thiocarbamates, of which tolnaftate (Fig. 10.22J) is an example, also inhibit squalene epoxidase. Tolnaftate inhibits this enzyme from *C. albicans*, but is inactive against whole cells, presumably because of its inability to penetrate the cell wall. Tolnaftate is used topically in the treatment or prophylaxis of tinea.

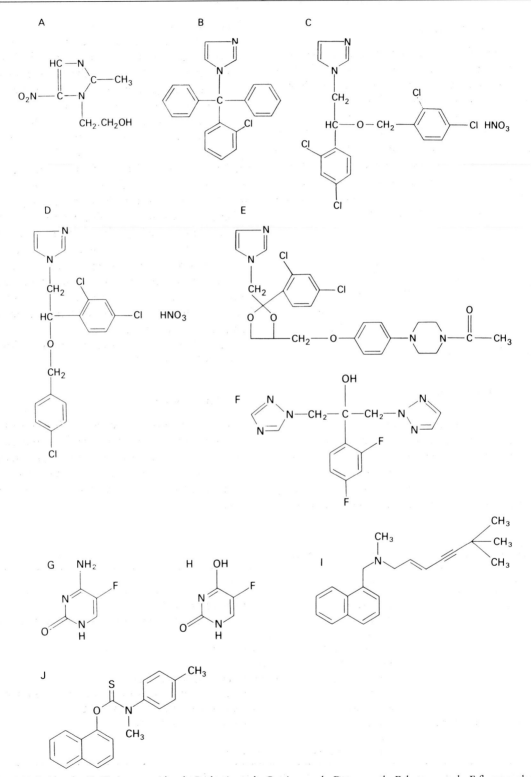

Fig. 10.22 Imidazoles (A–F): A, metronidazole; B, clotrimazole; C, miconazole; D, econazole; E, ketoconazole; F, fluconazole; G, flucytosine; H, 5-fluorouracil; I, terbinafine; J, tolnaftate.

13.12 Oxazolidinones

The oxazolidinones are a new class of synthetic antimicrobial agents. Produced in 1987, they were found to be active *in vitro* against antibiotic-susceptible and -resistant cocci and did not demonstrate cross-resistance with any other antibiotics.

Linezolid (Fig. 10.23), a totally synthetic 3-(fluorophenyl)-2-oxalidinone, was selected for use in clinical trials. It has subsequently been introduced into clinical medicine and appears to have a useful role to play. Already, however, linezolid-resistant MRSA strains have been described.

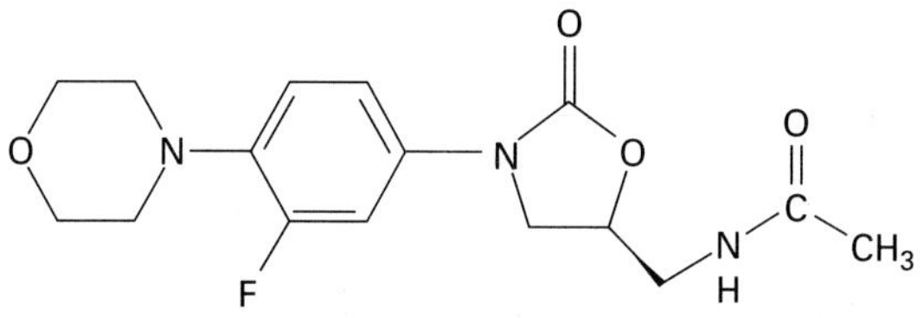

Fig. 10.23 Linezolid.

14 Antiviral drugs

Several compounds are known that are inhibitory to mammalian viruses in tissue culture, but only a few can be used in the treatment of human viral infections. The main problem in designing and developing antiviral agents is the lack of selective toxicity that is normally possessed by most compounds.

Viruses literally 'take over' the machinery of an infected human cell and thus an antiviral drug must be remarkably selectively toxic if it is to inhibit the viral particle without adversely affecting the human cell. Consequently, in comparison with antibacterial agents, very few inhibitors can be considered as being safe antiviral drugs, although the situation is improving. Possible sites of attack by antiviral agents include prevention of adsorption of a viral particle to the host cell, prevention of the intracellular penetration of the adsorbed virus, and inhibition of protein or nucleic acid synthesis (Chapter 5).

Genetic information for viral reproduction resides in its nucleic acid (DNA or RNA: see Chapter 5). The viral particle (virion) does not possess enzymes necessary for its own replication; after entry into the host cell, the virus uses the enzymes already present or induces the formation of new ones. Viruses replicate by synthesis of their separate components followed by assembly.

Antiviral drugs are considered below with a summary in Table 10.5.

14.1 Amantadines

Amantadine hydrochloride (Fig. 10.24A) does not prevent adsorption but inhibits viral penetration. It has a very narrow spectrum and is used prophylactically against infection with influenza A virus; it has no prophylactic value with other types of influenza virus.

Table 10.5 Examples of antiviral drugs and their clinical uses*

Group	Antiviral drug	Clinical uses
Nucleoside analogues	Idoxuridine	Skin including herpes labialis
	Ribavirin (tribavirin)	Severe respiratory syncytial virus bronchiolitis in infants and children
	Zidovudine	AIDS treatment
	Didanosine (DDI)	AIDS treatment
	Zalcitabine (DDC)	AIDS treatment
	Acyclovir (aciclovir)	Herpes simplex and varicella zoster
	Famciclovir	Cytomegalovirus infections in immunocompromised patients only
	Ganciclovir	Cytomegalovirus retinitis in patients with AIDS
Non-nucleoside analogues	Foscarnet	Prophylaxis: influenza A outbreak
	Amantadine	HIV
	Protease inhibitors	HIV infection

* For further information, see the current issue of the *British National Formulary*.

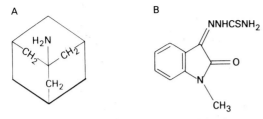

Fig. 10.24 A, Amantadine (used as the hydrochloride); B, methisazone.

14.2 Methisazone

Methisazone (Fig. 10.24B) inhibits DNA viruses (particularly vaccinia and variola) but not RNA viruses, and has been used in the prophylaxis of smallpox. It is now little used, especially as, according to the World Health Organization, smallpox has been eradicated.

14.3 Nucleoside analogues

Various nucleoside analogues have been developed that inhibit nucleic acid synthesis. Idoxuridine (2'-deoxy-5-iodouridine; IUdR; Fig. 10.25C) is a thymidine analogue which inhibits the utilization of thymidine (Fig. 10.25A) in the rapid synthesis of DNA that normally occurs in herpes-infected cells. Unfortunately, because of its toxicity, idoxuridine is unsuitable for systemic use and it is restricted to topical treatment of herpes-infected eyes. Other nucleoside analogues include the following: cytarabine (cytosine arabinoside; Ara-C; Fig. 10.25D) which has antineoplastic and antiviral properties and which has been employed topically to treat herpes keratitis resistant to idoxuridine; adenosine arabinoside (Ara-A; vidarabine); and ribavirin (1-β-D-ribofuranosyl-1,2,4-triazole-3, carboxamide; Fig. 10.25E) which has a broad spectrum of activity, inhibiting both RNA and DNA viruses. Vidarabine, in particular, has a high degree of selectivity against viral DNA replication and is primarily active against herpesviruses and some poxviruses. It may be used systemically or topically. It is related structurally to guanosine (Fig. 10.25B).

Human immunodeficiency virus (HIV) is a retrovirus, i.e. its RNA is converted in human cells by the enzyme reverse transcriptase to DNA, which is incorporated into the human genome and is responsible for producing new HIV particles. Zidovudine (azidothymidine, AZT; Fig. 10.25F) is a structural analogue of thymidine (Fig. 10.25A) and is used to treat AIDS patients. Zidovudine is converted in both infected and uninfected cells to the mono-, di- and eventually tri-phosphate derivatives. Zidovudine triphosphate, the active form, is a potent inhibitor of HIV replication, being mistaken for thymidine by reverse transcriptase. Premature chain termination of viral DNA ensues. However, AZT is relatively toxic because, as pointed out above, it is converted to the triphosphate by cellular enzymes and is thus also activated in uninfected cells.

2'3'-Dideoxycytidine (DDC, zalcitabine), a nucleoside analogue that also inhibits reverse transcriptase, is more active than zidovudine *in vitro*, and (unlike zidovudine) does not suppress erythropoiesis. DDC is not without toxicity, however, and a severe peripheral neurotoxicity, which is dose-related, has been reported. The chemical structures of DDC and of another analogue with similar properties, 2'3'-dideoxyinosine (DDI, didanosine), are presented in Fig. 10.25 (G, H, respectively).

Didanosine is a nucleoside reverse transcriptase inhibitor structurally related to inosine. It is converted intracellularly to dideoxyadenosine triphosphate. It acts against retroviruses, including HIV.

Aciclovir (acycloguanosine, Fig. 10.25I) is a novel type of nucleoside analogue that becomes activated only in herpes-infected host cells by a herpes-specific enzyme, thymidine kinase. This enzyme initiates conversion of aciclovir initially to a monophosphate and then to the antiviral triphosphate which inhibits viral DNA polymerase. The host cell polymerase is not inhibited to the same extent, and the antiviral triphosphate is not produced in uninfected cells. Ganciclovir (Fig. 10.25J) is up to 100 times more active than aciclovir against human cytomegalovirus (CMV) but is also much more toxic; it is reserved for the treatment of severe CMV in immunocompromised patients. Famciclovir is similar, being a pro-drug of penciclovir (an antiviral with similar activity to aciclovir) and valociclovir is a pro-drug ester of aciclovir.

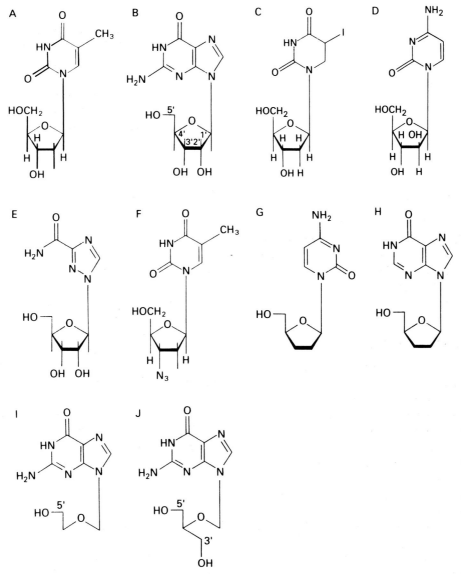

Fig. 10.25 Thymidine (A), guanosine (B) and some nucleoside analogues (C–J). C, idoxuridine; D, cytarabine; E, ribavirin; F, zidovudine (AZT); G, dideoxycytidine (DDC); H, dideoxyinosine (DDI); I, acyclovir; J, ganciclovir.

14.4 Non-nucleoside compounds

14.4.1 Phosphonoacetic acid and sodium phosphonoformate

Apart from the amantadines (section 14.1) and me-thisazone (section 14.2), various non-nucleoside drugs have shown antiviral activity. Two simple molecules with potent activity are phosphonoacetic acid (Fig. 10.26A) and sodium phosphonoformate (foscarnet, Fig. 10.26B). Phosphonoacetic acid has a high specificity for herpes simplex DNA synthesis, and has been shown to be non-mutagenic in experimental animals, but is highly toxic. Foscarnet inhibits herpes DNA polymerase, is non-toxic when applied to the skin and is a potentially useful agent in treating herpes simplex labialis (cold sores). It is

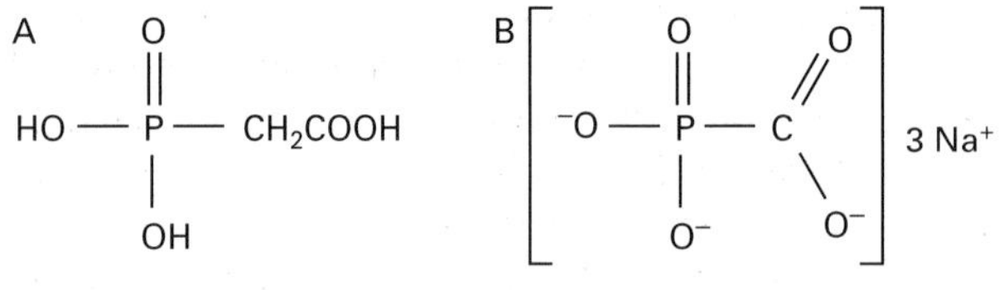

Fig. 10.26 A, Phosphonoacetic acid; B, sodium phosphonoformate (foscarnet).

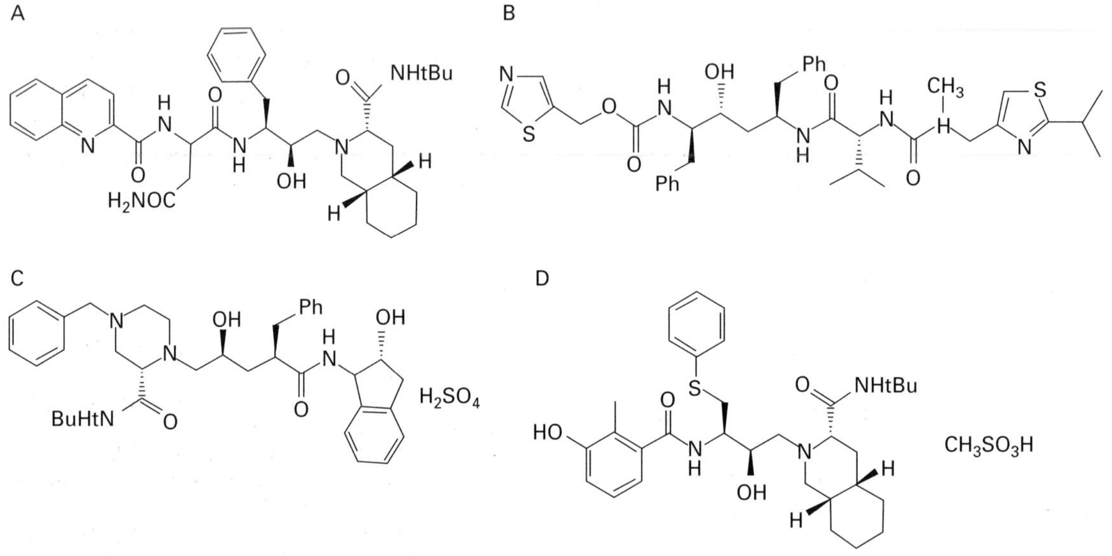

Fig. 10.27 HIV protease inhibitors: A, saquinavir; B, ritonavir; C, inidavir; D, nelfinavir.

used for cytomegalovirus retinitis in patients with AIDS in whom ganciclovir is inappropriate. Tetrahydroimidazobenzodiazepinone (TIBO) compounds have shown excellent activity *in vitro* against HIV reverse transcriptase in HIV type 1 (HIV-1) but not HIV-2 or other retroviruses.

14.4.2 Protease inhibitors

New antiviral agents have been based on virus-specific targets, especially the viral enzymes that are involved in the viral life cycle, i.e. responsible for the production of infectious viral particles. Research has focused on virus-encoded proteases that fulfil this role. Thus, specific inhibitors of HIV, herpesvirus and hepatitis C virus proteases are now known. Examples of clinically approved HIV pro-

tease inhibitors are saquinavir, ritonavir, indinavir and nelfinavir (Fig. 10.27A–D).

14.5 Interferons

Interferon is a low molecular weight protein, produced by virus-infected cells, that itself induces the formation of a second protein inhibiting the transcription of viral mRNA. Interferon is produced by the host cell in response to the virus particle, the viral nucleic acid and non-viral agents, including synthetic polynucleotides such as polyinosinic acid and polycytidylic acid (poly I:C). There are two types of interferon.

Type I interferons. These are acid-stable and comprise two major classes, leucocyte interferon (Le-IFN, IFN-α) released by stimulated leucocytes, and fibroblast interferon (F-IFN, IFN-β) released by stimulated fibroblasts.

Type II interferons. These are acid-labile and are also known as 'immune' (IFN-γ) interferons because they are produced by T lymphocytes (see Chapter 8) in the cellular immune system in response to specific antigens.

Type I interferons induce a virus-resistant state in human cells, whereas type II are more active in inhibiting growth of tumour cells.

Disappointingly low yields of F-IFN and Le-IFN are achieved from eukaryotic cells but recombinant DNA technology has been employed to produce interferon in prokaryotic cells (bacteria). This aspect is considered in more detail in Chapter 24.

sidered to be much fewer than originally thought. There is also the problem of a chemical or physical incompatibility between two drugs. Examples where combinations have an important role to play in antibacterial chemotherapy were provided earlier (sections 2.3 and 2.9) in which a β-lactamase inhibitor and an appropriate β-lactamase-labile penicillin form a single pharmaceutical product, and in section 8 (streptogramins). Further comment on drug combinations can be found in Chapter 14.

It must also be noted that a combination of two β-lactams does not necessarily produce a synergistic effect. Some antibiotics are excellent inducers of β-lactamase, and consequently a reduced response (antagonism) may be produced.

15 Drug combinations

A combination of two antibacterial agents may produce the following responses.

1 Synergism, where the joint effect is greater than the sum of the effects of each drug acting alone.

2 Additive effect, in which the combined effect is equal to the arithmetic sum of the effects of the two individual agents.

3 Antagonism (interference), in which there is a lesser effect of the mixture than that of the more potent drug action alone.

There are four possible justifications as to the use of antibacterial agents in combination.

1 The concept of clinical synergism, which may be extremely difficult to demonstrate convincingly. Even with trimethoprim plus sulphamethoxazole, where true synergism occurs *in vitro*, the optimum ratio of the two components may not always be present *in vivo*, i.e. at the site of infection in a particular tissue.

2 A wider spectrum of cover may be obtained, which may be (a) desirable as an emergency measure in life-threatening situations; or (b) of use in treating mixed infections.

3 The emergence of resistant organisms may be prevented. A classical example here occurs in combined antitubercular therapy (see earlier).

4 A possible reduction in dosage of a toxic drug may be achieved.

Indications for combined therapy are now con-

16 Further reading

Axelsen, P. H. (2002) *Essentials of Antimicrobial Pharmacology.* Humana Press, Totowa, NJ.

Bean, B. (1992) Antiviral therapy: current concepts and practices. *Clin Microbiol Rev,* 5, 146–182.

Bowden, K., Hants, N.V. & Watson, C.A. (1993) Structure-activity relationships of dihydrofolate reductase inhibitors. *J Chemother,* 5, 377–388.

Bugg, C.E., Carson, W.M. & Montgomery, J.A. (1993) Drugs by design. *Sci Am,* 269, 92–98.

British National Formulary. British Medical Association & Pharmaceutical Press, London. [The chapter on drugs used in the treatment of infections is a particularly useful section. New editions of the BNF appear at regular intervals]

Brown, A.G. (1981) New naturally occurring β-lactam antibiotics and related compounds. *J Antimicrob Chemother,* 7, 15–48.

Chopra, I. (1998) Research and development of antibacterial agents. *Curr Opinion Microbiol,* 1, 855–869.

Chopra, I., Hawkey, P.M. & Hinton, M. (1992) Tetracyclines, molecular and clinical aspects. *J Antimicrob Chemother,* 29, 245–277.

Cowan, M.M. (1999) Plant products as antimicrobial agents. *Clin Microbiol Rev,* 12, 564–582.

De Clerq, E. (1997) In search of a selective antiviral chemotherapy. *Clin Microbiol Rev,* 10, 674–693.

Finch, R.G., Greenwood, D., Norrby, R. & Whitley, R. (2002) *Antibiotic and Chemotherapy,* 8th edn. Churchill Livingstone, London and Edinburgh.

Hamilton-Miller, J.M.T. (1991) From foreign pharmacopoeias: 'new' antibiotics from old? *J Antimicrob Chemother,* 27, 702–705.

Hooper, D.C. & Wolfson, J.S. (1993) *Quinolone Antimicrobial Agents,* 2nd edn. American Society for Microbiology, Washington.

Hunter, P.A., Darby, G.K. & Russell, N.J. (1995) *Fifty Years of Antimicrobials: Past Perspectives and Future Trends*. 53rd Symposium of the Society for General Microbiology. Cambridge University Press, Cambridge.

Kuntz, I.D. (1992) Structure-based strategies for drug design and discovery. *Science*, **257**, 1079–1082.

Patick, A.K. & Potts, K.E. (1998) Protease inhibitors as antiviral agents. *Clin Microbiol Rev*, **11**, 614–627.

Power, E.G.M. & Russell, A.D. (1998) Design of antimicrobial chemotherapeutic agents. In: Smith, H.J., ed. *Introduction to Principles of Drug Design*, 3rd edn. Wright, Bristol.

Reeves, D.S. & Howard, A.J. (1991) New macrolides — the respiratory antibiotics for the 1990s. *J Hosp Infect*, **19** (Suppl. A).

Russell, A.D. & Chopra, I. (1996) *Understanding Antibacterial Action and Resistance*, 2nd edn. Ellis Horwood, Chichester.

Sammes, P.G. (1997–1982) *Topics in Antibiotic Chemistry*, vols 1–5. Ellis Horwood, Chichester.

Shanson, D.C. (1999) *Microbiology in Clinical Practice*, 3rd edn. Wright, London.

Chapter 11

Laboratory evaluation of antimicrobial agents

JMB Smith

1 Introduction

As the range of microorganisms acquiring re-sistance to the presently available antimicrobial agents continues to increase, evaluation of the po-tential antimicrobial action and nature of the in-hibitory and lethal effects of established and novel therapeutic agents and biocides has re-surfaced as important laboratory procedures. A linkage be-tween biocide usage and antibiotic resistance po-tentially exists. In addition, the emergence of new infectious agents (e.g. prions) and the escalating occurrence of significant bloodborne viruses (e.g. human immunodeficiency viruses, hepatitis B and C) which may readily contaminate medical instru-ments or the environment has jolted into reality the need for suitable and proven liquid disinfecting and sterilizing agents. Clearly the availability and effica-cy of such chemical agents must be backed by ap-propriate laboratory data. The events of September

11, 2001, in New York and the subsequent threat of bioterrorism worldwide, together with the continu-ing problems of legionellosis and contaminated air-conditioning units, has also renewed interest and debate into the value of biocides in the environmen-tal control of microorganisms and microbial dis-eases. Tests for evaluating candidate antimicrobial agents to be used in human and animal medicine as well as environmental biocides are now significant laboratory considerations.

1.1 Definitions

Key terms such as disinfection, sterilization and preservation are defined in Chapter 17 but other terms are often employed to describe the antimicro-bial activity of agents. Hence, terms such as bio-cidal, bactericidal, virucidal and fungicidal describe a killing activity, whereas bacteriostatic and fungi-static refer to inhibition of growth of the organism

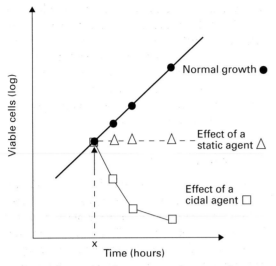

Fig. 11.1 Effect on the subsequent growth pattern of inhibitory (static Δ) or cidal (□) agents added at time X (the normal growth pattern is indicated by the ● line).

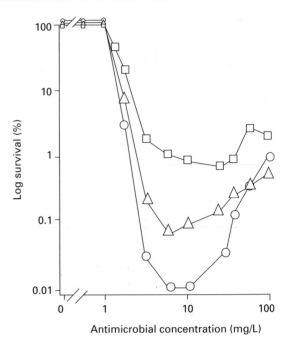

Fig. 11.2 Survival of *Enterococcus faecalis* exposed to a fluoroquinolone for 4 h at 37°C. Three initial bacterial concentrations were studied, 10^7 cfu/ml (□); 10^6 cfu/ml (Δ) and 10^5 cfu/ml (○). This clearly demonstrates a paradoxical effect (increasing antimicrobial concentrations past a critical level reveal decreased killing), and the effects of increased inoculum densities on subsequent killing (courtesy of Dr Z. Hashmi).

(Fig. 11.1). It must be remembered, however, that some microorganisms that appear to be dead and non-cultivable may be revived by appropriate methods, and that organisms incapable of multiplication may retain some enzymatic activity.

When evaluating the activity of antibacterial agents the terms minimum inhibitory concentration (MIC) and minimum bactericidal concentration (MBC) are commonly used. MIC refers to the minimum concentration of an antimicrobial agent that inhibits growth of the microorganism under test and is generally recorded in mg/L or μg/ml. With most cidal antimicrobials, the MIC and MBC are often near or equal in value, although with essentially static agents (e.g. tetracycline), the lowest concentration required to kill the microorganism (i.e. the MBC) is invariably many times the MIC and clinically unachievable without damage to the human host. Similar cidal terms can be applied to studies involving other microbes, e.g. minimum fungicidal concentration (MFC).

'Tolerance' is a term that implies the ability of some bacterial strains to survive, but not grow, at levels of antimicrobial agent that should normally be cidal. This applies' particularly to systems employing the cell wall active β-lactams and glycopep-

tides, and to Gram-positive bacteria such as streptococci. Normally, MIC and MBC levels in such tests should be similar (i.e. within one or two doubling dilutions); if the MIC/MBC ratio is 32 or greater, the term tolerance is used. Tolerance may in some way be related to the Eagle phenomenon (paradoxical effect), where increasing concentrations of antimicrobial result in less killing rather than the expected increase in cidal activity (see Fig. 11.2).

2 Factors affecting the antimicrobial activity of disinfectants

Laboratory tests for the evaluation of chemicals with potential antimicrobial activity must be scientifically based and ensure that the agent is safe and

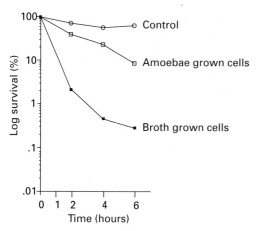

Fig. 11.3 Survival of stationary phase broth cultures of *Legionella pneumophila* and amoebae-grown *L. pneumophila* after exposure to 32 mg/L benzisothiazolone (Proxel) at 35°C in Ringer's solution. Adapted from Barker *et al.* (1992), *Appl Environ Microbiol*, 58, 2420–2425, with permission.

effective for its intended use. As shown by Krönig and Paul in the late 1890s, bacteria exposed to a cidal agent do not die simultaneously but in an orderly sequence, and attempts at applying the kinetics of pure chemical reactions to microbe/disinfectant interactions are often unrewarding. However, the antimicrobial/microorganism interaction is influenced by a variety of factors that may be related to natural (intrinsic) features of the microorganism involved and the chemical and physical environment in which tests are carried out. More expansive accounts concerning the dynamics of disinfection, relating largely to Chick's pioneering work with phenol in the early 20th century, can be readily accessed (see Further reading section).

2.1 Innate (natural) resistance of microorganisms

Microorganisms vary tremendously in their susceptibility to chemical disinfectants. Prions, bacterial endospores and mycobacteria possess the most innate resistance, while many vegetative bacteria and some viruses appear highly susceptible (see Chapter 17). In addition, microorganisms adhering to surfaces as biofilms or present within other cells (e.g. legionellae within amoebae), may reveal a marked

increase in resistance to disinfectants and biocides (Fig. 11.3). Therefore, when evaluating new disinfectants, a suitable range of microorganisms and environmental conditions must be included in tests. The European suspension test (prEN 12054) for hospital-related studies includes *Pseudomonas aeruginosa*, *Escherichia coli*, *Staphylococcus aureus* and *Enterococcus hirae*.

2.2 Microbial density

As many disinfectants require adsorption to the microbial cell surface prior to killing, dense cell populations may sequester all the available disinfectant before all cells are affected. Thus, from a practical point of view, the larger the number of microorganisms present, the longer it takes a disinfectant to complete killing of all cells. For instance, using identical test conditions, it has been shown that 10 spores of the anthrax bacillus (*Bacillus anthracis*) were destroyed in 30 minutes, while it took 3 hours to kill 100 000 (10^5) spores. The implications of washing and cleaning of objects (which removes most of the microorganisms) before disinfection, thus becomes obvious. However, when evaluating disinfectants in the laboratory, it must be remembered that unlike sterilization, kill curves with disinfectants may not be linear and the rate of killing may decrease at lower cell numbers (Fig. 11.3). Hence a 3-log killing may be more rapidly achieved with 10^8 than 10^4 cells. Cell numbers must, therefore, be standardized in disinfectant efficacy (suspension) tests and agreement reached on the degree of killing required over a stipulated time interval (see Table 11.1).

Table 11.1 Methods of recording viable cells remaining after exposure of an initial population of 1 000 000 (10^6) CFU to a cidal agent

Viable count remaining (CFU)	Log survival (%)	Log killing	% killing
100 000 (10^5)	10	1-log	90
10 000 (10^4)	1	2-log	99
1000 (10^3)	0.1	3-log	99.9
100 (10^2)	0.01	4-log	99.99
10 (10^1)	0.001	5-log	99.999

2.3 Disinfectant concentration and exposure time

The effects of concentration or dilution of the active ingredient on the activity of a disinfectant are of major importance. Apart from iodophors, the more concentrated a disinfectant, the greater its efficacy, and the shorter the time necessary to destroy the microorganism, i.e. there is an exponential relationship between potency and concentration. Therefore, a graph plotting the $\log_{10}$ of a death time (i.e. the time required to kill a standard inoculum) against the $\log_{10}$ of the concentration is usually a straight line, the slope of which is the concentration exponent (η). Expressed as an equation:

$$\eta = \frac{(\text{Log death time at concentration } C_2) -(\text{Log death time at concentration } C_1)}{\text{Log } C_1 - C_2}$$

Thus η can be obtained from experimental data either graphically or by substitution in the above equation (see Table 11.2).

Table 11.2 Concentration exponents, η, for some disinfectant substances

Antimicrobial agent	η
Hydrogen peroxide	0.5
Silver nitrate	0.9–1.0
Mercurials	0.03–3.0
Iodine	0.9
Crystal violet	0.9
Chlorhexidine	2
Formaldehyde	1
QACs	0.8–2.5
Acridines	0.7–1.9
Formaldehyde donors	0.8–0.9
Bronopol	0.7
Polymeric biguanides	1.5–1.6
Parabens	2.5
Sorbic acid	2.6–3.2
Potassium laurate	2.3
Benzyl alcohol	2.6–4.6
Aliphatic alcohols	6.0–12.7
Glycolmonophenyl ethers	5.8–6.4
Glycolmonoalkyl ethers	6.4–15.9
Phenolic agents	4.0–9.9

QAC, quaternary ammonium compound.

It is clear that dilution does not affect the cidal attributes of all disinfectants in a similar manner. Mercuric chloride with a concentration exponent of 1 will be reduced by the power of 1 on dilution, and a threefold dilution means the disinfectant activity will be reduced by the value 3^1, or to a third of its original activity. Phenol, however, has a concentration exponent of 6, so a threefold dilution in this case will mean a decrease in activity of 3^6 or 729 times less active than the original.

2.4 Physical and chemical factors

Known and proven influences include temperature, pH and water hardness.

2.4.1 Temperature

Within limits, the cidal activity of most disinfectants increases as the temperature rises. As the temperature is increased in arithmetical progression the rate (velocity) of disinfection increases in geometrical progression. Results may be expressed quantitatively by means of a temperature coefficient, either the temperature coefficient per degree rise in temperature (θ), or the coefficient per 10° rise (the Q_{10} value) (Hugo & Russell, 1998). As shown by Koch working with phenol and anthrax (*Bacillus anthracis*) spores over 120 years ago, raising the temperature of phenol from 20°C to 30°C increased the killing activity by a factor of 4 (the Q_{10} value).

θ may be calculated from the equation:

$$\theta^{(T_1 - T_2)} = t_1/t_2$$

Where t_1 is the extinction time at $T_1°$C, and t_2 the extinction at $T_2°$C (i.e. $T_1 + 1$°C).

Q_{10} values may be calculated easily by determining the extinction time at two temperatures differing exactly by 10°C. Then:

$$Q_{10} = \frac{\text{Time to kill at } T°}{\text{Time to kill at } (T + 10)°}$$

It is also possible to plot the rate of kill against the temperature.

While the value for Q_{10} of chemical and enzyme-catalysed reactions lies in a narrow range (between 2 and 3), values for disinfectants vary widely, e.g. 4

for phenol, 45 for ethanol, and almost 300 for ethylene glycol monoethyl ether. Clearly, relating chemical reaction kinetics to disinfection processes is potentially dangerous. Most laboratory tests involving disinfectant-like chemicals are now standardized to 20°C, i.e. around ambient room temperatures.

2.4.2 pH

Effects of pH on antimicrobial activity can be complex. As well as influencing the survival and rate of growth of the microorganism under test, changes in pH may affect the potency of the agent and its ability to combine with cell surface sites. If the agent is an acid or a base, its degree of ionization will depend on the pH. With some antimicrobials (e.g. phenols, acetic acid, benzoic acid), the non-ionized molecule is the active state and alkaline pHs which favour the formation of ions of such compounds will decrease the activity. Others (e.g. glutaraldehyde, quaternary ammonium compounds— QACs) reveal increased cidal activity as the pH rises and are best used under alkaline conditions. Adherence to cell surfaces is essential for the activity of many disinfectants; increasing the external pH renders cell surfaces more negatively charged and enhances the binding of cationic compounds such as chlorhexidine and QACs.

2.4.3 Divalent cations

Divalent cations (e.g. Mg^{2+}, Ca^{2+}) present in hard water may also interact with the microbial cell surface and block disinfectant adsorption sites necessary for activity. On the other hand, cationic compounds may disrupt the outer membrane of Gram-negative bacteria and facilitate their own entry.

2.5 Presence of extraneous organic material

It has long been known that the cidal activity of many antimicrobial agents is seriously impaired under 'dirty' conditions. Some of the original laboratory assays employed dried human faeces or yeast to mimic the effects of blood, pus or faeces on disinfectant activity. This is particularly true of the

halogen disinfectants (e.g. sodium hypochlorite) where the disinfectant reacts with the organic matter to form inactive complexes. It also seems that organic material may adhere to the microbial cell surface and block adsorption sites necessary for disinfectant activity. For practical purposes and to mirror potential in-use situations, disinfectants should be evaluated under both clean and dirty conditions. The latter usually includes the addition of albumin, although sheep blood or mucin have also been suggested.

3 Evaluation of liquid disinfectants

3.1 General

Phenol coefficient tests were developed in the early 20th century when typhoid fever was a significant public health problem and phenolics were used to disinfect contaminated utensils and other inanimate objects. Details of such tests can be found in earlier editions of this book. However, as non-phenolic disinfectants became more widely available, tests that more closely paralleled the conditions under which disinfectants were being used (e.g. blood spills) and which included a more diverse range of microbial types (e.g. viruses, bacteria, fungi, protozoa) were developed. Evaluation of a disinfectant's efficacy was based on its ability to kill microbes, i.e. its cidal activity, under environmental conditions mimicking as closely as possible real life situations. As an essential component of each test was a final viability assay, removal or neutralization of any residual disinfectant became a significant consideration.

Around 1970, Kelsey, Sykes and Maurer developed the so-called 'capacity-use dilution test' which measured the ability of a disinfectant at an appropriate in-use concentration to kill successive additions of a bacterial culture. Results were reported simply as pass or fail and not a numerical cipher (coefficient). Tests employed disinfectants diluted in clean hard water and in water containing organic material ('dirty' conditions), with the final recovery broth containing 3% Tween 80 as a neutralizer. Such tests were applicable for use with a wide variety of disinfectants (see Kelsey & Maurer, 1974).

191

However, it soon became apparent that the greatest information concerning the fate of microbes exposed to a disinfectant was obtainable by counting the number of viable cells remaining after exposure of a standard suspension of cells to the disinfectant for a given time interval—suspension tests. Viable counting is a technique used in many branches of pure and applied microbiology. Assessment of the number of viable microbes remaining after exposure allows the killing or cidal activity of the disinfectant to be expressed in a variety of ways, e.g. percentage kill (e.g. 99.999%), as a $\log_{10}$ reduction in numbers (e.g. 5-log killing), or by $\log_{10}$ survival expressed as a percentage. Examples of results are shown in Table 11.1.

Unfortunately, standardization of the methodology to be employed in these efficacy tests has proved difficult, if not impossible, to obtain, as has consensus on what level of killing represents a satisfactory and/or acceptable result. It must be stressed however, that unlike tests involving chemotherapeutic agents where the major aim is to establish antimicrobial concentrations that inhibit growth (i.e. MICs), disinfectant tests require determinations of appropriate cidal levels.

Levels of killing required over a given time interval tend to vary depending on the regulatory authority concerned. While a 5-log killing of bacteria (starting with 10^6 CFU/ml) has been suggested for suspension tests, some authorities require a 6-log killing in simulated use tests. With viruses, a 4-log killing tends to be an acceptable result, while with prions it has been recommended that a titre loss of 10^4 prions should be regarded as an indication of appropriate disinfection provided that there has been adequate prior cleaning. With simulated use tests, cleaning followed by appropriate disinfection should result in a prion titre loss of at least 10^7.

3.2 Antibacterial disinfectant efficacy tests

Various regulatory authorities in Europe (e.g. European Standard or Norm, EN; British Standards, BS; Germany, DGHM; France, AFNOR) and North America (e.g. Food and Drug Administration, FDA; Environmental Protection Authority, EPA; Association of Official Analytical Chemists, AOAC) have been associated with attempts to produce some form of standardization with disinfectant tests. Perhaps the most readily accessible and recent guide to the methodology of possible bactericidal, tuberculocidal, fungicidal and virucidal disinfectant efficacy tests, is that of Kampf and colleagues (2002). This publication summarizes and provides references to various EN procedures (e.g. prEN 12054). Whatever method used, however, it should generate results that are amenable to statistical analysis.

3.2.1 Suspension tests

While varying to some degree in their methodology, most of the proposed procedures tend to employ a standard suspension of the microorganism in water containing albumin (dirty conditions) and appropriate dilutions of the disinfectant—so-called 'suspension tests'. Tests are carried out at a set temperature (usually around room temperature or 20°C), and at a selected time interval samples are removed and viable counts are performed following neutralization of any disinfectant remaining in the sample. Neutralization or inactivation of residual disinfectant can be carried out by dilution, or by addition of specific agents (see Table 11.3). Using viable counts, it is possible to calculate the concentration of disinfectant required to kill 99.999% of the original suspension. Thus 10 survivors from an original population of 10^6 (1 000 000) cells represents a 99.999% or 5-log kill. As bacteria may initially decline in numbers in diluents devoid of additional disinfectant, results from tests incorporating disinfectant-treated cells can be compared with results from simultaneous tests involving a non-disinfectant-containing system (untreated cells). The bactericidal effect B_E can then be expressed as:

$$B_E = \log N_C - \log N_D$$

where N_C and N_D represent the final number of CFU/ml remaining in the control and disinfectant series, respectively.

Unfortunately, viable count procedures carry the proviso that one colony develops from one cell or one colony-forming unit (CFU). Such techniques are, therefore, not ideal for disinfectants (e.g. QACs such as cetrimide) that promote clumping in bacter-

Table 11.3 Neutralizing agents for some antimicrobial agents[a]

Antimicrobial agent	Neutralizing and/or inactivating agent[b]
Alcohols	None (dilution)
Alcohol-based hand gels	Tween 80, saponin, histidine and lecithin
Amoxycillin	β-Lactamase from *Bacillus cereus*[c]
Antibiotics (most)	None (dilution, membrane filtration[d], resin adsorption[e])
Benzoic acid	Dilution or Tween 80[f]
Benzyl penicillin	β-Lactamase from *Bacillus cereus*
Bronopol	Cysteine hydrochloride
Chlorhexidine	Lubrol W and egg lecithin *or* Tween 80 and lecithin (Letheen)
Formaldehyde	Ammonium ions
Glutaraldehyde	Glycine
Halogens	Sodium thiosulphate
Hexachlorophane	Tween 80
Mercurials	Thioglycollic acid (-SH compounds)
Phenolics	Dilution or Tween 80
QACs	Lubrol W and lecithin *or* Tween 80 and lecithin (Letheen)
Sulphonamides	*p*-Aminobenzoic acid

[a] Other than dilution—adapted from Hugo & Russell (1998).
[b] D/E neutralizing media—adequate for QACs, phenols, iodine and chlorine compounds, mecurials, formaldehyde and glutaraldehyde (see Rutala, 1999).
[c] Other appropriate enzymes can be considered—e.g. inactivating or modifying enzymes for chloramphenicol and aminoglycosides, respectively.
[d] Filter microorganisms onto membrane, wash, transfer membrane to growth medium.
[e] Resins for the absorption of antibiotics from fluids are available.
[f] Tween 80 (polysorbate 80).

ial suspensions, although the latter problem may be overcome by adding non-ionic surface active agents to the diluting fluid.

3.2.2 In-use and simulated use tests

Apart from suspension tests, in-use testing of used medical devices, and simulated use tests involving instruments or surfaces deliberately contaminated with an organic load and the appropriate test microorganism have been incorporated into disinfectant testing protocols. An example is the in-use test first enunciated by Maurer in 1972. It is used to determine whether the disinfectant in jars, buckets or other containers in which potentially contaminated material (e.g. lavatory brushes) has been placed contain living microorganisms, and in what numbers. A small volume of fluid is withdrawn from the in-use container, neutralized in a large volume of a suitable diluent and viable counts are performed on the resulting suspension. Two plates are involved in viable count investigations—one of which is incubated for 3 days at 32°C (rather than 37°C, as bacteria damaged by disinfectants recover more rapidly at lowered temperatures), and the other for 7 days at room temperature. Growth of one or two colonies per plate can be ignored (a disinfectant is not usually a sterilant), while 10 or more colonies would suggest poor and unsatisfactory cidal action.

Simulated use tests involve deliberate contamination of instruments, inanimate surfaces, or even skin surfaces, with a microbial suspension. This may either be under clean conditions or may utilize a diluent containing organic (e.g. albumin) material—dirty condition. After being left to dry, the contaminated surface is exposed to the test disinfectant for an appropriate time interval. The microbes are then removed (e.g. by rubbing with a sterile swab), resuspended in suitable neutralizing medium, and assessed for viability as for suspension tests. New products are often compared with a known comparator compound (e.g. 1 minute application of 60% v/v 2-propanol for hand disinfection products—see EN1500) to show increased efficacy of the novel product.

3.2.3 Problematic bacteria

Mycobacteria are hydrophobic in nature and it may be difficult to prepare homogeneous suspensions devoid of undue cell clumping. As *Mycobacterium tuberculosis* is very slow growing, a saprophytic rapidly growing species such as *Mycobacterium terrae* can be substituted in tests (as representative of *M. tuberculosis*).

Apart from vegetative bacterial cells, spores can also be used as the inoculum in tests. In such cases, incubation of plates for the final viability determination should be continued for several days to allow for germination and growth.

Compared with suspended (planktonic) cells, bacteria on surfaces as biofilms are invariably phenotypically more resistant to antimicrobial agents. With biofilms, suspension tests can be modified to involve biofilms produced on small pieces of an appropriate glass or metal substrate, or on the bottom of microtitre tray wells. After being immersed in, or exposed to the disinfectant solution for the appropriate time interval, the cells from the biofilm are removed, e.g. by sonication, and resuspended in a suitable neutralizing medium. Viable counts are then performed on the resulting planktonic cells.

Some important environmental bacteria survive in nature as intracellular parasites of other microbes, e.g. *Legionella pneumophila* within the protozoan *Acanthamoeba polyphaga*. Biocide activity is significantly reduced against intracellular legionellae (see Fig. 11.3). Disinfectant tests involving such bacteria should therefore be conducted both on planktonic bacteria and on suspensions involving amoebae-containing bacteria. With the latter, the final bacterial viable counts are performed after suitable lysis of the protozoan host. The legionellae/protozoal situation may also be complicated by the fact that the microbes often occur as biofilms.

3.3 Other microbe disinfectant tests

Suspension-type efficacy tests can also be performed on other microbes, e.g. fungi, viruses, using similar techniques to that described above for bacteria, although significant differences obviously occur in parts of the tests.

3.3.1 Antifungal (fungicidal) tests

Perhaps the main problem with fungi concerns the question of what to use as the inoculum. Unicellular yeasts can be treated as for bacteria, but whether to use spores (which may be more resistant than the vegetative mycelium) or pieces of hyphae with the filamentous moulds, has yet to be fully resolved. Spore suspensions (in saline containing the wetting agent Tween 80) obtained from 7-day-old cultures

are presently recommended. What fungus, e.g. yeast or mould, to use as the test microbe is also debatable, and will clearly vary depending on the perceived use for the disinfectant under test. Spore suspensions of at least 10^6 CFU/ml have been recommended. Viable counts are performed on suitable media (e.g. malt extract agar) with incubation at 20°C for 48 hours or longer. EN 1275 regulations for fungicidal activity require a minimum reduction in viability by a factor of 10^4 within 60 minutes; test fungi were *Candida albicans* and *Aspergillus niger*.

3.3.2 Antiviral (virucidal) tests

The testing of disinfectants for virucidal activity is not easy; viruses are obligate intracellular parasites and are unable to grow in artificial culture media. They require some other system employing living cells. Suggested test viruses include rotavirus, adenovirus, poliovirus, herpes simplex viruses, human immunodeficiency virus, pox viruses and papovavirus, although extension of this list to include additional bloodborne viruses such as hepatitis B and C, and significant animal pathogens (e.g. foot and mouth disease virus) could be argued. Appropriate facilities for handling such pathogens are essential.

Briefly, the virus is grown in an appropriate cell line that is then mixed with water containing an organic load and the disinfectant under test. After the appropriate time, residual viral infectivity is determined using a tissue culture/plaque assay or other system (e.g. animal host, molecular assay for some specific viral component). Such procedures are costly and time-consuming, and must be appropriately controlled to exclude factors such as disinfectant killing of the cell system or test animal. A reduction of infectivity by a factor of 10^4 has been regarded as evidence of acceptable virucidal activity (prEN 14476). For viruses which cannot be grown in the laboratory (e.g. hepatitis B), naturally infected cells/tissues must be used.

3.3.3 Prion disinfection tests

Prions are a unique class of pathogen, devoid of an agent-specific nucleic acid (DNA or RNA). Infection is associated with the abnormal isoform of a host cellular protein called prion protein (PrP^c). Prions exhibit high resistance to conventional chemical and physical decontamination methods — most studies have been done with tissue homogenates, which may offer some protective role. Hence the importance of a prior cleaning procedure before any attempted disinfection process.

Current prion disinfection assays are slow, laborious and costly — they employ 'contaminated' test tissue homogenates (prion 'strain' and concentration variable, possible disinfectant inactivation), test animals which serve to assess the viability of treated tissue, with the log decrease being calculated from incubation period assays rather than from end-point titrations.

While most disinfectants are inadequate for the elimination of prion infectivity, agents such as sodium hydroxide and sodium hypochlorite have been shown to be effective (Chapter 17).

4 Evaluation of solid disinfectants

Solid disinfectants usually consist of a disinfectant substance diluted by an inert powder. Phenolic substances adsorbed onto kieselguhr form the basis of many disinfectant powders, while another widely used solid disinfectant is sodium dichloroisocyanurate. Other disinfectant or antiseptic powders used in medicine include acriflavine and compounds with antifungal activity such as zinc undecenoate or salicylic acid mixed with talc. These disinfectants may be evaluated by applying them to suitable test organisms growing on a solid agar medium. Discs may be cut from the agar and subcultured for enumeration of survivors. Inhibitory activity is evaluated by dusting the powders onto the surface of seeded agar plates, using the inert diluents as a control. The extent of growth is then observed following incubation.

5 Evaluation of air disinfectants

A number of important infectious diseases are spread via microbial contamination of the air. This cross-infection can occur in a variety of situations — hospitals, cinemas, aeroplanes — while maintenance of a microbe-free environment is important for many aseptic procedures. The microorganisms themselves may be contained in aerosols, or may occur as airborne particles liberated from some environmental source, e.g. decaying vegetation. While the microorganisms can be killed by suitable radiation (e.g. UV), it is often more practical to use some form of chemical vapour or aerosol to kill them.

As shown by Robert Koch in 1881, the numbers of viable bacteria present in air can be assessed by simply exposing plates of solid nutrient media to the air. Any bacteria that fall onto the plates can then be detected following a suitable period of incubation. These gravitational methods are obviously applicable to many microorganisms, but present problems with viruses.

However, more meaningful data can be obtained if force rather than gravity is used to collect airborne particles. A stream of air can be directed onto the surface of a nutrient agar plate (impaction; slit sampler) or bubbled through an appropriate buffer or culture medium (liquid impingement). Various commercial impactor samplers are available. Filtration sampling, where the air is passed through a porous membrane, which is then cultured, can also be used.

For experimental evaluation of potential air disinfectants, bacterial or fungal airborne 'suspensions' can be created in a closed chamber, and then exposed to the disinfectant, which may be in the form of radiation, chemical vapour or aerosol. The airborne microbial population is then sampled at regular intervals using an appropriate forced-air apparatus such as the slit sampler. With viruses, the air can be bubbled through a suitable liquid medium, which is then subjected to some appropriate virological assay system. In all cases, problems arise in producing a suitable airborne microbial 'suspension' and in neutralizing residual disinfectant, which may remain in the air.

Solar heating, which can result in a 7-log reduction in viable bacteria over 6 hours, is a possible disinfection consideration for developing countries.

6 Evaluation of preservatives

Preservatives are widely employed in the cosmetic and pharmaceutical industries as well as in a variety of other manufacturing industries. While the inhibitory or cidal activity of the chemical to be used as the preservative can be evaluated using an appropriate *in vitro* test system (see sections 3.2.1 and 8.1.2) its continued activity when combined with the other ingredients in the final manufactured product must be established. Problems clearly exist with some products, where partitioning into various phases may result in the absence of preservative in one of the phases e.g. oil-in-water emulsions where the preservative may partition only into the oily phase, allowing any contaminant microorganisms to flourish in the aqueous phase. In addition, one or more of the components may inactivate the preservative. Some sort of simulated-use challenge test involving the final product is, therefore, required in addition to direct potency testing of the pure preservative. In the challenge test, the final preserved product is deliberately inoculated with a suitable environmental microorganism which may be fungal, e.g. candida, or bacterial, e.g. *Staphylococcus aureus, Escherichia coli, Pseudomonas aeruginosa*. For preparations with a high sucrose content, the osmophilic yeast *Zygosaccharomyces rouxii* is a consideration. The subsequent survival (inhibition), death or growth of the inoculum is then assessed using viable count techniques. Different performance criteria are laid down for injectable and ophthalmic preparations, topical preparations and oral liquid preparations in the *British Pharmacopoeia* and *European Pharmacopoeia*, which should be consulted for full details of the experimental procedures to be used.

In some instances, the range and/or spectrum of preservation can be extended by using more than one preservative at a time. Thus a combination of parabens (*p*-hydroxybenzoic acid) with varying water solubilities may protect both the aqueous and oil phases of an emulsion, while a combination of Germall 115 and parabens results in a preservative system with both antibacterial (Germall 115) and antifungal (parabens) activity.

7 Rapid evaluation procedures

In most of the tests mentioned above, results are not available until visible microbial growth occurs (at least in the controls). This usually takes 24 hours or more. Can the process be accelerated? While the answer is basically yes, only a few 'rapid' methods for detecting microbial viability or growth are presently employed in assessing the efficacy of antimicrobials (see Hugo & Russell, 1998). These include epifluorescent and bioluminescence techniques. The former relies on the fact that when exposed to the vital stain acridine orange and viewed under UV light, viable cells fluoresce green or greenish yellow, while dead cells appear orange.

With tests involving liquid systems the early growth of viable cells can be assessed by some light-scattering processes while blood culture techniques have classically used the production of CO_2 as an indicator of bacterial metabolism and growth. In addition, the availability of molecular techniques, such as quantitative PCR, may be useful in demonstrating the presence or growth of microorganisms that are slow or difficult to culture under usual laboratory conditions, e.g. viruses. This may obviate the need to neutralize residual disinfectant with some assays.

8 Evaluation of potential chemotherapeutic antimicrobials

Unlike tests for the evaluation of disinfectants where determination of cidal activity is of paramount importance, tests involving potential chemotherapeutic agents (antibiotics) invariably have as their main focus determination of MIC.

8.1 Tests for bacteriostatic activity

The historical gradient plates, ditch-plate and cup-plate techniques (see Hugo & Russell, 1998) have been replaced by more quantitative techniques such as disc diffusion (Fig. 11.4), broth and agar dilution, and E-tests (Fig. 11.5). All employ chemically defined media (e.g. Mueller-Hinton or Iso-Sensitest) at a pH of 7.2–7.4, and in the case of solid media, agar plates of defined thickness.

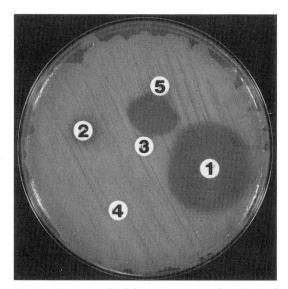

Fig. 11.4 Disc test with inhibition zones around two (1, 2) of five discs. While the zone around disc 1 is clear and easy to measure, that around disc 2 is indistinct. While none of the antimicrobials in discs 3, 4 or 5 appear to inhibit the bacterium, synergy (as evidenced by inhibition of growth between the discs) is evident with the antimicrobials in discs 3 and 5. Slight antagonism of the drug in disc 1 by that in disc 3 is evident.

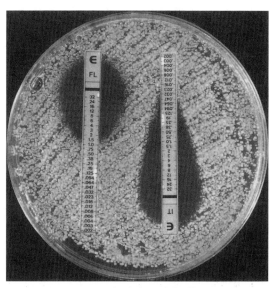

Fig. 11.5 E-test on an isolate of *Candida albicans*. Inhibition zone edges are distinct and the MICs for itraconazole (IT) and fluconazole (FL) (0.064 mg/L and 1.5 mg/L, respectively) are easily decipherable.

Regularly updated guidelines have been provided by the National Committee for Clinical Laboratory Standards (NCCLS) and are widely used in many countries, although the British Society for Antimicrobial Chemotherapy has produced its own guidelines and testing procedures (see Further reading section).

8.1.1 Disc tests

These are really modifications of the earlier cup or ditch-plate procedures where filter-paper discs impregnated with the antimicrobial replace the antimicrobial-filled cups or wells. For disc tests, standard suspensions (e.g. 0.5 McFarland standard) of log phase growth cells are prepared and inoculated onto the surface of appropriate agar plates to form a lawn. Commercially available filter-paper discs containing known concentrations of antimicrobial agent (it is possible to prepare your own discs for use with novel drugs) are then placed on the dried lawn and the plates are incubated aerobically at 35°C for 18 hours. The density of bacteria inoculated onto the plate should produce just confluent growth after incubation. Any zone of inhibition occurring around the disc is then measured, and after comparison with known standards, the bacterium under test is identified as susceptible or resistant to that particular antibiotic. For novel agents, these sensitivity parameters are only available after extensive clinical investigations are correlated with laboratory-generated data. Disc tests are basically qualitative, although it is possible to get some information on the degree of activity depending on the zone size (Fig. 11.6).

Although there are subtle variations of the disc test used in some countries, the basic principles behind the tests remain similar and are based on the original work of Bauer and colleagues. Some techniques employ a control bacterial isolate on each plate so that comparisons between zone sizes around the test and control bacterium can be ascertained (i.e. a disc potency control). Provided that discs are maintained and handled as recommended by the manufacturer, the value of such controls becomes debatable and probably unnecessary. Con-

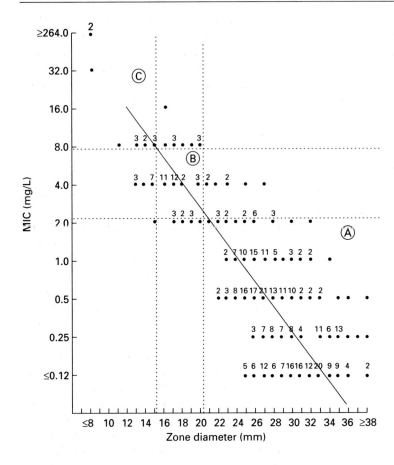

Fig. 11.6 A scattergram and regression line analysis correlating zone diameters and MICs. The breakpoints of susceptible (MIC ≤ 2.0 mg/L, zone diameter ≥ 21 mm) and resistant (MIC ≥ 8.0 mg/L, zone ≤ 15 mm) are shown by the dotted lines. For a complete correlation between MICs and zone diameter, all susceptible, intermediate and resistant isolates should fall in boxes A, B and C, respectively. Errors (correlations outside these boxes) occur (courtesy of Dr Z. Hashmi).

trol strains of bacteria are available which should have inhibition zones of a given diameter with stipulated antimicrobial discs. Use of such controls endorses the suitability of the methods (e.g. medium, inoculum density, incubation conditions) employed. For slow-growing microorganisms, the incubation period can be extended.

Problems arise with disc tests where the inoculum density is inappropriate (e.g. too low resulting in an indistinct edge to the inhibition zone following incubation), or where the edge is obscured by the sporadic growth of cells within the inhibition zone, i.e. the initial inoculum although pure contains cells expressing varying levels of susceptibility — so-called heterogeneity. As the distance from the disc increases, there is a logarithmic reduction in the antimicrobial concentration; the result is that small differences in zone diameter with antimicrobials

(e.g. vancomycin) which diffuse poorly through solid media may represent significantly different MICs. Possible synergistic or antagonistic combinations of antimicrobials can often be detected using disc tests (Fig. 11.4).

8.1.2 Dilution tests

These usually employ liquid media but can be modified to involve solid media. Doubling dilutions — usually in the range 0.12–256 mg/L — of the antimicrobial under test are prepared in a suitable broth medium, and a volume of log phase cells is added to each dilution to result in a final cell density of around 5×10^5 CFU/ml. After incubation at 35°C for 18 hours, the concentration of antimicrobial contained in the first clear tube is read as the MIC. Needless to say, dilution tests require a number of controls, e.g. sterility control, growth control, and the simultaneous testing of a bacterial strain with known MIC to show that the dilution series is correct.

Endpoints with dilution tests are usually sharp and easily defined, although 'skipped' wells (inhibition in a well with growth either side) and 'trailing' (a gradual reduction in growth over a series of wells) may be encountered. The latter is especially evident with antifungal tests (see below).

Nowadays, the dilution test for established antimicrobials has been simplified by the commercial availability of 96-well microtitre plates which have appropriate antimicrobial dilutions frozen or lyophilized onto wells in the plate. The appropriate antibacterial suspension (in 200–400-μl volumes) is simply added to each well, the plate is incubated as before, and the MIC is read.

Dilution tests can also be carried out using a series of agar plates containing known antimicrobial concentrations. Appropriate bacterial suspensions are inoculated onto each plate and the presence or absence of growth is recorded after suitable incubation.

Most clinical laboratories now employ agar dilution breakpoint testing methods. These are essentially truncated agar dilution MIC tests employing only a small range of antimicrobial concentrations around the critical susceptible/resistant cut off levels.

Many automated identification and sensitivity testing machines now utilize a liquid (broth) variant of the agar breakpoint procedure. Similar breakpoint antimicrobial concentrations are used with the presence or absence of growth being recorded by some automated procedure (e.g. light-scattering, colour change) after a suitable incubation period.

8.1.3 E-tests

Perhaps the most convenient and presently accepted method of determining bacterial MICs, however, is the E (Epsilometer)-test. Basically this is performed in a similar manner to the disc test except that nylon strips that have a linear gradient of antimicrobial lyophilized on one side are used instead of the filter-paper impregnated antimicrobial discs. On the other side of the nylon strip are a series

of lines and figures denoting MIC values (Fig. 11.5). The nylon strips are placed antimicrobial side down on the freshly prepared bacterial lawn and, after incubation, the MIC is determined by noting where the ellipsoid (pear-shaped) inhibition zone crosses the strip (Fig. 11.5). For most microorganisms, there appears to be excellent correlation between dilution and E-test MIC results.

8.1.4 Problematic bacteria

With some of the emerging antimicrobial-resistant bacterial pathogens, e.g. vancomycin-resistant enterococci (VRE), methicillin-resistant *Staphylococcus aureus* (MRSA), vancomycin-intermediate *S. aureus* (VISA), the standard methodology described above may fail to detect the resistant phenotype. This is due to a variety of factors including heterogeneous expression of resistance (e.g. MRSA, VISA), poor agar diffusion of the antimicrobial (e.g. vancomycin) and slow growth of resistant cells (e.g. VISA). Disc tests are unsuitable for VRE that should have MICs determined by E-test or dilution techniques. With MRSA, a heavier inoculum should be used in tests and 2–4% additional salt (NaCl) included in the medium with incubation for a full 48 hours. Reducing the incubation temperature to 30°C may also facilitate detection of the true MIC value. Although 100% of MRSA cells may contain resistance genes, the phenotype may only be evident in a small percentage of cells under the usual conditions employed in sensitivity tests. Expression is enhanced at lower temperatures and at higher salt concentrations. With VISA, MIC determinations require incubation for a full 24 hours or more because of the slower growth rate of resistant cells.

8.2 Tests for bactericidal activity

Minimum bactericidal concentration (MBC) testing is required for the evaluation of novel antimicrobials. The MBC is the lowest concentration (in mg/L) of antimicrobial that results in ≥99.9% killing of the bacterium under test. The 99.9% cutoff is an arbitrary *in vitro* value with 95% confidence limits that has uncertain clinical relevance.

MBCs are determined by spreading 0.1-ml

(100-µl) volumes of all clear (no growth) tubes from a dilution MIC test onto separate agar plates (residual antimicrobial in the 0.1-ml sample is 'diluted' out over the plate). After incubation at 35°C overnight (or longer for slow-growing bacteria), the numbers of colonies growing on each plate are recorded. The first concentration of drug that produces <50 colonies after subculture is considered the MBC. This is based on the fact that with MICs, the initial bacterial inoculum should result in about 5×10^5 CFU/ml. Inhibition, but not killing of this inoculum, should therefore result in the growth of 50 000 bacteria from the 0.1-ml sample. A 99.9% (3-log) kill would result in no more than 50 colonies on the subculture plate. With most modern antibacterial drugs, the concentration that inhibits growth is very close to the concentration that produces death, e.g. within one or two dilutions. In general, only MICs are determined for such drugs.

8.3 Tests for fungistatic and fungicidal activity

As fungi have become more prominent human pathogens, techniques for investigating the susceptibility of isolates to the growing number of antifungal agents have been developed. These have been largely based on the established bacterial techniques (disc, dilution, E-test) mentioned above, with the proviso that the medium used is different (e.g. use of RPMI 1640 plus 2% dextrose) and that the inoculum density (yeast cells or spores) used is reduced (c. 10^4 CFU/ml). With yeast disc and E-tests, a lawn producing just separated/distinct colonies is preferable to confluent growth (see Fig. 11.5). Addition of methylene blue (0.5 µg/ml) to media may improve the clarity of inhibition zone edges. Problems of 'tailing' or 'trailing' in dilution tests, and indistinct inhibition zone edges are often seen in tests involving azoles and yeasts and appear in some way related to the type of buffer employed in the growth medium. However, their presence has prompted studies into evaluating the use of other techniques as an indicator of significant fungistasis — e.g. 50% reduction in growth (rather than complete inhibition) as the endpoint, use of a dye (e.g. Alamar blue) colour change to indicate growth, and sterol (ergosterol) quantitation. Most

of these are presently outside the scope of most routine laboratories.

As with MBC estimations, minimum fungicidal concentration (MFC) evaluation is an extension of the MIC test. At the completion of the MIC test (e.g. 72 hours for filamentous fungi), 20 µl are subcultured onto a suitable growth medium from each optically clear microtitre tray well and the growth control well. These plates are then incubated at 35°C until growth is evident on the growth control subculture (24–48 hours). The MFC is the lowest drug concentration showing no growth or fewer than 3 colonies per plate to obtain approximately 99–99.5% killing activity.

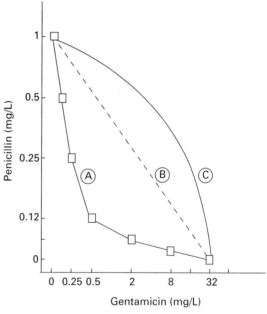

Fig. 11.7 Diagrammatic representation of MIC values obtained with two synergistic antimicrobials, penicillin and gentamicin. The resulting graph or isobologram (A) is obtained by linking MIC values for each drug alone and in various dilution combinations. The MIC values for penicillin and gentamicin alone are 1.0 mg/L and 32 mg/L, respectively. The slope of the isobologram for purely additive or antagonistic combinations is shown by B and C, respectively.

8.4 Evaluation of possible synergistic antimicrobial combinations

The potential interaction between two antimicrobials can be demonstrated using a variety of laboratory procedures, e.g. 'checkerboard' MIC assays where the microorganism is exposed to varying dilutions of each drug alone and in combination, disc diffusion tests (see Fig. 11.4) and kinetic kill curve assays. With the former, results can be plotted in the form of a figure called an isobologram (see Fig. 11.7).

8.4.1 Kinetic kill curves

In the case of kill curves, the microorganism is inoculated into tubes containing a single concentration of each antimicrobial alone, the same concentrations of each antimicrobial in combination, and no antimicrobial — i.e. four tubes. All tubes are then incubated and viable counts are performed at regular intervals on each system. With results plotted on semi-logarithmic paper, synergy is defined as a >100-fold increase in killing of the combination compared with either drug alone. Antagonism is defined as at least a 100-fold decrease in killing of the combination when compared with the most active agent alone, while an additive or autonomous combined effect results in a <10-fold change from that seen with the most active single drug. Both chemotherapeutic agents and disinfectants are amenable to kill curve assays.

9 Further reading

Buttner, M. P., Willeke K. & Grinshpun S. A. (2002) Sampling and analysis of airborne microorganisms. In: *Manual of Environmental Microbiology* (editor in chief C. J. Hurst), 2nd edn, pp. 814–826. ASM Press, Washington.

Espinel-Ingroff, A., Chaturvedi, V., Fothergill, A. & Rinaldi, M.G. (2002) Optimal testing conditions for determining MICs and minimum fungicidal concentrations of new and established antifungal agents for uncommon molds: NCCLS collaborative study. *J Clin Microbiol*, **40**, 3776–3781.

Hugo, W. B. & Russell, A. D. (1998) Evaluation of non-antibiotic antimicrobial agents. In: *Pharmaceutical Microbiology* (eds W.B. Hugo & A.D. Russell), 6th edn, pp. 229–255. Blackwell Science, Oxford.

Kampf, G., Rudolf, M., Labadie, J-C. & Barrett, S. P. (2002) Spectrum of antimicrobial activity and user acceptability of the hand disinfectant agent Sterillium ® Gel. *J Hosp Infect*, **52**, 141–147.

Kelsey, J. C. & Maurer, I. M. (1974) An improved Kelsey-Sykes test for disinfectants. *Pharm J*, **30**, 528–530.

Koneman, E. W., Allen, S. D., Janda, W. M., Schreckenberger, P. C. & Winn, W. C. (1997) Antimicrobial susceptibility testing. In: *Color Atlas and Textbook of Diagnostic Microbiology*, 5th edn, pp. 785–856. Lippincott-Raven, Philadelphia.

National Committee for Clinical Laboratory Standards (1997) Reference method for broth dilution antifungal susceptibility testing of yeasts; approved standard. NCCLS document M27-A, Wayne, PA.

National Committee for Clinical Laboratory Standards (2000) Methods for dilution antimicrobial susceptibility tests for bacteria that grow aerobically; approved standard, 5th edn. NCCLS document M7-A5, Wayne, PA.

National Committee for Clinical Laboratory Standards (2000) Performance standards for antimicrobial disk susceptibility tests; approved standard, 7th edn. NCCLS document M2-A7, Wayne, PA.

National Committee for Clinical Laboratory Standards (2002) Reference method for broth dilution antifungal susceptibility testing of filamentous fungi; approved standard. NCCLS document M38-A, Wayne, PA.

Russell, A. D., Furr, J. R. & Maillard, J-Y. (1997) Microbial susceptibility and resistance to biocides. *ASM News*, **63**, 481–487.

Rutala, W. A. (1999) Selection and use of disinfectants in healthcare. In: *Hospital Epidemiology and Infection Control* (ed. C. G. Mayhall), 2nd edn, pp. 1161–1187. Lippincott Williams & Wilkins, Philadelphia.

Rutala, W. A. & Weber, D. J. (2001) Creutzfeldt-Jakob Disease: recommendations for disinfection and sterilization. *Clin Infect Dis*, **32**, 1348–1356.

Walsh, S. E., Maillard, J-Y., Russell, A. D., Catrenich, C. E., Charbonneau, D. L. & Bartolo, R.G. (2003) Development of bacterial resistance to several biocides and effects on antibiotic susceptibility. *J Hosp Infect*, **55**, 98–107.

Widmer, A. F. & Frei, R. (1999) Decontamination, disinfection, and sterilization. In: *Manual of Clinical Microbiology* (eds P. R. Murray, E. J. Baron, M. A. Pfaller, F. C. Tenover & R. H. Yolken), 7th edn, pp. 138–164. ASM Press, Washington.

Chapter 12
Mechanisms of action of antibiotics and synthetic anti-infective agents

Peter Lambert

1 Introduction

The antibiotics and synthetic anti-infective agents described in Chapter 10 are used to treat infections caused by bacteria, fungi and protozoa. Most exert a highly selective toxic action upon their target microbial cells but have little or no toxicity towards mammalian cells. They can therefore be administered at concentrations sufficient to kill or inhibit the growth of infecting organisms without damaging mammalian cells. By comparison, the disinfec-

tants, antiseptics and preservatives described in Chapter 17 are too toxic for systemic treatment of infections. Figure 12.1 illustrates the five broad target areas of the major groups of antibiotics and synthetic agents used to treat microbial infections. Note that most of the agents are selective antibacterials, relatively few agents are available for treatment of fungal or protozoal infections. Study of the mechanism of action reveals the basis for the selective toxicity.

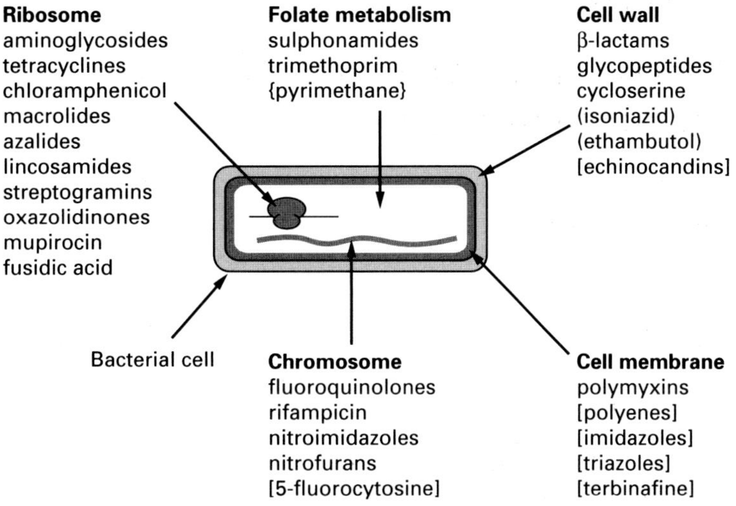

Ribosome
aminoglycosides
tetracyclines
chloramphenicol
macrolides
azalides
lincosamides
streptogramins
oxazolidinones
mupirocin
fusidic acid

Folate metabolism
sulphonamides
trimethoprim
{pyrimethane}

Cell wall
β-lactams
glycopeptides
cycloserine
(isoniazid)
(ethambutol)
[echinocandins]

Fig. 12.1 Schematic diagram of a typical bacterial cell showing the sites of action of the major classes of antibiotics and antimicrobial agents used to treat infections. Agents listed without brackets are used to treat bacterial infections. Agents used against mycobacterial, fungal or protozoal infections are indicated by the use of (), [] and {} brackets, respectively.

Bacterial cell

Chromosome
fluoroquinolones
rifampicin
nitroimidazoles
nitrofurans
[5-fluorocytosine]

Cell membrane
polymyxins
[polyenes]
[imidazoles]
[triazoles]
[terbinafine]

2 The microbial cell wall

2.1 Peptidoglycan biosynthesis in bacteria and its inhibition

Peptidoglycan is a vital component of the cell wall of virtually all bacteria. About 50% of the weight of the wall of Gram-positive bacteria is peptidoglycan, smaller amounts occur in mycobacterial walls (30%) and Gram-negative bacterial cell walls (10–20%). It is a macromolecule composed of sugar (glycan) chains cross-linked by short peptide chains (Fig. 12.2). The glycan chains contain alternating units of N-acetylmuramic acid and N-acetylglucosamine. Each N-acetylmuramic acid contains a short peptide substituent made up of four amino acids (the stem peptides). A key feature of peptidoglycan is the occurrence of the D-isomers of some amino acids in the stem peptides (particularly D-alanine and D-glutamic acid) and unusual amino acids such as meso-diaminopimelic acid which are not found in proteins. Cross-linking of the stem peptides may involve either a direct peptide bond between the fourth amino acid on one chain and the third amino acid on an adjacent chain or in some organisms the linkage may involve a short peptide bridge between the same amino acids on the stem peptides. The precise composition of peptidoglycan varies between different organisms but the overall structure is the same.

In all cases the peptidoglycan plays a vital role, it is responsible for maintaining the shape and mechanical strength of the bacterial cell. If it is damaged in any way, or its synthesis is inhibited, then the shape of the cells becomes distorted and they will eventually burst (lyse) due to the high internal osmotic pressure. Mammalian cells do not possess a cell wall and contain no other macromolecules resembling peptidoglycan. Consequently antibiotics which interfere with the synthesis and assembly of peptidoglycan show excellent selective toxicity.

2.1.1 D-Cycloserine

D-Cycloserine interferes with one of the early stages of synthesis of peptidoglycan involving the assembly of the dipeptide D-alanyl-D-alanine. This occurs inside the cytoplasm and involves a racemase enzyme which converts L-alanine to D-alanine and a ligase which couples two D-alanines together (Fig. 12.2). Both of these enzymes are inhibited by D-cycloserine, which bears some structural similarities to D-alanine. The antibiotic binds to the pyridoxal phosphate co-factor of the enzymes, effectively preventing them from forming D-alanyl-D-alanine. Subsequent stages of peptidoglycan synthesis, involving coupling of the dipeptide to three other amino acids on UDP-N-acetylmuramic acid, are therefore blocked. Note that initially the

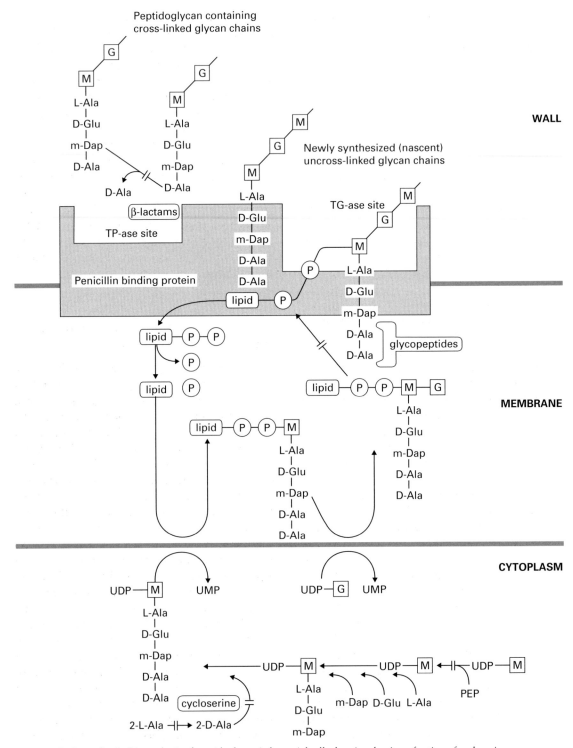

Fig. 12.2 Pathway for the biosynthesis of peptidoglycan in bacterial cells showing the sites of action of cycloserine, glycopeptide and β-lactam antibiotics.

peptide contains five amino acids, terminating in D-alanyl-D-alanine. The terminal D-alanine is removed on insertion into the cell wall.

2.1.2 *Glycopeptides — vancomycin and teicoplanin*

The peptidoglycan macromolecule is assembled in the cell wall by enzymes (transglycosylases and transpeptidases) located on the outer face of the cytoplasmic membrane. To reach the assembly site the precursors, which are synthesized in the cytoplasm, must cross the cell membrane. They do this linked to a lipid, undecaprenylphosphate, which acts as a carrier molecule, cycling between the inner and outer faces of the membrane. The biochemical details of this process are outlined in Fig. 12.2. Antibiotics interfering with this stage of peptidoglycan synthesis have been identified, e.g. bacitracin, but they have not found major applications in the treatment of infections.

The glycopeptides vancomycin and teicoplanin act at the stage where the peptidoglycan precursors are inserted into the cell wall by the transglycosylase enzyme on the outer face of the cell membrane. This enzyme assembles a growing glycan chain that is not initially cross-linked to the existing peptidoglycan in the cell wall. The linear glycan chain is assembled by the transglycosylase by sequential transfer of the growing chain to each molecule of the lipid intermediate carrier as it crosses the cell membrane. Glycopeptides block this process by binding, not to the enzyme itself, but to the peptidoglycan precursor, specifically to the D-alanyl-D-alanine portion. The presence of the bulky glycopeptides on each D-alanyl-D-alanine residue prevents extension of the linear glycan peptide in the cell wall by denying access of the transglycosylases to the substrate. Binding involves formation of a network of five hydrogen bonds between amino acid residues on the glycopeptide antibiotics and D-alanyl-D-alanine. Resistance to this unusual mechanism of enzyme inhibition can result from alteration in the D-alanyl-D-alanine substrate to D-alanyl-D-lactate, which occurs in glycopeptide (e.g. vancomycin)-resistant enterococci (VRE). Vancomycin does not penetrate the cell membrane of bacteria and is thought to bind to the disaccharide-pentapeptides on the outer face of the cytoplasmic membrane. It has been suggested that two vancomycin molecules form a back-to-back dimer which bridges between pentapeptides on separate glycan chains, thus preventing further peptidoglycan assembly. Teicoplanin also binds tightly to the D-alanyl-D-alanine region of the peptidoglycan precursor. However, as a lipoglycopeptide it may act slightly differently to vancomycin, by locating itself in the outer face of the cytoplasmic membrane and binding the pentapeptide as the precursors are transferred through the membrane. Glycopeptides must cross the cell wall to reach the outer face of the cell membrane where transglycosylation takes place. They are too large to penetrate the outer membrane of most Gram-negative bacteria and are consequently used for treatment of serious Gram-positive infections.

2.1.3 β-*Lactams — penicillins, cephalosporins, carbapenems and monobactams*

The final stage of peptidoglycan assembly is the cross-linking of the linear glycan strands assembled by transglycosylation to the existing peptidoglycan in the cell wall. This reaction is catalysed by transpeptidase enzymes, which are also located on the outer face of the cell membrane. They first remove the terminal D-alanine residue from each stem peptide on the newly synthesized glycan chain. The energy released from breaking the peptide bond between the two alanines is used in the formation of a new peptide bond between the remaining D-alanine on the stem peptide and a free amino group present on the third amino acid of the stem peptides in the existing cross-linked peptidoglycan. In many organisms, including *Escherichia coli*, this acceptor amino group is supplied by the amino acid diaminopimelic acid. In other organisms, e.g. *Staphylococcus aureus*, the acceptor amino group is supplied by the amino acid lysine. Although there is considerable variation in the composition of the peptide cross-link among different species of bacteria, the essential transpeptidation mechanism is the same. Therefore, virtually all bacteria can be inhibited by interference with this group of enzymes.

The β-lactam antibiotics inhibit transpeptidases

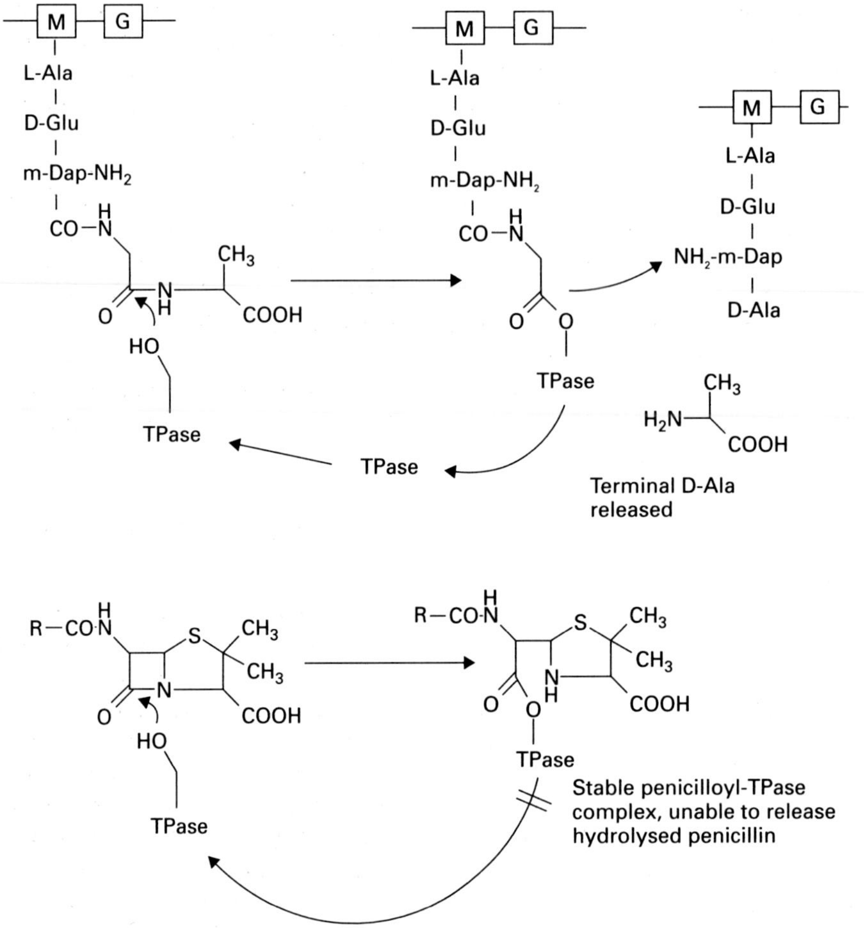

Fig. 12.3 The action of transpeptidase (TPase) with its natural substrate (upper) and penicillin G (lower). The OH group on a serine residue at the active site of the TPase attacks the peptide bond between the terminal D-alanyl-D-alanine in the peptidoglycan precursor, releasing the terminal D-alanine and forming a new peptide cross-link with existing peptidoglycan in the cell wall. Penicillin G blocks this process by forming a stable penicilloyl-TPase complex.

by acting as alternative substrates. They mimic the D-alanyl-D-alanine residues and react covalently with the transpeptidases (Fig. 12.3). The β-lactam bond (common to all members of the β-lactam antibiotics) is broken but the remaining portion of the antibiotic is not released immediately. The half-life for the transpeptidase–antibiotic complex is of the order of 10 minutes; during this time the enzyme cannot participate in further rounds of peptidoglycan assembly by reaction with its true substrate. The vital cross-linking of the peptidoglycan is therefore blocked while other aspects of cell growth

continue. The cells become deformed in shape and eventually burst through the combined action of a weakened cell wall, high internal osmotic pressure and the uncontrolled activity of autolytic enzymes in the cell wall. Penicillins, cephalosporins, carbapenems and monobactams all inhibit peptidoglycan cross-linking through interaction of the common β-lactam ring with the transpeptidase enzymes. However, there is considerable variation in the morphological effects of different β-lactams owing to the existence of several types of transpeptidase. The transpeptidase enzymes are usually referred to as penicillin-binding proteins (PBPs) because they can be separated and studied after reaction with ^{14}C-labelled penicillin. This step is necessary because there are very few copies of each enzyme present in a cell. They are usually separated according to their size by electrophoresis and are numbered PBP1, PBP2, etc. starting from the highest molecular weight species. In Gram-negative bacteria most of the high molecular weight transpeptidases also possess transglycosylase activity, i.e. they have a dual function in the final stages of peptidoglycan synthesis with the transglycosylase and transpeptidase activities located in separate regions of the protein structures. Furthermore, the different transpeptidases have specialized functions in the cell; all cross-link peptidoglycan but some are involved with maintenance of cell integrity, some regulate cell shape and others produce new cross wall between elongating cells, securing chromosome segregation prior to cell division. The varying sensitivity of the PBPs towards different β-lactams helps to explain the range of morphological effects observed on treated bacteria. For example, penicillin G (benzylpenicillin), ampicillin and cephaloridine are particularly effective in causing rapid lysis of Gram-negative bacteria such as *E. coli*. These antibiotics act primarily upon PBP 1B, the major transpeptidase of the organism. Other β-lactams have little activity against this PBP, e.g. mecillinam binds preferentially to PBP2 and it produces a pronounced change in the cells from a rod shape to an oval form. Many of the cephalosporins, e.g. cephalexin, cefotaxime and ceftazidime, bind to PBP3 resulting in the formation of elongated, filamentous cells. The lower molecular weight PBPs, 4, 5 and 6, do not possess transpeptidase activity. These are carboxypeptidases, which remove the terminal D-alanine from the pentapeptides on the linear glycans in the cell wall but do not catalyse the cross-linkage. Their role in the cells is to regulate the degree of cross-linking by denying the D-alanyl-D-alanine substrate to the transpeptidases but they are not essential for cell growth. Up to 90% of the amount of antibiotic reacting with the cells may be consumed in inhibiting the carboxypeptidases, with no lethal consequences to the cells.

Gram-positive bacteria also have multiple transpeptidases, but fewer than Gram-negatives.

Shape changes are less evident than with Gram-negative rod-shaped organisms. Cell death follows lysis of the cells mediated by the action of endogenous autolytic enzymes (autolysins) present in the cell wall which are activated following β-lactam action. Autolytic enzymes able to hydrolyse peptidoglycan are present in most bacterial walls, they are needed to re-shape the wall during growth and to aid cell separation during division. Their activity is regulated by binding to wall components such as the wall and membrane teichoic acids. When peptidoglycan assembly is disrupted through β-lactam action, some of the teichoic acids are released from the cells, which are then susceptible to attack by their own autolysins.

2.1.4 β-Lactamase inhibitors — clavulanic acid, sulbactam and tazobactam

Expression of β-lactamase enzymes is the most important mechanism through which organisms become resistant to β-lactams. The majority of the enzymes have a serine residue at their active site and bear structural and mechanistic similarities to the carboxypeptidases from which they are thought to have evolved. Unlike the transpeptidases and carboxypeptidases, the β-lactamases hydrolyse β-lactam antibiotics very efficiently, releasing fragments of the antibiotics rapidly instead of remaining bound to the ring-opened forms for several minutes. A number of successful inhibitors, including clavulanic acid, sulbactam and tazobactam have been developed for use in combination with susceptible β-lactams (amoxycillin, ampicillin and piperacillin, respectively), protecting them from inactivation by the β-lactamases. The inhibitors are hydrolysed by the β-lactamases in the same manner as susceptible β-lactam antibiotics, the β-lactam ring being broken by attack by a serine residue in the active site of the enzyme. Instead of undergoing rapid release from the active site serine, the inhibitors remain bound and undergo one of several different fates. It is thought that the hydrolysed inhibitors can interact with a second enzyme residue in the active site of the β-lactamase, forming a covalently cross-linked, irreversibly inhibited complex.

2.2 Mycolic acid and arabinogalactan biosynthesis in mycobacteria

The cell walls of mycobacteria contain an arabino-galactan polysaccharide in addition to the peptido-glycan, plus a variety of high molecular weight lipids, including the mycolic acids, glycolipids, phospholipids and waxes. The lipid-rich nature of the mycobacterial wall is responsible for the characteristic acid-fastness on staining and serves as a penetration barrier to many antibiotics. Isoniazid and ethambutol have long been known as specific antimycobacterial agents, exerting no activity towards other bacteria, but their mechanisms of action have only recently been established.

2.2.1 Isoniazid

Isoniazid interferes with mycolic acid synthesis by inhibiting an enoyl reductase (InhA) which forms part of the fatty acid synthase system in mycobacteria. Mycolic acids are produced by a diversion of the normal fatty acid synthetic pathway in which short-chain (16 carbon) and long-chain (24 carbon) fatty acids are produced by addition of 7 or 11 malonate extension units from malonyl coenzyme A to acetyl coenzyme A. InhA inserts a double bond into the extending fatty acid chain at the 24 carbon stage. The long-chain fatty acids are further extended and condensed to produce the 60–90 carbon β-hydroxymycolic acids which are important components of the mycobacterial cell wall. Isoniazid is converted inside the mycobacteria to a free radical species by a catalase peroxidase enzyme, KatG. The active free radicals then attack and inhibit the enoyl reductase, InhA, by covalent attachment to the active site.

2.2.2 Ethambutol

Ethambutol is thought to block assembly of the arabinogalactan polysaccharide by inhibition of an arabinotransferase enzyme. Cells treated with ethambutol accumulate the isoprenoid intermediate decaprenylarabinose, which supplies arabinose units for assembly in the arabinogalactan polymer.

2.3 Echinocandins—caspofungin

Caspofungin is the first member of the echinocandin group of antifungal agents to be developed for treatment of serious fungal infections. It interferes with the synthesis of the β-1,3-D-glucan polymer in the fungal cell wall. Without the glucan polymer, the integrity of the fungal cell wall is compromised, yeast cells lose their rigidity and become like protoplasts; the effect is especially pronounced in *Candida* species.

3 Protein synthesis

3.1 Protein synthesis and its selective inhibition

Figure 12.4 outlines the process of protein synthesis involving the ribosome, mRNA, a series of aminoacyl transfer RNA (tRNA) molecules (at least one for each amino acid) and accessory protein factors involved in initiation, elongation and termination. As the process is essentially the same in prokaryotic (bacterial) and eukaryotic cells (i.e. higher organisms and mammalian cells) it is surprising that there are so many selective agents which act in this area (see Fig. 12.1).

Bacterial ribosomes are smaller than their mammalian counterparts. They consist of one 30S and one 50S subunit (the S suffix denotes the size, which is derived from the rate of sedimentation in an ultracentrifuge). The 30S subunit comprises a single strand of 16S rRNA and over 20 different proteins that are bound to it. The larger 50S subunit contains two single strands of rRNA (23S and 5S) together with over 30 different proteins. The subunits pack together to form an intact 70S ribosome. The equivalent subunits for mammalian ribosomes are 40S and 60S making an 80S ribosome. Some agents exploit subtle differences in structure between the bacterial and mammalian ribosomes. The macrolides, azalides and chloramphenicol act upon the 50S subunits in bacteria but not the 60S subunits of mammalian cells. By contrast, the tetracyclines derive their selective action through active uptake by microbial cells and only limited penetration of mammalian cells. They are equally active against both kinds of ribosomes by binding to the

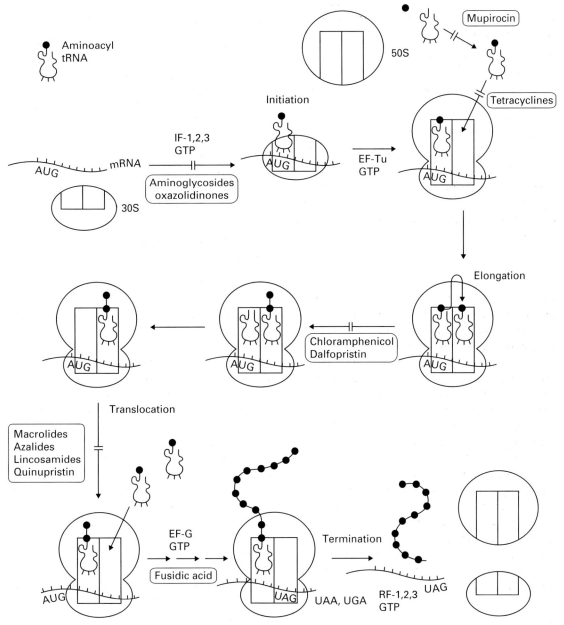

Fig. 12.4 Outline of the process of protein synthesis (translation of messenger RNA) in bacterial cells. The four stages of synthesis are shown: initiation, elongation, translocation and termination with the sites of action of antibiotics. AUG is the start codon on messenger RNA (mRNA) specifying the first amino acid in bacterial proteins, N-formylmethionine. UAG, UAA and UGA are termination codons specifying no amino acid. 30S and 50S are the subunits of the ribosome. Other protein factors involved in protein synthesis are initiation factors (IF-1, 2, 3), elongation factors (EF-Tu and EF-G) and release factors (RF-1, 2, 3).

respective 30S and 40S subunits but insufficient drug enters mammalian cells to block protein synthesis.

3.2 Aminoglycoside-aminocyclitol antibiotics

Most of the information on the mechanisms of action of aminoglycoside-aminocyclitol (AGAC) antibiotics comes from studies with streptomycin. One effect of AGACs is to interfere with the initiation and assembly of the bacterial ribosome (Fig. 12.4). During assembly of the initiation complex, N-formylmethionyl-tRNA (fmet-tRNA) binds initially to the ribosome binding site on the untranslated 5′ end of the mRNA together with the 30S ribosomal subunit. Three protein initiation factors (designated IF-1, 2 and 3) and a molecule of guanosine triphosphate (GTP) are involved in positioning the fmet-tRNA on the AUG start codon of mRNA. IF-1 and IF-3 are then released from the complex, GTP is hydrolysed to guanosine diphosphate (GDP) and released with IF-2 as the 50S subunit joins the 30S subunit and mRNA to form a functional ribosome. The fmet-tRNA occupies the peptidyl site (P site) leaving a vacant acceptor site (A site) to receive the next aminoacyl-tRNA specified by the next codon on the mRNA. Streptomycin binds tightly to one of the protein components of the 30S subunit. Binding of the antibiotic to the protein, which is the receptor for IF-3, prevents initiation and assembly of the ribosome.

Streptomycin binding to the 30S subunit also distorts the shape of the A site on the ribosome and interferes with the positioning of the aminoacyl-tRNA molecules during peptide chain elongation. Streptomycin, therefore, exerts two effects: inhibition of protein synthesis by freezing the initiation complex, and misreading of the codons through distortion of the 30S subunit. Simple blockage of protein synthesis would be bacteriostatic rather than bactericidal. As streptomycin and the other AGACs exert a potent lethal action it seems that the formation of toxic, non-functional proteins through misreading of the codons on mRNA is a more likely mechanism of action. This can be demonstrated with cell-free translation systems in which isolated bacterial ribosomes are supplied with artificial mRNA template such as polyU or polyC and all the other factors, including aminoacyl-tRNAs needed for protein synthesis.

In the absence of an AGAC the ribosomes will produce the artificial polypeptides, polyphenylalanine (as specified by the codon UUU) or polyproline (as specified by the codon CCC). However, when streptomycin is added, the ribosomes produce a mixture of polythreonine (codon ACU) and polyserine (codon UCU). The misreading of the codons does not appear to be random: U is read as A or C and C is read as A or U. If such misreading occurs in whole cells the accumulation of non-functional or toxic proteins would eventually prove fatal to the cells. There is some evidence that the bacterial cell membrane is damaged when the cells attempt to excrete the faulty proteins.

The effectiveness of the AGACs is enhanced by their active uptake by bacteria, which proceeds in three phases. First, a rapid uptake occurs within a few seconds of contact, which represents binding of the positively charged AGAC molecules to the negatively charged surface of the bacteria. This phase is referred to as the energy-independent phase (EIP) of uptake. In the case of Gram-negative bacteria the AGACs damage the outer membrane causing release of some lipopolysaccharide, phospholipid and proteins but this is not directly lethal to the cells. Second, there follows an energy-dependent phase of uptake (EDP I) lasting about 10 minutes, in which the AGAC is actively transported across the cytoplasmic membrane. A second energy-dependent phase (EDP II) which leads to further intracellular accumulation follows after some AGAC has bound to the ribosomes in the cytoplasm. Although the precise details of uptake by EDP I and EDP II are not clear, both require organisms to be growing aerobically. Anaerobes do not take up AGACs by EDP I or EDP II and are consequently resistant to their action.

3.3 Tetracyclines

This group of antibiotics is actively transported into bacterial cells, possibly as the magnesium complex, achieving a 50-fold concentration inside the cells. Mammalian cells do not actively take up the tetracyclines (small amounts enter by diffusion alone) and it is this difference in uptake that determines the selective toxicity. Resistance to the tetracyclines is usually associated with failure of the active uptake system or with an active efflux pump, which removes the drug from the cells before it can interfere with ribosome function. Other resistance mechanisms involve ribosomal protection and modification. Protein synthesis by both bacterial and mammalian ribosomes is inhibited by the tetracyclines in cell-free systems. The action is upon the smaller subunit. Binding of just one molecule of tetracycline to the bacterial 30S subunit occurs at a site involving the 3′ end of the 16S rRNA, a number of associated ribosomal proteins and magnesium ions. The effect is to block the binding of aminoacyl-tRNA to the A site of the ribosome and halt protein synthesis. Tetracyclines are bacteriostatic rather than bactericidal, consequently they should not be used in combination with β-lactams, which require cells to be growing and dividing to exert their lethal action.

3.4 Chloramphenicol

Of the four possible optical isomers of chloramphenicol, only the D-*threo* form is active. This antibiotic selectively inhibits protein synthesis in bacterial ribosomes by binding to the 50S subunit in the region of the A site involving the 23S rRNA. The normal binding of the aminocyl-tRNA in the A site is affected by chloramphenicol in such a way that the peptidyl transferase cannot form a new peptide bond with the growing peptide chain on the tRNA in the P site. Studies with aminocyl-tRNA fragments containing truncated tRNA chains suggest that the shape of the region of tRNA closest to the amino acid is distorted by chloramphenicol. The altered orientation of this region of the aminoacyl-tRNA in the A site is sufficient to prevent peptide bond formation. Chloramphenicol has a broad spectrum of activity, which covers Gram-positive and Gram-negative bacteria, mycoplasmas, rickettsia and chlamydia. It has the valuable property of penetrating into mammalian cells and is, therefore, the drug of choice for treatment of intracellular pathogens, including *Salmonella typhi*, the causative organism of typhoid. Although it does not inhibit 80S ribosomes, the 70S ribosomes of mammalian mitochondria are sensitive and therefore some inhibition occurs in rapidly growing mammalian cells with high mitochondrial activity.

3.5 Macrolides and azalides

Erythromycin is a member of the macrolide group of antibiotics; it selectively inhibits protein synthesis in a broad range of bacteria by binding to the 50S subunit. The site at which it binds is close to that of chloramphenicol and involves the 23S rRNA. Resistance to chloramphenicol and erythromycin can occur by methylation of different bases within the same region of the 23S rRNA. The sites are, therefore, not identical but binding of one antibiotic prevents binding of the other. Unlike chloramphenicol, erythromycin blocks translocation. This is the process by which the ribosome moves along the mRNA by one codon after the peptidyl transferase reaction has joined the peptide chain to the aminoacyl-tRNA in the A site. The peptidyl-tRNA is moved (translocated) to the P site, vacating the A site for the next aminocyl-tRNA. Energy is derived by hydrolysis of GTP to GDP by an associated protein elongation factor, EF-G. By blocking the translocation process, erythromycin causes release of incomplete polypeptides from the ribosome. It is assumed that the azalides, such as azithromycin, have a similar action to the macrolides. The azalides have improved intracellular penetration over the macrolides and are resistant to the metabolic conversion which reduces the serum half-life of erythromycin.

3.6 Lincomycin and clindamycin

These agents bind selectively to a region of the 50S ribosomal subunit close to that of chloramphenicol and erythromycin. They block elongation of the peptide chain by inhibition of peptidyl transferase.

3.7 Streptogramins — quinupristin and dalfopristin

The two unrelated streptogramins, quinupristin and dalfopristin, are used in combination (in a 30 : 70 ratio) to treat infections caused by staphylococci and enterococci (including MRSA and VRE). Their action is synergistic, and is generally bactericidal compared with either agent used alone or compared with antibiotics in the macrolide group. The main target is the bacterial 50S ribosome, with the formulation acting to inhibit protein synthesis. The agents bind sequentially to the 50S subunit; dalfopristin alters the shape of the subunit so that more quinupristin can bind. Dalfopristin blocks an early step in protein synthesis by forming a bond with the ribosome, preventing elongation of the peptide chain by the peptidyl transferase. Quinupristin blocks a later step by preventing the extension of peptide chains and causing incomplete chains to be released. The overall effect is to block elongation.

3.8 Oxazolidinones — linezolid

Oxazolidinones such as linezolid act at the early stage of protein synthesis, preventing the formation of the initiation complex between the 30S subunit, mRNA and fmet-tRNA.

3.9 Mupirocin

The target of mupirocin is one of a group of enzymes which couple amino acids to their respective tRNAs for delivery to the ribosome and incorporation into protein. The particular enzyme inhibited by mupirocin is involved in producing isoleucyl-tRNA. The basis for the inhibition is a structural similarity between one end of the mupirocin molecule and isoleucine. Protein synthesis is halted when the ribosome encounters the isoleucine codon through depletion of the pool of isoleucyl-tRNA.

3.10 Fusidic acid

This steroidal antibiotic does not act upon ribosome itself, but upon one of the associated elongation factors, EF-G. This factor supplies energy for translocation by hydrolysis of GTP and GDP. Another elongation factor, EF-Tu, promotes binding of aminoacyl-tRNA molecules to the A site through binding and hydrolysis of GTP. Both EF-G and EF-Tu have overlapping binding sites on the ribosome. Fusidic acid binds the EF-G:GDP complex to the ribosome after one round of translocation has taken place. This prevents further incorporation of aminoacyl-tRNA by blocking the binding of EF-Tu:GTP. Fusidic acid owes its selective antimicrobial action to active uptake by bacteria and exclusion from mammalian cells. The equivalent elongation factor in mammalian cells, EF-2, is susceptible to fusidic acid in cell-free systems.

4 Chromosome function and replication

4.1 Basis for the selective inhibition of chromosome replication and function

As with protein synthesis, the mechanisms of chromosome replication and function are essentially the same in prokaryotes and eukaryotes. There are, however, important differences in the detailed functioning and properties in the enzymes involved and these differences are exploited by a number of agents as the basis of selective inhibition. The microbial chromosome is large in comparison with the cell that contains it (approximately 500 times the length of *E. coli*). It is, therefore, wound into a compact, supercoiled form inside the cell. During replication the circular double helix must be unwound to allow the DNA polymerase enzymes to synthesize new complimentary strands. The shape of the chromosome is manipulated by the cell by the formation of regions of supercoiling. Positive supercoiling (coiling in the same sense as the turns of the double helix) makes the chromosome more compact. Negative supercoiling (generated by twisting the chromosome in the opposite sense to the helix) produces localized strand separation which is required both for replication and transcription. In a bacterium such as *E. coli* four different topoisomerase enzymes are responsible for maintaining the shape of DNA during cell division. They act by cutting one or both of the DNA strands, they remove and generate supercoiling, then reseal the strands. Their activity is essential for the microbial cell to relieve the complex tangling of the chromosome (both knotting and chain link formation) which results from progression of the replication fork around the circular chromosome. Type I topoisomerases cut one strand of DNA and pass the other strand through the gap before resealing. Type II enzymes cut both strands and pass another double helical section of the DNA through the gap before resealing. In *E. coli* topoisomerases I and III are both type I enzymes while topoisomerases II and IV are type II enzymes. Topoisomerase II (also known as DNA gyrase) and topoisomerase IV are essential enzymes which are inhibited by the fluoro-quinolone group of antimicrobials. Topoisomerase II is responsible for introducing negative supercoils into DNA and for relieving torsional stress, which accumulates ahead of sites of transcription and replication. Topoisomerase IV provides a potent decatenating (unlinking) activity that removes links and knots generated behind the replication fork.

The basic sequence of events for microbial chromosome replication is described below.

4.1.1 Synthesis of precursors

Purines, pyrimidines and their nucleosides and nucleoside triphosphates are synthesized in the cytoplasm. At this stage the antifolate drugs (sulphonamides and dihydrofolate reductase inhibitors) act by interfering with the synthesis and recycling of the co-factor dihydrofolic acid (DHF). Thymidylic acid (2-deoxy-thymidine monophosphate, dTMP) is an essential nucleotide precursor of DNA synthesis. It is produced by the enzyme thymidylate synthetase by transfer of a methyl group from tetrahydrofolic acid (THF) to the uracil base on uridylic acid (2-deoxyuridine monophosphate, dUMP) (Fig. 12.5). THF is converted to DHF in this process and must be reverted to THF by the enzyme dihydrofolate reductase (DHFR) before

the cycle can be repeated. By inhibiting DHFR, the antifolates effectively block the production of dTMP and hence DNA synthesis.

The antifungal agent 5-fluorocytosine also interferes with these early stages of DNA synthesis. Through conversion to the nucleoside triphosphate it subsequently blocks thymidylic acid production through inhibition of the enzyme thymidylate synthetase (Fig. 12.6).

The antiviral nucleosides aciclovir and ganciclovir are also converted to their respective nucleoside triphosphates in the cytoplasm of infected cells. They proceed to inhibit viral DNA replication either by inhibition of the DNA polymerase or by incorporation into DNA with subsequent termination of chain extension. Finally the anti-HIV drug AZT acts in an analogous manner, being converted to the corresponding triphosphate and inhibiting viral RNA synthesis by the HIV reverse transcriptase.

4.1.2 Unwinding of the chromosome

As described in section 4.1 the DNA double helix must unwind to allow access of the polymerase enzymes to produce two new strands of DNA. This is facilitated by topoisomerase I (DNA gyrase) which is the target of the fluoroquinolones. Some agents interfere with the unwinding of the chromosome by physical obstruction. These include the acridine dyes, of which the topical antiseptic proflavine is the most familiar, and the antimalarial acridine mepacrine. They prevent strand separation by

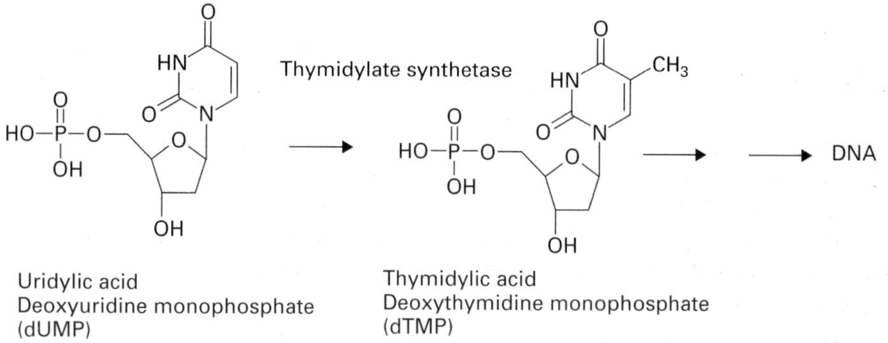

Uridylic acid
Deoxyuridine monophosphate
(dUMP)

Thymidylic acid
Deoxythymidine monophosphate
(dTMP)

DNA

Fig. 12.5 Conversion of uridylic acid to thymidylic acid by the enzyme thymidylate synthetase, a vital early stage in the synthesis of DNA.

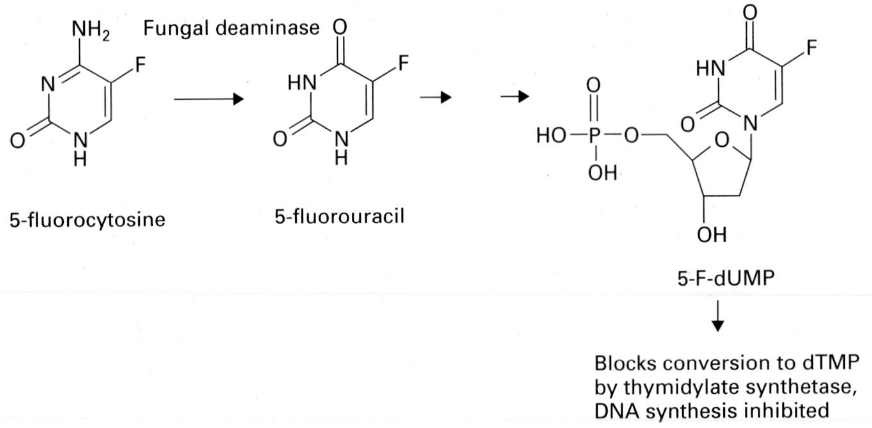

Fig. 12.6 Conversion of the antifungal agent 5-fluorocytosine (5-FC) to 5-fluorouracil by a deaminase enzyme inside fungal cells and subsequent inhibition of fungal DNA synthesis through inhibition of thymidylate synthetase.

insertion (intercalation) between base pairs from each strand, but exhibit very poor selective toxicity.

4.1.3 Replication of DNA strands

The unwound DNA strands are kept unfolded during replication by binding a protein called Albert's protein. A series of enzymes produce new strands of DNA using each of the separated strands as templates. One strand is produced continuously. The other is produced in a series of short strands called Okazaki fragments that are joined by a DNA ligase. The entire process is carefully regulated with proofreading stages to check that each nucleotide is correctly incorporated as specified by the template sequence. There are no therapeutic agents yet known which interfere directly with the DNA polymerases.

4.1.4 Transcription

The process of transcription, the copying of a single strand of mRNA sequence using one strand of the chromosome as a template, is carried out by RNA polymerase. This is a complex of four proteins (2 α, 1 β and 1 β' subunits) which make up the core enzyme. Another small protein, the σ factor, joins the core enzyme, which binds to the promoter region of the DNA preceding the gene that is to be transcribed. The correct positioning and orientation of the polymerase is obtained by recognition of specific marker sites on the DNA at positions −10 and −35 nucleotide bases before the initiation site for transcription. The σ factor is responsible for recognition of the initiation signal for transcription and the core enzyme possesses the activity to join the nucleotides in the sequence specified by the gene. Mammalian genes possess an analogous RNA polymerase but there are sufficient differences in structure to permit selective inhibition of the microbial enzyme by the semisynthetic rifamycin antibiotics rifampicin and rifabutin.

4.2 Fluoroquinolones

The fluoroquinolones selectively inhibit topoisomerases II and IV, which are not found in mammalian cells. The enzymes, both tetramers comprising two A and two B subunits, are capable of catalysing a variety of changes in DNA topology. The topoisomerases bind to the chromosome at points where two separate double-stranded regions cross. This can be at a supercoiled region, a knotted or a linked (catenane) region. The A subunits (gyrA for topoisomerase II and parC for topoisomerase

IV) cut both DNA strands on one chain with a 4 base pair stagger; the other chain is passed through the break which is then re-sealed. The B subunits (gyrB for topoisomerase II and parE for topoisomerase IV) derive energy for the reaction by hydrolysis of ATP. The precise details of the interaction are not clear but it appears that the fluoroquinolones do not simply eliminate enzyme function, they actively poison the cells by trapping the topoisomerases as drug–enzyme–DNA complexes in which double-strand DNA breaks are held together by the enzyme protein alone. The enzymes are unable to reseal the DNA with the result that the chromosome in treated cells becomes fragmented. The number of fragments (approximately 100 per cell) is comparable to the number of supercoils in the chromosome. The action of the fluoroquinolones probably triggers secondary responses in the cells which are responsible for death. One notable morphological effect of fluoroquinolone treatment of Gram-negative rod-shaped organisms is the formation of filaments. In Gram-positive cocci topoisomerase IV may be the more important target for fluoroquinolone action.

4.3 Nitroimidazoles (metronidazole, tinidazole) and nitrofurans (nitrofurantoin)

These agents also cause DNA strand breakage but by a direct chemical action rather than by inhibition of a topoisomerase. Metronidazole is active only against anaerobic organisms. The nitro group of metronidazole is converted to a nitronate radical by the low redox potential within cells. The activated metronidazole then attacks the DNA, producing strand breakage. Another nitroimidazole, tinidazole, and the nitrofuran nitrofurantoin are thought to act in a similar manner.

4.4 Rifampicin and rifabutin

The action of rifampicin is upon the β subunit of RNA polymerase. Binding of just one molecule of rifampicin inhibits the initiation stage of transcription in which the first nucleotide is incorporated in the RNA chain. Once started, transcription itself is not inhibited. It has been suggested that the structure of rifampicin resembles that of two adenosine nucleotides in RNA; this may form the basis of the binding of the antibiotic to the β subunit. One problem is the rapid development of resistance in organisms due to alterations in the amino acids comprising one particular region of the β subunit. These changes do not affect the activity of the polymerase but render it insensitive to rifampicin. The action of rifampicin is specific for the microbial RNA polymerase, the mammalian version being unaffected. Rifabutin, which has enhanced activity against *Mycobacterium avium* complex, is thought to act in the same way as rifampicin.

4.5 5-Fluorocytosine (5-FC)

This antifungal agent inhibits DNA synthesis at the early stages involving production of the nucleotide thymidylic acid (TMP). 5-FC is converted by a deaminase inside fungi to 5-fluorouracil then to the corresponding nucleoside triphosphate, 5-fluorodeoxyuridine monophosphate (5-F-dUMP) which then acts as an inhibitor of thymidylate synthetase (Fig. 12.6). This enzyme normally produces thymidylic acid (TMP) from deoxyuridine monophosphate (dUMP) by addition of a methyl group (supplied by a folate co-factor, section 4.1.1) to the 5 position of the uracil ring. As this position is blocked by the fluoro group in 5-FC, the phosphate acts as an inhibitor of the enzyme. 5-FC can be considered as a pro-drug; it has the value of being taken up by fungi as the nucleoside, whereas the active triphosphate produced inside the cells would not be taken up because of its negative charge. Although 5-FC is an important antifungal agent in the treatment of life-threatening infections, resistance can occur due to active efflux of the drug from the cells before it can inhibit DNA synthesis.

5 Folate antagonists

5.1 Folate metabolism in microbial and mammalian cells

Folic acid is an important co-factor in all living cells. In the reduced form, tetrahydrofolate (THF), it

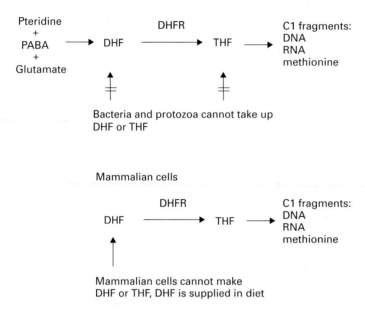

Fig. 12.7 Pathways of folate metabolism and use in microbial cells (upper) and mammalian cells (lower). Bacterial and protozoal cells must synthesize dihydrofolic acid (DHF) from *p*-aminobenzoic acid (PABA). DHF is converted to tetrahydrofolic acid (THF) by the enzyme dihydrofolate reductase (DHFR). THF supplies single carbon units for various pathways including DNA, RNA and methionine synthesis. Mammalian cells do not make DHF, it is supplied from the diet, conversion to THF occurs via a DHFR enzyme as in microbial cells.

functions as a carrier of single carbon fragments, which are used in the synthesis of adenine, guanine, thymine and methionine (Fig. 12.7). One important folate-dependent enzyme is thymidylate synthetase, which produces TMP by transfer of the methyl group from THF to UMP. In this and other folate-dependent reactions THF is converted to dihydrofolic acid (DHF), which must be reduced back to THF before it can participate again as a carbon fragment carrier. The enzyme responsible for the reduction of DHF to THF is dihydrofolate reductase (DHFR) which uses the nucleotide NADPH$_2$ as a co-factor. Bacteria, protozoa and mammalian cells all possess DHFR but there are sufficient differences in the enzyme structure for inhibitors such as trimethoprim and pyrimethamine to inhibit the bacterial and protozoal enzymes selectively without damaging the mammalian form. In the case of protozoa such as the *Plasmodium* species responsible for malaria, the DHFR is a double enzyme which also contains the thymidylate synthetase activity.

There is another fundamental difference between folate utilization in microbial and mammalian cells (Fig. 12.7). Bacteria and protozoa are unable to take up exogenous folate and must synthesize it themselves. This is carried out in a series of reactions involving first the synthesis of dihydropteroic acid from one molecule each of pteridine and *p*-aminobenzoic acid (PABA). Glutamic acid is then added to form DHF, which is reduced by DHFR to THF. Mammalian cells do not make their own DHF, instead they take it up from dietary nutrients and convert it to THF using DHFR.

5.2 Sulphonamides

Sulphonamides (e.g. sulphamethoxazole and dapsone) are structural analogues of PABA (Fig. 12.8). They competitively inhibit the incorporation of PABA into dihydropteroic acid and there is some evidence for their incorporation into false folate analogues, which inhibit subsequent metabolism. The presence of excess PABA will reverse the inhibitory action of sulphonamides, as will thymine, adenine, guanine and methionine. However these nutrients are not normally available at the site of infections for which the sulphonamides are used.

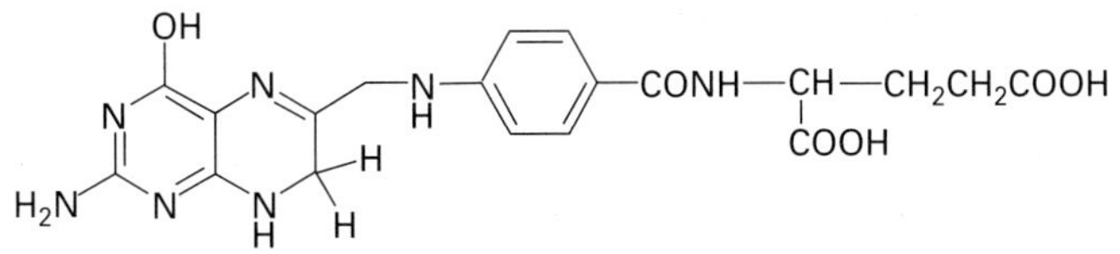

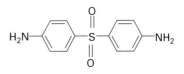

Dihydrofolic acid (DHF)

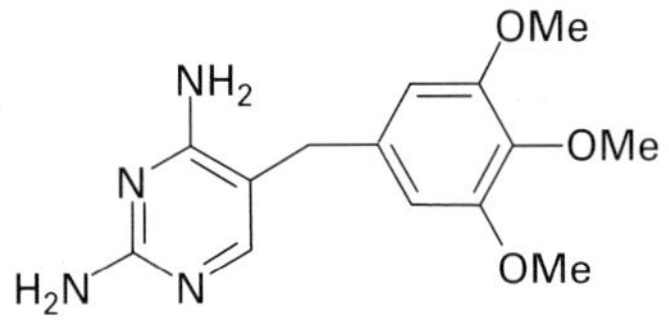

Trimethoprim (antibacterial)

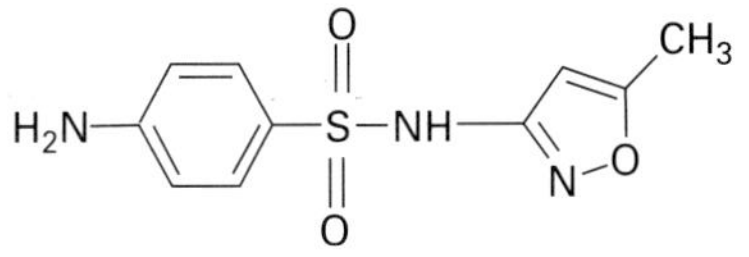

Sulphamethoxazole (antibacterial)

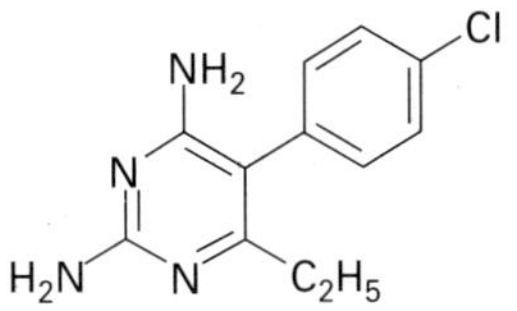

Pyrimethamine (antimalarial)

Dapsone (antimalarial, antileprotic)

Fig. 12.8 Structural relationships between dihydrofolate reductase inhibitors (trimethoprim and pyrimethamine), sulphonamides (sulphamethoxazole and dapsone) and dihydrofolic acid.

5.3 DHFR inhibitors — trimethoprim and pyrimethamine

Trimethoprim is a selective inhibitor of bacterial DHFR. The bacterial enzyme is several thousand times more sensitive than the mammalian enzyme. Pyrimethamine, likewise, is a selective inhibitor of plasmodial DHFR. Both are structural analogues of the dihydropteroic acid portion of the DHF substrate (Fig. 12.8). Crystal structures of the bacterial, plasmodial and mammalian DHFRs, each containing either bound substrate or the inhibitors, have been determined by X-ray diffraction studies. These show how inhibitors fit tightly into the active site normally occupied by the DHF substrate, forming a pattern of strong hydrogen bonds with amino acid residues and water molecules lining the site. Another DHFR is proguanil, a guanidine-containing pro-drug which is metabolized in the liver to cycloguanil, an active selective inhibitor of plasmodial DHFR. Methotrexate is a potent DHFR inhibitor that has an analogous structure to the whole DHF molecule, including the glutamate residue. It has no selectivity towards microbial DHFR and cannot, therefore, be used to treat infec-tions; however, it is widely used as an anticancer agent. A derivative of methotrexate that is used for treatment of *Pneumocystis carinii* infections in AIDS patients is trimetrexate. Although it is very toxic to mammalian cells, simultaneous administration of leucovorin (formyl-THF or folinic acid) as an alternative source of folate which cannot be taken up by the organism protects host tissues. DHFR inhibitors can be used in combination with a sulphonamide to achieve a double interference with folate metabolism. Suitable combinations with matching pharmacokinetic properties are sulphamethoxazole with trimethoprim (the antibacterial co-trimoxazole) and dapsone with pyrimethamine (the antimalarial Maloprim).

6 The cytoplasmic membrane

6.1 Composition and susceptibility of membranes to selective disruption

The integrity of the cytoplasmic membrane is vital for the normal functioning of all cells. Bacterial membranes do not contain sterols and in this

217

respect differ from membranes of fungi and mammalian cells. Fungal membranes contain predominantly ergosterol as the sterol component whereas mammalian cells contain cholesterol. Gram-negative bacteria contain an additional outer-membrane structure that provides a protective penetration barrier to potentially harmful substances, including many antibiotics. The outer membrane has an unusual asymmetric structure in which phospholipids occupy the inner face and the lipopolysaccharide (LPS) occupies the outer face. The outer membrane is attached to the peptidoglycan by proteins and lipoproteins. The stability of all membranes is maintained by a combination of non-covalent interactions between the constituents involving ionic, hydrophobic and hydrogen bonding. The balance of these interactions can be disturbed by the intrusion of molecules (membrane-active agents) which destroy the integrity of the membrane, thereby causing leakage of cytoplasmic contents or impairment of metabolic functions associated with the membrane. Most membrane-active agents that function in this way, e.g. the alcohols, quaternary ammonium compounds and bisbiguanides (considered in Chapters 17 and 18) have very poor selectivity. They cannot be used systemically because of their damaging effects upon mammalian cells; instead they are used as skin antiseptics, disinfectants and preservatives. A few agents can be used therapeutically: the polymyxins (colistin), which act principally upon the outer membrane of Gram-negative bacteria, and the antifungal polyenes, which act upon fungal membranes. Other antifungal agents, the imidazoles, triazoles and terbinafine act by blocking the synthesis of ergosterol, the major sterol present in fungal membranes (see also Chapter 4).

6.2 Polymyxins

Polymyxin E (colistin) is used in the treatment of serious Gram-negative bacterial infections, particularly those caused by *Pseudomonas aeruginosa*. It binds tightly to the lipid A component of LPS in the outer membrane of Gram-negative bacteria. The outer leaflet of the membrane structure is distorted, segments of which are released and the permeability barrier is destroyed. The polymyxin molecules can then penetrate to the cytoplasmic membrane where they bind to phospholipids, disrupt membrane integrity, and cause irreversible leakage of cytoplasmic components. Their detergent-like properties are a key feature of this membrane-damaging action, which is similar to that of quaternary ammonium compounds. The high affinity of colistin for LPS is an advantage in the treatment of *P. aeruginosa* lung infections where neutralization of the endotoxic action of LPS released from the organisms may help to reduce inflammation. With increasing resistance to the major groups of antibiotics, some multiresistant organisms (e.g. *Acinetobacter* species) remain sensitive only to membrane-active agents such as colistin.

6.3 Polyenes

Amphotericin B and nystatin are the most commonly used members of this group of antifungal agents. They derive their action from their strong affinity towards sterols, particularly ergosterol. The hydrophobic polyene region binds to the hydrophobic sterol ring system within fungal membranes. In so doing, the hydroxylated portion of the polyene is pulled into the membrane interior, destabilizing the structure and causing leakage of cytoplasmic constituents. It is possible that polyene molecules associate together in the membrane to form aqueous channels. The pattern of leakage is progressive, with small metal ions such as K^+ leaking first, followed by larger amino acids and nucleotides. The internal pH of the cells falls as K^+ ions are released, macromolecules are degraded and the cells are killed. The selective antifungal activity of the polyenes is poor, depending on the higher affinity for ergosterol than cholesterol. Kidney damage is a major problem when polyenes are used systemically to treat severe fungal infections. The problem can be reduced, but not eliminated by administration of amphotericin as a lipid complex or liposome.

6.4 Imidazoles and triazoles

The azole antifungal drugs act by inhibiting the synthesis of the sterol components of the fungal membrane (see also Chapter 4). They are inhibitors

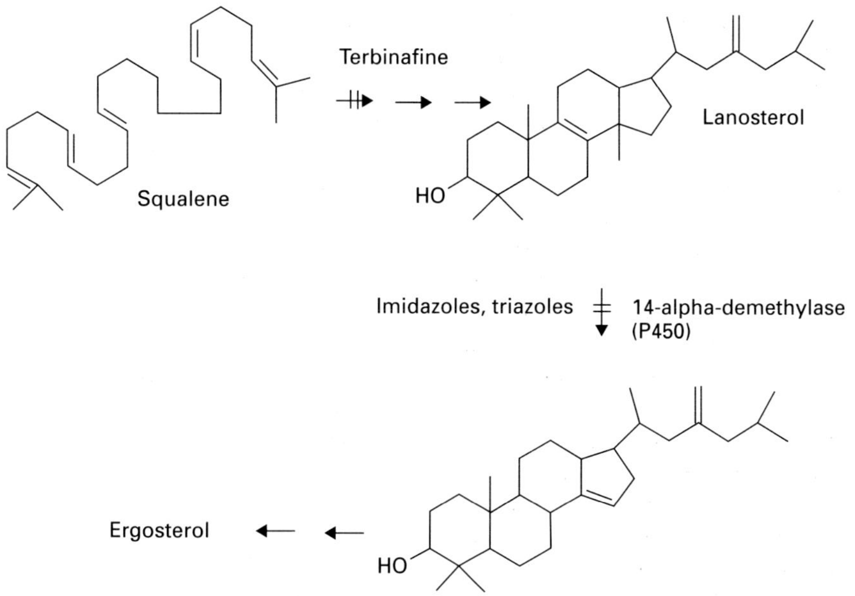

Fig. 12.9 Pathway for synthesis of the essential fungal sterol ergosterol and the sites of inhibition by the antifungal agents terbinafine, imidazoles and triazoles.

of one step in the complex pathway of ergosterol synthesis involving the removal of a methyl group from lanosterol (Fig. 12.9). The 14α-demethylase enzyme responsible is dependent upon cytochrome P-450. The imidazoles and triazoles cause rapid defects in fungal membrane integrity due to reduced levels of ergosterol, with loss of cytoplasmic constituents leading to similar effects to the polyenes. The azoles are not entirely specific for fungal ergosterol synthesis and have some action upon mammalian sterol metabolism, for example they reduce testosterone synthesis.

6.5 Terbinafine

This synthetic antifungal agent inhibits the enzyme squalene epoxidase at an early stage in fungal sterol biosynthesis. Acting as a structural analogue of squalene, terbinafine causes the accumulation of this unsaturated hydrocarbon, and a decrease in ergosterol in the fungal cell membrane (Fig. 12.9).

7 Further reading

Amyes, S. G. B, Thompson, C., Miles, R. & Tillotson, G. (1996) *Antimicrobial Chemotherapy, Theory, Practice and Problems*. Martin Dunitz, London.

Franklin, T. J. & Greenwood, D. (2000) *Antimicrobial Chemotherapy*, 4th edn. Oxford University Press, Oxford.

Franklin, T. J. & Snow, G. A. (1989) *Biochemistry of Antimicrobial Action*, 4th edn. Chapman & Hall, London.

Loll, P. J. & Axelsen P. H. (2000) The structural biology of molecular recognition by vancomycin. *Annu Rev Biophys Biomol Struct*, **29**, 265–289.

Russell, A. D. & Chopra, I. (1990) *Understanding Antibacterial Action and Resistance*. Ellis Horwood, New York.

van Heijenoort, J. (2001) Formation of the glycan chains in the synthesis of bacterial peptidoglycan. *Glycobiology*, **11**, 25R-36R.

Williams, R. A. D., Lambert, P. A. & Singleton, P. (1996) *Antimicrobial Drug Action*. Bios, Oxford.

Young, K. D. (2001) Approaching the physiological functions of penicillin-binding proteins in *Escherichia coli*. *Biochimie*, **83**, 99–102.

Chapter 13
Bacterial resistance to antibiotics

Anthony Smith

1 Introduction

It is both a cliché and a truism to state that antibiotic resistance has been around for as long as antibiotics have been used to treat infection. Indeed, the origin of antibiotic resistance extends much further back in evolutionary terms and reflects the attack and counter-attack of complex microbial flora in order to establish ecological niches and survive. It is true to say that early treatment failures with antibiotics did not represent a significant clinical problem because other classes of agents, with different cellular targets, were available. It is the emergence of multiple resistance, i.e. resistance to several types of antibiotic agent, that is causing major problems in the clinic today. Several factors drove this situation in the 1970s and 1980s, including the introduction of extended-spectrum agents and advances in medical techniques, for example, in organ transplantation and cancer chemotherapy. The net result has been a huge selective pressure in favour of multiply resistant species. Coupled with this, there has been a sharp decline in the introduc-

tion of agents acting on new cellular targets over the last 30 years compared with the 20-year period following World War II. There are a number of resistant organisms causing concern at present. Notable Gram-positive organisms include methicillin-resistant *Staphylococcus aureus* (MRSA) and coagulase-negative staphylococci, glycopeptide-intermediate sensitivity *S. aureus* (GISA), vancomycin-resistant *Enterococcus* (VRE) species and penicillin-resistant *Streptococcus pneumoniae*. Concerns among the Gram-negative organisms include multidrug-resistant *Pseudomonas aeruginosa*, *Stenotrophomonas maltophilia* and *Acinetobacter baumannii* and members of the Enterobacteriaceae with extended-spectrum β-lactamases. Multidrug resistance in the acid-fast bacilli *Mycobacterium tuberculosis* and *M. avium* complex pose major health threats worldwide.

2 Origins of resistance

Some bacteria are said to have *innate* resistance

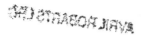

against antibiotics and this typically reflects variations in the structure of their cell envelope. These will be identified in subsequent sections on resistance mechanisms. Resistance or reduced susceptibility may also be *phenotypic*, resulting from adaptation to growth within a specific environment. A characteristic of such phenotypic resistance is reversion to antibiotic susceptibility upon subculture in conventional laboratory media and failure to isolate genotypic resistant mutants (section 17). The origins of antibiotic resistance genes are unclear; however, studies using clincal isolates collected before the introduction of antibiotics demonstrated susceptibility, although conjugative plasmids (section 16.1) were present. Resistance can be achieved by horizontal acquisition of resistance genes, mobilized via insertion sequences, transposons and conjugative plasmids, by recombination of foreign DNA into the chromosome, or by mutations in different chromosomal loci. Given that it is only 60 years since the introduction of antibiotics, mutation of common ancestral genes could not be the only resistance mechanism. Many resistance genes will have derived from the diverse gene pool present in environmental microorganisms, most likely produced as protective mechanisms by antibiotic-producing organisms. Genetic exchange is likely to arise in soil and the general environment as well as the gut of humans and animals. Rapid mutation can occur and there is clearly a heavy selective pressure resulting from the overuse of antibiotics in medical practice. Agricultural and veterinary use of antibiotics also makes an important and unhelpful contribution. The mutation process is not a static event and a complex network of factors influences the rate and type of mutants that can be selected under antibiotic selective pressure. Antibiotic concentration, physiological conditions such as nutrient availability and stress can each regulate mutation rates. The structure of a gene is relevant to mutability. Size is not the main factor, as not every mutation in a gene that encodes an antibiotic target leads to resistance. Resistance only occurs by mutations which are both permissive (that is, not lethal or leading to an unacceptable reduction in 'fitness' or ability to cause infection) and able to produce a resistance phenotype. The probability that such a mutation arises will be proportional to the number of target sites within the gene. In *Escherichia coli*, mutations in the *gyrA* gene, encoding the GyrA subunit of topoisomerase II and leading to fluoroquinolone resistance (section 8) have been identified in at least seven locations, whereas mutational changes in only three positions in the *parC* gene, encoding a subunit of topoisomerase IV, have been observed. As a consequence, the prediction that the mutation rate would be higher in *gyrA* than *parC* is correct. Such observations and predictions cannot be extrapolated to other organisms. Indeed, the opposite is true for fluoroquinolone resistance in *S. pneumoniae*.

3 Mechanisms of resistance

Resistance to antimicrobial agents typically occurs by one or more of the following mechanisms:
1 Inactivation of the drug
2 Alteration of the target
3 Reduced cellular uptake
4 Increased efflux.

In this chapter, resistance will be examined by agent, but attention will be drawn to mechanisms which can permit resistance to multiple, chemically different agents. This is most commonly associated with efflux and this will be described in section 16.4.

4 Resistance to β-lactam antibiotics

β-Lactam antibiotics act by inhibiting the carboxy/transpeptidase or penicillin-binding proteins (PBPs) involved in the late stages of peptidoglycan biosynthesis. Although introduced nearly 60 years ago, β-lactam antibiotics still represent the most widely used class of agents in the clinic today. Resistance to many β-lactam agents is common and is most often caused by β-lactamases or by mutation in the PBPs resulting in reduced affinity. Reduced uptake and efflux are also seen, but they are less significant.

4.1 β-Lactamases

A number of different β-lactamases have been de-

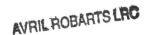

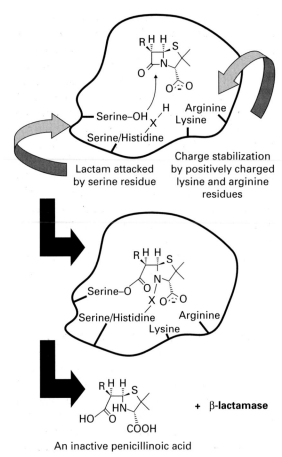

Fig. 13.1 General scheme for inhibition of β-lactam-type antibiotics by β-lactamase.

scribed, but all share the feature of catalysing the ring-opening of the β-lactam moiety (Fig. 13.1). Thus, the structural homology with the terminal D-Ala-D-Ala of maturing peptidoglycan, shared by all β-lactam antibiotics, is lost.

β-Lactamases may be chromosomal or plasmid-borne, inducible or constitutive, and for this reason their terminology can be confusing. A number of classification systems have been proposed, including classes A–D based on peptide sequence. Classes A, C and D have a serine at the active site, whereas class B enzymes have four zinc atoms at their active site and these are also called metallo-β-lactamases. Class A enzymes are highly active against benzylpenicillin, class B β-lactamases are effective against penicillins and cephalosporins. Class C en-

zymes are usually inducible, but mutation can lead to overexpression. Class D is composed of the OXA-type enzymes, which can hydrolyse oxacillin. Increasing resistance to β-lactam agents, mainly by β-lactamase, prompted the discovery and introduction of agents with greater β-lactam stability such as cephalosporins, carbapenems and monobactams. Resistance first appeared in organisms such as *Enterobacter cloacae* and *Pseudomonas aeruginosa*, due to mutations causing overproduction of the class C chromosomal AmpC β-lactamase. Subsequently, in the late 1980s, resistance occurred in organisms such as *Klebsilla pneumoniae* and *Escherichia coli* that lack an inducible AmpC enzyme. Resistance was found to be mediated by plasmids encoding extended-spectrum β-lactamases (ESBLs). These arose from mutational development of more limited-spectrum β-lactamases such as TEM and SHV that either increased the size of the active site pocket or altered its binding characteristics to allow the larger cephalosporins to enter and be broken down. TEM derivatives predominate, possibly favoured by the use of ceftazidime and other slowly penetrating cephalosporins. These mutations also increase the binding of clavulanic acid and so these ESBLs remain susceptible to inhibition by this and other β-lactamase inhibitors such as sulbactam and tazobactam, which are generally ineffective against class C β-lactamases.

Continuing use of the third-generation cephalosporins and the introduction of β-lactamase inhibitor combinations (clavulanate with amoxycillin or ticarcillin, sulbactam with ampicillin, and tazobactam with piperacillin; see section 4.2) resulted in the appearance of plasmids encoding class C β-lactamases. After several unconfirmed reports, the first proof that a class C β-lactamase had been captured on a plasmid came in 1990 when transmissible resistance to α-methoxy and oxyimino-β-lactams was shown to be mediated by an enzyme whose gene was 90% identical to the *ampC* gene of *E. cloacae*. They have subsequently been found worldwide. Strains with plasmid-mediated AmpC enzymes are typically resistant to aminopenicillins (ampicillin or amoxycillin), carboxypenicillins (carbenicillin or ticarcillin) and ureidopenicillins (piperacillin). The enzymes also provide resistance to the oxyimino cephalosporins (ceftazidime, cefo-

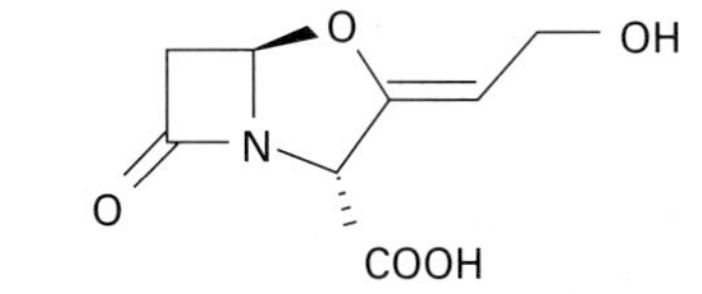

Clavulanic acid

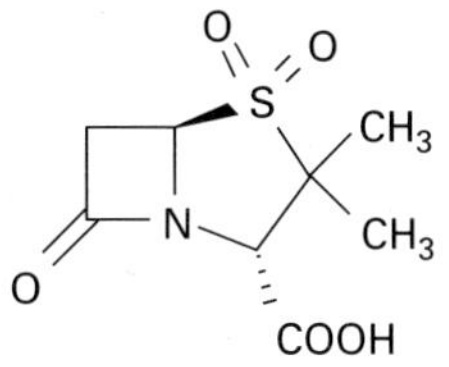

Sulbactam

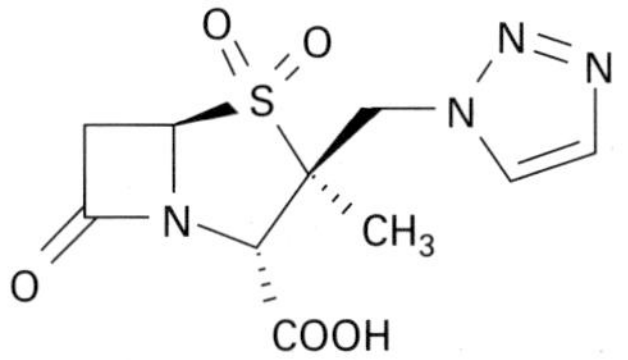

Tazobactam

Fig. 13.2 Structures of β-lactamase inhibitors.

taxime, ceftriaxone) and the 7-α-methoxy group (cefoxitin, cefmetazole and moxalactam) as well as the monobactam aztreonam.

4.2 β-Lactamase inhibitors

In addition to introducing agents with increased stability to β-lactamase inhibition, β-lactamase inhibitors including clavulanic acid, sulbactam and tazobactam have been developed (Fig. 13.2). Clavulanic acid is produced by a streptomyces and is a suicide inhibitor of β-lactamases from a number of Gram-negative and Gram-positive organisms. These β-lactamase inhibitors do not have any significant antimicrobial activity against bacterial transpeptidases, but their combination with a β-lactam antibiotic (see above) has extended the clinical usefulness of the latter.

4.3 Altered penicillin-binding proteins (PBPs) and methicillin-resistant *Staphylococcus aureus*

Altered PBPs are responsible for reduced sensitivity

to β-lactam agents by *Streptococcus pneumoniae* (PBP1a, PBP2b and PBP2x) and *Haemophilus influenzae* (PBP3A and PBP3b), but by far the most clinically significant example is methicillin-resistant *Staphylococcus aureus* (MRSA). By the early 1950s, the acquisition and spread of plasmid-encoded β-lactamases had blunted the effectiveness of penicillin for treating *S. aureus* infections such as boils, carbuncles, pneumonia, endocarditis and osteomyelitis. The β-lactamase-stable agent methicillin was introduced in 1959, but by 1960, methicillin-resistant strains were identified. This was the result of *S. aureus* acquiring the *mecA* gene, which encodes an altered PBP gene, PBP2a. The *mecA* gene is chromosomal and expression is either constitutive or inducible, but not by methicillin. PBP2a has low affinity for most β-lactam antibiotics.

5 Resistance to glycopeptide antibiotics

Vancomycin and teicoplanin are the two glycopeptides used clinically. They bind the terminal D-alanyl-D-alanine side-chains of peptidoglycan and prevent cross-linking in a number of Gram-positive organisms. They are not active against Gram-negative organisms due to the presence of the outer membrane. Vancomycin use increased dramatically in response to the increasing incidence of MRSA and resistance was first reported in the enterococci in 1988. Vancomycin-resistant enterococci (VRE) now account for more than 20% of all enterococcal infections. Resistance is greatest amongst *E. faecium* strains, but significant numbers of the more clinically significant *E. faecalis* are also resistant. Five types of resistance, VanA to VanE have now been reported. Phenotypic VanA resistance is the most common and confers high-level resistance to vancomycin and teicoplanin. VanA resistance is mediated by a seven gene cluster on the transposable genetic element Tn*1546* (Fig. 13.3).

Resistance to vancomycin is via a sensor histidine kinase (VanS) and a response regulator (VanR). VanH encodes a D-lactate dehydrogenase/α-keto acid reductase and generates D-lactate, which is the substrate for VanA, a D-Ala-D-Lac ligase. The result is cell wall precursors terminating in D-Ala-D-

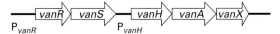

Fig. 13.3 Organization of vancomycin resistance gene cluster.

Lac to which vancomycin binds with very low affinity. This change in affinity is mediated by one hydrogen bond. The complex formed between vancomycin and D-Ala-D-Ala is stabilized by five hydrogen bonds, whereas only four hydrogen bonds can form between vancomycin and D-Ala-D-Lac and the complex is unstable (Fig. 13.4). Further, VanX encodes a D-Ala-D-Ala dipeptidase which can modify endogenous D-Ala-D-Ala precursors. Recent genetic analysis has identified close homology between this cluster and genes present in the vancomycin-producing organism *Amycolatopsis orientalis*, suggesting that selective pressure has forced genes originally present to protect antibiotic-producing organisms to jump to other species. VanB resistance is also acquired and the peptidoglycan precursor is again D-Ala-D-Lac, but isolates often remain susceptible to teicoplanin. VanC resistance is intrinsic and chromosomally encoded in some enterococcal species such as *E. gallinarum* and the peptidoglycan precursor is D-Ala-D-Ser. Less is known of VanD and VanE resistance, but both are acquired. VanD uses D-Ala-D-Lac and VanE uses D-Ala-D-Ser.

5.1 MRSA and reduced glycopeptide susceptibility

There is major concern that high-level, VanA-type resistance could transfer to staphylococci, particularly MRSA. Experimental transfer of the enterococcal VanA system to *S. aureus* on the skin of mice has been reported, but other mechanisms resulting in intermediate-level resistance occur in clinical isolates. In the 1960s and 1970s MRSA was not feared because several other treatment options existed, including use of tetracyclines, macrolides and aminoglycosides. But multiple resistance was accumulating and by the 1980s empiric therapy of staphylococcal infections, particularly nosocomial sepsis, was changed to the glycopeptide antibiotic

vancomycin. MRSA levels were rising and the early 1990s saw a major increase in vancomycin use. The inevitable consequence of the selective pressure was the isolation in 1997 of the first *S. aureus* strain with reduced susceptibility to vancomycin and teicoplanin (vancomycin MIC = 8 μg/ml). At the beginning of the 21st century, MRSA is responsible for up to 25% of nosocomial infections in the USA and reports of community-acquired MRSA infections are increasing. While reports of 'superbugs' resistant to all known antibiotics abound, it is important to distinguish between reduced susceptibility and resistance, recognizing that there are conflicting definitions of resistance and resistance breakpoints. Strains with MIC values <4 μg/ml are considered sensitive, 8–16 μg/ml intermediate and >32 μg/ml resistant. Thus the acronyms VISA (vancomycin-intermediate *S. aureus*) and GISA (glycopeptide-insensitive *S. aureus*) are used to denote strains with vancomycin or teicoplanin MICs of 8 μg/ml, whereas VRSA (vancomyin-resistant *S. aureus*) is reserved for strains with MIC values >32 μg/ml. The mechanism of glycopeptide resistance is poorly understood, but strains show longer doubling times and decreased susceptibility to lysostaphin. Increased quantities of PBP2 and PBP2′ and cell wall precursors are presumed to trap vancomycin, while amidation of glutamine residues in cell wall muropeptides reduces the cross-linking and consequently the number of vancomycin target molecules.

6 Resistance to aminoglycoside antibiotics

The aminoglycosides are hydrophilic sugars possessing a number of amino and hydroxy substituents. The amine groups are protonated at biological pH and it is the polycationic nature of the molecules that affords them their affinity for nucleic acids, particularly the acceptor (A) site of 16S ribosomal RNA. Aminoglycoside binding to the A site interferes with the accurate recognition of cognate tRNA by rRNA during translation and may also perturb translocation of the tRNA from the A site to the peptidyl-tRNA site (P site). While high-level resistance in aminoglycoside-producing microorganisms is by methylation of the rRNA, this

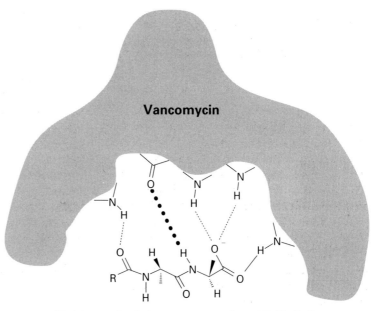

Stable complex between vancomycin and D-Ala-D-Ala

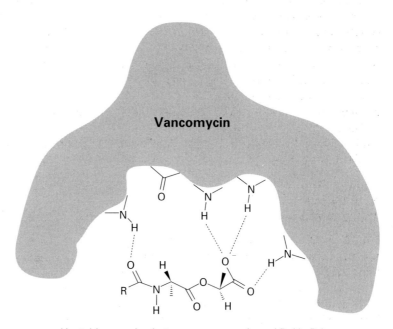

Fig. 13.4 Mechanism of high-level vancomycin resistance. Hydrogen bonds are denoted by dashed lines. The key hydrogen bond present in the stable complex with D-Ala-D-Ala, but missing in the unstable complex with D-Ala-D-Lac, is shown in heavy type.

Unstable complex between vancomycin and D-Ala-D-Lac

is NOT the mechanism of resistance in previously susceptible strains. The most common mechanism for clinical aminoglycoside resistance is their structural modification by enzymes expressed in resistant organisms, which compromises their ability to interact with rRNA. There are three classes of these enzymes: aminoglycoside phosphatases (APHs), aminoglycoside nucleotidyltransferases (ANTs) and aminoglycoside acetyltransferases (AACs). Within each class, there are enzymes with differing

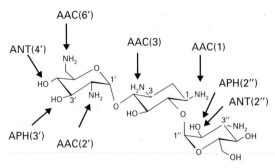

Fig. 13.5 Structure of kanamycin B showing system of ring numbering and sites of action of some aminoglycoside-modifying enzymes. AAC, aminoglycoside acetyltransferase; ANT, aminoglycoside nucleotidyltransferase and APH, aminoglycoside phosphotransferase.

specificities around the sugars. There are four ANTs [ANT(6), ANT(4′), ANT(3″) and ANT(2″)], seven APHs [APH(3′), APH(2″), APH(3″), APH(6), APH(9), APH(4) and APH(7″)] and four AACs [AAC(2′), AAC(6′), AAC(1) and AAC(3)]. There is also a bifunctional enzyme, AAC(6′)-AAC(2″). Aminoglycosides are typically susceptible to attack by multiple enzymes (Fig. 13.5). Attempts to circumvent these modifying enzymes have centred on structural modifications. Examples include tobramycin which lacks the 3′-hydroxyl group and is thus not a substrate for APH(3′) and amikacin which has an acylated N-1 group and is not a substrate for several modifying enzymes. Other strategies are exemplified by experimental compounds such as 3′-oxo-kanamycin. This molecule is a substrate for APH(3′), but the phosphorylation product is unstable and regenerates the original antibiotic.

7 Resistance to tetracycline antibiotics

Chlortetracycline and oxytetracycline were discovered in the late 1940s and studies of representative populations before their widespread use suggests that emergence of resistance is a relatively modern event. More than 60% of *Shigella flexneri* isolates are resistant to tetracycline; resistant isolates of *Salmonella enterica* serovar *typhimurium* are becoming more common and among Gram-positive species, approximately 90% of MRSA strains and 60% of multiply resistant *Streptococcus pneumoniae* are now tetracycline-resistant. The major mechanisms of resistance are efflux and ribosomal protection. One exception is the *tet(X)* gene that encodes an enzyme which modifies and inactivates the tetracycline molecule, although this does not appear to be clinically significant. The Tet efflux proteins belong to the major facilitator superfamily (MFS). These proteins exchange a proton for a tetracycline–cation (usually Mg^{2+}) complex, reducing the intracellular drug concentration and protecting the target ribosomes in the cell. In Gram-negative bacteria, the efflux determinants comprise divergently oriented efflux and repressor proteins that share overlapping promoter and operator regions. In the absence of a tetracycline–Mg^{2+} complex, the repressor protein binds and blocks transcription of both genes. Drug binding alters the conformation of the repressor so that it can no longer bind the DNA operator region and block transcription. This method of regulation probably applies to all of the Gram-negative efflux systems including *tet(A)*, *tet(C)*, *tet(D)*, *tet(E)*, *tet(G)* and *tet(H)*.

No repressor proteins have been identified in the Gram-positive *tet(K)* or *tet(L)* genes and regulation of plasmid-borne tetracycline resistance appears to be by translational attenuation, involving stem-loop mRNA structures and tetracycline-induced unmasking of the ribosome binding site permitting translation of the efflux protein. Regulation of chromosomal *tet(L)* expression involves tetracycline-promoted stalling of the ribosomes during translation of early codons of the leader peptide, which allows re-initiation of translation at the ribosome binding site for the structural gene. Ribosomal protection is mediated by cytoplasmic proteins that inhibit tetracycline and also confer resistance to doxycycline and minocycline. These proteins share homology with the elongation factors EF-Tu and EF-G, and expression of Tet(M) and Tet(O) proteins appears to be regulated. A 400-bp region upstream from the coding region for *tet(O)* is needed for full expression, but the mechanism(s) has not been characterized. The widespread emergence of efflux- and ribosome protection-based resistance to first- and second-generation

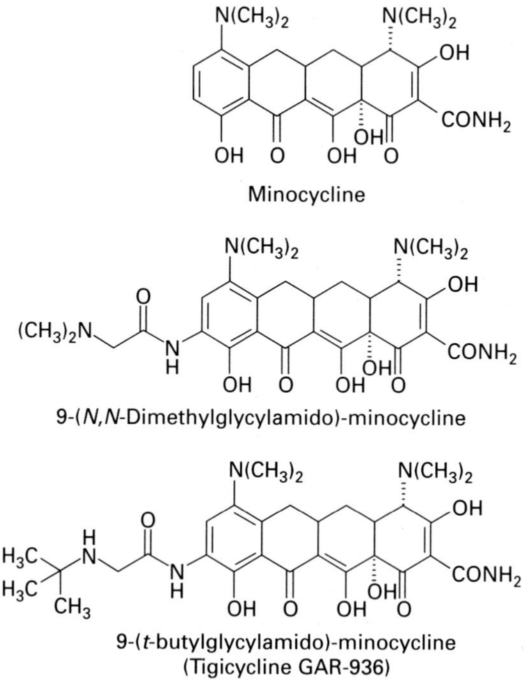

Fig. 13.6 Structural modifications at the 9 position of the tetracycline antibiotic minocycline conferring increased stability against resistance mechanisms.

tetracyclines has prompted the development of the 9-glycinyltetracyclines (9-glycylcyclines). 9-Amino-acylamido derivatives of minocycline have similar activity to earlier compounds; however, when the acyl group is modified to include an *N,N*-dialkylamine or 9-*t*-butyl-glycylamido moiety (Fig. 13.6), antimicrobial activity is retained and the compounds are active against strains containing *tet* genes responsible for resistance by efflux and ribosomal protection.

8 Resistance to fluoroquinolone antibiotics

Fluoroquinolones bind and inhibit two bacterial topoisomerase enzymes: DNA gyrase (topoisomerase II) which is required for DNA supercoiling, and topoisomerase IV which is required for strand separation during cell division. DNA gyrase tends to be the major target in Gram-negative bacteria,

whereas both topoisomerases are inhibited in Gram-positive bacteria. Each topoisomerase is termed a heterotetramer, being composed of two copies of two different subunits designated A and B. The A and B subunits of DNA gyrases are encoded by *gyrA* and *gyrB*, respectively, whilst topoisomerase IV is encoded by *parC* and *parE* (*grlA* and *grlB* in *S. aureus*). Mutations in *gyrA*, particularly involving substitution of a hydroxyl group with a bulky hydrophobic group, induce conformational changes such that the fluoroquinolone can no longer bind. Mutations have also been detected in the B subunit, but these are probably less important. Alterations involving Ser80 and Glu84 of *S. aureus grlA* and Ser79 and Asp83 of *S. pneumoniae parC* have led to quinolone resistance. Like GyrB, mutations in ParE leading to resistance are not common. While changes in GyrA and ParC give resistance to the older fluoroquinolones, MIC values do not always rise above clinically defined breakpoints for newer agents such as gemifloxacin and moxifloxacin.

Topoisomerases are located in the cytoplasm and thus fluoroquinolones must cross the cell envelope to reach their target. Changes in outer-membrane permeability have been associated with resistance in Gram-negative bacteria, but permeability does not appear to be an issue with Gram-positive species. Efflux, however, does make a contribution to resistance, mainly low level, in both Gram-positive and Gram-negative bacteria. The NorA-mediated efflux system in *S. aureus* was characterized in 1990. It is expressed weakly in wild-type strains and resistance is thought to occur via mutations leading to increased expression of *norA*. NorA is a member of the major facilitator superfamily and homologues are also present in *Streptococcus pneumoniae* and *Bacillus* sp. There is a tendency for it to be more effective for hydrophilic fluoroquinolones, but there is no strict correlation. Fluoroquinolones are now being used for treating *Mycobacterium avium* and multidrug-resistant *M. tuberculosis* and efflux-mediated resistance has been identified. A number of efflux pumps have been identified among Gram-negative bacteria, including AcrA in *E. coli*, which is regulated in part by the multiple antibiotic resistance (Mar) operon (section 16.3).

9 Resistance to macrolide, lincosamide and streptogramin (MLS) antibiotics

Although chemically distinct, members of the MLS group of antibiotics all inhibit bacterial protein synthesis by binding to a target site on the ribosome. Gram-negative bacteria are intrinsically resistant due to the permeability barrier of the outer membrane, and three resistance mechanisms have been described in Gram-positive bacteria. Target modification, involving adenine methylation of domain V of the 23S ribosomal RNA, is the most common mechanism. The adenine-N^6-methyltransferase, encoded by the *erm* gene, results in resistance to erythromycin and other macrolides (including the azalides), as well as the lincosamides and group B streptogramins. Streptogramin A-type antibiotics are unaffected and streptogramin A/B combinations remain effective. Expression of the *erm* gene may be constitutive or inducible. When expression is inducible, resistance is seen only against 14- and 15-membered macrolides; lincosamide and streptogramin antibiotics remain active. Telithromycin (Fig. 13.7), the first of a new class of ketolide agents in the MLS family, does not induce MLS resistance and also retains activity against domain V-modified ribosomes and inhibition of protein synthesis through strong interaction with domain II. The second resistance mechanism is efflux. Expression of the *mef* gene confers resistance to macrolides only, whereas *msr* expression results in resistance to macrolides and streptogramins. Efflux-mediated resistance of *S. aureus* to streptogramin A antibiotics is also conferred by *vga* and *vgaB* gene products. A third resistance mechanism, involving ribosomal mutation, has been reported in a small number of clinical isolates of *S. pneumoniae*.

10 Resistance to chloramphenicol

Chloramphenicol inhibits protein synthesis by binding the 50S ribosomal subunit and preventing the peptidyltransferase step. Decreased outer-membrane permeability and active efflux have been identified in Gram-negative bacteria; however, the major resistance mechanism is drug inactivation by chloramphenicol acetyltransferase. This occurs in

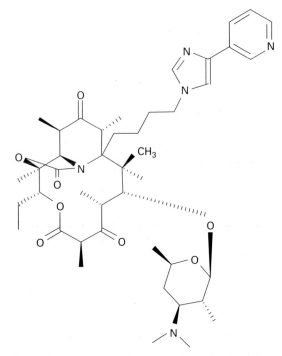

Fig. 13.7 Structure of telithromycin, a ketolide macrolide antibiotic that retains activity against 23S domain V modified ribosomal RNA.

both Gram-positive and Gram-negative species, but the *cat* genes, typically found on plasmids, share little homology.

11 Resistance to the oxazolidinone antibiotics

Linezolid is the first of a new class of oxazolidinone antimicrobials with a novel target in protein synthesis. Linezolid does not interfere with translation initiation at the stage of mRNA binding or formation of 30S pre-initiation complexes, rather it involves binding the 50S rRNA. Its affinity for 50S rRNA from Gram-positive bacteria is twice that for the corresponding molecule in Gram-negative bacteria and as such linezolid has been approved for treating various Gram-positive infections, including MRSA. Resistance is appearing, although rare at present. Mutation in the central loop of domain V of the component 23S rRNA subunit appears to be the main mechanism, including a G2576T mutation in three isolates of linezolid-resistant MRSA.

12 Resistance to trimethoprim

Trimethoprim competitively inhibits dihydrofolate reductase (DHFR) and resistance can be caused by overproduction of host DHFR, mutation in the structural gene for DHFR and acquisition of the *dfr* gene encoding a resistant form. There are at least 15 DHFR enzyme types based on sequence homology and acquisition of *dfr* genes encoding alternative DHFR of type I, II or V is the most common mechanism of trimethoprim resistance among the Enterobacteriaceae.

13 Resistance to mupirocin

Nasal carriage of MRSA strains has been identified as an important target for infection control protocols aimed at reducing spread and acquisition. Mupirocin (pseudomonic acid A) is an effective topical antimicrobial used in MRSA eradication. It is an analogue of isoleucine that competitively binds isoleucyl-tRNA synthetase (IRS) and inhibits protein synthesis. Low-level resistance (MIC 4–256 µg/ml) is usually due to mutation of the host IRS, whereas high-level resistance (MIC >512 µg/ml) is due to acquisition of a distinct IRS that is less sensitive to inhibition. The *mupA* gene, typically carried on transferable plasmids, is found in *S. aureus* and coagulase-negative staphylococci, and encodes an IRS with only 30% homology to the mupirocin-sensitive form.

14 Resistance to peptide antibiotics — polymyxin

Many peptide antibiotics have been described and can be broadly classified as non-ribosomally synthesized peptides; they include the polymyxins, bacitracins and gramicidins as well as the glycopeptides (section 5) and the ribosomally synthesized peptides such as the antimicrobial peptides of the innate immune system. Polymyxins and other cationic antimicrobial peptides have a self-promoted uptake across the cell envelope and perturb the cytoplasmic membrane barrier. Addition of a 4-amino-4-deoxy-L-arabinose (L-Ara4N) moiety to the phosphate groups on the lipid A component of Gram-negative lipopolysaccharide has been implicated in resistance to polymyxin. Details of the pathway for L-Ara4N biosynthesis from UDP glucuronic acid, encoded by the *pmr* operon, are emerging.

15 Resistance to anti-mycobacterial therapy

The nature of mycobacterial infections, particularly tuberculosis, means that chemotherapy differs from other infections. Organisms tend to grow slowly (long generation time) in a near dormant state with little metabolic activity. Hence, a number of the conventional antimicrobial targets are not suitable. Isoniazid is bactericidal, reducing the count of aerobically growing organisms. Pyrazinamide is active only at low pH, making it well suited to killing organisms within necrotic foci early in infection, but less useful later on when these foci have reduced in number. Rifampicin targets slow-growing organisms. Resistance mechanisms have now been described and multiple resistance poses a serious threat to health. Current treatment regimens do result in a high cure rate and the combination of agents makes it highly unlikely that there will be a spontaneous resistant isolate to all the components. Problems most commonly occur in patients who receive inadequate therapy which provides a serious selection advantage. Resistance can occur to single agents and subsequently to multiple agents. Resistance to rifampicin arises from mutation in the beta subunit of RNA polymerase encoded by *rpoB* and resistant isolates show decreased growth rates. Modification of the catalase gene *katG* results in resistance to isoniazid, mainly by reduced or absent catalase activity. Catalase activity is absolutely required to convert isoniazid to the active hydrazine derivative. Interestingly, animal model studies suggest that *M. tuberculosis* strains in which the *katG* gene is inactivated are attenuated compared with wild-type strains. Low-level rifampicin resistance can be obtained by point mutations in *inhA* leading to its overexpression. Pyrazinamide is a pro-drug requiring pyrazinamidase to produce the active pyrazinoic acid. Most cases of resistance are due to mutations in the pyrazinamidase gene (*pncA*), but gene inactivation by the insertion sequence IS*6110* has been reported. Streptomycin resistance can arise through mutations in *rrs* and *rpsL* which affect streptomycin binding. However, these account for only half of the resistant isolates, so further resistance mechanisms await definition. Ethambutol resistance has been noted in *M. tuberculosis* and other species such as *M. smegmatis*. Ethambutol inhibits the polymerization of arabinan in the arabinogalactan and lipoarabinomannan of the mycobacterial cell wall and one of its likely targets is the family of arabinosyltransferases encoded by the *emb* locus. Missense mutations in the *embB* gene in this locus confer resistance to ethambutol.

16 Multiple drug resistance

16.1 R-factors

Several issues of multiple drug resistance have already been raised in this chapter. Notable examples are MRSA, which can harbour both small cryptic plasmids and larger plasmids encoding resistance to antiseptics, disinfectants, trimethoprim, penicillin, gentamicin, tobramycin and kanamycin, and multidrug-resistant *M. tuberculosis*. Of equal concern are instances where isolates can become resistant to multiple, chemically distinct agents in a single biological event. One of the earliest examples was in Japan in 1959. Previously sensitive *E. coli* became resistant to multiple antibiotics through acquisition of a conjugative plasmid (R-factor) from resistant *Salmonella* and *Shigella* isolates. A number of R-factors have now been characterized including RP4, encoding resistance to ampicillin, kanamycin, tetracycline and neomycin, found in *P. aeruginosa* and other Gram-negative bacteria; R1, encoding resistance to ampicillin, kanamycin, sulphonamides, chloramphenicol and streptomycin, found in Gram-negative bacteria and pSH6, encoding resistance to gentamicin, trimethoprim and kanamycin, found in *S. aureus*.

16.2 Mobile gene cassettes and integrons

Many Gram-negative resistance genes are located in gene cassettes. One or more of these cassettes can be integrated into a specific position on the chromosome termed an integron. More than 60 cassettes have been identified, each comprising only a promotor-less single gene (usually antibiotic resistance) and a 59-base element forming a specific recombination site. This recombination site confers mobility because it is recognized by specific recombinases encoded by integrons that catalyse integration of the cassette into a specific site within the integron. Thus, integrons are genetic elements that recognize and capture multiple mobile gene cassettes. As the gene typically lacks a promoter, expression is dependent on correct orientation into the integron to supply the upstream promoter. Four classes of integron have been identified, although only one member of class 3 has been described and class 4 integrons are limited to *Vibrio cholerae*. Analysis of the resistant *Shigella* strains isolated in Japan has shown that some of the conjugative plasmids included an integron with one or two integrated cassettes.

16.3 Chromosomal multiple-antibiotic resistance (Mar) locus

The multiple-antibiotic resistance (*mar*) locus was first described in *Escherichia coli* by Stuart Levy and colleagues at Tufts University and has since been recognized in other enteric bacteria. The locus consists of two divergently transcribed units, *marC* and *marRAB*. Little is known of *marC* and *marB*; however, *marR* encodes a repressor of the operon, and *marA* encodes a transcriptional activator affecting expression of more than 60 genes. Increased expression of the *MarRAB* operon resulting from mutations in *marO* or *marR*, or from inactivation of MarR following exposure to inducing agents such as salicylate, leads to the Mar phenotype. This phenotype is characterized by resistance to structurally unrelated antibiotics, organic solvents, oxidative stress and chemical disinfectants. A number of effector mechanisms have been identified, including increased expression of the *acrAB-tolC* multidrug efflux system (section 16.4) and the *soxRS* regulon.

16.4 Multidrug efflux pumps

Whereas some efflux pumps excrete only one drug or class of drugs, a multidrug efflux pump can excrete a wide range of compounds where there is often little or no chemical similarity between the substrates. One common characteristic may be agents with a significant hydrophobic domain. For this reason, hydrophilic compounds such as the aminoglycoside antibiotics are not exported by these systems. A distinction needs to be drawn between those efflux systems, typically in Gram-positive bacteria, that pump their substrate across the cytoplasmic membrane, such as the QacA and Smr pumps which both export quaternary ammonium compounds and basic dyes, and those which efflux across the cytoplasmic and outer membranes of Gram-negative bacteria. There are some examples of single membrane systems in Gram-negative bacteria, such as the EmrE protein in *E. coli*, but they are not of great clinical significance. The majority of Gram-negative pumps span both membranes and include the AcrAB-TolC system in *E. coli* and the MexAB-OprM system in *P. aeruginosa*. Genomic analyses are revealing numerous homologues. Using the MexAB-OprM system as the prototypic example (Fig. 13.8), MexA is the linker protein and MexB is in the cytoplasmic membrane. MexB is a resistance-nodulation-division (RND) family member and is predicted to be a proton antiporter with 12 membrane-spanning α-helices. OprM shows homology with outer-membrane channels of systems thought to export such diverse molecules as nodulation signals and alkaline proteases. Mutations in regulatory genes such as *nalB* cause overexpression of MexAB-OprM and consequently multidrug resistance. MexB is a proton antiporter and efflux by this and other members of the RND family is energized by proton motive force. This contrasts with mammalian multidrug efflux pumps (MDR) that are powered by ATP hydrolysis.

17 Clinical resistance — MIC values, breakpoints, phenotype and outcome

The resistance mechanisms described in this chapter typically lead to an increase in MIC value,

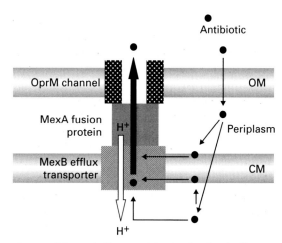

Fig. 13.8 Schematic diagram of the MexAB-OprM efflux pump from *Pseudomonas aeruginosa*. (Kindly supplied by K. Poole.)

although it should be remembered that this does not always equate with clinical failure. If the MIC value remains below the breakpoint value, which can itself be difficult to determine, then the antibiotic will remain effective in the clinic. But such arguments assume that MIC values, which are typically determined when the isolate is growing in complex, sensitivity-test broth, equate with the sensitivity of the organism when growing in the many subtly different environments encountered during infection *in vivo*. Unfortunately, the antibiotic literature contains numerous examples of treatment failures despite apparent sensitivity in the test tube and this resistance is referred to as being phenotypic. Put in other words, resistance is a consequence of the adaptation of the organism to grow and survive within the *in vivo* environment and subculture into conventional laboratory growth medium rarely shows the existence of resistant mutants. There are several key factors at play here, particularly slow/no growth, nutrient depletion and mode of growth. There are numerous papers showing a tendency for nutrient depletion, that is restricted or non-availability of an important nutrient, and slow/no growth to be associated with reduced susceptibility to antibiotics and biocides.

There is now increasing concern over the role played by microbial biofilms in infection. These include the well-known examples of medical device-related infections, such as those associated with artificial joints, prosthetic heart valves and catheters. Many chronic infections, not related to medical devices, are also due to bacteria either not growing and relatively dormant or growing slowly as biomasses or adherent biofilms on mucosal surfaces. A bacterial biofilm is typically defined as a population of cells growing as a consortium on a surface and enclosed in a complex exopolymer matrix. Commonly in the wider environment but less so in infections, the population is mixed and also of heterogeneous physiologies. Growth as a biofilm almost always leads to a large increase in resistance to antimicrobial agents, including antibiotics, biocides and preservatives, compared with cultures grown in suspension (planktonic) in conventional liquid media, but there is no generally agreed mechanism to account for this resistance. Although there is general acceptance that there are numerous planktonic phenotypes, many papers refer to 'the biofilm phenotype', implicitly assuming (wrongly) that there is only one. Those same parameters known to influence planktonic physiology and antibiotic susceptibility, including growth rate and/or specific nutrient limitation, also apply to biofilm physiology and antibiotic susceptibility. The general resistance of biofilms is clearly phenotypic. The well characterized resistance mechanisms described above — lack of antibiotic penetration, inactivation, efflux and repair — make contributions in some circumstances. However, compelling evidence that they are uniquely responsible for biofilm resistance is lacking. Reduced growth rate probably has an involvement, particularly in that it is associated with responses to stress. During stress responses, key structures are protected and cellular processes close down to a state of dormancy, and it has been proposed that exceptional vegetative cell dormancy is the basic explanation of biofilm resistance.

18 Concluding comments

It has been said that in the early years of the 21st century we are in an interim between the first antibiotic era, exemplified by the β-lactams, macrolides, tetracyclines, aminoglycosides and fluoroquinolones, and a second era of new agents directed against targets waiting to be revealed by genomics and proteomics research. In this interim, the goals must be to reduce antibiotic usage and encourage the return of a susceptible human commensal flora. Finally, it must be remembered that antibiotics are not man's invention. Microorganisms have used them in attack and counter-attack against each other for billions of years. Our efforts over the last 60 years seem trivial in comparison.

19 Further reading

Alekshun, M. N. & Levy, S. B. (1999) The *mar* regulon: multiple resistance to antibiotics and other toxic chemicals. *Trends Microbiol*, 7, 410–413.

Chopra, I. & Roberts, M. (2001) Tetracycline antibiotics: mode of action, applications, molecular biology, and epidemiology of bacterial resistance. *Microbiol Mol Biol Rev*, 65, 232–260.

Fluit, A. C., Visser, M. R. & Schmitz, F. J. (2001) Molecular detection of antimicrobial resistance. *Clin Microbiol Rev*, 14, 836–871.

Gillespie, S. H. (2002) Evolution of drug resistance in *Mycobacterium tuberculosis*: clinical and molecular perspective. *Antimicrob Agents Chemother*, 46, 267–274.

Kotra, L. P., Haddad, J. & Mobashery, S. (2000) Aminoglycosides: perspectives on mechanism of action and resistance and strategies to counter resistance. *Antimicrob Agents Chemother*, 44, 3249–3256.

Martinez, J. L. & Baquero, F. (2000) Mutation frequencies and antibiotic resistance. *Antimicrob Agents Chemother*, 44, 1771–1777.

Murray, B. E. (2000) Vancomycin-resistant enterococcal infections. *N Engl J Med*, 342, 710–721.

Nikaido, H. (1996) Multidrug efflux pumps of gram-negative bacteria. *J Bacteriol* 178, 5853–5859.

Philippon, A., Arlet, G. & Jacoby, G. A. (2002) Plasmid-determined AmpC-type β-lactamases. *Antimicrob Agents Chemother*, 46, 1–11.

Recchia, G. D. & Hall, R. M. (1997) Origins of the mobile gene cassettes found in integrons. *Trends Microbiol*, 5, 389–394.

Chapter 14
Clinical uses of antimicrobial drugs

Roger Finch

1 Introduction

The worldwide use of antimicrobial drugs continues to rise; in 2000 these agents accounted for an expenditure of approximately £25 billion. In the UK prescribing in general practice accounts for approximately 90% of all antibiotics and largely involves oral and topical agents. Hospital use accounts for the remaining 10% of antibiotic prescribing with a much heavier use of injectable agents. Although this chapter is concerned with the clinical use of antimicrobial drugs, it should be remembered that these agents are also extensively used in veterinary practice and, to a diminishing extent, in animal husbandry as growth promoters. In humans the therapeutic use of anti-infectives has revolutionized the management of most bacterial infections, many parasitic and fungal diseases and, with the availability of aciclovir and a growing number of anti-retroviral agents (see Chapters 5 and 10), selected herpesvirus infections and human immunodeficiency virus (HIV) infection, respectively. Although originally used for the treatment of established bacterial infections, antibiotics have proved useful in the prevention of infection in various high-risk circumstances; this applies especially to patients undergoing various surgical procedures where peri-operative antibiotics have significantly reduced postoperative infectious complications.

The advantages of effective antimicrobial chemotherapy are self-evident, but this has led to a significant problem in ensuring that they are always appropriately used. Surveys of antibiotic use have demonstrated that more than 50% of antibiotic prescribing can be inappropriate; this may reflect prescribing in situations where antibiotics are either ineffective, such as viral infections, or that the selected agent, its dose, route of administration or duration of use are inappropriate. Of particular concern is the unnecessarily prolonged use of antibiotics for surgical prophylaxis. Apart from being wasteful of health resources, prolonged use encourages superinfection by drug-resistant organisms and unnecessarily increases the risk of adverse drug reactions. Thus, it is essential that the clinical use of these agents be based on a clear understanding of the principles that have evolved to ensure safe, yet effective, prescribing.

Further information about the properties of antimicrobial agents described in this chapter can be found in Chapter 10.

2 Principles of use of antimicrobial drugs

2.1 Susceptibility of infecting organisms

Drug selection should be based on knowledge of its activity against infecting microorganisms. Selected organisms may be predictably susceptible to a particular agent, and laboratory testing is therefore rarely performed. For example, *Streptococcus pyogenes* is uniformly sensitive to penicillin. In contrast, the susceptibility of many Gram-negative enteric bacteria is less predictable and laboratory guidance is essential for safe prescribing. The susceptibility of common bacterial pathogens and widely prescribed antibiotics is summarized in Table 14.1. It can be seen that, although certain bacteria are susceptible *in vitro* to a particular agent, use of that drug may be inappropriate, either on pharmacological grounds or because other less toxic agents are preferred.

2.2 Host factors

In vitro susceptibility testing does not always predict clinical outcome. Host factors play an important part in determining outcome and this applies particularly to circulating and tissue phagocytic activity. Infections can progress rapidly in patients suffering from either an absolute or functional deficiency of phagocytic cells. This applies particularly to those suffering from various haematological malignancies, such as the acute leukaemias, where phagocyte function is impaired both by the disease and also by the use of potent cytotoxic drugs which destroy healthy, as well as malignant, white cells. Under these circumstances it is essential to select agents that are bactericidal, as bacteriostatic drugs, such as the tetracyclines or sulphonamides, rely on host phagocytic activity to clear bacteria. Widely used bactericidal agents include the aminoglycosides, broad-spectrum penicillins, the cephalosporins and quinolones (see Chapter 10).

In some infections the pathogenic organisms are located intracellularly within phagocytic cells and, therefore, remain relatively protected from drugs that penetrate cells poorly, such as the penicillins and cephalosporins. In contrast, erythromycin, rifampicin and the fluoroquinolones readily penetrate phagocytic cells. Legionnaires' disease is an example of an intracellular infection and is treated with erythromycin with or without rifampicin.

2.3 Pharmacological factors

Clinical efficacy is also dependent on achieving satisfactory drug concentrations at the site of the infection; this is influenced by the standard pharmacological factors of absorption, distribution, metabolism and excretion. If an oral agent is selected, gastrointestinal absorption should be satisfactory. However, it may be impaired by factors such as the presence of food, drug interactions (including chelation), or impaired gastrointestinal function either as a result of surgical resection or malabsorptive states. Although effective, oral absorption may be inappropriate in patients who are vomiting or have undergone recent surgery; under these circumstances a parenteral agent will be required and has the advantage of providing rapidly effective drug concentrations.

Antibiotic selection also varies according to the anatomical site of infection. Lipid solubility is of importance in relation to drug distribution. For example, the aminoglycosides are poorly lipid-soluble and although achieving therapeutic concentrations within the extracellular fluid compartment, penetrate the cerebrospinal fluid (CSF) poorly. Likewise the presence of inflammation may affect drug penetration into the tissues. In the presence of meningeal inflammation, β-lactam agents achieve satisfactory concentrations within the CSF, but as the inflammatory response subsides drug concentrations fall. Hence it is essential to maintain sufficient dosaging throughout the treatment of bacterial meningitis. Other agents such as chloramphenicol are little affected by the presence or absence of meningeal inflammation.

Therapeutic drug concentrations within the bile duct and gall bladder are dependent upon biliary excretion. In the presence of biliary disease, such as gallstones or chronic inflammation, the drug

Table 14.1 Sensitivity of selected bacteria to common antibacterial agents

	Staphylococcus aureus (pen. sensitive)	*Staphylococcus aureus* (pen. resistant)	*Streptococcus pyogenes* and *Streptococcus pneumoniae*	*Enterococcus*	*Cl. perfringens*	*Neisseria gonorrhoeae*	*Neisseria meningitidis*	*Haemophilus influenzae*	*Escherichia coli*	*Klebsiella spp.*	*Proteus spp.* (indole-negative)	*Proteus spp.* (indole-positive)	*Serratia spp.*	*Salmonella spp.*	*Shigella spp.*	*Pseudomonas spp.*	*Bacteroides fragilis*	Other *Bacteroides spp.*	*Chlamydia spp.*	*Mycoplasma pneumoniae*	*Rickettsia spp.*
Penicillin V/G	+	R	+*	+	+	+*	+	±	R	R	R	R	R	R	R	R	R	+	R	R	R
Methicillin, flucloxacillin	+	+*	+	R	(±)	(±)	(±)	R	R	R	R	R	R	R	R	R	R	(±)	R	R	R
Ampicillin, amoxicillin	+	R	+*	+	+	+*	+	±	±	R	+	R	R	±	±	R	R	+	R	R	R
Ticarcillin	(+)	R	(+)	R	+	(+)	+	(±)	±	±	+	+	±	(±)	(±)	+*	±	±	R	R	R
Cefazolin	+	+*	+	R	(±)	(±)	(±)	+	+	±	+	R	R	(±)	(±)	R	R	+	R	R	R
Cefamandole, cefuroxime	+	+	+	R	+	(±)	+	+	+	±	+	R	±	(±)	(±)	R	R	±	R	R	R
Cefoxitin	+	+	+	R	+	(±)	+	+	+	+	+	+	+	(±)	(±)	R	+	+	R	R	R
Cefotaxime, ceftriaxone	+	+	+	R	+	+	+	+	+	+	+	+	+	(±)	(±)	±	R/±	R/+	R	R	R
Ceftazidime	+	+	+	R		+	+	+	+	+	+	+	+	(±)	(±)	+	±	±	R	R	R
Erythromycin	+	+	+	+	±	(±)	(±)	±	R	R	R	R	R	R	R	R	±	+	+	+	+
Clindamycin	+*	+*	+*	R	+*	+	R	R	R	R	R	R	R	(±)	(±)	R	+	+	R	R	+
Tetracyclines	+*	+*	±	+	+	+	+	+*	+	±	±	±	+*	+*	+	R	+	±	+	+	+
Chloramphenicol	+	+	+	±	+	+	+	+	+	±	+	±	+	+	+	R	+	+	+	R	+
Ciprofloxacin	±	±	R	R	R	+	+	+	+	+	+	+	+	+	+	(+)	R	R	R	R	R
Gentamicin, tobramycin, amikacin, netilmicin	+	+	R	±	(±)	±	±	±	+	+*	+	+	+*	(±)	(±)	+*	R	R	R	R	R
Sulphonamides	+	+	±	±	(±)	±	±	±	±	±	±	±	R	±	±	R	R	R	+	R	R
Trimethoprim–sulphamethoxazole	+	+	+	+	R	+	+	+	+	+	+	+	R	+	+	R	R	R	+	R	R

+, Sensitive; R, resistant; ±, some strains resistant; ( ), not appropriate therapy; *, rare strains resistant.

concentration may fail to reach therapeutic levels. In contrast, drugs that are excreted primarily via the liver or kidneys may require reduced dosaging in the presence of impaired renal or hepatic function. The malfunction of excretory organs may not only risk toxicity from drug accumulation, but will also reduce urinary concentration of drugs excreted primarily by glomerular filtration. This applies to the aminoglycosides and the urinary antiseptics nalidixic acid and nitrofurantoin, where therapeutic failure of urinary tract infections may complicate severe renal failure.

2.4 Drug resistance

Drug resistance may be a natural or an acquired characteristic of a microorganism. This may result from impaired cell wall or cell envelope penetration, enzymatic inactivation, altered binding sites or active extrusion from the cell as a result of efflux mechanisms (Chapter 13). Acquired drug resistance may result from mutation, adaptation or gene transfer. Spontaneous mutations occur at low frequency, as in the case of *Mycobacterium tuberculosis* where a minority population of organisms is resistant to isoniazid. In this situation the use of isoniazid alone will eventually result in overgrowth by this subpopulation of resistant organisms.

Genetic resistance may be chromosomal or transferable on transposons or plasmids. Plasmid-mediated resistance has been increasingly recognized among Gram-negative enteric pathogens. By the process of conjugation (Chapter 13), resistance plasmids may be transferred between bacteria of the same and different species and also different genera. Such resistance can code for multiple antibiotic resistance. For example, the penicillins, cephalosporins, chloramphenicol and the aminoglycosides are all subject to enzymatic inactivation, which may be plasmid-mediated. Knowledge of the local epidemiology of resistant pathogens within a hospital, and especially within high-dependency areas such as intensive care units, is invaluable in guiding appropriate drug selection.

2.4.1 Multidrug resistance

In recent years multidrug resistance has increased among certain pathogens. These include *Staphylococcus aureus*, enterococci and *M. tuberculosis*. *Staph. aureus* resistant to methicillin is known as methicillin-resistant *Staph. aureus* (MRSA). These strains are resistant to many antibiotics and have been responsible for major epidemics worldwide, usually in hospitals where they affect patients in high-dependency units such as intensive care units, burns units and cardiothoracic units. MRSA have the ability to colonize staff and patients and to spread readily among them. Several epidemic strains are currently circulating in the UK. The glycopeptides vancomycin or teicoplanin and the oxazolidinone linezolid are the currently recommended agents for treating patients infected with these organisms.

Another serious resistance problem is that of drug-resistant enterococci. These include *Enterococcus faecalis* and, in particular, *E. faecium*. Resistance to the glycopeptides has again been a problem among patients in high-dependency units. Four different phenotypes are recognized (VanA, VanB, VanC and VanD). The VanA phenotype is resistant to both glycopeptides, while the others are sensitive to teicoplanin but demonstrate high (VanB) or intermediate (VanC) resistance to vancomycin; VanD resistance has only recently been described and remains uncommon. Those fully resistant to the glycopeptides are increasing in frequency and causing great concern as they are essentially resistant to almost all antibiotics.

Tuberculosis is on the increase after decades in which the incidence had been steadily falling. Drug-resistant strains have emerged largely among inadequately treated or non-compliant patients. These include the homeless, alcoholic, intravenous drug abusing and immigrant populations. Resistance patterns vary but increasingly include rifampicin and isoniazid. Furthermore, outbreaks of multidrug-resistant tuberculosis have been increasingly reported from a number of hospital centres in the USA and more recently Europe, including the UK. These infections have occasionally spread to health-care workers and are giving rise to considerable concern.

The underlying mechanisms of resistance are considered in Chapter 13.

2.5 Drug combinations

Antibiotics are generally used alone, but may on occasion be prescribed in combination. Combining two antibiotics may result in synergism, indifference or antagonism. In the case of synergism, microbial inhibition is achieved at concentrations below that for each agent alone and may prove advantageous in treating relatively insusceptible infections such as enterococcal endocarditis, where a combination of penicillin and gentamicin is synergistically active. Another advantage of synergistic combinations is that it may enable the use of toxic agents where dose reductions are possible. For example, meningitis caused by the fungus *Cryptococcus neoformans* responds to an abbreviated course of amphotericin B when it is combined with 5-flucytosine, thereby reducing the risk of toxicity from amphotericin B.

Combined drug use is occasionally recommended to prevent resistance emerging during treatment. For example, treatment may fail when fusidic acid is used alone to treat *Staph. aureus* infections, because resistant strains develop rapidly; this is prevented by combining fusidic acid with flucloxacillin. Likewise, tuberculosis is initially treated with a minimum of three agents, such as rifampicin, isoniazid and pyrazinamide; again drug resistance is prevented, which may result if either agent is used alone.

The most common reason for using combined therapy is in the treatment of confirmed or suspected mixed infections where a single agent alone will fail to cover all pathogenic organisms. This is the case in serious abdominal sepsis where mixed aerobic and anaerobic infections are common and the use of metronidazole in combination with either an aminoglycoside or a broad-spectrum cephalosporin is essential. Finally, drugs are used in combination in patients who are seriously ill and about whom uncertainty exists concerning the microbiological nature of their infection. This initial 'blind therapy' frequently includes a broad-spectrum penicillin or cephalosporin in combination with an aminoglycoside. The regimen should be modified in the light of subsequent microbiological information.

2.6 Adverse reactions

Regrettably, all chemotherapeutic agents have the potential to produce adverse reactions with varying degrees of frequency and severity, and these include hypersensitivity reactions and toxic effects. These may be dose-related and predictable in a patient with a history of hypersensitivity or a previous toxic reaction to a drug or its chemical analogues. However, many adverse events are idiosyncratic and therefore unpredictable.

Hypersensitivity reactions range in severity from fatal anaphylaxis, in which there is widespread tissue oedema, airway obstruction and cardiovascular collapse, to minor and reversible hypersensitivity reactions such as skin eruptions and drug fever. Such reactions are more likely in those with a history of hypersensitivity to the drug, and are more frequent in patients with previous allergic diseases such as childhood eczema or asthma. It is important to question patients closely concerning hypersensitivity reactions before prescribing, as it precludes the use of all compounds within a class, such as the sulphonamides or tetracyclines, while cephalosporins should be used with caution in patients who are allergic to penicillin because these agents are structurally related. They should be avoided entirely in those who have had a previous severe hypersensitivity reaction to penicillin.

Drug toxicity is often dose-related and may affect a variety of organs or tissues. For example, the aminoglycosides are both nephrotoxic and ototoxic to varying degrees; therefore, dosaging should be individualized and the serum assayed, especially where renal function is abnormal, to avoid toxic effects and non-therapeutic drug concentrations. An example of dose-related toxicity is chloramphenicol-induced bone marrow suppression. Chloramphenicol interferes with the normal maturation of bone marrow stem cells and high concentrations may result in a steady fall in circulating red and white cells and also platelets. This effect is generally reversible with dose reduction or drug withdrawal. This dose-related toxic reaction of chloramphenicol should be contrasted with idiosyncratic bone marrow toxicity which is unrelated to dose and occurs at a much lower frequency of approximately 1:40 000 and is frequently irreversible, ending fatally. Toxic effects may also be genetically determined. For example, peripheral neuropathy may occur in those who are slow acetylators of isoniazid, while haemolysis occurs in those deficient in the red cell enzyme glucose-6-phosphate dehydrogenase, when treated with sulphonamides or primaquine.

2.7 Superinfection

Anti-infective drugs not only affect the invading organism undergoing treatment but also have an impact on the normal bacterial flora, especially of the skin and mucous membranes. This may result in microbial overgrowth of resistant organisms with subsequent superinfection. One example is the common occurrence of oral or vaginal candidiasis in patients treated with broad-spectrum agents such as ampicillin or tetracycline. A more serious example is the development of pseudomembranous colitis from the overgrowth of toxin-producing strains of *Clostridium difficile* present in the bowel flora following the use of clindamycin and other broad-spectrum antibiotics. This condition is managed by drug withdrawal and oral vancomycin. Rarely, colectomy (excision of part or whole of the colon) may be necessary for severe cases.

2.8 Chemoprophylaxis

An increasingly important use of antimicrobial agents is that of infection prevention, especially in relationship to surgery. Infection remains one of the most important complications of many surgical procedures, and the recognition that peri-operative antibiotics are effective and safe in preventing this complication has proved a major advance in surgery. The principles that underlie the chemoprophylactic use of antibacterials relate to the predictability of infection for a particular surgical procedure, both in terms of its occurrence, microbial aetiology and susceptibility to antibiotics. Therapeutic drug concentrations present at the operative site at the time of surgery rapidly reduce the number of potentially infectious organisms and prevent wound sepsis. If prophylaxis is delayed to the postoperative period then efficacy is markedly impaired. It is important that chemopro-

phylaxis be limited to the peri-operative period, the first dose being administered approximately 1 hour before surgery for injectable agents and repeated for a maximum of two to three repeat doses postoperatively. Prolonging chemoprophylaxis beyond this period is not cost-effective and increases the risk of adverse drug reactions and superinfection. One of the best examples of the efficacy of surgical prophylaxis is in the area of large bowel surgery. Before the widespread use of chemoprophylaxis, postoperative infection rates for colectomy were often 30% or higher; these have now been reduced to around 5%.

Chemoprophylaxis has been extended to other surgical procedures where the risk of infection may be low but its occurrence has serious consequences. This is especially true for the implantation of prosthetic joints or heart valves. These are major surgical procedures and although infection may be infrequent its consequences are serious and on balance the use of chemoprophylaxis is cost-effective.

Examples of chemoprophylaxis in the non-surgical arena include the prevention of endocarditis with amoxicillin in patients with valvular heart disease undergoing dental surgery, and the prevention of secondary cases of meningococcal meningitis with rifampicin among household contacts of an index case.

3 Clinical use

The choice of antimicrobial chemotherapy is initially dependent on the clinical diagnosis. Under some circumstances the clinical diagnosis implies a microbiological diagnosis which may dictate specific therapy. For example, typhoid fever is caused by *Salmonella typhi*, which is generally sensitive to chloramphenicol, co-trimoxazole and ciprofloxacin. However, for many infections, establishing a clinical diagnosis implies a range of possible microbiological causes and requires laboratory confirmation from samples collected, preferably before antibiotic therapy is begun. Laboratory isolation and susceptibility testing of the causative agent establish the diagnosis with certainty and make drug selection more rational. However, in many circumstances, especially in general practice, microbiological documentation of an infection is not possible. Hence knowledge of the usual microbiological cause of a particular infection and its susceptibility to antimicrobial agents is essential for effective drug prescribing. The following section explores a selection of the problems associated with antimicrobial drug prescribing for a range of clinical conditions.

3.1 Respiratory tract infections

Infections of the respiratory tract are among the commonest of infections, and account for much consultation in general practice and a high percentage of acute hospital admissions. They are divided into infections of the upper respiratory tract, involving the ears, throat, nasal sinuses and the trachea, and the lower respiratory tract (LRT), where they affect the airways, lungs and pleura.

3.1.1 Upper respiratory tract infections

Acute pharyngitis presents a diagnostic and therapeutic dilemma. The majority of sore throats are caused by a variety of viruses; fewer than 20% are bacterial and hence potentially responsive to antibiotic therapy. However, antibiotics are widely prescribed and this reflects the difficulty in discriminating streptococcal from non-streptococcal infections clinically in the absence of microbiological documentation. Nonetheless, *Strep. pyogenes* is the most important bacterial pathogen and this responds to oral penicillin. However, up to 10 days' treatment is required for its eradication from the throat. This requirement causes problems with compliance as symptomatic improvement generally occurs within 2–3 days.

Although viral infections are important causes of both otitis media and sinusitis, they are generally self-limiting. Bacterial infections may complicate viral illnesses, and are also primary causes of ear and sinus infections. *Streptococcus pneumoniae* and *Haemophilus influenzae* are the commonest bacterial pathogens. Amoxicillin is widely prescribed for these infections as it is microbiologically active, penetrates the middle ear and sinuses, is well tolerated and has proved effective.

3.1.2 Lower respiratory tract infections

Infections of the LRT include pneumonia, lung abscess, bronchitis, bronchiectasis and infective complications of cystic fibrosis. Each presents a specific diagnostic and therapeutic challenge, which reflects the variety of pathogens involved and the frequent difficulties in establishing an accurate microbial diagnosis. The laboratory diagnosis of LRT infections is largely dependent upon culturing sputum. Unfortunately this may be contaminated with the normal bacterial flora of the upper respiratory tract during expectoration. In hospitalized patients, the empirical use of antibiotics before admission substantially diminishes the value of sputum culture and may result in overgrowth by non-pathogenic microbes, thus causing difficulty with the interpretation of sputum culture results. Alternative diagnostic samples include needle aspiration of sputum directly from the trachea or of fluid within the pleural cavity. Blood may also be cultured and serum examined for antibody responses or microbial antigens. In the community, few patients will have their LRT infection diagnosed microbiologically and the choice of antibiotic is based on clinical diagnosis.

Pneumonia. The range of pathogens causing acute pneumonia includes viruses, bacteria and, in the immunocompromised host, parasites and fungi. Table 14.2 summarizes these pathogens and indicates drugs appropriate for their treatment. Clinical assessment includes details of the evolution of the infection, any evidence of a recent viral infection, the age of the patient and risk factors such as corticosteroid therapy or pre-existing lung disease. The extent of the pneumonia, as assessed clinically or by X-ray, is also important.

Streptococcus pneumoniae remains the commonest cause of pneumonia and still responds well to penicillin despite a global increase in isolates showing reduced susceptibility to this agent. In addition, a number of atypical infections may cause pneumonia and include *Mycoplasma pneumoniae*, *Legionella pneumophila*, psittacosis and occasionally Q fever. With psittacosis there may be a history of contact with parrots or budgerigars; while Legionnaires' disease has often been acquired during hotel holidays in the Mediterranean area. The

Table 14.2 Microorganisms responsible for pneumonia and the therapeutic agent of choice

Pathogen	Drug(s) of choice
Streptococcus pneumoniae	Penicillin
Staphylococcus aureus	Flucloxacillin ± fusidic acid
Haemophilus influenzae	Cefotaxime or ciprofloxacin
Klebsiella pneumoniae	Cefotaxime ± gentamicin
Pseudomonas aeruginosa	Gentamicin ± ceftazidime
Mycoplasma pneumoniae	Erythromycin or tetracycline
Legionella pneumophila	Erythromycin ± rifampicin
Chlamydia psittaci	Tetracycline
Mycobacterium tuberculosis	Rifampicin + isoniazid + ethambutol + pyrazinamide*
Herpes simplex, varicella/zoster	Aciclovir
Candida spp.	Fluconazole
Aspergillus spp.	Amphotericin B
Anaerobic bacteria	Penicillin or metronidazole

* Reduce to two drugs after 6–8 weeks.

atypical pneumonias, unlike pneumococcal pneumonia, do not respond to penicillin. Legionnaires' disease is treated with erythromycin and, in the presence of severe pneumonia, rifampicin is added to the regimen. Mycoplasma infections are best treated with either erythromycin or tetracycline, while the latter drug is indicated for both psittacosis and Q fever.

Lung abscess. Destruction of lung tissue may lead to abscess formation and is a feature of aerobic Gram-negative bacillary and *Staph. aureus* infections. In addition, aspiration of oropharyngeal secretion can lead to chronic low-grade sepsis with abscess formation and the expectoration of foul-smelling sputum that characterizes anaerobic sepsis. The latter condition responds to high-dose penicillin, which is active against most of the normal oropharyngeal flora, while metronidazole may be appropriate for strictly anaerobic infections. In the case of aerobic Gram-negative bacillary sepsis, aminoglycosides, with or without a broad-spectrum cephalosporin, are the agents of choice. Acute staphylococcal pneumonia is an extremely serious infection and requires treatment with high-dose flucloxacillin alone or in combination with fusidic acid.

Cystic fibrosis. Cystic fibrosis is a multi-system, congenital abnormality that often affects the lungs and results in recurrent infections, initially with *Staph. aureus*, subsequently with *H. influenzae* and eventually leads on to recurrent *Pseudomonas aeruginosa* infection. The last organism is associated with copious quantities of purulent sputum that are extremely difficult to expectorate. *Ps. aeruginosa* is a co-factor in the progressive lung damage that is eventually fatal in these patients. Repeated courses of antibiotics are prescribed and although they have improved the quality and longevity of life, infections caused by *Ps. aeruginosa* are difficult to treat and require repeated hospitalization and administration of parenteral antibiotics such as an aminoglycoside, either alone or in combination with an antipseudomonal penicillin or cephalosporin. The dose of aminoglycosides tolerated by these patients is often higher than in normal individuals and is associated with larger volumes of distribution for these and other agents. Some benefit may also be obtained from inhaled aerosolized antibiotics. Unfortunately drug resistance may emerge and makes drug selection more dependent upon laboratory guidance.

3.2 Urinary tract infections

Urinary tract infection is a common problem in both community and hospital practice. Although occurring throughout life, infections are more common in pre-school girls and women during their childbearing years, although in the elderly the sex distribution is similar. Infection is predisposed by factors that impair urine flow. These include congenital abnormalities, reflux of urine from the bladder into the ureters, kidney stones and tumours and, in males, enlargement of the prostate gland. Bladder catheterization is an important cause of urinary tract infection in hospitalized patients.

3.2.1 Pathogenesis

In those with structural or drainage problems the risk exists of ascending infection to involve the kidney and occasionally the bloodstream. Although structural abnormalities may be absent in women of childbearing years, infection can become recurrent, symptomatic and extremely distressing. Of greater concern is the occurrence of infection in the pre-school child, as normal maturation of the kidney may be impaired and may result in progressive damage which presents as renal failure in later life.

From a therapeutic point of view, it is essential to confirm the presence of bacteriuria (a condition in which there are bacteria in the urine), as symptoms alone are not a reliable method of documenting infection. This applies particularly to bladder infection, where the symptoms of burning micturition (dysuria) and frequency can be associated with a variety of non-bacteriuric conditions. Patients with symptomatic bacteriuria should always be treated. However, the necessity to treat asymptomatic bacteriuric patients varies with age and the presence or absence of underlying urinary tract abnormalities. In the pre-school child it is essential to treat all urinary tract infections and maintain the urine in a sterile state so that normal kidney maturation can proceed. Likewise in pregnancy there is a risk of infection ascending from the bladder to involve the kidney. This is a serious complication and may result in premature labour. Other indications for treating asymptomatic bacteriuria include the presence of underlying renal abnormalities such as stones, which may be associated with repeated infections caused by *Proteus* spp.

3.2.2 Drug therapy

The antimicrobial treatment of urinary tract infection presents a number of interesting challenges. Drugs must be selected for their ability to achieve high urinary concentrations and, if the kidney is involved, adequate tissue concentrations. Safety in childhood or pregnancy is important as repeated or prolonged medication may be necessary. The choice of agent will be dictated by the microbial aetiology and susceptibility findings, because the latter can vary widely among Gram-negative enteric bacilli, especially in patients who are hospitalized. Table 14.3 shows the distribution of bacteria causing urinary tract infection in the community and in hospitalized patients. The greater tendency towards infections caused by *Klebsiella* spp. and *Ps. aeruginosa* should be noted as antibiotic sensitivity

Table 14.3 Urinary tract infection — distribution of pathogenic bacteria in the community and hospitalized patients

Organism	Community (%)	Hospital (%)
Escherichia coli	75	55
Proteus mirabilis	10	13
Klebsiella or *Enterobacter* spp.	4	18
Enterococci	6	5
Staphylococcus epidermidis	5	4
Pseudomonas aeruginosa	–	5

is more variable for these pathogens. Drug resistance has increased substantially in recent years and has reduced the value of formerly widely prescribed agents such as the sulphonamides and ampicillin.

Uncomplicated community-acquired urinary tract infection presents few problems with management. Drugs such as trimethoprim, ciprofloxacin and ampicillin are widely used. Cure rates are close to 100% for ciprofloxacin, about 80% for trimethoprim and about 50% for ampicillin — to which resistance has been steadily increasing. Treatment for 3 days is generally satisfactory and is usually accompanied by prompt control of symptoms. Single-dose therapy with amoxicillin 3 g has also been shown to be effective in selected individuals. Alternative agents include nitrofurantoin, nalidixic acid and norfloxacin, although these are not as well tolerated. Oral cephalosporins and co-amoxiclav are also used.

It is important to demonstrate the cure of bacteriuria with a repeat urine sample collected 4–6 weeks after treatment, or sooner should symptoms fail to subside. Recurrent urinary tract infection is an indication for further investigation of the urinary tract to detect underlying pathology that may be surgically correctable. Under these circumstances it also is important to maintain the urine in a sterile state. This can be achieved with repeated courses of antibiotics, guided by laboratory sensitivity data. Alternatively, long-term chemoprophylaxis for periods of 6 months to control infection by either prevention or suppression is widely used. Trimethoprim is the most commonly prescribed chemoprophylactic agent and is given as a single nightly dose. This achieves high urinary concentrations throughout the night and generally ensures a sterile urine. Nitrofurantoin is an alternative agent.

Infection of the kidney demands the use of agents that achieve adequate tissue as well as urinary concentrations. As bacteraemia (a condition in which there are bacteria circulating in the blood) may complicate infection of the kidney, it is generally recommended that antibiotics be administered parenterally. Although ampicillin was formerly widely used, drug resistance is now common and agents such as cefotaxime or ciprofloxacin are often preferred, because the aminoglycosides, although highly effective and preferentially concentrated within the renal cortex, carry the risk of nephrotoxicity.

Infections of the prostate tend to be persistent, recurrent and difficult to treat. This is in part due to the more acid environment of the prostate gland, which inhibits drug penetration by many of the antibiotics used to treat urinary tract infection. Agents that are basic in nature, such as erythromycin, achieve therapeutic concentrations within the gland but unfortunately are not active against the pathogens responsible for bacterial prostatitis. Trimethoprim, however, is a useful agent as it is preferentially concentrated within the prostate and is active against many of the causative pathogens. It is important that treatment be prolonged for several weeks, as relapse is common.

3.3 Gastrointestinal infections

The gut is vulnerable to infection by viruses, bacteria, parasites and occasionally fungi. Virus infections are the most prevalent but are not susceptible to chemotherapeutic intervention. Bacterial infections are more readily recognized and raise questions concerning the role of antibiotic management. Parasitic infections of the gut are beyond the scope of this chapter.

Bacteria cause disease of the gut as a result of either mucosal invasion or toxin production or a combination of the two mechanisms, as summarized in Table 14.4. Treatment is largely directed at replacing and maintaining an adequate intake of fluid and electrolytes. Antibiotics are generally not recommended for infective gastroenteritis, but deserve consideration where they have been

Table 14.4 Bacterial gut infections — pathogenic mechanisms

Origin	Site of infection	Mechanism
Campylobacter jejuni	Small and large bowel	Invasion
Salmonella spp.	Small and large bowel	Invasion
Shigella spp.	Large bowel	Invasion ± toxin
Escherichia coli		
enteroinvasive	Large bowel	Invasion
enterotoxigenic	Small bowel	Toxin
Clostridium difficile	Large bowel	Toxin
Staphylococcus aureus	Small bowel	Toxin
Vibrio cholerae	Small bowel	Toxin
Clostridium perfringens	Small bowel	Toxin
Yersinia spp.	Small and large bowel	Invasion
Bacillus cereus	Small bowel	Invasion ± toxin
Vibrio parahaemolyticus	Small bowel	Invasion + toxin

demonstrated to abbreviate the acute disease or to prevent complications including prolonged gastrointestinal excretion of the pathogen where this poses a public health hazard.

It should be emphasized that most gut infections are self-limiting. However, attacks can be severe and may result in hospitalization. Antibiotics are used to treat severe *Campylobacter* and *Shigella* infections; erythromycin and ciprofloxacin, respectively, are the preferred agents. Such treatment abbreviates the disease and eliminates gut excretion in *Shigella* infection. However, in severe *Campylobacter* infection the data are currently equivocal, although the clinical impression favours the use of erythromycin for severe infections. The role of antibiotics for *Campylobacter* and *Shigella* infections should be contrasted with gastrointestinal salmonellosis, for which antibiotics are contraindicated as they do not abbreviate symptoms, are associated with more prolonged gut excretion and introduce the risk of adverse drug reactions. However, in severe salmonellosis, especially at extremes of age, systemic toxaemia and bloodstream infection can occur and under these circumstances treatment with either ciprofloxacin or trimethoprim is appropriate.

Typhoid and paratyphoid fevers (known as enteric fevers), although acquired by ingestion of salmonellae, *Sal. typhi* and *Sal. paratyphi*, respectively, are largely systemic infections and antibiotic therapy is mandatory; ciprofloxacin is now the drug of choice although trimethoprim or chloramphenicol are satisfactory alternatives. Prolonged gut excretion of *Sal. typhi* is a well-known complication of typhoid fever and is a major public health hazard in developing countries. Treatment with ciprofloxacin or high dose ampicillin can eliminate the gall bladder excretion which is the major site of persistent infection in carriers. However, the presence of gallstones reduces the chance of cure.

Cholera is a serious infection causing epidemics throughout Asia. Although a toxin-mediated disease, largely controlled with replacement of fluid and electrolyte losses, tetracycline has proved effective in eliminating the causative vibrio from the bowel, thereby abbreviating the course of the illness and reducing the total fluid and electrolyte losses.

Traveller's diarrhoea may be caused by one of many gastrointestinal pathogens (Table 14.4). However, enterotoxigenic *Escherichia coli* is the most common pathogen. While it is generally short-lived, traveller's diarrhoea can seriously mar a brief period abroad, be it for holiday or business purposes. Although not universally accepted, the use of short-course trimethoprim or quinolone such as norfloxacin can abbreviate an attack in patients with severe disease.

3.4 Skin and soft tissue infections

Infections of the skin and soft tissue commonly follow traumatic injury to the epithelium but occasionally may be bloodborne. Interruption of the integrity of the skin allows ingress of micro-organisms to produce superficial, localized infections which on occasion may become more deep-seated and spread rapidly through tissues. Skin trauma complicates surgical incisions and accidents, including burns. Similarly, prolonged immobilization can result in pressure damage to skin from impaired blood flow. It is most commonly seen in patients who are unconscious.

Microbes responsible for skin infection often arise from the normal skin flora, which includes

Staph. aureus. In addition *Strep. pyogenes*, *Ps. aeruginosa* and anaerobic bacteria are other recognized pathogens. Viruses also affect the skin and mucosal surfaces, either as a result of generalized infection or localized disease as in the case of herpes simplex. The latter is amenable to antiviral therapy in selected patients, although for the majority of patients, virus infections of the skin are self-limiting.

Strep. pyogenes is responsible for a range of skin infections: impetigo is a superficial infection of the epidermis which is common in childhood and is highly contagious; cellulitis is a more deep-seated infection which spreads rapidly through the tissues to involve the lymphatics and occasionally the bloodstream; erysipelas is a rapidly spreading cellulitis commonly involving the face, which characteristically has a raised leading edge due to lymphatic involvement. Necrotizing fasciitis is a more serious, rapidly progressive infection of the skin and subcutaneous structures including the fascia and musculature. Despite early diagnosis and high-dose intravenous antibiotics, this condition is often life-threatening and may require extensive surgical debridement of devitalized tissue and even limb amputation to ensure survival. A fatal outcome is usually the result of profound toxaemia and bloodstream spread. Penicillin is the drug of choice for all these infections although in severe instances parenteral administration is appropriate. The use of topical agents, such as tetracycline, to treat impetigo may fail as drug resistance is now recognized.

Staph. aureus is responsible for a variety of skin infections which require therapeutic approaches different from those of streptococcal infections. Staphylococcal cellulitis is indistinguishable clinically from streptococcal cellulitis and responds to flucloxacillin, but generally fails to respond to penicillin owing to penicillinase (β-lactamase) production. *Staph. aureus* is an important cause of superficial, localized skin sepsis which varies from small pustules to boils and occasionally to a more deeply invasive, suppurative skin abscess known as a carbuncle. Antibiotics are generally not indicated for these conditions. Pustules and boils settle with antiseptic soaps or creams and often discharge spontaneously, whereas carbuncles frequently require surgical drainage. *Staph. aureus* may also cause postoperative wound infections, sometimes associated with retained suture material, and settles once the stitch is removed. Antibiotics are only appropriate in this situation if there is extensive accompanying soft tissue invasion.

Anaerobic bacteria are characteristically associated with foul-smelling wounds. They are found in association with surgical incisions following intra-abdominal procedures and pressure sores, which are usually located over the buttocks and hips where they become infected with faecal flora. These infections are frequently mixed and include Gram-negative enteric bacilli, which may mask the presence of underlying anaerobic bacteria. The principles of treating anaerobic soft tissue infection again emphasize the need for removal of all foreign and devitalized material. Antibiotics such as metronidazole or clindamycin should be considered where tissue invasion has occurred.

The treatment of infected burn wounds presents a number of peculiar facets. Burns are initially sterile, especially when they involve all layers of the skin. However, they rapidly become colonized with bacteria whose growth is supported by the protein-rich exudate. Staphylococci, *Strep. pyogenes* and, particularly, *Ps. aeruginosa* frequently colonize burns and may jeopardize survival of skin grafts and occasionally, and more seriously, result in bloodstream invasion. Treatment of invasive *Ps. aeruginosa* infections requires combined therapy with an aminoglycoside, such as gentamicin or tobramycin, and an antipseudomonal agent, such as ceftazidime or piperacillin. This produces high therapeutic concentrations which generally act in a synergistic manner. The use of aminoglycosides in patients with serious burns requires careful monitoring of serum concentrations to ensure that they are therapeutic yet non-toxic, as renal function is often impaired in the days immediately following a serious burn. Excessive sodium loading may complicate the use of large doses of antipseudomonal penicillins such as piperacillin.

3.5 Central nervous system infections

The brain, its surrounding covering of meninges and the spinal cord are subject to infection, which is generally bloodborne but may also complicate neurosurgery, penetrating injuries or direct spread from infection in the middle ear or nasal sinuses. Viral meningitis is the most common infection but is generally self-limiting. Occasionally destructive forms of encephalitis occur; an example is herpes simplex encephalitis. Bacterial infections include meningitis and brain abscesses and carry a high risk of mortality, while in those who recover, residual neurological damage or impairment of intellectual function may follow. This occurs despite the availability of antibiotics active against the responsible bacterial pathogens. Fungal infections of the brain, although rare, are increasing in frequency, particularly among immunocompromised patients who either have underlying malignant conditions or are on potent cytotoxic drugs.

The treatment of bacterial infections of the central nervous system highlights a number of important therapeutic considerations. Bacterial meningitis is caused by a variety of bacteria although their incidence varies with age. In the neonate, *E. coli* and group B streptococci account for the majority of infections, while in the pre-school child *H. influenzae* was the commonest pathogen before the introduction of a highly effective vaccine. *Neisseria meningitidis* has a peak incidence between 5 and 15 years of age, while pneumococcal meningitis is predominantly a disease of adults.

Penicillin is the drug of choice for the treatment of group B streptococcal, meningococcal and pneumococcal infections but, as discussed earlier, CSF concentrations of penicillin are significantly influenced by the intensity of the inflammatory response. To achieve therapeutic concentrations within the CSF, high dosages are required, and in the case of pneumococcal meningitis should be continued for 10–14 days. Resistance among *Strep. pneumoniae* to penicillin has increased worldwide. When causing meningitis, treatment is increasingly unsuccessful. Alternative agents include ceftriaxone and meropenem.

Resistance of *H. influenzae* to ampicillin has increased in the past two decades and varies geographically. Thus, it can no longer be prescribed with confidence as initial therapy, and cefotaxime or ceftriaxone are now the preferred alternatives. However, once laboratory evidence for β-lactamase activity is excluded, ampicillin can be safely substituted.

E. coli meningitis carries a mortality of greater than 40% and reflects both the virulence of this organism and the pharmacokinetic problems of achieving adequate CSF antibiotic levels. The broad-spectrum cephalosporins such as cefotaxime, ceftriaxone or ceftazidime have been shown to achieve satisfactory therapeutic levels and are the agents of choice to treat Gram-negative bacillary meningitis. Treatment again must be prolonged for periods ranging from 2 to 4 weeks.

Brain abscess presents a different therapeutic challenge. An abscess is locally destructive to the brain and causes further damage by increasing intracranial pressure. The infecting organisms are varied but those arising from middle ear or nasal sinus infection are often polymicrobial and include anaerobic bacteria, micro-aerophilic species and Gram-negative enteric bacilli. Less commonly, a pure *Staph. aureus* abscess may complicate blood-borne spread. Brain abscess is a neurosurgical emergency and requires drainage. However, antibiotics are an important adjunct to treatment. The polymicrobial nature of many infections demands prompt and careful laboratory examination to determine optimum therapy. Drugs are selected not only on their ability to penetrate the blood–brain barrier and enter the CSF but also on their ability to penetrate the brain substance. Metronidazole has proved a valuable alternative agent in such infections, although it is not active against micro-aerophilic streptococci, which must be treated with high-dose benzylpenicillin. The two are often used in combination. Chloramphenicol is an alternative agent.

3.6 Fungal infections

Fungal infections are divided into superficial or deep-seated infections. Superficial infections affect the skin, nails or mucosal surfaces of the mouth or genital tract. In contrast, deep-seated fungal diseases may target the lung or disseminate via the bloodstream to organs such as the brain, spleen, liver or skeletal system.

The fungal infections of the skin and nails include *Tinea pedis* (athlete's foot), *T. capitis* and *T.*

Table 14.5 Treatment recommendations for selected deep-seated fungal infections

Infection	Preferred treatment	Alternative treatment
Candida spp.	Fluconazole	Amphotericin B
Cryptococcus neoformans	Fluconazole	Amphotericin B ± flucytosine
Aspergillus spp.	Amphotericin B	Itraconazole
Mucormycosis	Amphotericin B	–

carporis (ringworm), *Candida* intertrigo (usually groin and submammary regions) and pityriasis (*Malassezia*). A variety of topical and systemic antifungal agents are available. The imidazole class of drugs includes clotrimazole and miconazole, which are highly effective topically. Systemic antifungals used to treat superficial fungal infections include griseofulvin and terbinafine, which is an allylamine. Both agents are ineffective in the treatment of deep-seated fungal infections that may be caused by yeasts (*Cryptococcus neoformans*), yeast-like fungi (*Candida* spp.) or the filamentous fungi (*Aspergillus* spp). These produce a variety of syndromes for which different antifungal agents are indicated (Table 14.5). The polyenes include amphotericin B, which after many years remains the agent of choice for the treatment of a wide variety of life-threatening fungal diseases which often complicate cancer chemotherapy, organ transplantation and immunodeficiency diseases, such as AIDS. Nephrotoxicity is common but can be avoided by careful dosaging or the use of liposomal formulations. The other major class of systemic antifungals is the triazoles, which include fluconazole and itraconazole. These are extremely well tolerated but may interact with a number of drugs and drug classes such as the sulphonylureas, antihistamines and lipid-lowering agents among others.

3.7 Medical device-associated infections

A wide variety of medical devices are increasingly used in clinical practice. These range from vasculature and urinary catheters, prosthetic joints and heart valves, shunts and stents for improving the flow of CSF, blood or bile according to their site of use, to intracardiac patches and vascular pumps. Unfortunately infection is the most frequent complication of their use and may result in the need to replace or remove the device, sometimes with potentially life-threatening and fatal consequences.

Infections are often caused by organisms arising from the normal skin flora, which gain access at the time of insertion of the device. *Staph. epidermidis* is among the most frequent of isolates. Following attachment to the surface of the device, the organisms undergo multiplication with the formation of extracellular polysaccharide material (glycocalyx) which contains slowly replicating cells to form a biofilm. Microorganisms within a biofilm are less vulnerable to attack by host defences (phagocytes, complement and antibodies) and are relatively insusceptible to antibiotic therapy despite the variable ability of drugs to penetrate the biofilm.

Management approaches have therefore emphasized the need for prevention through the addition of good sterile technique at the time of insertion. Manufacturers have also responded by using materials and creating surface characteristics of implanted materials inclement to microbial attachment. Likewise the use of prophylactic antibiotics at the time of insertion of deep-seated devices such as joint and heart valve prostheses has further reduced the risk of infection. Once a medical device becomes infected, management is difficult. Treatment with agents such as flucloxacillin, vancomycin and most recently linezolid is often unsuccessful and the only course of action is to remove the device.

4 Antibiotic policies

4.1 Rationale

The plethora of available antimicrobial agents presents both an increasing problem of selection to the prescriber and difficulties for the diagnostic laboratory as to which agents should be tested for susceptibility. Differences in antimicrobial activity among related compounds are often of minor importance but can occasionally be of greater significance and may be a source of confusion to the non-specialist. This applies particularly to large classes of drugs,

such as the penicillins and cephalosporins, where there has been an explosion in the availability of new agents in recent years. Guidance, in the form of an antibiotic policy, has a major role to play in providing the prescriber with a range of agents appropriate to his/her needs and should be supported by laboratory evidence of susceptibility to these agents.

In recent years, increased awareness of the cost of medical care has led to a major review of various aspects of health costs. The pharmacy budget has often attracted attention as, unlike many other hospital expenses, it is readily identifiable in terms of cost and prescriber. Thus, an antibiotic policy is also seen as a means whereby the economic burden of drug prescribing can be reduced or contained. There can be little argument with the recommendation that the cheaper of two compounds should be selected where agents are similar in terms of efficacy and adverse reactions. Likewise, generic substitution is also desirable provided that there is bioequivalence. It has become increasingly impractical for pharmacists to stock all the formulations of every antibiotic currently available, and here again an antibiotic policy can produce significant savings by limiting the amount of stock held. A policy based on a restricted number of agents also enables price reduction on purchasing costs through competitive tendering. The above activities have had a major influence on containing or reducing drug costs, although these savings have often been lost as new and often expensive preparations become available, particularly in the field of biological and anticancer therapy.

Another increasingly important argument in favour of an antibiotic policy is the occurrence of drug-resistant bacteria within an institution. The presence of sick patients and the opportunities for the spread of microorganisms can produce outbreaks of hospital infection. The excessive use of selected agents has been associated with the emergence of drug-resistant bacteria which have often caused serious problems within high-dependency areas, such as intensive care units or burns units where antibiotic use is often high. One oft-quoted example is the occurrence of a multiple antibiotic-resistant *K. aerogenes* within a neurosurgical intensive care unit in which the organism became resistant to all currently available anti-biotics and was associated with the widespread use of ampicillin. By prohibiting the use of all antibiotics, and in particular ampicillin, the resistant organism rapidly disappeared and the problem was resolved.

Currently the most important hospital-acquired pathogen is methicillin-resistant *Staph. aureus*, which is responsible for a range of serious infections such as pneumonia, postoperative wound infection and skin infections which may in turn be complicated by bloodstream spread. The use of vancomycin and teicoplanin has escalated as a consequence, and in turn has been linked to the emergence of vancomycin-resistant enterococci.

In formulating an antibiotic policy, it is important that the susceptibility of microorganisms be monitored and reviewed at regular intervals. This applies not only to the hospital as a whole, but to specific high-dependency units in particular. Likewise general practitioner samples should also be monitored. This will provide accurate information on drug susceptibility to guide the prescriber as to the most effective agent.

4.2 Types of antibiotic policies

There are a number of different approaches to the organization of an antibiotic policy. These range from a deliberate absence of any restriction on prescribing to a strict policy whereby all anti-infective agents must have expert approval before they are administered. Restrictive policies vary according to whether they are mainly laboratory-controlled, by employing restrictive reporting, or whether they are mainly pharmacy-controlled, by restrictive dispensing. In many institutions it is common practice to combine the two approaches.

4.2.1 Free prescribing policy

The advocates of a free prescribing policy argue that strict antibiotic policies are both impractical and limit clinical freedom to prescribe. It is also argued that the greater the number of agents in use the less likely it is that drug resistance will emerge to any one agent or class of agents. However, few would support such an approach, which is generally an argument for mayhem.

4.2.2 Restricted reporting

Another approach that is widely practised in the UK is that of restricted reporting. The laboratory, largely for practical reasons, tests only a limited range of agents against bacterial isolates. The agents may be selected primarily by microbiological staff or following consultation with their clinical colleagues. The antibiotics tested will vary according to the site of infection, as drugs used to treat urinary tract infections often differ from those used to treat systemic disease.

There are specific problems regarding the testing of certain agents such as the cephalosporins, where the many different preparations have varying activity against bacteria. The practice of testing a single agent to represent first-generation, second-generation or third-generation compounds is questionable, and with the new compounds susceptibility should be tested specifically to that agent. By selecting a limited range of compounds for use, sensitivity testing becomes a practical consideration and allows the clinician to use such agents with greater confidence.

4.2.3 Restricted dispensing

As mentioned above, the most Draconian of all antibiotic policies is the absolute restriction of drug dispensing pending expert approval. The expert opinion may be provided by either a microbiologist or infectious disease specialist. Such a system can only be effective in large institutions where staff are available 24 hours a day. This approach is often cumbersome, generates hostility and does not necessarily create the best educational forum for learning effective antibiotic prescribing.

A more widely used approach is to divide agents into those approved for unrestricted use and those for restricted use. Agents on the unrestricted list are appropriate for the majority of common clinical situations. The restricted list may include agents where microbiological sensitivity information is essential, such as for vancomycin and certain aminoglycosides. In addition, agents that are used infrequently but for specific indications, such as parenteral amphotericin B, are also restricted in use. Other compounds that may be expensive and used for specific indications, such as broad-spectrum β-lactams in the treatment of *Ps. aerugi-nosa* infections, may also be justifiably included on the restricted list. Items omitted from the restricted or unrestricted list are generally not stocked, although they can be obtained at short notice as necessary.

Such a policy should have a mechanism whereby desirable new agents are added as they become available and is most appropriately decided at a therapeutics committee. Policing such a policy is best effected as a joint arrangement between senior pharmacists and microbiologists. This combined approach of both restricted reporting and restricted prescribing is extremely effective and provides a powerful educational tool for medical staff and students faced with learning the complexities of modern antibiotic prescribing. In some hospitals 'Antibiotic Teams' have emerged to advise and educate staff while monitoring compliance with prescribing policies as well as ensuring good standards of patient management.

5 Further reading

Cohen, J. & Powderley, D. (2003) *Infectious Diseases*, 2nd edn. Mosby, Philadelphia.

Finch, R. G. (2001) Antimicrobial therapy: principles of use. *Medicine*, 29, 35–40.

Finch, R. G., Greenwood, D., Norrby, R. & Whitley, R. (2002) *Antibiotic and Chemotherapy*, 8th edn. Churchill Livingstone, Edinburgh.

Greenwood, D. (2000) *Antimicrobial Chemotherapy*, 4th edn. Oxford University Press, Oxford.

Mandell, G. L., Douglas, R. G. & Bennett, J. E. (2000) *Principles and Practice of Infectious Diseases*, 5th edn. Churchill Livingstone, Philadelphia.

Part 3

Microbiological Aspects of Pharmaceutical Processing

Chapter 15

Ecology of microorganisms as it affects the pharmaceutical industry

Elaine Underwood

1 Introduction

The microbiological quality of pharmaceutical products is influenced by the environment in which they are manufactured and by the materials used in their formulation. With the exception of preparations which are terminally sterilized in their final container, the microflora of the final product may represent the contaminants from the raw materials, from the equipment with which it was made, from the atmosphere, from the person operating the process or from the final container into which it was packed. Some of the contaminants may be pathogenic while others may grow even in the presence of preservatives and spoil the product. Any microorganisms that are destroyed by in-process heat treatment may still leave cell residues which may be toxic or pyrogenic (Chapter 3), as the pyrogenic fraction, lipid A, which is present in the cell wall is not destroyed under the same conditions as the organisms.

In parallel with improvements in manufacturing technology there have been developments in Good Manufacturing Practices to minimize contamination by a study of the ecology of microorganisms, the hazards posed by them and any points in the process which are critical to their control. This approach has been distilled into the concept of Hazard Analysis of Critical Control Points (HACCP), with the objective of improving the microbiological safety of the product in a cost-effective manner, which has been assisted by the development of rapid methods for the detection of microorganisms.

2 Atmosphere

2.1 Microbial content

Air is not a natural environment for the growth and reproduction of microorganisms, as it does not contain the necessary amount of moisture and nutrients in a form that can be utilized. However, almost any sample of untreated air contains suspended bacteria, moulds and yeasts, but to survive they must be able to tolerate desiccation and the continuing dry state. Microorganisms commonly isolated from air are the spore-forming bacteria *Bacillus* spp. and *Clostridium* spp., the non-sporing bacteria *Staphylococcus* spp., *Streptococcus* spp. and *Corynebacterium* spp., the moulds *Penicillium* spp., *Cladosporium* spp., *Aspergillus* spp. and *Mucor* spp., as well as the yeast *Rhodotorula* spp.

The number of organisms in the atmosphere depends on the activity in the environment and the amount of dust that is disturbed. An area containing working machinery and active personnel will have a higher microbial count than one with a still atmosphere, and the air count of a dirty, untidy room will be greater than that of a clean room. The microbial air count is also influenced by humidity. A damp atmosphere usually contains fewer organisms than a dry one, as the contaminants are carried down by the droplets of moisture. Thus, the air in a cold store is usually free from microorganisms and air is less contaminated during the wet winter months than in the drier summer months.

Microorganisms are carried into the atmosphere suspended on particles of dust, skin or clothing, or in droplets of moisture or sputum following talking, coughing or sneezing. The size of the particles to which the organisms are attached, together with the humidity of the air, determines the rate at which they will settle out. Bacteria and moulds not attached to suspended matter will settle out slowly in a quiet atmosphere. The rate of settling out will depend upon air current caused by ventilation, air extraction systems, convection currents above heat sources and the activity in the room.

The microbial content of the air may be increased during the handling of contaminated materials during dispensing, blending and their addition to formulations. In particular, the use of starches and some sugars in the dry state may increase the mould count. Some packaging components, e.g. card and paperboard, have a microflora of both moulds and bacteria, and this is often reflected in high counts around packaging machines.

Common methods for checking the microbiological quality of air include the following:

1 The exposure of Petri dishes containing a nutrient agar to the atmosphere for a given length of time. This relies upon microorganisms or dust particles bearing them settling on the surface.
2 The use of an air-sampling machine which draws a measured volume of air from the environment and impinges it on a nutrient agar surface on either a Petri dish, a plastic strip or a membrane filter which may then be incubated with a nutrient medium. This method provides valuable information in areas of low microbial contamination, particularly if the sample is taken close to the working area.

The type of formulation being prepared determines the microbiological standard of the air supply required and the hazard it poses. In areas where products for injection and ophthalmic use which cannot be terminally sterilized by moist heat are being manufactured, the air count should be very low and regarded as a critical control point in the process, as although these products are required to pass a test for sterility (Chapter 20), the test itself is destructive, and therefore only relatively few samples are tested. An unsatisfactory air count may lead to the casual contamination of a few containers and may be undetected by the test for sterility. In addition, if the microbiological air quality is identified as a critical point, it may also give an early warning of potential contamination and permit timely correction. The manufacture of liquid or semi-solid preparations for either oral or topical use requires a clean environment for both the production and filling stages. While many formulations are adequately protected by chemical preservatives or a pH unfavourable to airborne bacteria that may settle in them, preservation against mould spores is more difficult to achieve.

2.2 Reduction of microbial count

The microbial count of air may be reduced by filtration, chemical disinfection and to a limited extent by ultraviolet (UV) light. Filtration is the most commonly used method and filters may be made of a variety of materials such as cellulose, glass wool, fibreglass mixtures or polytetrafluorethylene (PTFE) with resin or acrylic binders. There are standards in both the UK and USA for the quality of moving air, in the UK there is a grading system from

A to D and in the USA, six classes from class 1 to class 100 000. For the most critical aseptic work, it may be necessary to remove all particles in excess of 0.1 µm in size using a high efficiency particulate air (HEPA) filter, but for many operations a standard of < 100 particles per 3.5 litres (1.0 ft^3) of 0.5 µm or larger (grade A in the UK — class 100 in the USA) is adequate. Such fine filtration is usually preceded by a coarse filter stage, or any suspended matter is removed by passing the air through an electrostatic field. To maintain efficiency, all air filters must be kept dry, as microorganisms may be capable of movement along continuous wet films and may be carried through a damp filter.

Filtered air may be used to purge a complete room, or it may be confined to a specific area and incorporate the principle of laminar flow, which permits operations to be carried out in a gentle current of sterile air. The direction of the airflow may be horizontal or vertical, depending on the type of equipment being used, the type of operation and the material being handled. It is important that there is no obstruction between the air supply and the exposed product, as this may result in the deflection of microorganisms or particulate matter from a non-sterile surface and cause contamination. Airflow gauges are essential to monitor that the correct flow rate is obtained in laminar flow units and in complete suites to ensure that a positive pressure from clean to less clean areas is always maintained.

The integrity of the air-filtration system must be checked regularly, and the most common method is by counting the particulate matter both in the working area and across the surface of the filter. For systems which have complex ducting or where the surfaces of the terminal filters are recessed, smoke tests using a chemical of known particulate size may be introduced just after the main fan and monitored at each outlet. The test has a twofold application, as both the terminal filter and any leaks in the ducting can be checked. These methods are useful in conjunction with those for determining the microbial air count as given earlier.

Chemical disinfectants are limited in their use as air sterilants because of their irritant properties when sprayed. However, some success has been achieved with atomized propylene glycol at a concentration of 0.05–0.5 mg/L and quaternary ammonium compounds (QACs) at 0.075% may be used. For areas that can be effectively sealed off for fumigation purposes, formaldehyde gas at a concentration of 1–2 mg/L of air at a relative humidity of 80–90% is effective.

UV irradiation at wavelengths between 240 and 280 nm (2400 and 2800 Å) is used to reduce bacterial contamination of air, but it is only active at a relatively short distance from the source. Bacteria and mould spores, particularly those with heavily pigmented spore coats, are often resistant to such treatment. It is however, useful if used in combination with air filtration.

2.3 Compressed air

Compressed air has many applications in the manufacture of pharmaceutical products. A few examples of its uses are the conveyance of powders and suspension, providing aeration for some fermentations and as a power supply for the reduction of particle size by impaction. Unless it is sterilized by filtration or a combination of heat and filtration, microorganisms present will be introduced into the product. The microbial content of compressed air may be assessed by bubbling a known volume through a nutrient liquid and either filtering through a membrane, which is then incubated with a nutrient agar and a total viable count made, or the microbial content may be estimated more rapidly using techniques developed to detect changes in physical or chemical characteristics in the nutrient liquid.

3 Water

The microbial ecology of water is of great importance in the pharmaceutical industry owing to its multiple uses as a constituent of many products as well as for various washing and cooling processes. Two main aspects are involved: the quality of the raw water and any processing it receives and the distribution system. Both should be taken into consideration when reviewing the hazards to the finished product and any critical control points.

Microorganisms indigenous to fresh water include *Pseudomonas* spp., *Alcaligenes* spp., *Flavobacterium* spp., *Chromobacter* spp. and *Serratia* spp. Such bacteria are nutritionally undemanding and often have a relatively low optimum growth temperature. Bacteria which are introduced as a result of soil erosion, heavy rainfall and decaying plant matter include *Bacillus subtilis*, *B. megaterium*, *Enterobacter aerogenes* and *Enterobacter cloacae*. Contamination by sewage results in the presence of *Proteus* spp., *Escherichia coli* and other enterobacteria, *Streptococcus faecalis* and *Clostridium* spp. Bacteria which are introduced as a result of animal or plant debris usually die as a result of the unfavourable conditions.

An examination of stored industrial water supplies showed that 98% of the contaminants were Gram-negative bacteria; other organisms isolated were *Micrococcus* spp., *Cytophaga* spp., yeast, yeast-like fungi and actinomycetes.

3.1 Raw or mains water

The quality of the water from the mains supply varies with both the source and the local authority, and while it is free from known pathogens and from faecal contaminants such as *E. coli*, it may contain other microorganisms. When the supply is derived from surface water the flora is usually more abundant and faster-growing than that of supplies from a deep-water source such as a well or spring. This is due to surface waters receiving both microorganisms and nutrients from soil and sewage while water from deep sources has its microflora filtered out. On prolonged storage in a reservoir, water-borne organisms tend to settle out, but in industrial storage tanks the intermittent throughput ensures that, unless treated, the contents of the tank serve as a source of infection. The bacterial count may rise rapidly in such tanks during summer months and reach 10^5–10^6 per ml.

One of the uses of mains water is for washing chemicals used in pharmaceutical preparations to remove impurities or unwanted by-products of a reaction, and although the bacterial count of the water may be low, the volume used is large and the material being washed may be exposed to a considerable number of bacteria.

The microbial count of the mains water will be reflected in both softened and deionized water which may be prepared from it.

3.2 Softened water

This is usually prepared by either a base-exchange method using sodium zeolite, by a lime-soda ash process, or by the addition of sodium hexametaphosphate. In addition to the bacteria derived from the mains water, additional flora of *Bacillus* spp. and *Staphylococcus aureus* may be introduced into systems which use brine for regeneration and from the chemical filter beds which, unless treated, can act as a reservoir for bacteria.

Softened water is often used for washing containers before filling with liquid or semi-solid preparations and for cooling systems. Unless precautions are taken, the microbial count in a cooling system or jacketed vessel will rise rapidly and if faults develop in the cooling plates or vessel wall, contamination of the product may occur.

3.3 Deionized or demineralized water

Deionized water is prepared by passing mains water through anion and cation exchange resin beds to remove the ions. Thus, any bacteria present in the mains water will also be present in the deionized water, and beds which are not regenerated frequently with strong acid or alkali are often heavily contaminated and add to the bacterial content of the water. This problem has prompted the development of resins able to resist microbiological contamination. One such resin, a large-pore, strong-base, macroreticular, quaternary ammonium anion exchange resin which permits microorganisms to enter the pore cavity and then electrostatically binds them to the cavity surface, is currently being marketed. The main function is a final cleaning bed downstream of conventional demineralizing columns.

Deionized water is used in pharmaceutical formulations, for washing containers and plant, and for the preparation of disinfectant solutions.

3.4 Distilled water

As it leaves the still, distilled water is free from

microorganisms, and contamination occurs as a result of a fault in the cooling system, the storage vessel or the distribution system. The flora of contaminated distilled water is usually Gram-negative bacteria and as it is introduced after a sterilization process, it is often a pure culture. A level of organisms up to 10^6 per ml has been recorded.

Distilled water is often used in the formulation of oral and topical pharmaceutical preparations and a low bacterial count is desirable. It is also used after distillation with a specially designed still, often made of glass, for the manufacture of parenteral preparations and a post-distillation heat sterilization stage is commonly included in the process. Water for such preparations is often stored at 80°C to prevent bacterial growth and the production of pyrogenic substances which accompany such growth.

3.5 Water produced by reverse osmosis

Water produced by reverse osmosis (RO) is forced by an osmotic pressure through a semi-permeable membrane which acts as a molecular filter. The diffusion of solubles dissolved in the water is impeded, and those with a molecular weight in excess of 250 do not diffuse at all. The process, which is the reverse of the natural process of osmosis, thus removes microorganisms and their pyrogens. Post-RO contamination may occur if the plant after the membrane, the storage vessel or the distribution system is not kept free from microorganisms.

3.6 Distribution system

If microorganisms colonize a storage vessel, it then acts as a microbial reservoir and contaminates all water passing through it. It is therefore important that the contents of all storage vessels are tested regularly. Reservoirs of microorganisms may also build up in booster pumps, water meters and unused sections of pipeline. Where a high positive pressure is absent or cannot be continuously maintained, outlets such as cocks and taps may permit bacteria to enter the system.

An optimum system for reducing the growth of microbial flora is one that ensures a constant recirculation of water at a positive pressure through a ring-main without 'dead-legs' (areas which due to their location are not regularly used) and only very short branches to the take-off points. In addition there should be a system to re-sterilize the water, usually by membrane filtration or UV light treatment, just before return to the main storage tank.

Some plumbing materials used for storage vessels, pipework and jointing may support microbial growth. Some plastics, in particular plasticized polyvinylchlorides and resins used in the manufacture of glass-reinforced plastics, have caused serious microbiological problems when used for water storage and distribution systems. Both natural and synthetic rubbers used for washers, O-rings and diaphragms are susceptible to contamination if not sanitized regularly. For jointing, packing and lubricating materials, PTFE and silicone-based compounds are superior to those based on natural products such as vegetable oils or fibres and animal fats, and petroleum-based compounds.

3.7 Disinfection of water

Three methods are used for treating water, namely chemicals, filtration or light.

3.7.1 Chemical treatment

Chemical treatment is applicable usually to raw, mains and softened water, but is also used to treat the storage and distribution systems of distilled and deionized water and of water produced by reverse osmosis (section 3.5).

Sodium hypochlorite and chlorine gas are the most common agents for treating the water supply itself, and the concentration employed depends both upon the dwell time and the chlorine demand of the water. For most purposes a free residual chlorine level of 0.5–5 ppm is adequate. For storage vessels, pipelines, pumps and outlets a higher level of 50–100 ppm may be necessary, but it is usually necessary to use a descaling agent before disinfection in areas where the water is hard. Distilled, deionized and RO systems and pipelines may be treated with sodium hypochlorite or 1% formaldehyde solution. With deionized systems it is usual to exhaust the resin beds with brine before sterilization with formaldehyde to prevent its inactivation to paraformaldehyde. If only local contamination occurs, live steam is often effective in eradicating it. During chemical sterilization it is important that no 'dead-legs' remain untreated and that all instruments such as water meters are treated.

3.7.2 *Filtration*

Membrane filtration is useful where the usage is moderate and a continuous circulation of water can be maintained. Thus, with the exception of that drawn off for use, the water is continually being returned to the storage tank and refiltered. As many waterborne bacteria are small, it is usual to install a 0.22-μm pore-size membrane as the terminal filter and to use coarser prefilters to prolong its life. Membrane filters require regular sterilization to prevent microbial colonization and 'grow through'. They may be treated chemically with the remainder of the storage/distribution system or removed and treated by moist heat. The latter method is usually the most successful for heavily contaminated filters.

3.7.3 *Light*

UV light at a wavelength of 254 nm is useful for the disinfection of water of good optical clarity. Such treatment has an advantage over chemical disinfection as there is no odour or flavour problem and, unlike membrane filters, it is not subject to microbial colonization. One of the newer technologies suitable for disinfecting water is UV-rich high intensity light pulses in which 30% of the energy is at wavelengths of <300 nm, with pulse durations of 10^6 to 10^1 seconds and a density from 0.1 to 50 J/cm^2. The siting of the distribution system is important, as any insanitary fittings downstream of the unit will recontaminate the water. Industrial in-line units with sanitary type fittings which replace part of the water pipeline are manufactured.

3.7.4 *Microbial checks*

One of the most useful techniques for checking the microbial quality of water is by membrane filtration, as this permits the concentration of a small number of organisms from a large volume of water. When chlorinated water supplies are tested it is necessary to add an inactivating agent such as sodium thiosulphate. Although an incubation temperature of 37°C may be necessary to recover some pathogens or faecal contaminants from water, many indigenous species fail to grow at this temperature, and it is usual to incubate at 20–26°C for their detection.

4 Skin and respiratory tract flora

4.1 Microbial transfer from operators

Microorganisms may be transferred to pharmaceutical preparations from the process operator. This is undesirable in the case of tablets and powders, and may result in spoilage of solutions or suspensions, but in the case of parenteral preparations it may have serious consequences for the patient. Of the natural skin flora organisms, *Staph. aureus* is perhaps the most undesirable. It is common on the hands and face and, as it resides in the deep layers of the skin, it is not eliminated by washing. Other bacteria present are *Sarcina* spp. and diphtheroids, but occasionally Gram-negative rods such as *Acinetobacter* spp. and *Alcaligenes* spp. achieve resident status in moist regions. In the fatty and waxy sections of the skin, lipophilic yeast are often present, *Pityrosporum ovale* on the scalp and *P. orbiculare* on glabrous skin. Various dermatophytic fungi such as *Epidermophyton* spp., *Microsporon* spp. and *Trichophyton* spp. may be present. Ear secretions may also contain saprophytic bacteria.

Bacteria other than the natural skin flora may be transferred from the operator as a result of poor personal hygiene, such as faecal organisms from the anal region or bacteria from a wound. Open wounds without clinical manifestation of bacterial growth often support pathogenic bacteria and *Staph. aureus* has been found in 20%. Other contaminants include micrococci, enterococci, α-haemolytic and non-haemolytic streptococci, *Clostridium* spp., *Bacillus* spp. and Gram-negative intestinal bacteria. *Clostridium perfringens* in such circumstances is usually present as a saprophyte and dies fairly rapidly. Wounds showing signs of infection may support *Staph. aureus*, *Strep. pyogenes*, enterococci, coliforms, *Proteus* spp. and *Pseudomonas aeruginosa*.

The nasal passages may contain large numbers of

Staph. aureus and a limited number of *Staph. albus*, while the nasopharynx is often colonized by streptococci of the viridans group, *Strep. salivarius* or *Neisseria pharynges*. Occasionally, pathogens such as *Haemophilus influenzae* and *Klebsiella pneumoniae* may be present. The most common organisms secreted during normal respiratory function and speech are saprophytic streptococci of the viridans group.

The hazard of the transfer of microorganisms from humans to pharmaceutical preparations may be reduced by comprehensive training in personal hygiene coupled with regular medical checks to prevent carriers of pathogenic organisms from coming in contact with any product.

4.2 Hygiene and protective clothing

Areas designed for the manufacture of products intended for injection and eye or ear preparations usually have washing facilities with foot-operated taps, antiseptic soap and hot-air hand driers at the entrance to the suite, which must be used by all process operators. For the manufacture of such products it is also necessary for the operators to wear sterilized clothing including gowns, trousers, boots, hoods, face masks and gloves. For the production of products for oral and topical use, staff should be made to wash their hands before entering the production area. The requirements for protective clothing are usually less stringent but include clean overalls, hair covering and gloves, and where possible, face masks are an advantage.

5 Raw materials

Raw materials account for a high proportion of the microorganisms introduced during the manufacture of pharmaceuticals, and the selection of materials of a good microbiological quality aids in the control of contamination levels in both products and the environment. It is, however, common to have to accept raw materials which have some non-pathogenic microorganisms present and an assessment must be made as to the risk of their survival to spoil the finished product by growing in the presence of a preservative system, or the efficacy of an in-process treatment stage to destroy or remove

them. Whatever the means of prevention of growth or survival by chemical or in-process treatment, it should be regarded as critical and controlled accordingly.

Untreated raw materials that are derived from a natural source usually support an extensive and varied microflora. Products from animal sources such as gelatine, desiccated thyroid, pancreas and cochineal may be contaminated with animal-borne pathogens. For this reason some statutory bodies such as the British Pharmacopoeia require freedom of such materials from *Escherichia coli* and *Salmonella* spp. at a stated level before they can be used in the preparation of pharmaceutical products. The microflora of materials of plant origin such as gum acacia and tragacanth, agar, powdered rhubarb and starches may arise from that indigenous to plants and may include bacteria such as *Erwinia* spp., *Pseudomonas* spp., *Lactobacillus* spp., *Bacillus* spp. and streptococci, moulds such as *Cladosporium* spp., *Alternaria* spp. and *Fusarium* spp. and non-mycelated yeasts, or those introduced during cultivation. For example, the use of untreated sewage as a fertilizer may result in animal-borne pathogens such as *Salmonella* spp. being present. Some refining processes modify the microflora of raw materials, for example drying may concentrate the level of spore-forming bacteria and some solubilizing processes may introduce waterborne bacteria such as *E. coli*.

Synthetic raw materials are usually free from all but incidental microbial contamination.

The storage condition of raw materials, particularly hygroscopic substances, is important, and as a minimum water activity (A_w) of 0.70 is required for osmophilic yeasts, 0.80 for most spoilage moulds and 0.91 for most spoilage bacteria, precautions should be taken to ensure that dry materials are held below these levels. Some packaging used for raw materials, such as unlined paper sacks, may absorb moisture and may itself be subject to microbial deterioration and so contaminate the contents. For this reason polythene-lined sacks are preferable. Some liquid or semi-solid raw materials contain preservatives, but others such as syrups depend upon osmotic pressure to prevent the growth of osmophiles, which are often present. With this type of material it is important that they are held at a constant temperature, as any variation may result in evaporation of some of the water content followed by condensation and dilution of the surface layers to give an A_w value which may permit the growth of osmophiles and spoil the syrup.

The use of natural products with a high non-pathogenic microbial count is possible if a sterilization stage is included either before or during the manufacturing process.

Such sterilization procedures (see also Chapter 20) may include heat treatment, filtration, irradiation, recrystallization from a bactericidal solvent such as an alcohol, or for dry products where compatible, ethylene oxide gas. If the raw material is only a minor constituent and the final product is adequately preserved either by lack of A_w, chemically or by virtue of its pH, sugar or alcohol content, an in-process sterilization stage may not be necessary. If, however, the product is intended for parenteral or ophthalmic use a sterilization stage is essential.

The handling of contaminated raw materials as described previously may increase the airborne contamination level, and if there is a central dispensing area precautions may be necessary to prevent airborne cross-contamination, as well as that from infected measuring and weighing equipment. This presents a risk for all materials but in particular those stored in the liquid state where contamination may result in the bulk being spoiled.

6 Packaging

Packaging material has a dual role and acts both to contain the product and to prevent the entry of microorganisms or moisture which may result in spoilage, and it is therefore important that the source of contamination is not the packaging itself. The microflora of packaging materials is dependent upon both its composition and storage conditions. This, and a consideration of the type of pharmaceutical product to be packed, determine whether a sterilization treatment is required.

Glass containers are sterile on leaving the furnace, but are often stored in dusty conditions and packed for transport in cardboard boxes. As a result they may contain mould spores of *Penicillium* spp., *Aspergillus* spp. and bacteria such as *Bacillus*

spp. It is commonplace to either airblow or wash glass containers to remove any glass spicules or dust which may be present, and it is often advantageous to include a disinfection stage if the product being filled is a liquid or semi-solid preparation. Plastic bottles that are either blow- or injection-moulded have a very low microbial count and may not require disinfection. They may, however, become contaminated with mould spores if they are transported in a non-sanitary packaging material such as unlined cardboard.

Packaging materials that have a smooth, impervious surface, free from crevices or interstices, such as cellulose acetate, polyethylene, polypropylene, polyvinylchloride, and metal foils and laminates, all have a low surface microbial count. Cardboard and paperboard, unless treated, carry mould spores of *Cladosporium* spp., *Aspergillus* spp. and *Penicillium* spp. and bacteria such as *Bacillus* spp. and *Micrococcus* spp.

Closure liners of pulpboard or cork, unless specially treated with a preservative, foil or wax coating, are often a source of mould contamination for liquid or semi-solid products. A closure with a plastic flowed-in liner is less prone to introduce or support microbial growth than one stuck in with an adhesive, particularly if the latter is based on a natural product such as casein. If required, closures can be sterilized by either formaldehyde or ethylene oxide gas.

In the case of injectables and ophthalmic preparations which are manufactured aseptically but do not receive a sterilization treatment in their final container the packaging has to be sterilized. Dry heat at 170°C is often used for vials and ampoules. Containers and closures may also be sterilized by moist heat, chemicals and irradiation, but consideration of the destruction or removal of bacterial pyrogens may be necessary. Regardless of the type of sterilization, the process must be validated and critical control points must be established.

7 Buildings

7.1 Walls and ceilings

Moulds are the most common flora of walls and ceilings and the species usually found are *Cladospo-*

rium spp., *Aspergillus* spp., particularly *A. niger* and *A. flavus*, *Penicillium* spp. and *Aureobasidium* (*Pullularia*) spp. They are particularly common in poorly ventilated buildings with painted walls. The organisms derive most of their nutrients from the plaster onto which the paint has been applied and a hard gloss finish is more resistant than a softer, matt one. The addition of up to 1% of a fungistat such as pentachlorophenol, 8-hydroxyquinoline or salicylanilide is an advantage. To reduce microbial growth, all walls and ceilings should be smooth, impervious and washable and this requirement is met by cladding with a laminated plastic. In areas where humidity is high, glazed bricks or tiles are the optimal finish, and where a considerable volume of steam is used, ventilation at ceiling level is essential. For areas where aseptic filling operations are carried out it is an advantage to have a false ceiling with the services for lighting and ventilation sited above it to minimize particulate matter in the environment. It is important that the joint between the false ceiling and the room below is well sealed.

To aid cleaning, all electrical cables and ducting for other services should be installed deep in cavity walls where they are accessible for maintenance but do not collect dust. All pipes that pass through walls should be sealed flush to the surface.

7.2 Floors and drains

To minimize microbial contamination, all floors should be easy to clean, impervious to water and laid on a flat surface. In some areas it may be necessary for the floor to slope towards a drain, in which case the gradient should be such that no pools of water form. Any joints in the floor, necessary for expansion, should be adequately sealed. The floor-to-wall junction should be coved.

The finish of the floor usually relates to the process being carried out and in an area where little moisture or product is liable to be spilt, polyvinyl chloride welded sheeting may be satisfactory, but in wet areas or where frequent washing is necessary, brick tiles, sealed concrete or a hard ground and polished surface like terrazzo is superior. In areas where acid or alkaline chemicals or cleaning fluids are applied, a resistant sealing and jointing material must be used. If this is neglected

the surface becomes pitted and porous and readily harbours microorganisms.

Where floor drainage channels are necessary they should be open if possible, shallow and easy to clean. Connections to drains should be outside areas where sensitive products are being manufactured and, where possible, drains should be avoided in areas where aseptic operations are being carried out. If this cannot be avoided, they must be fitted with effective traps, preferably with electrically operated heat-sterilizing devices.

7.3 Doors, windows and fittings

To prevent dust from collecting, all ledges, doors and windows should fit flush with walls. Doors should be well fitting to reduce the entry of microorganisms, except where a positive air pressure is maintained. Ideally, all windows in manufacturing areas should serve only to permit light entry and should not be used for ventilation. In areas where aseptic operations are carried out, an adequate air-control system, other than windows, is essential.

Overhead pipes in all manufacturing areas should be sited away from equipment to prevent condensation and possible contaminants from falling into the product. Unless neglected, stainless steel pipes support little microbial growth, but lagged pipes present a problem and unless they are regularly treated with a disinfectant they will support mould growth.

8 Equipment

Each piece of equipment used to manufacture or pack pharmaceuticals has its own peculiar area where microbial growth may be supported, and knowledge of its weak points may be built up by regular tests for contamination. The type and extent of growth will depend on the source of the contamination, the nutrients available and the environmental conditions, in particular the temperature and pH.

The following points are common to many pieces of plant and serve as a general guide to reduce the risk of microbial colonization.

1 All equipment should be easy to dismantle and clean.

2 All surfaces that are in contact with the product should be smooth, continuous and free from pits, with all sharp corners eliminated and junctions rounded or coved. All internal welding should be polished out and there should be no dead ends. All contact surfaces require routine inspection for damage, particularly those of lagged equipment, and double-walled and lined vessels, as any cracks or pinholes in the surface may allow the product to seep into an area where it is protected from cleaning and sterilizing agents, and where microorganisms may grow and contaminate subsequent batches of product.

3 There should be no inside screw threads and all outside threads should be readily accessible for cleaning.

4 Coupling nuts on all pipework and valves should be capable of being taken apart and cleaned.

5 Agitator blades and the shaft should preferably be of one piece and be accessible for cleaning. If the blades are bolted onto the shaft, the product may become entrained between the shaft and blades and support microorganisms. If the shaft is packed into a housing and this fitting is within a manufacturing vessel it also may act as a reservoir of microorganisms.

6 Mechanical seals are preferable to packing boxes as packing material is usually difficult to sterilize and often requires a lubricant which may gain access to the product. The product must also be protected from lubricant used on other moving parts.

7 Valves should be of a sanitary design, and all contact parts must be treated during cleaning and sanitation, and a wide variety of plug type valves are available for general purpose use. For aseptically manufactured and filled products valves fitted with steam barriers are available. If diaphragm valves are used, it is essential to inspect the diaphragm routinely. Worn diaphragms can permit seepage of the product into the seat of the valve, where it is protected from cleaning and sterilizing agents and may act as a growth medium for microorganisms. In addition, if diaphragm valves are used in a very wet area, a purpose-made cover may be useful to prevent access of water and potential microbial growth occurring under the diaphragm.

8 All pipelines should slope away from the product source and all process and storage vessels should be self-draining. Run-off valves should be as near to the tank as possible and sampling through them should be avoided, as any nutrient left in the valve may encourage microbial growth which could contaminate the complete batch. A separate sampling cock or hatch is preferable.

9 If a vacuum exhaust system is used to remove the air or steam from a vessel, it is necessary to clean and disinfect all fittings regularly. This prevents residues which may be drawn into them from supporting microbial growth, which may later be returned to the vessel in the form of condensate and contaminate subsequent batches of product. If air is bled back into the vessel it should be passed through a sterilizing filter.

10 If any filters or straining bags made from natural materials such as canvas, muslin or paper are used, care must be taken to ensure that they are cleaned and sterilized regularly to prevent the growth of moulds such as *Cladosporium* spp., *Stachybotrys* spp. and *Aureobasidium* (*Pullularia*) *pullulans*, which utilize cellulose and would impair them.

8.1 Pipelines

The most common materials used for pipelines are stainless steel, glass and plastic, and the latter may be rigid or flexible. Continuous sections of pipework are often designed to be cleaned and sterilized in place by the flow of cleansing and sterilizing agents at a velocity of not less than 1.5 m/s through the pipe of the largest diameter in the system. The speed of flow coupled with a suitable detergent removes microorganisms by a scouring action. To be successful, stainless steel pipes must be welded to form a continuous length and must be polished internally to eliminate any pits or crevices that would provide a harbour for microorganisms. However, as soon as joints and cross-connections are introduced they provide a harbour for microorganisms, particularly behind rubber or teflon O-rings. In the case of plastic pipes, bonded joints can form an area where microorganisms are protected from cleaning and sterilizing agents.

The 'in-place' cleaning system described for pipelines may also be used for both plate and tubular types of heat exchange units, pumps and some homogenizers. However, valves and all T-piece fittings for valves and temperature and pressure gauges may need to be cleaned manually. Tanks and reaction vessels may be cleaned and sterilized automatically by rotary pressure sprays, which are sited at a point in the vessel where the maximum area of wall may be treated. If spray balls are incorporated into a system that re-uses the cleansing-in-place (CIP) fluids, then it may be necessary to incorporate a filter to remove particles which may block the pores of the spray ball. Fixtures such as agitators, pipe inlets, outlets and vents may have to be cleaned manually. The nature of many products or the plant design often renders cleaning in place impracticable and the plant has to be dismantled for cleaning and sterilizing.

8.2 Cleansing

There are several cleansing agents available to suit the product to be removed, and the agents include acids, alkalis and anionic, cationic and non-ionic detergents. The agent selected must fulfil the following criteria.

1 It must suit the surface to be cleaned and not cause corrosion.
2 It must remove the product without leaving a residue.
3 It must be compatible with the water supply.

Sometimes a combined cleansing and sterilizing solution is desirable, in which case the two agents must be compatible.

8.3 Disinfection and sterilization

Equipment may be sterilized or disinfected by heat, chemical disinfection or a combination of both. Many tanks and reaction vessels are sterilized by steam under pressure, and small pieces of equipment and fittings may be autoclaved, but it is important that the steam has access to all surfaces. Equipment used to manufacture and pack dry powder is often sterilized by dry heat. Chemical disinfectants commonly include sodium hypochlorite and organochlorines at 50–100 ppm free residual chlorine, QACs (0.1–0.2%), 70% (v/v) ethanol in water and 1% (v/v) formaldehyde solution. The method of disinfection may be total immersion for small objects or by spraying the internal surfaces of larger equipment. When plant is dismantled for cleaning and sterilizing, all fittings such as couplings, valves, gaskets and O-rings also require treatment. The removal of chemical disinfectants is very important in fermentation processes where residues may affect sensitive cultures.

All disinfection and sterilization processes for equipment should be validated, for preference using a microbiological challenge with an organism of appropriate resistance to the disinfectant, sterilant or sterilizing conditions. Once the required log reduction of the challenge organism has been achieved, physical and/or chemical parameters can be set which form the critical control points for the process.

8.4 Microbial checks

Either as part of an initial validation or as an ongoing exercise, the efficacy of CIP systems can be checked by plating out a sample of the final rinse water with a nutrient agar, or by swab tests. Swabs may be made of either sterile cotton wool or calcium alginate. The latter is used in conjunction with a diluent containing 1% sodium hexametaphosphate which dissolves the swab and releases the organisms removed from the equipment; these organisms may then be plated out with a nutrient agar or alternative methods of evaluation may be used. Swabs are useful for checking the cleanliness of curved pieces of equipment, pipes, orifices, valves and connections, but unless a measuring guide is used the results cannot be expressed quantitatively. Such measurement can be made by pressing a nutrient agar against a flat surface. The agar is usually poured into specially designed Petri dishes or contact plates, or is in the form of a disc sliced from a cylinder of a solid nutrient medium. The nutrient agar or plate or section, when incubated, replicates the contamination on the surface tested. As this technique leaves a nutrient residue on the surface tested, the equipment must be washed and resterilized before use. The development of methods for the rapid detection of microorganisms has advantages over more traditional methods if quantitative results are used as part of a critical control programme, but not all methods lend themselves to identifying the contaminant, and it may be necessary to use a combination of methods if qualitative determinations are required.

9 Cleaning equipment and utensils

The misuse of brooms and mops can substantially increase the microbial count of the atmosphere by raising dust or by splashing with waterborne contaminants. To prevent this, either a correctly designed vacuum cleaner or a broom made of synthetic material, which is washed regularly, may be used. Hospital trials have shown that, when used, a neglected dry mop redistributes microorganisms which it has picked up, but a neglected wet mop redistributes many times the number of organisms it picked up originally, because it provides a suitable environment for their growth. In order to maintain mops and similar non-disposable cleaning equipment in a good hygienic state, it was found to be necessary first to wash and then to boil or autoclave the items, and finally to store them in a dry state. Disinfectant solutions were found to be inadequate.

Many chemical disinfectants (see also Chapter 17), in particular the halogens, some phenolics and QACs, are inactivated in the presence of organic matter and it is essential that all cleaning materials such as buckets and fogging sprays are kept clean. Halogens rapidly deteriorate at their use-dilution levels and QACs are liable to become contaminated with *Ps. aeruginosa* if stored diluted. For such reasons it is preferable to store the bulk of the disinfectant in a concentrated form and to dilute it to the use concentration only as required.

10 Further reading

Anderson, J. D. & Cox, C. S. (1967) Microbial survival. In: *Airborne Microbes* (eds P.H. Gregory & J.L. Monteith), pp. 203–226. Seventeenth Symposium of the Society for General Microbiology. Cambridge University Press, Cambridge.

Burman, N .P. & Colbourne, J. S. (1977) Techniques for the assessment of growth of microorganisms on plumbing materials used in contact with potable water supplies. *J Appl Bacteriol*, **43**, 137–144.

Chambers, C. W. & Clarke, N. A. (1968) Control of bacteria in non-domestic water. *Adv Appl Microbiol*, **8**, 105–143.

Collings, V. G. (1964) The freshwater environment and its significance in industry. *J Appl Bacteriol*, **27**, 143–150.

Denyer, S. P. & Baird, R. M. (1990) *Guide to Microbiological Control in Pharmaceuticals*. Ellis Horwood, Chichester.

Favero, M. S., McDade, J. J., Robertson, J. A., Hoffman, R. V. & Edward, R. W. (1968) Microbiological sampling of surfaces. *J Appl Bacteriol*, **31**, 336–343.

Gould, G. W. (1999) *New and Emerging Technologies, Disinfection, Preservation and Sterilization*, pp. 767–776. Blackwell Science, Oxford.

Gregory, P. H. (1973) *Microbiology of the Atmosphere*, 2nd edn. Leonard Hill, London.

Maurer, I. M. (1985) *Hospital Hygiene*, 3rd edn. Edward Arnold, London.

Nishannon, A. & Pokja, M. S. (1977) Comparative studies of microbial contamination of surfaces by the contact plate and swab methods. *J Appl Bacteriol*, **42**, 53–63.

Packer, M. E. & Litchfield, J. H. (1972) *Food Plant Sanitation*. Chapman & Hall, London.

Russell, A. D., Hugo, W. B. & Ayliffe, G. A. J. (1998) *Principles and Practice of Disinfection, Preservation and Sterilization*, 3rd edn. Blackwell Scientific, Oxford.

Skinner, F. A. & Carr, F. G. (1974) *The Normal Microbial Flora of Man*. Society for Applied Bacteriology Symposium No. 5. Academic Press, London.

Underwood, E. (1998) Good manufacturing practice. In: *Principles and Practice of Disinfection, Preservation and Sterilization* (eds A.D. Russell, W.B. Hugo & G.A.J. Ayliffe), 3rd edn. Blackwell Scientific, Oxford.

Chapter 16
Microbial spoilage, infection risk and contamination control

Rosamund Baird

1 Introduction

Pharmaceutical products used in the prevention, treatment and diagnosis of disease contain a wide variety of ingredients, often in quite complex physicochemical states. Such products must not only meet current pharmaceutical Good Manufacturing Practice (GMP) requirements for quality, safety and efficacy, but also must be stable and sufficiently elegant to be acceptable to patients.

Products made in the pharmaceutical industry today must meet high microbiological specifications, i.e. if not sterile, they are expected to have no more than a minimal microbial population at the time of product release.

Nevertheless, from time to time a few rogue products with an unacceptable level and type of contamination will occasionally escape the quality assurance net. The consequences of such contamination may be serious and far-reaching on several accounts, particularly if contaminants have had the opportunity to multiply to high levels. Firstly, the product may be spoiled, rendering it unfit for use through chemical and physicochemical deterioration of the formulation. Spoilage and subsequent wastage of individual batches usually results in major financial problems for the manufacturer through direct loss of faulty product. Secondly, the threat of litigation and the unwanted, damaging publicity of recalls may have serious economic implications for the manufacturer. Thirdly, inadvertent use of contaminated products may present a potential health hazard to patients, perhaps resulting in outbreaks of medicament-related infections, and ironically therefore contributing to the spread of disease. Most commonly, heavy contamination of product with opportunist pathogens, such as *Pseudomonas* spp., has resulted in the spread of nosocomial (hospital-acquired) infections in compromised patients; less frequently, low levels of contamination with pathogenic organisms, such as *Salmonella*, have attracted considerable attention, as have products contaminated with toxic microbial metabolites. The consequences of microbial contamination in pharmaceutical products are discussed in more detail below.

2 Spoilage—chemical and physicochemical deterioration of pharmaceuticals

Microorganisms form a major part of the natural recycling processes for biological matter in the environment. As such, they possess a wide variety of degradative capabilities, which they are able to exert under relatively mild physicochemical conditions. Mixed natural communities are often far more effective co-operative biodeteriogens than the individual species alone, and sequences of attack of complex substrates occur where initial attack by one group of microorganisms renders them susceptible to further deterioration by secondary, and subsequent, microorganisms. Under suitable environmental selection pressures, novel degradative pathways may emerge with the capability to attack newly introduced synthetic chemicals (xenobiotics). However, the rates of degradation of materials released into the environment can vary greatly, from half-lives of hours (phenol) to months ('hard' detergents) to years (halogenated pesticides).

The overall rate of deterioration of a chemical will depend upon: its molecular structure; the physicochemical properties of a particular environment; the type and quantity of microbes present; and whether the metabolites produced can serve as sources of usable energy and precursors for the biosynthesis of cellular components, and hence the creation of more microorganisms.

Pharmaceutical formulations may be considered as specialized micro-environments and their susceptibility to microbial attack can be assessed using conventional ecological criteria. Some naturally occurring ingredients are particularly sensitive to attack, and a number of synthetic components, such as modern surfactants, have been deliberately constructed to be readily degraded after disposal into the environment. Crude vegetable and animal drug extracts often contain a wide assortment of microbial nutrients besides the therapeutic agents. This, combined with frequently conducive and unstable physicochemical characteristics, leaves many formulations with a high potential for microbial attack, unless steps are taken to minimize it.

2.1 Pharmaceutical ingredients susceptible to microbial attack

Therapeutic agents. Through spoilage, active drug constituents may be metabolized to less potent or chemically inactive forms. Under laboratory conditions, it has been shown that a variety of microorganisms can metabolize a wide assortment of drugs, resulting in loss of activity. Materials as diverse as alkaloids (morphine, strychnine, atropine), analgesics (aspirin, paracetamol), thalidomide, barbiturates, steroid esters and mandelic acid can be metabolized and serve as substrates for growth. Indeed the use of microorganisms to carry out subtle transformations on steroid molecules forms the basis of the commercial production of potent therapeutic steroidal agents (see Chapter 25). In practice, reports of drug destruction in medicines are less frequent. There have, however, been some notable exceptions: the metabolism of atropine in eyedrops by contaminating fungi; inactivation of penicillin injections by β-lactamase-producing bacteria (see Chapters 10 and 13); steroid metabolism in damp tablets and creams by fungi; microbial hydrolysis of aspirin in suspension by esterase-producing bacteria; and chloramphenicol deactivation in an oral medicine by a chloramphenicol acetylase-producing contaminant.

Surface-active agents. Anionic surfactants, such as the alkali metal and amine soaps of fatty acids, are generally stable due to the slightly alkaline pH of the formulations, although readily degraded once diluted into sewage. Alkyl and alkylbenzene sulphonates and sulphate esters are metabolized by ω-oxidation of their terminal methyl groups followed by sequential β-oxidation of the alkyl chains and fission of the aromatic rings. The presence of chain branching involves additional α-oxidative processes. Generally, ease of degradation decreases with increasing chain length and complexity of branching of the alkyl chain.

Non-ionic surfactants, such as alkylpolyoxyethylene alcohol emulsifiers, are readily metabolized by a wide variety of microorganisms. Increasing chain lengths and branching again decrease ease of attack. Alkylphenol polyoxyethylene alcohols are similarly attacked, but are significantly more resistant. Lipolytic cleavage of the fatty acids from sorbitan esters, polysorbates and sucrose esters is often followed by degradation of the cyclic nuclei, producing numerous small molecules readily utilizable for microbial growth. Ampholytic surfactants, based on phosphatides, betaines and alkylamino-substituted amino acids, are an increasingly important group of surfactants and are generally reported to be reasonably biodegradable. The cationic surfactants used as antiseptics and preservatives in pharmaceutical applications are usually only slowly degraded at high dilution in sewage. Pseudomonads have been found growing readily in quaternary ammonium antiseptic solutions, largely at the expense of other ingredients such as buffering materials, although some metabolism of the surfactant has also been observed.

Organic polymers. Many of the thickening and suspending agents used in pharmaceutical formulations are subject to microbial depolymerization by specific classes of extracellular enzymes, yielding nutritive fragments and monomers. Examples of

such enzymes, with their substrates in parentheses are: amylases (starches), pectinases (pectins), cellulases (carboxymethylcelluloses, but not alkylcelluloses), uronidases (polyuronides such as in tragacanth and acacia), dextranases (dextrans) and proteases (proteins). Agar (a complex polysaccharide) is an example of a relatively inert polymer and, as such, is used as a support for solidifying microbiological culture media. The lower molecular weight polyethylene glycols are readily degraded by sequential oxidation of the hydrocarbon chain, but the larger congeners are rather more recalcitrant. Synthetic packaging polymers such as nylon, polystyrene and polyester are extremely resistant to attack, although cellophane (modified cellulose) is susceptible under some humid conditions.

Humectants. Low molecular weight materials such as glycerol and sorbitol are included in some products to reduce water loss and may be readily metabolized unless present in high concentrations (see section 2.3.3).

Fats and oils. These hydrophobic materials are usually attacked extensively when dispersed in aqueous formulations such as oil-in-water emulsions, aided by the high solubility of oxygen in many oils. Fungal attack has been reported in condensed moisture films on the surface of oils in bulk, or where water droplets have contaminated the bulk oil phase. Lipolytic rupture of triglycerides liberates glycerol and fatty acids, the latter often then undergoing β-oxidation of the alkyl chains and the production of odiferous ketones. While the microbial metabolism of pharmaceutical hydrocarbon oils is rarely reported, this is a problem in engineering and fuel technology when water droplets have accumulated in oil storage tanks and subsequent fungal colonization has catalysed serious corrosion.

Sweetening, flavouring and colouring agents. Many of the sugars and other sweetening agents used in pharmacy are ready substrates for microbial growth. However, some are used in very high concentrations to reduce water activity in aqueous products and inhibit microbial attack (see section 2.3.3). At one time, a variety of colouring agents (such as tartrazine and amaranth) and flavouring agents (such as peppermint water) were kept as stock solutions for extemporaneous dispensing purposes but they frequently supported the growth of *Pseudomonas* spp., including *Ps. aeruginosa*. Such stock solutions should now be preserved or freshly made as required by dilution of alcoholic solutions which are much less susceptible to microbial attack.

Preservatives and disinfectants. Many preservatives and disinfectants can be metabolized by a wide variety of Gram-negative bacteria, although most commonly at concentrations below their effective 'use' levels. Growth of pseudomonads in stock solutions of quaternary ammonium antiseptics and chlorhexidine has resulted in infection of patients. *Pseudomonas* spp. have metabolized 4-hydroxybenzoate ester preservatives contained in eye-drops and caused serious eye infections, and have also metabolized the preservatives in oral suspensions and solutions. In selecting suitable preservatives for formulation, a detailed knowledge of the properties of such agents, their susceptibility to contamination and limitations clearly provides invaluable information.

2.2 Observable effects of microbial attack on pharmaceutical products

Microbial contaminants usually need to attack formulation ingredients and create substrates necessary for biosynthesis and energy production before they can replicate to levels where obvious spoilage becomes apparent. Thus, for example, 10^6 microbes will have an overall degradative effect around 10^6 times faster than one cell. However, growth and attack may well be localized in surface moisture films or very unevenly distributed within the bulk of viscous formulations such as creams. Early indications of spoilage are often organoleptic, with the release of unpleasant smelling and tasting metabolites such as 'sour' fatty acids, 'fishy' amines, 'bad eggs', bitter, 'earthy' or sickly tastes and smells. Products may become unappealingly discoloured by microbial pigments of various shades. Thickening and suspending agents such as tragacanth, acacia or carboxymethylcellulose can be depolymerized resulting in loss of viscosity, and sedimentation of suspended ingredients. Alternatively, microbial polymerization of sugars and surfactant molecules can produce slimy, viscous masses in

syrups, shampoos and creams, and fungal growth in creams has produced 'gritty' textures. Changes in product pH can occur depending on whether acidic or basic metabolites are released, and become so modified as to permit secondary attack by microbes previously inhibited by the initial product pH. Gaseous metabolites may be seen as trapped bubbles within viscous formulations.

When a complex formulation such as an oil-in-water emulsion is attacked, a gross and progressive spoilage sequence may be observed. Metabolism of surfactants will reduce stability and accelerate 'creaming' of the oil globules. Lipolytic release of fatty acids from oils will lower pH and encourage coalescence of oil globules and 'cracking' of the emulsion. Fatty acids and their ketonic oxidation products will provide a sour taste and unpleasant smell, while bubbles of gaseous metabolites may be visible, trapped in the product, and pigments may discolour it (see Fig. 16.1).

2.3 Factors affecting microbial spoilage of pharmaceutical products

By understanding the influence of environmental parameters on microorganisms, it may be possible to manipulate formulations to create conditions which are as unfavourable as possible for growth and spoilage, within the limitations of patient acceptability and therapeutic efficacy. Furthermore, the overall characteristics of a particular formulation will indicate its susceptibility to attack by various classes of microorganisms.

2.3.1 *Types and size of contaminant inoculum*

Successful formulation of products against microbial attack involves an element of prediction. An understanding of where and how the product is to be used, and the challenges it must face during its life, will enable the formulator to build-in as much protection as possible against microbial attack. When failures inevitably occur from time to time, knowledge of the microbial ecology and careful identification of contaminants can be most useful in tracking down the defective steps in the design or production process.

Low levels of contaminants may not cause appre-

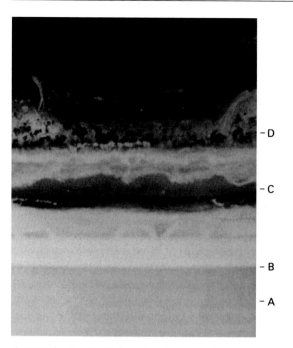

Fig. 16.1 Section (×1.5) through an inadequately preserved olive oil, oil-in-water, emulsion in an advanced state of microbial spoilage showing: A, discoloured, oil-depleted, aqueous phase; B, oil globule-rich creamed layer; C, coalesced oil layer from 'cracked' emulsion; D, fungal mycelian growth on surface. Also present are a foul taste and evil smell!

ciable spoilage, if unable to replicate in a product; however, an unexpected surge in the contaminant bioburden may present an unacceptable challenge to the designed formulation. This could arise if, for example: raw materials were unusually contaminated; there was a lapse in the plant-cleaning protocol; a biofilm detached itself from within supplying pipework; or the product had been grossly misused during administration. Inoculum size alone is not always a reliable indicator of likely spoilage potential. Low levels of aggressive pseudomonads in a weakly preserved solution may suggest a greater risk than tablets containing fairly high numbers of fungal and bacterial spores.

When an aggressive microorganism contaminates a medicine, there may be an appreciable lag period before significant spoilage begins, the duration of which decreases disproportionately with increasing contaminant loading. As there is usually a considerable delay between manufacture and administration of factory-made medicines, growth and attack could ensue during this period unless additional steps were taken to prevent it. On the other hand, for extemporaneously dispensed formulations some control can be provided by specifying short shelf-lives, for example 2 weeks.

The isolation of a particular microorganism from a markedly spoiled product does not necessarily mean that it was the initiator of the attack. It could be a secondary opportunist contaminant which had overgrown the primary spoilage organism once the physicochemical properties had been favourably modified by the primary spoiler.

2.3.2 Nutritional factors

The simple nutritional requirements and metabolic adaptability of many common spoilage microorganisms enable them to utilize many formulation components as substrates for biosynthesis and growth. The use of crude vegetable or animal products in a formulation provides an additionally nutritious environment. Even demineralized water prepared by good ion-exchange methods will normally contain sufficient nutrients to allow significant growth of many waterborne Gram-negative bacteria such as *Pseudomonas* spp. When such contaminants fail to survive, it is unlikely to be the result of nutrient limitation in the product but due to other, non-supportive, physicochemical or toxic properties.

Acute pathogens require specific growth factors normally associated with the tissues they infect but which are often absent in pharmaceutical formulations. They are thus unlikely to multiply in them, although they may remain viable and infective for an appreciable time in some dry products where the conditions are suitably protective.

2.3.3 Moisture content: water activity (A_w)

Microorganisms require readily accessible water in appreciable quantities for growth to occur. By measuring a product's water activity (A_w), it is possible to obtain an estimate of the proportion of uncomplexed water that is available in the formulation to support microbial growth, using the formula: $A_w =$ vapour pressure of formulation/vapour pressure of water under similar conditions.

The greater the solute concentration, the lower is the water activity. With the exception of halophilic bacteria, most microorganisms grow best in dilute solutions (high A_w) and, as solute concentration rises (lowering A_w), growth rates decline until a minimal growth-inhibitory A_w, is reached. Limiting A_w values are of the order of: Gram-negative rods, 0.95; staphylococci, micrococci and lactobacilli, 0.9; and most yeasts, 0.88. Syrup-fermenting osmotolerant yeasts have spoiled products with A_w levels as low as 0.73, while some filamentous fungi such as *Aspergillus glaucus* can grow at 0.61.

The A_w of aqueous formulations can be lowered to increase resistance to microbial attack by the addition of high concentrations of sugars or polyethylene glycols. However, even Syrup BP (67% sucrose; $A_w = 0.86$) has failed occasionally to inhibit osmotolerant yeasts and additional preservation may be necessary. With a continuing trend towards the elimination of sucrose from medicines, alternative solutes, such as sorbitol and fructose, have been investigated which are not thought to encourage dental caries. A_w can also be reduced by drying, although the dry, often hygroscopic medicines (tablets, capsules, powders, vitreous 'glasses') will require suitable packaging to prevent resorption of water and consequent microbial growth (Fig. 16.2).

Tablet film coatings are now available which greatly reduce water vapour uptake during storage while allowing ready dissolution in bulk water. These might contribute to increased microbial stability during storage in particularly humid climates, although suitable foil strip packing may be more effective, albeit more expensive.

Condensed water films can accumulate on the surface of otherwise 'dry' products such as tablets or bulk oils following storage in damp atmospheres with fluctuating temperatures, resulting in sufficiently high localized A_w to initiate fungal growth. Condensation similarly formed on the surface of viscous products such as syrups and creams, or exuded by syneresis from hydrogels, may well permit surface yeast and fungal spoilage.

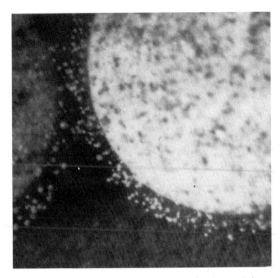

Fig. 16.2 Fungal growth on a tablet which has become damp (raised A_w) during storage under humid conditions. Note the sparseness of mycelium, and conidiophores. The contaminant is thought to be a *Penicillium* sp.

2.3.4 *Redox potential*

The ability of microbes to grow in an environment is influenced by its oxidation-reduction balance (redox potential), as they will require compatible terminal electron acceptors to permit their respiratory pathways to function. The redox potential even in fairly viscous emulsions may be quite high due to the appreciable solubility of oxygen in most fats and oils.

2.3.5 *Storage temperature*

Spoilage of pharmaceuticals could occur potentially over the range of about −20°C to 60°C, although it is much less likely at the extremes. The particular storage temperature may selectively determine the types of microorganisms involved in spoilage. A deep freeze at −20°C or lower is used for long-term storage of some pharmaceutical raw materials and short-term storage of dispensed total parenteral nutrition (TPN) feeds prepared in hospitals. Reconstituted syrups and multi-dose eye-drop packs are sometimes dispensed with the instruction to 'store in a cool place' such as a domestic fridge (8°–12°C), partly to reduce the risk of growth of contaminants inadvertently introduced during use. Conversely, Water for Injections (EP) should be held at 80°C or above after distillation and before packing and sterilization to prevent possible regrowth of Gram-negative bacteria and the release of endotoxins.

2.3.6 pH

Extremes of pH prevent microbial attack. Around neutrality bacterial spoilage is more likely, with reports of pseudomonads and related Gram-negative bacteria growing in antacid mixtures, flavoured mouthwashes and in distilled or demineralized water. Above pH 8 (e.g. with soap-based emulsions) spoilage is rare. In products with low pH levels (e.g. fruit juice-flavoured syrups with a pH 3–4), mould or yeast attack is more likely. Yeasts can metabolize organic acids and raise the pH to levels where secondary bacterial growth can occur. Although the use of low pH adjustment to preserve foodstuffs is well established (e.g. pickling, coleslaw, yoghurt), it is not practicable to make deliberate use of this for medicines.

2.3.7 Packaging design

Packaging can have a major influence on microbial stability of some formulations in controlling the entry of contaminants during both storage and use. Considerable thought has gone into the design of containers to prevent the ingress of contaminants into medicines for parenteral administration, owing to the high risks of infection by this route. Self-sealing rubber wads must be used to prevent microbial entry into multi-dose injection containers (Chapter 19) following withdrawals with a hypodermic needle. Wide-mouthed cream jars have now been replaced by narrow nozzles and flexible screw-capped tubes, thereby removing the likelihood of operator-introduced contamination during use of the product. Where medicines rely on their low A_w to prevent spoilage, packaging such as strip foils must be of water vapour-proof materials with fully efficient seals. Cardboard outer packaging and labels themselves can become substrates for microbial attack under humid conditions, and preservatives are often included to reduce the risk of damage.

2.3.8 Protection of microorganisms within pharmaceutical products

The survival of microorganisms in particular environments is sometimes influenced by the presence of relatively inert materials. Thus, microbes can be more resistant to heat or desiccation in the presence of polymers such as starch, acacia or gelatin. Adsorption onto naturally occurring particulate material may aid establishment and survival in some environments. There is a belief, but limited hard evidence, that the presence of suspended particles such as kaolin, magnesium trisilicate or aluminium hydroxide gel may influence contaminant longevity in those products containing them, and that the presence of some surfactants, suspending agents and proteins can increase the resistance of microorganisms to preservatives, over and above their direct inactivating effect on the preservative itself.

3 Hazard to health

Nowadays, it is well recognized that the inadvertent use of a contaminated pharmaceutical product may also present a potential health hazard to the patient. Although isolated outbreaks of medicament-related infections had been reported since the early part of the 20th century, it was only in the 1960s and 1970s that the significance of this contamination to the patient was more fully understood.

Inevitably, the infrequent isolation of true pathogens, such as *Salmonella* spp. and the reporting of associated infections following the use of products contaminated with these organisms (tablets, pancreatin and thyroid extract), have attracted considerable attention. More often, the isolation of common saprophytic and non-fastidious opportunist contaminants with limited pathogenicity to healthy individuals has presented a significant challenge to compromised patients.

Gram-negative contaminants, particularly *Pseudomonas* spp. which have simple nutritional requirements and can multiply to significant levels in aqueous products, have been held responsible for numerous outbreaks of infection. For example, while the intact cornea is quite resistant to infection, it offers little resistance to pseudomonads and

Table 16.1 Contaminants found in pharmaceutical products

Year	Product	Contaminant
1907	Plague vaccine	*Clostridium tetani*
1943	Fluorescein eye-drops	*Pseudomonas aeruginosa*
1946	Talcum powder	*Clostridium tetani*
1948	Serum vaccine	*Staphylococcus aureus*
1955	Chloroxylenol disinfectant	*Pseudomonas aeruginosa*
1966	Thyroid tablets	*Salmonella muenchen*
1966	Antibiotic eye ointment	*Pseudomonas aeruginosa*
1966	Saline solution	*Serratia marcescens*
1967	Carmine powder	*Salmonella cubana*
1967	Hand cream	*Klebsiella pneumoniae*
1969	Peppermint water	*Pseudomonas aeruginosa*
1970	Chlorhexidine-cetrimide antiseptic solution	*Pseudomonas cepacia*
1972	Intravenous fluids	*Pseudomonas, Erwinia* and *Enterobacter* spp.
1972	Pancreatin powder	*Salmonella agona*
1977	Contact lens solution	*Serratia* and *Enterobacter* spp.
1981	Surgical dressings	*Clostridium* spp.
1982	Iodophor solution	*Pseudomonas aeruginosa*
1983	Aqueous soap	*Pseudomonas stutzeri*
1984	Thymol mouthwash	*Pseudomonas aeruginosa*
1986	Antiseptic mouthwash	Coliforms

related bacteria when scratched, or damaged by irritant chemicals; loss of sight has frequently occurred following the use of poorly designed ophthalmic solutions which had become contaminated by *Pseudomonas aeruginosa* and even supported its active growth. Pseudomonads contaminating 'antiseptic' solutions have infected the skin of badly burnt patients, resulting in the failure of skin grafts and subsequent death from Gram-negative septicaemia. Infections of eczematous skin and respiratory infections in neonates have been traced to ointments and creams contaminated with Gram-negative bacteria. Oral mixtures and antacid suspensions can support the growth of Gram-negative bacteria and serious consequences have resulted following their inadvertent administration to patients who were immunocompromised as a result of antineoplastic chemotherapy. Growth of Gram-negative bacteria in bladder washout solutions has been held responsible for painful infections. In more recent times, *Pseudomonas* contamination of parenteral nutritional fluids during their aseptic compounding in the hospital pharmacy caused the death of several children in the same hospital.

Fatal viral infections resulting from the use of contaminated human tissue or fluids as components of medicines are well recorded. Examples of this include human immunodeficiency virus (HIV) infection of haemophiliacs by contaminated and inadequately treated factor VIII products made from pooled human blood, and Creutzfeldt–Jakob disease (CJD) from injections of human growth hormone derived from human pituitary glands, some of which were infected.

Pharmaceutical products of widely differing forms are known to be susceptible to contamination with a variety of microorganisms, ranging from true pathogens to a motley collection of opportunist pathogens (see Table 16.1). Disinfectants, antiseptics, powders, tablets and other products providing an inhospitable environment to invading contaminants are known to be at risk, as well as products with more nutritious components, such as creams and lotions with carbohydrates, amino acids, vitamins and often appreciable quantities of water.

The outcome of using a contaminated product may vary from patient to patient, depending on the type and degree of contamination and how the product is to be used. Undoubtedly, the most serious effects have been seen with contaminated injected products where generalized bacteraemic shock and in some cases death of patients have been reported. More likely, a wound or sore in broken skin may become locally infected or colonized by the contaminant; this may in turn result in extended hospital bed occupancy, with ensuing economic consequences. It must be stressed, however, that the majority of cases of medicament-related infections are probably not recognized or reported as such. Recognition of these infections presents its own problems. It is a fortunate hospital physician who can, at an early stage, recognize contamination shown as a cluster of infections of rapid onset, such as that following the use of a contaminated intravenous fluid in a hospital ward. The chances of a general practitioner recognizing a medicament-related infection of insidious onset, perhaps spread over several months, in a diverse group of patients in the community, are much more remote. Once recognized, of course, there is a moral obligation to withdraw the offending product; subsequent investigations of the incident therefore become retrospective.

3.1 Microbial toxins

Gram-negative bacteria contain lipopolysaccharides (endotoxins) in their outer cell membranes (Chapter 19); these can remain in an active condition in products even after cell death and some can survive moist heat sterilization. Although inactive by the oral route, endotoxins can induce a number of physiological effects if they enter the bloodstream via contaminated infusion fluids, even in nanogram quantities, or via diffusion across membranes from contaminated haemodialysis solutions. Such effects may include fever, activation of the cytokine system, endothelial cell damage, all leading to septic and often fatal febrile shock.

The acute bacterial toxins associated with food poisoning episodes are not commonly reported in pharmaceutical products, although aflatoxin-producing aspergilli have been detected in some vegetable ingredients. However, many of the metabolites of microbial deterioration have quite

unpleasant tastes and smell even at low levels, and would deter most patients from using such a medicine.

4 Sources and control of contamination

4.1 In manufacture

Regardless of whether manufacture takes place in industry (Chapter 15) or on a smaller scale in the hospital pharmacy, the microbiological quality of the finished product will be determined by the formulation components used, the environment in which they are manufactured and the manufacturing process itself. As discussed in Chapter 21, quality must be built into the product at all stages of the process and not simply inspected at the end of manufacture: (i) raw materials, particularly water and those of natural origin, must be of a high microbiological standard; (ii) all processing equipment should be subject to planned preventive maintenance and should be properly cleaned after use to prevent cross-contamination between batches; (iii) cleaning equipment should be appropriate for the task in hand and should be thoroughly cleaned and properly maintained; (iv) manufacture should take place in suitable premises, supplied with filtered air, for which the environmental requirements vary according to the type of product being made; (v) staff involved in manufacture should not only have good health but also a sound knowledge of the importance of personal and production hygiene; and (vi) the end-product requires suitable packaging which will protect it from contamination during its shelf-life and is itself free from contamination.

4.1.1 Hospital manufacture

Manufacture in hospital premises raises certain additional problems with regard to contamination control.

4.1.1.1 Water

Mains water in hospitals is frequently stored in large roof tanks, some of which may be relatively inaccessible and poorly maintained. Water for pharmaceutical manufacture requires some further treatment, usually by distillation, reverse osmosis (Chapter 15) or deionization or a combination of these, depending on the intended use of water. Such processes need careful monitoring, as does the microbiological quality of the water after treatment. Storage of water requires particular care, as some Gram-negative opportunist pathogens can survive on traces of organic matter present in treated water and will readily multiply to high numbers at room temperature. Water should therefore be stored at a temperature in excess of 80°C and circulated in the distribution system at a flow rate of 1–2 m/s to prevent the build-up of bacterial biofilms in the piping.

4.1.1.2 Environment

The microbial flora of the hospital pharmacy environment is a reflection of the general hospital environment and the activities undertaken there. Free-living opportunist pathogens, such as *Ps. aeruginosa*, can normally be found in wet sites, such as drains, sinks and taps. Cleaning equipment, such as mops, buckets, cloths and scrubbing machines, may be responsible for distributing these organisms around the pharmacy; if stored wet they provide a convenient niche for microbial growth, resulting in heavy contamination of equipment. Contamination levels in the production environment may, however, be minimized by observing good manufacturing practices, by installing heating traps in sink U-bends, thus destroying one of the main reservoirs of contaminants, and by proper maintenance and storage of equipment, including cleaning equipment. Additionally, cleaning of production units by contractors should be carried out to a pharmaceutical specification.

4.1.1.3 Packaging

Sacking, cardboard, card liners, corks and paper are unsuitable for packaging pharmaceuticals, as they are heavily contaminated, for example with bacterial or fungal spores. These have now been replaced by non-biodegradable plastic materials. In the past, packaging in hospitals has been frequently re-used for economic reasons. Large numbers of containers may be returned to the pharmacy, bringing with them microbial contaminants introduced during use in the wards. Particular problems have

been encountered with disinfectant solutions where residues of old stock have been 'topped up' with fresh supplies, resulting in the issue of contaminated solutions to wards. Re-usable containers must therefore be thoroughly washed and dried, and never refilled directly.

Another common practice in hospitals is the repackaging of products purchased in bulk into smaller containers. Increased handling of the product inevitably increases the risk of contamination, as shown by one survey when hospital-repacked items were found to be contaminated twice as often as those in the original pack (Public Health Laboratory Service Report, 1971).

4.2 In use

Pharmaceutical manufacturers may justly argue that their responsibility ends with the supply of a well-preserved product of high microbiological standard in a suitable pack and that the subsequent use, or indeed abuse, of the product is of little concern to them. Although much less is known about how products become contaminated during use, their continued use in a contaminated state is clearly undesirable, particularly in hospitals where it could result in the spread of cross-infection. All multi-dose products are vulnerable to contamination during use. Regardless of whether products are used in hospital or in the community environment, the sources of contamination are the same, but opportunities for observing it are greater in the former. Although the risk of contamination during product use has been much reduced in recent years, primarily through improvements in packaging and changes in nursing practices, it is nevertheless salutary to reflect upon past reported case histories.

4.2.1 Human sources

During normal usage, patients may contaminate their medicine with their own microbial flora; subsequent use of such products may or may not result in self-infection (Fig. 16.3).

Topical products are considered to be most at risk, as the product will probably be applied by hand thus introducing contaminants from the resident skin flora of staphylococci, *Micrococcus* spp.

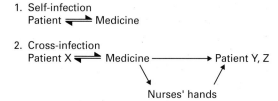

1. Self-infection
   Patient ⇌ Medicine

2. Cross-infection
   Patient X ⇌ Medicine ⟶ Patient Y, Z
                    ↘   ↗
                    Nurses' hands

Fig. 16.3 Mechanisms of contamination during use of medicinal products.

and diphtheroids but also perhaps transient contaminants, such as *Pseudomonas*, which would normally be removed with effective hand-washing. Opportunities for contamination may be reduced by using disposable applicators for topical products or by giving oral products by disposable spoon.

In hospitals, multi-dose products, once contaminated, may serve as a vehicle of cross-contamination or cross-infection between patients. Zinc-based products packed in large stockpots and used in the treatment and prevention of bed-sores in long-stay and geriatric patients were reportedly contaminated during use with *Ps. aeruginosa* and *Staphylococcus aureus*. If unpreserved, these products permit multiplication of contaminants, especially if water is present either as part of the formulation, for example in oil/water (o/w) emulsions, or as a film in w/o emulsions which have undergone local cracking, or as a condensed film from atmospheric water. Appreciable numbers of contaminants may then be transferred to other patients when the product is re-used. Clearly the economics and convenience of using stockpots need to be balanced against the risk of spreading cross-infection between patients and the inevitable increase in length of the patients' stay in hospital. The use of stockpots in hospitals has noticeably declined over the past two decades or so.

A further potential source of contamination in hospitals is the nursing staff responsible for medicament administration. During the course of their work, nurses' hands become contaminated with opportunist pathogens which are not part of the normal skin flora but which are easily removed by thorough hand-washing and drying. In busy wards, hand-washing between attending to patients may be overlooked and contaminants may subsequently be transferred to medicaments during administration. Hand lotions and creams used to prevent chapping of nurses' hands may similarly become contaminated, especially when packaged in multi-dose containers and left at the side of the hand-basin, frequently without lids. The importance of thorough hand-washing in the control of hospital cross-infection cannot be overemphasized. Hand lotions and creams should be well preserved and, ideally, packaged in disposable dispensers. Other effective control methods include the supply of products in individual patient's packs and the use of non-touch techniques for medicament administration.

4.2.2 *Environmental sources*

Small numbers of airborne contaminants may settle in products left open to the atmosphere. Some of these will die during storage, with the rest probably remaining at a static level of about 10^2–10^3 colony forming units (CFU) per g or per ml. Larger numbers of waterborne contaminants may be accidentally introduced into topical products by wet hands or by a 'splash-back mechanism' if left at the side of a basin. Such contaminants generally have simple nutritional requirements and, following multiplication, levels of contamination may often exceed 10^6 CFU per g or per ml. This problem is encountered particularly when the product is stored in warm hospital wards or in hot steamy bathroom cupboards at home. Products used in hospitals as soap substitutes for bathing patients are particularly at risk and soon not only become contaminated with opportunist pathogens such as *Pseudomonas* spp., but also provide conditions conducive to their multiplication. The problem is compounded by stocks kept in multi-dose pots for use by several patients in the same ward over an extended period of time.

The indigenous microbial population is quite different in the home and in hospitals. Pathogenic organisms are found much more frequently in the latter and consequently are isolated more often from medicines used in hospital. Usually, there are fewer opportunities for contamination in the home, as patients are generally issued with individual supplies in small quantities.

4.2.3 Equipment sources

Patients and nursing staff may use a range of applicators (pads, sponges, brushes and spatulas) during medicament administration, particularly for topical products. If re-used, these easily become contaminated and may be responsible for perpetuating contamination between fresh stocks of product, as has indeed been shown in studies of cosmetic products. Disposable applicators or swabs should therefore always be used.

In hospitals today a wide variety of complex equipment is used in the course of patient treatment. Humidifiers, incubators, ventilators, resuscitators and other apparatus require proper maintenance and decontamination after use. Chemical disinfectants used for this purpose have in the past, through misuse, become contaminated with opportunist pathogens, such as *Ps. aeruginosa*, and ironically have contributed to, rather than reduced, the spread of cross-infection in hospital patients. Disinfectants should only be used for their intended purpose and directions for use must be followed at all times.

5 The extent of microbial contamination

Most reports of medicament-borne contamination in the literature tend to be anecdotal in nature, referring to a specific product and isolated incident. Little information is available on the overall risk of products becoming contaminated and causing patient infections when subsequently used. Such information is considered invaluable not only because it may indicate the effectiveness of existing practices and standards, but also because the value of potential improvements in patient quality can be balanced against the inevitable cost of such processes.

5.1 In manufacture

Investigations carried out by the Swedish National Board of Health in 1965 revealed some startling findings on the overall microbiological quality of non-sterile products immediately after manufacture. A wide range of products was routinely found to be contaminated with *Bacillus subtilis*, *Staph. albus*, yeasts and moulds, and in addition large numbers of coliforms were found in a variety of tablets. Furthermore, two nationwide outbreaks of infection in Sweden were subsequently traced to the inadvertent use of contaminated products. Two hundred patients were involved in an outbreak of salmonellosis, caused by thyroid tablets contaminated with *Salmonella bareilly* and *Sal. muenchen*; and eight patients had severe eye infections following the use of a hydrocortisone eye ointment contaminated with *Ps. aeruginosa*. The results of this investigation had a profound effect on the manufacture of all medicines; not only were they then used as a yardstick to compare the microbiological quality of non-sterile products made in other countries, but also as a baseline upon which international standards could be founded.

Under the subsequent Medicines Act 1968, pharmaceutical products made in industry were expected to conform to microbiological and chemical quality specifications. The majority of products have since been shown to conform to a high standard, although spot checks have occasionally revealed medicines of unacceptable quality and so necessitated product recall. By contrast, pharmaceutical products made in hospitals were much less rigorously controlled, as shown by several surveys in the 1970s in which significant numbers of preparations were found to be contaminated with *Ps. aeruginosa*. In 1974, however, hospital manufacture also came under the terms of the Medicines Act and, as a consequence, considerable improvements were subsequently seen not only in the conditions and standard of manufacture, but also in the chemical and microbiological quality of finished products. Hospital manufacturing operations were later rationalized. Economic constraints caused a critical evaluation of the true cost of these activities. Competitive purchasing from industry in many cases produced cheaper alternatives, and small-scale manufacturing was largely discouraged. Where licensed products were available, NHS policy dictated that these were to be purchased from a commercial source and not made locally.

Removal of Crown immunity from the NHS in 1991 meant that manufacturing operations in hospitals were then subject to the full licensing provisions of the Medicines Act 1968, i.e. hospital pharmacies intending to manufacture were required to obtain a manufacturing licence and to comply fully with the EC Guide to Good Pharmaceutical Manufacturing Practice (Anon, 1992, revised in 1997 and 2002). Among other requirements, this included the provision of appropriate environmental manufacturing conditions and associated environmental monitoring. Subsequently, the Medicines Control Agency (MCA) issued guidance in 1992 on certain manufacturing exemptions, by virtue of the product batch size or frequency of manufacture. The need for extemporaneous dispensing of 'one-off' special formulae continued in hospital pharmacies, although this work was largely transferred from the dispensing bench to dedicated preparative facilities with appropriate environmental control. Today hospital manufacturing is concentrated on the supply of bespoke products from a regional centre or small-scale specialist manufacture of those items currently unobtainable from industry. Re-packing of commercial products into more convenient pack sizes is still, however, common practice.

5.2 In use

Higher rates of contamination are invariably seen in products after opening and use and, among these, medicines used in hospitals are more likely to be contaminated than those used in the general community. The Public Health Laboratory Service Report of 1971 expressed concern at the overall incidence of contamination in non-sterile products used on hospital wards (327 of 1220 samples) and the proportion of samples found to be heavily contaminated (18% in excess of 10^4 CFU per g or per ml). Notably, the presence of *Ps. aeruginosa* in 2.7% of samples (mainly oral alkaline mixtures) was considered to be highly undesirable.

By contrast, medicines used in the home are not only less often contaminated but also contain lower levels of contaminants and fewer pathogenic organisms. Generally, there are fewer opportunities for contamination here because individual patients use smaller quantities. Medicines in the home may, however, be hoarded and used for extended periods of time. Additionally, storage conditions may be unsuitable and expiry dates ignored; thus problems

other than those of microbial contamination may be seen in the home.

6 Factors determining the outcome of a medicament-borne infection

Although impossible to quantify, the use of contaminated medicines has undoubtedly contributed to the spread of cross-infection in hospitals; undeniably, such nosocomial (hospital-acquired) infections have also extended the length of stay in hospital with concomitant costs. A patient's response to the microbial challenge of a contaminated medicine may be diverse and unpredictable, perhaps with serious consequences. Clinical reactions may not be evident in one patient, yet in another these may be indisputable, illustrating one problem in the recognition of medicament-borne infections. Clinical reactions may range from inconvenient local infections of wounds or broken skin, caused possibly from contact with a contaminated cream, to gastrointestinal infections from the ingestion of contaminated oral products, to serious widespread infections such as a bacteraemia or septicaemia, possibly resulting in death, as caused by the administration of contaminated infusion fluids. Undoubtedly, the most serious outbreaks of infection have been seen in the past where contaminated products have been injected directly into the bloodstream of patients whose immunity is already compromised by their underlying disease or therapy.

The outcome of any episode is determined by a combination of several factors, among which the type and degree of microbial contamination, the route of administration and the patient's resistance are of particular importance.

6.1 Type and degree of microbial contamination

Microorganisms that contaminate medicines and cause disease in patients may be classified as true pathogens or opportunist pathogens. Pathogenic organisms like *Clostridium tetani* and *Salmonella* spp. rarely occur in products, but when present cause serious problems. Wound infections and several cases of neonatal death have resulted from use of talcum powder containing *Cl. tetani*. Outbreaks of salmonellosis have followed the inadvertent ingestion of contaminated thyroid and pancreatic powders. On the other hand, opportunist pathogens like *Ps. aeruginosa*, *Klebsiella*, *Serratia* and other free-living organisms are more frequently isolated from medicinal products and, as their name suggests, may be pathogenic if given the opportunity. The main concern with these organisms is that their simple nutritional requirements enable them to survive in a wide range of pharmaceuticals, and thus they tend to be present in high numbers, perhaps in excess of 10^6–10^7 CFU/g or CFU/ml. The product itself, however, may show no visible sign of contamination. Opportunist pathogens can survive in disinfectants and antiseptic solutions that are normally used in the control of hospital cross-infection, but which, when contaminated, may even perpetuate the spread of infection. Compromised hospital patients, i.e. the elderly, burned, traumatized or immunosuppressed, are considered to be particularly at risk from infection with these organisms, whereas healthy patients in the general community have given little cause for concern.

The critical dose of microorganisms that will initiate an infection is largely unknown and varies not only between species but also within a species. Animal and human volunteer studies have indicated that the infecting dose may be reduced significantly in the presence of trauma or foreign bodies or if accompanied by a drug having a local vasoconstrictive action.

6.2 The route of administration

As stated previously, contaminated products injected directly into the bloodstream or instilled into the eye cause the most serious problems. Intrathecal and epidural injections are potentially hazardous procedures. In practice, epidural injections are frequently given through a bacterial filter. Injectable and ophthalmic solutions are often simple solutions and provide Gram-negative opportunist pathogens with sufficient nutrients to multiply during storage; if contaminated, a bioburden of 10^6 CFU as well as the production of endotoxins should be expected. Total parenteral nutrition fluids, formulated for individual patients'

nutritional requirements, can also provide more than adequate nutritional support for invading contaminants. *Ps. aeruginosa*, the notorious contaminant of eye-drops, has caused serious ophthalmic infections, including the loss of sight in some cases. The problem is compounded when the eye is damaged through the improper use of contact lenses or scratched by fingernails or cosmetic applicators.

The fate of contaminants ingested orally in medicines may be determined by several factors, as is seen with contaminated food. The acidity of the stomach may provide a successful barrier, depending on whether the medicine is taken on an empty or full stomach and also on the gastric emptying time. Contaminants in topical products may cause little harm when deposited on intact skin. Not only does the skin itself provide an excellent mechanical barrier, but few contaminants normally survive in competition with its resident microbial flora. Skin damaged during surgery or trauma or in patients with burns or pressure sores may, however, be rapidly colonized and subsequently infected by opportunist pathogens. Patients treated with topical steroids are also prone to local infections, particularly if contaminated steroid drugs are inadvertently used.

6.3 Resistance of the patient

A patient's resistance is crucial in determining the outcome of a medicament-borne infection. Hospital patients are more exposed and susceptible to infection than those treated in the general community. Neonates, the elderly, diabetics and patients traumatized by surgery or accident may have impaired defence mechanisms. People suffering from leukaemia and those treated with immunosuppressants are most vulnerable to infection; there is an undeniable case for providing all medicines in a sterile form for these patients.

7 Preservation of medicines using antimicrobial agents: basic principles

7.1 Introduction

An antimicrobial 'preservative' may be included in a formulation to minimize the risk of spoilage and preferably to kill low levels of contaminants introduced during storage or repeated use of a multidose container. However, where there is a low risk of contamination, as with tablets, capsules and dry powders, the inclusion of a preservative may be unnecessary. Preservatives should never be added to mask poor manufacturing processes.

The properties of an ideal preservative are well recognized: a broad spectrum of activity and a rapid rate of kill; selectivity in reacting with the contaminants and not the formulation ingredients; non-irritant and non-toxic to the patient; and stable and effective throughout the life of the product.

Unfortunately, the most active antimicrobial agents are often non-selective in action, inter-reacting significantly with formulation ingredients as well as with patients and microorganisms. Having excluded the more toxic, irritant and reactive agents, those remaining generally have only modest antimicrobial efficacy, and there are now no preservatives considered sufficiently non-toxic for use in highly sensitive areas, e.g. for injection into central nervous system tissues or for use within the eye. A number of microbiologically effective preservatives used in cosmetics have caused a significant number of cases of contact dermatitis, and are thus precluded from use in pharmaceutical creams. Although a rapid rate of kill may be preferable, this may only be possible for relatively simple aqueous solutions such as eye-drops or injections. For physicochemically complex systems such as emulsions and creams, inhibition of growth and a slow rate of killing may be all that can be realistically achieved.

In order to maximize preservative efficacy, it is essential to have an appreciation of those parameters that influence antimicrobial activity.

7.2 Effect of preservative concentration, temperature and size of inoculum

Changes in the efficacy of preservatives vary exponentially with changes in concentration. The effect of changes in concentration (concentration exponent, η, Chapter 11) varies with the type of agent. For example, halving the concentration of phenol ($\eta = 6$) gives a 64-fold (2^6) reduction in killing activity, while a similar dilution for chlorhexidine ($\eta = 2$)

reduces the activity by only fourfold (2^2). Changes in preservative activity are also seen with changes in product temperature, according to the temperature coefficient, Q_{10}. Thus, a reduction in temperature from 30°C to 20°C could result in a significantly reduced rate of kill for *Escherichia coli*, fivefold in the case of phenol ($Q_{10} = 5$) and 45-fold in the case of ethanol ($Q_{10} = 45$). If both temperature and concentration vary concurrently, the situation is more complex; however, it has been suggested that if a 0.1% chlorocresol ($\eta = 6$, $Q_{10} = 5$) solution completely killed a suspension of *E. coli* at 30°C in 10 minutes, it would require around 90 minutes to achieve a similar effect if stored at 20°C and if slight overheating during production had resulted in a 10% loss in the chlorocresol concentration (other factors remaining constant).

Preservative molecules are used up as they inactivate microorganisms and as they interact non-specifically with significant quantities of contaminant 'dirt' introduced during use. This will result in a progressive and exponential decline in the efficiency of remaining preservative. Preservative 'capacity' is a term used to describe the cumulative level of contamination that a preserved formulation can tolerate before becoming so depleted as to become ineffective. This will vary with preservative type and complexity of formulation.

7.3 Factors affecting the 'availability' of preservatives

Most preservatives interact in solution to some extent with many of the commonly used formulation ingredients via a number of weak bonding attractions as well as with any contaminants present. Unstable equilibria may form in which only a small proportion of total preservative present is 'available' to inactivate the relatively small microbial mass; the resulting rate of kill may be far lower than might be anticipated from the performance of simple aqueous solutions. However, 'unavailable' preservative may still contribute to the general irritancy of the product. It is commonly believed that where the solute concentrations are very high, and A_w is appreciably reduced, the efficiency of preservatives is often significantly reduced and they may be virtually inactive at very low A_w. The practice of including preservatives in very low A_w products such as tablets and capsules is ill advised, as it only offers minimal protection for the dry tablets; should they become damp, they would be spoiled for other, non-microbial, reasons.

7.3.1 Effect of product pH

In the weakly acidic preservatives, activity resides primarily in the unionized molecules and they only have significant efficacy at pHs where ionization is low. Thus, benzoic and sorbic acids ($pK_a = 4.2$ and 4.75, respectively) have limited preservative usefulness above pH 5, while the 4(p)-hydroxybenzoate esters with their non-ionizable ester group and poorly ionizable hydroxyl substituent (pK_a c. 8.5) have a moderate protective effect even at neutral pH levels. The activity of quaternary ammonium preservatives and chlorhexidine probably resides with their cations; they are effective in products of neutral pH. Formulation pH can also directly influence the sensitivity of microorganisms to preservatives (see Chapter 11).

7.3.2 Efficiency in multiphase systems

In a multiphase formulation, such as an oil-in-water emulsion, preservative molecules will distribute themselves in an unstable equilibrium between the bulk aqueous phase and (i) the oil phase by partition, (ii) the surfactant micelles by solubilization, (iii) polymeric suspending agents and other solutes by competitive displacement of water of solvation, (iv) particulate and container surfaces by adsorption and (v) any microorganisms present. Generally, the overall preservative efficiency can be related to the small proportion of preservative molecules remaining unbound in the bulk aqueous phase, although as this becomes depleted some slow re-equilibration between the components can be anticipated. The loss of neutral molecules into oil and micellar phases may be favoured over ionized species, although considerable variation in distribution is found between different systems.

In view of these major potential reductions in preservative efficacy, considerable effort has been directed to devise equations in which one might substitute variously derived system parameters (such as partition coefficients, surfactant and polymer binding constants and oil:water ratios) to obtain estimates of residual preservative levels in aqueous phases. Although some modestly successful predictions have been obtained for very simple laboratory systems, they have proved of limited practical value, as data for many of the required parameters are unavailable for technical grade ingredients or for the more complex commercial systems.

7.3.3 Effect of container or packaging

Preservative availability may be appreciably reduced by interaction with packaging materials. Phenolics, for example, will permeate the rubber wads and teats of multi-dose injection or eye-drop containers and also interact with flexible nylon tubes for creams. Quaternary ammonium preservative levels in formulations have been significantly reduced by adsorption onto the surfaces of plastic and glass containers. Volatile preservatives such as chloroform are so readily lost by the routine opening and closing of containers that their usefulness is somewhat restricted to preservation of medicines in sealed, impervious containers during storage, with short in-use lives once opened.

8 Quality assurance and the control of microbial risk in medicines

8.1 Introduction

Quality assurance (QA) encompasses a scheme of management which embraces all the procedures necessary to provide a high probability that a medicine will conform consistently to a specified description of quality (a formalized measure of fitness for its intended purpose). It includes formulation design and development (R&D), good pharmaceutical manufacturing practice (GPMP), as well as quality control (QC) and post-marketing surveillance. As many microorganisms may be hazardous to patients or cause spoilage of formulations under suitable conditions, it is necessary to perform a risk assessment of contamination for each product. At each stage of its anticipated life from raw materials to administration, a risk assessment should be made and strategies should be developed and calculated to reduce the overall risk(s) to acceptably low levels. Such risk assessments are complicated by uncertainties about the exact infective and spoilage hazards likely for many contaminants, and by difficulties in measuring their precise performance in complex systems. As the consequences of product failure and patient damage will inevitably be severe, it is usual for manufacturing companies to make worst-case presumptions and design strategies to cover them fully; lesser problems are also then encompassed. As it must be assumed that all microorganisms may be potentially infective for those routes of administration where the likelihood of infection from contaminants is high, then medicines to be given via these routes must be supplied in a sterile form, as is the case with injectable products. It must also be presumed that those administering medicines may not necessarily be highly skilled or motivated in contamination-control techniques; additional safeguards to control risks may be included in these situations. This may include detailed information on administration and even training, in addition to providing a high quality formulation.

8.2 Quality assurance in formulation design and development

The risk of microbial infection and spoilage arising from microbial contamination during manufacture, storage and use could be eliminated by presenting all medicines in sterile, impervious, single-dosage units. However, the high cost of this strategy restricts its use to situations where there is a high risk of consequent infection from any contaminants. Where the risk is assessed as much lower, less efficient but less expensive strategies are adopted. The high risk of infection by contaminants in parenteral medicines, combined with concerns about the systemic toxicity of preservatives almost always demands sterile single-dosage units. With eye-drops for domestic use the risks are perceived to be lower, and sterile multi-dose products with preservatives to combat the anticipated in-use contamination are accepted; sterile single-dose units are more common in hospitals where there is an increased risk of infection. Oral and topical routes of administration are generally perceived to present relatively low risks of

infection and the emphasis is more on the control of microbial content during manufacture and subsequent protection of the formulation from chemical and physicochemical spoilage.

As part of the design process, it is necessary to include features in the formulation and delivery system that provide as much suitable protection as possible against microbial contamination and spoilage. Owing to potential toxicity and irritancy problems, antimicrobial preservatives should only be considered where there is clear evidence of positive benefit. Manipulation of physicochemical parameters, such as A_w, the elimination of particularly susceptible ingredients, the selection of a preservative or the choice of container may individually and collectively contribute significantly to overall medicine stability. For 'dry' dosage forms where their very low A_w provides protection against microbial attack, the moisture vapour properties of packaging materials require careful examination.

Preservatives are intended to offer further protection against environmental microbial contaminants. However, as they are relatively non-specific in their reactivity (see section 7), it is difficult to calculate with any certainty what proportion of preservative added to all but the simplest medicine will be available for inactivating such contamination. Laboratory tests have been devised to challenge the product with an artificial bioburden. Such tests should form part of formulation development and stability trials to ensure that suitable activity is likely to remain throughout the life of the product. They are not normally used in routine manufacturing quality control.

Some 'preservative challenge tests' (preservative efficacy tests) add relatively large inocula of various laboratory cultures to aliquots of the product and determine their rate of inactivation by viable counting methods (single challenge tests), while others re-inoculate repeatedly at set intervals, monitoring the efficiency of inactivation until the system fails (multiple challenge test). This latter technique may give a better estimate of the preservative capacity of the system than the single challenge approach, but is both time-consuming and expensive. Problems arise when deciding whether the observed performance in such tests gives reliable predictions of real in-use efficacy. Although test organisms should bear some similarity in type and spoilage potential to those met in use, it is known that repeated cultivation on conventional microbiological media (nutrient agar, etc.) frequently results in reduced aggressiveness of strains. Attempts to maintain spoilage activity by inclusion of formulation ingredients in culture media gives varied results. Some manufacturers have been able to maintain active spoilage strains by cultivation in unpreserved, or diluted aliquots, of formulations.

The *British Pharmacopoeia* and the *European Pharmacopoeia* describe a single challenge preservative test that routinely uses four test organisms (two bacteria, a yeast and a mould), none of which has any significant history of spoilage potential and which are cultivated on conventional media. However, extension of the basic test is recommended in some situations, such as the inclusion of an osmotolerant yeast if it is thought such in-use spoilage might be a problem. Despite its accepted limitations and the cautious indications given as to what the tests might suggest about a formulation, the test does provide some basic, but useful indicators of likely in-use stability. UK Product Licence applications for preserved medicines must demonstrate that the formulation at least meets the preservative efficacy criteria of the *British Pharmacopoeia* or a similar test.

The concept of the D-value as used in sterilization technology (Chapter 20) has been applied to the interpretation of challenge testing. Expression of the rate of microbial inactivation in a preserved system in terms of a D-value enables estimation of the nominal time to achieve a prescribed proportionate level of kill. Problems arise, however, when trying to predict the behaviour of very low levels of survivors, and the method has its critics as well as its advocates.

8.3 Good pharmaceutical manufacturing practice (GPMP)

GPMP is concerned with the manufacture of medicines, and includes control of ingredients, plant construction, process validation, production and cleaning (see also Chapter 21). QC is that part of GPMP dealing with specification, documentation and assessing conformance to specification.

With traditional QC, a high reliance has been placed on testing samples of finished products to determine the overall quality of a batch. This practice can, however, result in considerable financial loss if non-compliance is detected only at this late stage, leaving the expensive options of discarding or re-working the batch. Additionally, some microbiological test methods have poor precision and/or accuracy. Validation can be complex or impossible, and interpretation of results can prove difficult. For example, although a sterility assurance level of less than one failure in 10^6 items submitted to a terminal sterilization process is considered acceptable, conventional 'tests for sterility' for finished products (such as that in the *European Pharmacopoeia*) could not possibly be relied upon to find one damaged but viable microbe within the 10^6 items, regardless of allowing for its cultivation with any precision (Chapter 20). Moreover, end-product testing will not prevent and may not even detect the isolated rogue processing failure.

It is now generally accepted that a high assurance of overall product quality can only come from a detailed specification, control and monitoring of *all* the stages that contribute to the manufacturing process. More realistic decisions about conformance to specification can then be made using information from *all* relevant parameters (parametric release method), not just from the results of selective testing of finished products. Thus, a more realistic estimate of the microbial quality of a batch of tablets would be achieved from a knowledge of specific parameters (such as the microbial bioburden of the starting materials, temperature records from granule drying ovens, the moisture level of the dried granules, compaction data, validation records for the foil strip sealing machine and microbial levels in the finished tablets), than from the contaminant content of the finished tablets alone. Similarly, parametric release is now accepted as an operational alternative to routine sterility testing for batch release of some finished sterile products. Through parametric release the manufacturer can provide assurance that the product is of the stipulated quality, based on the evidence of successful validation of the manufacturing process and review of the documentation on process monitoring carried out during manufacturing.

It may be necessary to exclude certain undesirable contaminants from starting materials, such as pseudomonads from bulk aluminium hydroxide gel, or to include some form of pre-treatment to reduce their bioburdens by irradiation, such as for ispaghula husk and spices. For biotechnology-derived drugs produced in human or animal tissue culture, considerable efforts are made to exclude cell lines contaminated with latent host viruses. Official guidelines to limit the risk of prion contamination in medicines require bovine-derived ingredients to be obtained from sources where bovine spongiform encephalopathy (BSE) is not endemic.

By considering manufacturing plant and its environs from an ecological and physiological viewpoint of microorganisms, it is possible not only to identify areas where contaminants may accumulate and even thrive to create hazards for subsequent production batches, but also to manipulate design and operating conditions in order to discourage such colonization. The ability to clean and dry equipment thoroughly is a very useful deterrent to growth. Design considerations should include the elimination of obscure nooks and crannies and the ability to be able to clean thoroughly in all areas. Some larger items of equipment now have cleaning-in-place (CIP) and sterilization-in-place (SIP) systems installed to improve decontamination capabilities.

It may be necessary to include intermediate steps within processing to reduce the bioburden and improve the efficiency of lethal sterilization cycles, or to prevent swamping of the preservative in a non-sterile medicine after manufacture. Some of the newer and fragile biotechnology-derived products may include chromatographic and/or ultrafiltration processing stages to ensure adequate reductions of viral contamination levels rather than conventional sterilization cycles.

In a validation exercise, it must be demonstrated that each stage of the system is capable of providing the degree of intended efficiency within the limits of variation for which it was designed. Microbial spoilage aspects of process validation might include examination of the cleaning system for its ability to remove deliberately introduced contamination. Chromatographic removal of viral contaminants would be validated by determining the log reduction achievable against a known titre of added viral particles.

8.4 Quality control procedures

While there is general agreement on the need to control total microbial levels in non-sterile medicines and to exclude certain species that have previously proved troublesome, the precision and accuracy of current methods for counting (or even detecting) some microbes in complex products are poor. Pathogens, present in low numbers, and often damaged by processing, can be very difficult to isolate. Products showing active spoilage can yield surprisingly low viable counts on testing; although present in high numbers, a particular organism may be neither pathogenic nor the primary spoilage agent, but may be relatively inert, e.g. ungerminated spores or a secondary contaminant which has outgrown the initiating spoiler. Unevenly distributed growth in viscous formulations will present serious sampling problems. The type of culture medium (even different batches of the same medium) and conditions of recovery and incubation may greatly influence any viable counts obtained from products.

An unresolved problem concerns the timing of sampling. Low levels of pseudomonads shortly after manufacture may not constitute a spoilage hazard if their growth is checked. However, if unchecked, high levels may well initiate spoilage.

The *European Pharmacopoeia* has introduced both quantitative and qualitative microbial standards for non-sterile medicines, which may become enforceable in some member states. It prescribes varying maximum total microbial levels and exclusion of particular species according to the routes of administration. The *British Pharmacopoeia* has now included these tests, but suggests that they should be used to assist in validating GPMP processing procedures and not as conformance standards for routine end-product testing. Thus, for a medicine to be administered orally, there should not be more than 10^3 aerobic bacteria or 10^2 fungi per gram or cm^3 of product, and there should be an absence of *Escherichia coli*. Higher levels may be permissible if the product contains raw materials of natural origin.

Most manufacturers perform periodic tests on their products for total microbial counts and the presence of known problem microorganisms; generally these are used for in-house confirmation of the continuing efficiency of their GPMP systems, rather than as conventional end-product conformance tests. Fluctuation in values, or the appearance of specific and unusual species, can warn of defects in procedures and impending problems.

In order to reduce the costs of testing and shorten quarantine periods, there is considerable interest in automated alternatives to conventional test methods for the detection and determination of microorganisms. Although not in widespread use at present, promising methods include electrical impedance, use of fluorescent dyes and epifluorescence, and the use of 'vital' stains. Considerable advances in the sensitivity of methods for estimating microbial adenosine triphosphate (ATP) using luciferase now allow the estimation of extremely low bioburdens. The recent development of highly sensitive laser scanning devices for detecting bacteria variously labelled with selective fluorescent probes enables the apparent detection even of single cells.

Endotoxin (pyrogen) levels in parenteral and similar products must be extremely low in order to prevent serious endotoxic shock on administration (Chapter 19). Formerly, this was checked by injecting rabbits and noting any febrile response. Most determinations are now performed using the *Limulus* test in which an amoebocyte lysate from the horseshoe crab (*Limulus polyphemus*) reacts specifically with microbial lipopolysaccharides to give a gel and opacity even at very high dilutions. A variant of the test using a chromogenic substrate gives a coloured end-point that can be detected spectroscopically. Tissue culture tests are under development where the ability of endotoxins to induce cytokine release is measured directly.

Sophisticated and very sensitive methods have been developed in the food industry for detecting many other microbial toxins. For example, aflatoxin detection in seedstuffs and their oils is performed by solvent extraction, adsorption onto columns containing antibodies selective for the toxin, and detection by exposure to ultraviolet light.

Although it would be unusual to test for signs of active physicochemical or chemical spoilage of products as part of routine product quality control procedures, this may occasionally be necessary in order to examine an incident of anticipated product failure, or during formulation development. Many volatile and unpleasant-tasting metabolites are generated during active spoilage which are readily apparent. Their characterization by HPLC or GC can be used to distinguish microbial spoilage from other, non-biological deterioration. Spoilage often results in physicochemical changes which can be monitored by conventional methods. Thus, emulsion spoilage may be followed by monitoring changes in creaming rates, pH changes, particle sedimentation and viscosity.

8.5 Post-market surveillance

Despite extensive development and a rigorous adherence to procedures, it is impossible to guarantee that a medicine will never fail under the harsh abuses of real-life conditions. A proper quality assurance system must include procedures for monitoring in-use performance and for responding to customer complaints. These must be meticulously followed up in great detail in order to decide whether carefully constructed and implemented schemes for product safety require modification to prevent the incident recurring.

9 Overview

Prevention is undoubtedly better than cure in minimizing the risk of medicament-borne infections. In manufacture the principles of good manufacturing practice must be observed, and control measures must be built in at all stages. Thus, initial stability tests should show that the proposed formulation can withstand an appropriate microbial challenge; raw materials from an authorized supplier should comply with in-house microbial specifications; environmental conditions appropriate to the production process should be subject to regular microbiological monitoring; and finally, end-product analysis should indicate that the product is microbiologically suitable for its intended use and conforms to accepted in-house and international standards.

Based on present knowledge, contaminants, by virtue of their type or number, should not present a potential health hazard to patients when used.

Contamination during use is less easily controlled. Successful measures in the hospital pharmacy have included the packaging of products as individual units, thereby discouraging the use of multi-dose containers. Unit packaging (one dose per patient) has clear advantages, but economic constraints have prevented this desirable procedure from being realized. Ultimately, the most fruitful approach is through the training and education of patients and hospital staff, so that medicines are used only for their intended purpose. The task of implementing this approach inevitably rests with the clinical and community pharmacists of the future.

10 Acknowledgement

With thanks to Edgar Beveridge who contributed a chapter on Spoilage and Preservation in earlier editions of this book.

11 Further reading

Anon. (1992) and (1997) *The Rules Governing Medicinal Products in the European Community*, Vol IV. Office for Official Publications of the EC.

Attwood, D. & Florence, A. T. (1983) *Surfactant Systems, Their Chemistry, Pharmacy and Biology*. Chapman & Hall, London.

Baines, A. (2000) Endotoxin testing. In: *Handbook of Microbiological Control: Pharmaceuticals and Medical Devices* (eds R.M. Baird, N.A. Hodges & S.P. Denyer), pp. 144–167. Taylor & Francis, London.

Baird, R. M. (1981) Drugs and cosmetics. In: *Microbial Biodeterioration* (ed. A.H. Rose), pp. 387–426. Academic Press, London.

Baird, R. M. (1985) Microbial contamination of pharmaceutical products made in a hospital pharmacy. *Pharm J*, **234**, 54–55.

Baird, R. M. (1985) Microbial contamination of non-sterile pharmaceutical products made in hospitals in the North East Regional Health Authority. *J Clin Hosp Pharm*, **10**, 95–100.

Baird, R. M. (2004) Sterility assurance: concepts, methods and problems. In: *Principles and Practice of Disinfection, Preservation and Sterilization* (eds A. Fraise, P. Lambert & J-Y. Maillard), 4th edn, pp. 526–539. Blackwell Scientific, Oxford.

Baird, R. M. & Shooter, R. A. (1976) *Pseudomonas aeruginosa* infections associated with the use of contaminated medicaments. *BMJ*, **2**, 349–350.

Baird, R. M., Brown, W. R. L. & Shooter, R. A. (1976) *Pseudomonas aeruginosa* in hospital pharmacies. *BMJ*, **1**, 511–512.

Baird, R. M., Elhag, K. M. & Shaw, E. J. (1976) *Pseudomonas thomasii* in a hospital distilled water supply. *J Med Microbial*, **9**, 493–495.

Baird, R. M., Parks, A. & Awad, Z. A. (1977) Control of *Pseudomonas aeruginosa* in pharmacy environments and medicaments. *Pharm J*, **119**, 164–165.

Baird, R. M., Crowden, C. A., O'Farrell, S. M. & Shooter, R. A. (1979) Microbial contamination of pharmaceutical products in the home. *J Hyg*, **83**, 277–283.

Baird, R. M. & Bloomfield, S. F. L. (1996) *Microbial Quality Assurance of Cosmetics, Toiletries and Non-sterile Pharmaceuticals*. Taylor & Francis, London.

Baird, R. M., Hodges, N. A. & Denyer, S. P. (2000). *Handbook of Microbiological Control: Pharmaceuticals and Medical Devices*. Taylor & Francis, London.

Bassett, D. C. J. (1971) Causes and prevention of sepsis due to Gram-negative bacteria: common sources of outbreaks. *Proc R Soc Med*, **64**, 980–986.

Brannan, D. K. (1995) Cosmetic preservation. *J Soc Cosmet Chem*, **46**, 199–220.

British Pharmacopoeia (2003) HMSO, London.

Crompton, D. O. (1962) Ophthalmic prescribing. *Australas J Pharm*, **43**, 1020–1028.

Denyer, S. P. & Baird, R. M. (1990). *Guide to Microbiological Control in Pharmaceuticals*. Ellis Horwood, London.

European Pharmacopoeia, 4th edn. (2002) EP Secretariat, Strasbourg.

Fraise, A., Lambert P. & Maillard, J-Y. (2004) *Principles and Practice of Disinfection, Preservation and Sterilization*, 4th edn. Blackwell Science, Oxford.

Gould, G. W. (1989) *Mechanisms of Action of Food Preservation Procedures*. Elsevier Science Publishers, Barking.

Hills, S. (1946) The isolation of *Cl. tetani* from infected talc. *N Z Med J*, **45**, 419–423.

Hugo, W. B. (1995) A brief history of heat, chemical and radiation preservation and disinfectants. *Int Biodet Biodeg*, **36**, 197–217.

Kallings, L. O., Ringertz, O., Silverstolpe, L. & Ernerfeldt, F. (1966) Microbiological contamination of medicinal preparations. 1965 Report to the Swedish National Board of Health. *Acta Pharm Suecica*, **3**, 219–228.

Maurer, I. M. (1985) *Hospital Hygiene*, 3rd edn. Edward Arnold, London.

Meers, P. D., Calder, M. W, Mazhar, M. M. & Lawrie, G. M. (1973) Intravenous infusion of contaminated dextrose solution: the Devonport incident. *Lancet*, **ii**, 1189–1192.

Morse, L. J., Williams, H. I., Grenn, F. P, Eldridge, E. F & Rotta, J. R. (1967) Septicaemia due to *Klebsiella pneumoniae* originating from a handcream dispenser. *N Engl J Med*, 277, 472–473.

Myers, G. E. & Pasutto, F. M. (1973) Microbial contamination of cosmetics and toiletries. *Can J Pharm Sci*, 8, 19–23.

Noble, W. C. & Savin, J. A. (1966) Steroid cream contaminated with *Pseudomonas aeruginosa*. *Lancet*, i, 347–349.

Parker, M. T. (1972) The clinical significance of the presence of microorganisms in pharmaceutical and cosmetic preparations. *J Soc Cosm Chem*, 23, 415–426.

Report of the Public Health Laboratory Service Working Party (1971) Microbial contamination of medicines administered to hospital patients. *Pharm J*, 207, 96–99.

Smart, R. & Spooner, D. F. (1972) Microbiological spoilage in pharmaceuticals and cosmetics. *J Soc Cosm Chem*, 23, 721–737.

Stebbing, L. (1993) *Quality Assurance: The Route to Efficiency and Competitiveness*, 2nd edn. Ellis Horwood, Chichester.

Chapter 17
Chemical disinfectants, antiseptics and preservatives

Sean Gorman and Eileen Scott

1 Introduction

Disinfectants, antiseptics and preservatives are chemicals that have the ability to destroy or inhibit the growth of microorganisms and that are used for this purpose.

Disinfectants. Disinfection is the process of removing microorganisms, including potentially pathogenic ones, from the surfaces of inanimate objects. The British Standards Institution further defines disinfection as not necessarily killing all microorganisms, but reducing them to a level ac-

ceptable for a defined purpose, for example, a level which is harmful neither to health nor to the quality of perishable goods. Chemical disinfectants are capable of different levels of action (Table 17.1). The term high level disinfection indicates destruction of all microorganisms but not necessarily bacterial spores; intermediate level disinfection indicates destruction of all vegetative bacteria including *Mycobacterium tuberculosis* but may exclude some viruses and fungi and implies little or no sporicidal activity; low level disinfection can destroy most vegetative bacteria, fungi and viruses,

Table 17.1 Levels of disinfection attainable

	Disinfection level		
	Low	Intermediate	High
Microorganisms killed	Most vegetative bacteria Some viruses Some fungi	Most vegetative bacteria including *M. tuberculosis* Most viruses including hepatitis B virus (HBV) Most fungi	All microorganisms unless extreme challenge or resistance exhibited
Microorganisms surviving	*M. tuberculosis* Bacterial spores Some viruses and prions	Bacterial spores Prions	Extreme challenge of resistant bacterial spores Prions

but this will not include spores and some of the more resistant microorganisms. Some high level disinfectants have good sporicidal activity and have been ascribed the name 'liquid chemical sterilant' or 'chemosterilant' to indicate that they can effect a complete kill of all microorganisms, as in sterilization.

Antiseptics. Antisepsis is defined as destruction or inhibition of microorganisms on living tissues having the effect of limiting or preventing the harmful results of infection. It is *not* a synonym for disinfection (British Standards Institution). The chemicals used are applied to skin and mucous membranes, therefore as well as having adequate antimicrobial activity they must not be toxic or irritating for skin. Antiseptics are mostly used to reduce the microbial population on the skin before surgery or on the hands to help prevent spread of infection by this route. Antiseptics are often lower concentrations of the agents used for disinfection.

Preservatives. These are included in pharmaceutical preparations to prevent microbial spoilage of the product and to minimize the risk of the consumer acquiring an infection when the preparation is administered. Preservatives must be able to limit proliferation of microorganisms that may be introduced unavoidably into non-sterile products such as oral and topical medications during their manufacture and use. In sterile products such as eye-drops and multi-dose injections preservatives should kill any microbial contaminants introduced inadvertently during use. It is essential that a preservative is not toxic in relation to the intended route of administration of the preserved preparation.

Preservatives therefore tend to be employed at low concentrations, and consequently levels of antimicrobial action also tend to be of a lower order than for disinfectants or antiseptics. This is illustrated by the *European Pharmacopoeia* requirements for preservative efficacy where a degree of bactericidal activity is necessary, although this should be obtained within a few hours or over several days of microbial challenge depending on the type of product to be preserved. Other terms are considered in Chapter 11.

There are around 250 chemicals that have been identified as active components of microbiocidal products in the European Union. The aim of this chapter is to introduce the range of chemicals in common use and to indicate their activities and applications.

2 Factors affecting choice of antimicrobial agent

Choice of the most appropriate antimicrobial compound for a particular purpose depends on:
- properties of the chemical agent
- microbiological challenge
- intended application
- environmental factors
- toxicity of the agent.

2.1 Properties of the chemical agent

The process of killing or inhibiting the growth of microorganisms using an antimicrobial agent is basically that of a chemical reaction and the rate and extent of this reaction will be influenced by the factors of concentration of chemical, temperature, pH and formulation. The influence of these factors on activity is considered in Chapter 11, and is referred to in discussing the individual agents. Tissue toxicity influences whether a chemical can be used as an antiseptic or preservative, and this limits the range of chemicals for these applications or necessitates the use of lower concentrations of the chemical. This is discussed further in section 2.5.

2.2 Microbiological challenge

The types of microorganism present and the levels of microbial contamination (the bioburden) both have a significant effect on the outcome of chemical treatment. If the bioburden is high, long exposure times or higher concentrations of antimicrobial may be required. Microorganisms vary in their sensitivity to the action of chemical agents. Some organisms, either because of their resistance to disinfection (for further discussion see Chapter 18) or because of their significance in cross-infection or nosocomial (hospital-acquired) infections, merit attention. Of particular concern is the significant increase in resistance to disinfectants resulting from microbial growth in biofilm form rather than free suspension. Microbial biofilms form readily on available surfaces, posing a serious problem for Hospital Infection Control Committees in advising suitable disinfectants for use in such situations.

The efficacy of an antimicrobial agent must be investigated by appropriate capacity, challenge and in-use tests to ensure that a standard is obtained which is appropriate to the intended use (Chapter 11). In practice, it is not usually possible to know which organisms are present on the articles being treated. Thus, it is necessary to categorize chemicals according to their antimicrobial capabilities and for the user to have an awareness of what level of antimicrobial action is required in a particular situation (Table 17.1).

2.2.1 Vegetative bacteria

At in-use concentrations, chemicals used for disinfection should be capable of killing most vegetative

bacteria within a reasonable contact period. This includes 'problem' organisms such as listeria, campylobacter, legionella, vancomycin-resistant enterococci (VRE) and methicillin-resistant *Staphylococcus aureus* (MRSA). Antiseptics and preservatives are also expected to have a broad spectrum of antimicrobial activity but at the in-use concentrations, after exerting an initial biocidal effect, their main function may be biostatic. Gram-negative bacilli, which are the main causes of nosocomial infections, are often more resistant than Gram-positive species. *Pseudomonas aeruginosa*, an opportunist pathogen (i.e. it is pathogenic if the opportunity arises; see also Chapter 7), has gained a reputation as the most resistant of the Gram-negative organisms. However, problems mainly arise when a number of additional factors such as heavily soiled articles or diluted or degraded solutions are involved.

2.2.2 Mycobacterium tuberculosis

M. tuberculosis (the tubercle bacillus) and other mycobacteria are resistant to many bactericides. Resistance is either (a) intrinsic, mainly due to reduced cellular permeability or (b) acquired, due to mutation or the acquisition of plasmids. Tuberculosis remains an important public health hazard, and indeed the annual number of tuberculosis cases is rising in many countries. The greatest risk of acquiring infection is from the undiagnosed patient. Equipment used for respiratory investigations can become contaminated with mycobacteria if the patient is a carrier of this organism. It is important to be able to disinfect the equipment to a safe level to prevent transmission of infection to other patients (Table 17.2).

2.2.3 Bacterial spores

Prions (section 2.2.7) are generally considered to be the infectious agents most resistant to chemical disinfectants and sterilization processes; strictly speaking, however, they are not microorganisms because they have no cellular structure nor do they contain nucleic acids. Of the conventional microorganisms, bacterial spores are the most resistant to chemical treatment. The majority of antimicrobial

Table 17.2 Antibacterial activity of commonly used disinfectants and antiseptics

Class of compound	Activity against		General level* of antibacterial activity
	Mycobacteria	*Bacterial spores*	
Alcohols			
Ethanol/isopropyl	+	–	Intermediate
Aldehydes			
Glutaraldehyde	+	+	High
Ortho-phthaldehyde	+	+	High
Formaldehyde	+	+	High
Biguanides			
Chlorhexidine	–	–	Intermediate
Halogens			
Hypochlorite/ chloramines	+	+	High
Iodine/iodophor	+	+	Intermediate, problems with *Ps. aeruginosa*
Peroxygens			
Peracetic acid	+	+	High
Hydrogen peroxide	+	+	High
Phenolics			
Clear soluble fluids	+	–	Intermediate
Chloroxylenol	–	–	Low
Bisphenols	–	–	Low, poor against *Ps. aeruginosa*
Quaternary ammonium compounds			
Benzalkonium	–	–	Intermediate
Cetrimide	–	–	Intermediate

*Activity will depend on concentration, time of contact, temperature, etc. (see Chapter 11) but these are activities expected if in-use concentrations were being employed.

agents have no useful sporicidal action in a pharmaceutical context. However, certain aldehydes, halogens and peroxygen compounds have excellent activity under controlled conditions and are sometimes used as an alternative to physical methods for sterilization of heat-sensitive equipment. In these circumstances, correct usage of the agent is of paramount importance, as safety margins are lower in comparison with physical methods of sterilization (Chapter 20).

The antibacterial activity of disinfectants and antiseptics is summarized in Table 17.2.

2.2.4 Fungi

The vegetative fungal form is often as sensitive as vegetative bacteria to antimicrobial agents. Fungal spores (conidia and chlamydospores; see Chapter 4) may be more resistant, but this resistance is of much lesser magnitude than for bacterial spores. The ability to rapidly destroy pathogenic fungi such as the important nosocomial pathogen, *Candida albicans,* filamentous fungi such as *Trichophyton mentagrophytes,* and spores of common spoilage moulds such as *Aspergillus niger* is put to advantage in many applications of use. Many disinfectants have good activity against these fungi (Table 17.3). In addition, ethanol (70%) is rapid and reliable against *Candida* species.

2.2.5 Viruses

Susceptibility of viruses to antimicrobial agents can depend on whether the viruses possess a lipid enve-

Table 17.3 Antifungal activity of disinfectants and antiseptics.

Antimicrobial agent	Time (min) to give >99.99% kill* of		
	Aspergillus niger	Trichophyton mentagrophytes	Candida albicans
Phenolic (0.36%)	<2	<2	<2
Chlorhexidine gluconate (0.02%, alcoholic)	<2	<2	<2
Iodine (1%, alcoholic)	<2	<2	<2
Povidone-iodine (10%, alcoholic and aqueous)	10	<2	<2
Hypochlorite (0.2%)	10	<2	5
Cetrimide (1%)	<2	20	<2
Chlorhexidine gluconate (0.05%) + cetrimide (0.5%)	20	>20	>2
Chlorhexidine gluconate (0.5%, aqueous)	20	>20	>2

* Initial viable counts were c. 1×10^6/ml in suspension test.

lope. Non-lipid viruses are frequently more resistant to disinfectants and it is also likely that such viruses cannot be readily categorized with respect to their sensitivities to antimicrobial agents. These viruses are responsible for many nosocomial infections, e.g. rotaviruses, picornaviruses and adenoviruses (see Chapter 5) and it may be necessary to select an antiseptic or disinfectant to suit specific circumstances. Certain viruses, such as Ebola and Marburg, which cause haemorrhagic fevers, are highly infectious and their safe destruction by disinfectants is of paramount importance. Hepatitis A is an enterovirus considered to be one of the most resistant viruses to disinfection.

There is much concern for the safety of personnel handling articles contaminated with pathogenic viruses such as hepatitis B virus (HBV) and human immunodeficiency virus (HIV) which causes AIDS (acquired immune deficiency syndrome). Disinfectants must be able to treat rapidly and reliably accidental spills of blood, body fluids or secretions from HIV-infected patients. Such spills may contain levels of HIV as high as 10^4 infectious units/ml. Fortunately, HIV is inactivated by most chemicals at in-use concentrations. However, the recommendation is to use high level disinfectants (Table 17.2) for decontamination of HIV- or HBV-infected reusable medical equipment. For patient-care areas cleaning and disinfection with intermediate level disinfectants is satisfactory. Flooding with a liquid germicide is only required when large spills of cultured or concentrated infectious agents have to be dealt with.

The virucidal activity of chemicals is difficult to determine in the laboratory. Tissue culture techniques are the most common methods for growing and estimating viruses; however, antimicrobial agents may also adversely affect the tissue culture.

2.2.6 Protozoa

Acanthamoeba spp. can cause acanthamoeba keratitis with associated corneal scarring and loss of vision in soft contact lens wearers. The cysts of this protozoan present a particular problem in respect of lens disinfection. The chlorine-generating systems in use are generally inadequate. Although polyhexamethylene biguanide shows promise as an acanthamoebicide, only hydrogen peroxide-based disinfection is considered completely reliable and consistent in producing an acanthamoebicidal effect.

2.2.7 Prions

Prions (small proteinaceous infectious particles) are a unique class of infectious agent causing spongiform encephalopathies such as bovine spongiform encephalopathy (BSE) in cattle and Creutzfeldt–Jakob disease (CJD) in humans. There is considerable concern about the transmission of these agents from infected animals or patients. Risk of infectivity is highest in brain, spinal cord and eye tissues. There are still many unknown factors regarding destruction of prions and they are considered resistant to most disinfectant procedures. For heat-resistant medical instruments that come into contact with high infectivity tissues or high-risk contacts, immersion in sodium hydroxide (1 N) or sodium hypochlorite (20 000 ppm available chlorine) for 1 hour is advised in WHO guidelines and this must be followed by further treatment including autoclaving, cleaning and routine sterilization.

2.3 Intended application

The intended application of the antimicrobial agent, whether for preservation, antisepsis or disinfection, will influence its selection and also affect its performance. For example, in medicinal preparations the ingredients in the formulation may antagonize preservative activity. The risk to the patient will depend on whether the antimicrobial is in close contact with a break in the skin or mucous membranes or is introduced into a sterile area of the body.

In disinfection of instruments, the chemicals used must not adversely affect the instruments, e.g. cause corrosion of metals, affect clarity or integrity of lenses, or change the texture of synthetic polymers. Many materials such as fabrics, rubber and plastics are capable of adsorbing certain disinfectants, e.g. quaternary ammonium compounds (QACs) are adsorbed by fabrics, while phenolics are adsorbed by rubber, the consequence of this being a reduction in the concentration of active compound. A disinfectant can only exert its effect if it is in contact with the item being treated. Therefore access to all parts of an instrument or piece of equipment is essential. For small items, total immersion in the disinfectant must also be ensured.

2.4 Environmental factors

Organic matter can have a drastic effect on antimicrobial capacity either by adsorption or chemical inactivation, thus reducing the concentration of active agent in solution or by acting as a barrier to the penetration of the disinfectant. Blood, body fluids, pus, milk, food residues or colloidal proteins, even present in small amounts, all reduce the effectiveness of antimicrobial agents to varying degrees, and some are seriously affected. In their normal habitats, microorganisms have a tendency to adhere to surfaces and are thus less accessible to the chemical agent. Some organisms are specific to certain environments and their destruction will be of paramount importance in the selection of a suitable agent, e.g. *Legionella* in cooling towers and non-potable water supply systems, *Listeria* in the dairy and food industry and HBV in blood-contaminated articles.

Dried organic deposits may inhibit penetration of the chemical agent. Where possible, objects to be disinfected should be thoroughly cleaned. The presence of ions in water can also affect activity of antimicrobial agents, thus water for testing biocidal activity can be made artificially 'hard' by addition of ions.

These factors can have very significant effects on activity and are summarized in Table 17.4.

2.5 Toxicity of the agent

In choosing an antimicrobial agent for a particular application some consideration must be given to its toxicity. Increasing concern for health and safety is reflected in the Control of Substances Hazardous to Health (COSHH) Regulations (1999) that specify the precautions required in handling toxic or potentially toxic agents. In respect of disinfectants these regulations affect, particularly, the use of phenolics, formaldehyde and glutaraldehyde. Toxic volatile substances, in general, should be kept in covered containers to reduce the level of exposure to irritant vapour and they should be used with an extractor facility. Limits governing the exposure of individuals to such substances are now listed, e.g. 0.7 mg/m^3 (0.2 ppm) glutaraldehyde for both short- and long-term exposure. Many disinfectants including the aldehydes, glutaraldehyde less so than formaldehyde, may affect the eyes, skin (causing contact dermatitis) and induce respiratory distress. Face protection and impermeable nitrile rubber gloves should be worn when using these agents. Table 17.4 lists the toxicity of many of the disinfectants in use and other concerns of toxicity are described below for individual agents.

Where the atmosphere of a workplace is likely to be contaminated, sampling and analysis of the at-

Table 17.4 Properties of commonly used disinfectants and antiseptics

Class of compound	Effect of organic matter	pH optimum	Toxicity and OES*	Other factors
Alcohols				
Ethanol	Slight		Avoid broken skin, eyes OES: 1000 ppm/1900 mg/m^3, 8 h only	Poor penetration, good cleansing properties, flammable
Isopropanol	Slight		OES: 500 ppm/1225 mg/m^3, 10 min; 400 ppm/980 mg/m^3, 8 h	
Aldehydes				
Glutaraldehyde	Slight	pH 8	Respiratory complaints and contact dermatitis reported Eyes, sensitivity OES: 0.2 ppm/0.7 mg/m^3, 10 min only	Non-corrosive, useful for heat-sensitive instruments Use in well-ventilated area. Gloves, goggles and apron worn for preparation
Formaldehyde	Moderate		Respiratory distress, dermatitis MEL: 2 ppm/2.5 mg/m^3, 10 min and 8 h	
Biguanides Chlorhexidine	Severe	pH 7–8	Avoid contact with eyes and mucous membranes Sensitivity may develop	Incompatible with soap and anionic detergents Inactivated by hard water, some materials and plastic
Chlorine compounds Hypochlorite	Severe	Acid/neutral pH	Irritation of skin, eyes and lungs OES: 1 ppm/3 mg/m^3, 10 min; 0.5 ppm/1.5 mg/m^3, 8 h	Corrosive to metals Dichloroisocyanurate likely to produce Cl gas when used to disinfect acidic urines
Hydrogen peroxide	Slight/moderate	Acid/neutral pH	May irritate skin and mucous membranes OES: 2 ppm/3 mg/m^3, 10 min; 1 ppm, 8 h	May develop high pressure in container
Iodine preparations	Severe	Acid pH	Eye irritation. Tincture or KI as Lugol's Iodine OES: 0.1 ppm/1 mg/m^3, 10 min only	May corrode metals
Phenolics				
Clear soluble fluids	Slight	Acid pH	Protect skin and eyes	Absorbed by rubber/plastic
Black/white fluids	Moderate/severe		Very irritant May irritate skin	Greatly reduced by dilution
Chloroxylenol	Severe		OES: 10 ppm/38 mg/m^3, 10 min; 5 ppm/19 mg/m^3, 8 h	Absorbed by rubber/plastic
QACs Cetrimide Benzalkonium chloride	Severe	Alkaline pH	Avoid contact with eyes	Incompatible with soap and anionic detergents Absorbed by fabrics

* Health and Safety Executive (1996).

OES, occupational exposure standard; MEL, maximum exposure limit. MELs are the time-weighted average upper limits of a substance permitted in the breathing zone of a person. OESs are the maximum concentrations of a substance in air to which individuals may be exposed during their working life and at which present knowledge indicates there will be no ill effects. They are often the same as 8-h MELs.

mosphere may need to be carried out on a periodic basis with a frequency determined by conditions.

3 Types of compound

The following section presents in alphabetical order by chemical grouping the agents most often employed for disinfection, antisepsis and preservation. This information is summarized in Table 17.5.

3.1 Acids and esters

Antimicrobial activity, within a pharmaceutical context, is generally found only in the organic acids. These are weak acids and will therefore dissociate incompletely to give the three entities HA, H^+ and A^- in solution. As the undissociated form, HA, is the active antimicrobial agent, the ionization constant, K_a, is important and the pK_a of the acid must be considered, especially in formulation of the agent.

3.1.1 Benzoic acid

This is an organic acid, C_6H_5COOH, which is included, alone or in combination with other preservatives, in many pharmaceuticals. Although the compound is often used as the sodium salt, the non-ionized acid is the active substance. A limitation on its use is imposed by the pH of the final product as the pK_a of benzoic acid is 4.2 at which pH 50% of the acid is ionized. It is advisable to limit use of the acid to preservation of pharmaceuticals with a maximum final pH of 5.0 and if possible < 4.0. Concentrations of 0.05–0.1% are suitable for oral preparations. A disadvantage of the compound is the development of resistance by some organisms, in some cases involving metabolism of the acid resulting in complete loss of activity. Benzoic acid also has some use in combination with other agents, salicylic acid for example, in the treatment of superficial fungal infections.

3.1.2 Sorbic acid

This compound is a widely used preservative as the acid or its potassium salt. The pKa is 4.8 and, as with benzoic acid, activity decreases with increasing pH and ionization. It is most effective at pH 4 or below. Pharmaceutical products such as gums, mucilages and syrups are usefully preserved with this agent.

3.1.3 Sulphur dioxide, sulphites and metabisulphites

Sulphur dioxide has extensive use as a preservative in the food and beverage industries. In a pharmaceutical context, sodium sulphite and metabisulphite or bisulphite have a dual role acting as preservatives and anti-oxidants.

3.1.4 Esters of p-hydroxybenzoic acid (parabens)

A series of alkyl esters (Fig. 17.1) of p-hydroxybenzoic acid was originally prepared to overcome the marked pH dependence on activity of the acids. These parabens, the methyl, ethyl, propyl and butyl esters, are less readily ionized, having pK_a values in the range 8–8.5, and exhibit good preservative activity even at pH levels of 7–8, although optimum activity is again displayed in acidic solutions. This broader pH range allows extensive and successful use of the parabens as pharmaceutical preservatives. They are active against a wide range of fungi but are less so against bacteria, especially the pseudomonads, which may utilize the parabens as a carbon source. They are frequently used as preservatives of emulsions, creams and lotions where two phases exist. Combinations of esters are most successful for this type of product in that the more water-soluble methyl ester (0.25%) protects the aqueous phase, whereas the propyl or butyl esters (0.02%) give protection to the oil phase. Such combinations are also considered to extend the range of activity. As inactivation of parabens occurs with non-ionic surfactants due care should be taken in formulation with both materials.

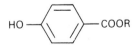

Fig. 17.1 p-Hydroxybenzoates (R is methyl, ethyl, propyl, butyl, or benzyl).

Table 17.5 Examples of the main antimicrobial groups as antiseptics, disinfectants and preservatives

Antimicrobial agent	Antiseptic activity		Disinfectant activity		Preservative activity	
	Concentration	Typical formulation/application	Concentration	Typical formulation/application	Concentration	Typical formulation/application
Acids and esters, e.g. benzoic acid, parabens					0.05–0.1% 0.25%	For oral and topical formulations
Alcohols, e.g. ethyl or isopropyl	50–90% in water	Skin preparation	50–90% in water	Clean surface preparation		
Aldehydes, e.g. glutaraldehyde	10%	Gel for warts	2.0%	Solution for instruments		
Biguanides, e.g. chlorhexidine† (gluconate, acetate, etc.)	0.02% 0.2% 0.5% (in 70% alcohol) 1.0% 4.0%	Bladder irrigation Mouthwash Skin preparation Dusting powder, cream dental gel Pre-operative scrub in surfactant	0.05% 0.5% (in 70% alcohol)	Storage of instruments, clean instrument disinfection (30 min) Emergency instrument disinfection (2 min)	0.0025% 0.01%	Solution for hard contact lenses Eye-drops
Chlorine, e.g. hypochlorite	≤0.5%avCl₂	Solution for skin and wounds	1–10%	Solution for surfaces and instruments		
Hydrogen peroxide	1.5% 3–6%	Stabilized cream Solution for wounds and ulcers, mouthwash	3.0%	Disinfection of soft contact lenses		
Iodine compounds, e.g. free iodine, povidone-iodine	1.0% 1.0% 2.5% 7.5% 10%	Aqueous or alcoholic (70%) solution Mouthwash Dry powder spray Scalp and skin cleanser Pre-operative scrub, fabric dressing	10.0%	Aqueous or alcoholic solution		
Phenolics, e.g. clear soluble phenolics, chloroxylenol	0.5% 1.3% 2.0%	Dusting powder Solution Skin cleanser	1–2%	Solution		
QACs, e.g. cetyltrimethyl ammonium bromide (cetrimide)	0.1% 0.5% 1.0%	Solution for wounds and burns Cream Skin solution	0.1% 1.0%	Storage of instruments Instruments (1 h)	0.01%	Eye-drops

* Also used in combination with other agents, e.g. chlorhexidine, iodine.
† Several forms available having $x\%$ chlorhexidine and $10x\%$ cetrimide.
QAC, quaternary ammonium compound.

3.2 Alcohols

3.2.1 Alcohols used for disinfection and antisepsis

The aliphatic alcohols, notably ethanol and isopropanol, are used for disinfection and antisepsis. They are bactericidal against vegetative forms, including *Mycobacterium* species, but are not sporicidal. Cidal activity drops sharply below 50% concentration. Alcohols have poor penetration of organic matter and their use is therefore restricted to clean conditions. They possess properties such as a cleansing action and volatility, are able to achieve a rapid and large reduction in skin flora and have been widely used for skin preparation before injection or other surgical procedures. The risk of transmission of infection due to poor hand hygiene has been attributed to lack of compliance with hand-washing procedures. An alcohol hand-rub offers a rapid easy-to-use alternative that is more acceptable to personnel and is increasingly being recommended for routine use. However, the contact time of an alcohol-soaked swab with the skin prior to venepuncture is so brief that it is thought to be of doubtful value.

Ethanol (CH_3CH_2OH) is widely used as a disinfectant and antiseptic. The presence of water is essential for activity, hence 100% ethanol is ineffective. Concentrations between 60% and 95% are bactericidal and a 70% solution is usually employed for the disinfection of skin, clean instruments or surfaces. At higher concentrations, e.g. 90%, ethanol is also active against most viruses, including HIV. Ethanol is also a popular choice in pharmaceutical preparations and cosmetic products as a solvent and preservative.

Isopropyl alcohol (isopropanol, $CH_3.CHOH.CH_3$) has slightly greater bactericidal activity than ethanol but is also about twice as toxic. It is less active against viruses, particularly non-enveloped viruses, and should be considered a limited-spectrum virucide. Used at concentrations of 60–70%, it is an acceptable alternative to ethanol for preoperative skin treatment and is also employed as a preservative for cosmetics.

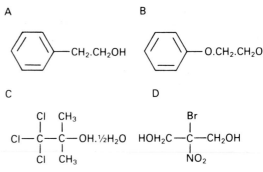

Fig. 17.2 Structural formulae of alcohols used in preserving and disinfection: A, 2-phenylethanol; B, 2-phenoxyethanol; C, chlorbutol (trichloro-*t*-butanol); D, bronopol (2-bromo-2-nitropropan-1,3-diol).

3.2.2 Alcohols as preservatives

The aralkyl alcohols and more highly substituted aliphatic alcohols (Fig. 17.2) are used mostly as preservatives. These include:

(1) Benzyl alcohol ($C_6H_5CH_2OH$). This has antibacterial and weak local anaesthetic properties and is used as an antimicrobial preservative at a concentration of 2%, although its use in cosmetics is restricted.

(2) Chlorbutol (chlorobutanol; trichlorobutanol; trichloro-*t*-butanol). Typical in-use concentration: 0.5%. It has been used as a preservative in injections and eye-drops. It is unstable, decomposition occurring at acid pH during autoclaving, while alkaline solutions are unstable at room temperature.

(3) Phenylethanol (phenylethyl alcohol; 2-phenylethanol). Typical in-use concentration: 0.25–0.5%. It is reported to have greater activity against Gram-negative organisms and is usually employed in conjunction with another agent.

(4) Phenoxyethanol (2-phenoxyethanol). Typical in-use concentration: 1%. It is more active against *Ps. aeruginosa* than against other bacteria and is usually combined with other preservatives such as the hydroxybenzoates to broaden the spectrum of antimicrobial activity.

(5) Bronopol (2-bromo-2-nitropropan-1,3-diol). Typical in-use concentration: 0.01–0.1%. It has a broad spectrum of antibacterial activity, including *Pseudomonas* species. The main limitation on the use of bronopol is that when exposed to light at

alkaline pH, especially if accompanied by an increase in temperature, solutions decompose, turning yellow or brown. A number of decomposition products including formaldehyde are produced. In addition, nitrite ions may be produced and react with any secondary and tertiary amines present forming nitrosamines, which are potentially carcinogenic.

3.3 Aldehydes

A number of aldehydes possess antimicrobial properties, including sporicidal activity, with glutaraldehyde the most widely used for disinfection. It is a highly effective biocide and its use as a 'chemosterilant' reflects this.

3.3.1 Glutaraldehyde

Glutaraldehyde (CHO(CH$_2$)$_3$CHO) has a broad spectrum of antimicrobial activity and rapid rate of kill, most vegetative bacteria being killed within a minute of exposure, although bacterial spores may require 3 hours or more. The latter depends on the intrinsic resistance of spores, which may vary widely. It has the further advantage of not being affected significantly by organic matter. The glutaraldehyde molecule possesses two aldehyde groupings which are highly reactive and their presence is an important component of biocidal activity. The monomeric molecule is in equilibrium with polymeric forms, and the physical conditions of temperature and pH have a significant effect on this equilibrium. At a pH of 8, biocidal activity is greatest but stability is poor due to polymerization. In contrast, acid solutions are stable but considerably less active, although as temperature is increased, there is a breakdown in the polymeric forms which exist in acid solutions and a concomitant increase in free active dialdehyde, resulting in better activity. In practice, glutaraldehyde is generally supplied as an acidic 2% or greater aqueous solution, which is stable on prolonged storage. This is then 'activated' before use by addition of a suitable alkalizing agent to bring the pH of the solution to its optimum for activity. The activated solution will have a limited shelf-life, in the order of 2 weeks, although more stable formulations are available. Glutaraldehyde

is employed mainly for the cold, liquid chemical sterilization of medical and surgical materials that cannot be sterilized by other methods. Endoscopes, including for example, arthroscopes, laparascopes, cystoscopes and bronchoscopes may be decontaminated by glutaraldehyde treatment. Times employed in practice for high level disinfection are often considerably less than the many hours recommended by manufacturers to achieve sterilization.

3.3.2 Ortho-*phthalaldehyde*

Ortho-phthalaldehyde (OPA) is a recent addition to the aldehyde group of high level disinfectants. This agent has demonstrated excellent activity in *in vitro* studies, showing superior mycobactericidal activity compared with glutaraldehyde. OPA has several other advantages over glutaraldehyde. It requires no activation, is not a known irritant to the eyes or nasal passages and has excellent stability over the pH range 3–9. Its use for disinfection of endoscopes appears promising.

3.3.3 Formaldehyde

Formaldehyde (HCHO) can be used in either the liquid or gaseous state for disinfection purposes. In the vapour phase it has been used for decontamination of isolators, safety cabinets and rooms; however, recent trends have been to combine formaldehyde vapour with low temperature steam (LTSF) for the sterilization of heat-sensitive items (Chapter 20). Formaldehyde vapour is highly toxic and potentially carcinogenic if inhaled, thus its use must be carefully controlled. It is not very active at temperatures below 20°C and requires a relative humidity of at least 70%. The agent is not supplied as a gas but either as a solid polymer, paraformaldehyde, or a liquid, formalin, which is a 34–38% aqueous solution. The gas is liberated by heating or mixing the solid or liquid with potassium permanganate and water. Formalin, diluted 1:10 to give 4% formaldehyde may be used for disinfecting surfaces. In general, however, solutions of either aqueous or alcoholic formaldehyde are too irritant for routine application to skin, while poor penetration and a tendency to polymerize on surfaces limit its use as a disinfectant for pharmaceutical purposes.

3.3.4 Formaldehyde-releasing agents

Various formaldehyde condensates have been developed to reduce the irritancy associated with formaldehyde while maintaining activity, and these are described as formaldehyde-releasing agents or masked-formaldehyde compounds.

Noxythiolin (N-hydroxy N-methylthiourea) is supplied as a dry powder and on aqueous reconstitution slowly releases formaldehyde and N-methylthiourea. The compound has extensive antibacterial and antifungal properties and is used both topically and in accessible body cavities as an irrigation solution and in the treatment of peritonitis. Polynoxylin (poly[methylenedi(hydroxymethyl) urea]) is a similar compound available in gel and lozenge formulations.

Taurolidine (bis-[1,1-dioxoperhydro-1,2,4-thiadiazinyl-4]methane) is a condensate of two molecules of the amino acid taurine and three molecules of formaldehyde. It is more stable than noxythiolin in solution and has similar uses. The activity of taurolidine is stated to be greater than that of formaldehyde.

3.4 Biguanides

3.4.1 Chlorhexidine and alexidine

Chlorhexidine is an antimicrobial agent first synthesized at Imperial Chemical Industries in 1954 in a research programme to produce compounds related to the biguanide antimalarial proguanil.

Compounds containing the biguanide structure could be expected to have good antibacterial effects, thus the major part of the proguanil structure is found in chlorhexidine. The chlorhexidine molecule, a bisbiguanide, is symmetrical. A hexamethylene chain links two biguanide groups, to each of which a para-chlorophenyl radical is bound (Fig. 17.3). A related compound is the bisbiguanide alexidine, which has use as an oral antiseptic and anti-plaque agent. Alexidine (Fig. 17.3A) differs from chlorhexidine (Fig. 17.3B) in that it possesses ethylhexyl end-groups.

Chlorhexidine base is not readily soluble in water, therefore the freely soluble salts, acetate, gluconate and hydrochloride are used in formulation. Chlorhexidine exhibits the greatest antibacterial activity at pH 7–8 where it exists exclusively as a dication. The cationic nature of the compound results in activity being reduced by anionic compounds including soap due to the formation of insoluble salts. Anions to be wary of include bicarbonate, borate, carbonate, chloride, citrate and phosphate with due attention being paid to the presence of hard water. Deionized or distilled water should preferably be used for dilution purposes. Reduction in activity will also occur in the presence of blood, pus and other organic matter. Chlorhexidine has widespread use, in particular as an antiseptic. It has significant antibacterial activity, although Gram-negative bacteria are less sensitive than Gram-positive organisms. A concentration of 1 : 2 000 000 prevents growth of, for example,

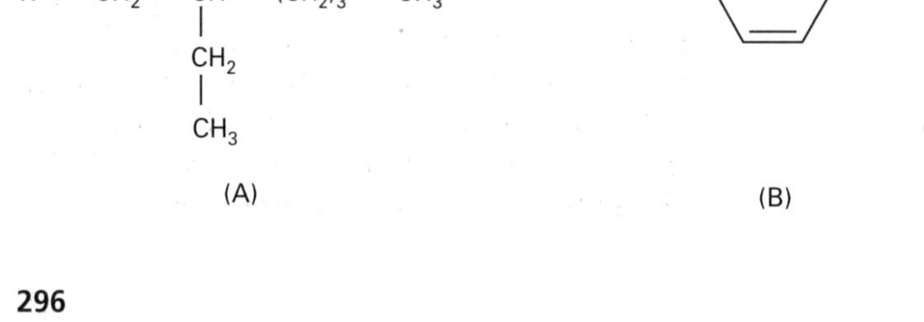

Fig. 17.3 Bisbiguanides: A, alexidine; B, chlorhexidine.

Staph. aureus, whereas a 1:50000 dilution prevents growth of *Ps. aeruginosa.* Reports of pseudomonad contamination of aqueous chlorhexidine solutions have prompted the inclusion of small amounts of ethanol or isopropanol. Chlorhexidine is ineffective at ambient temperatures against bacterial spores and *M. tuberculosis.* Limited antifungal activity has been demonstrated which unfortunately restricts its use as a general preservative. Skin sensitivity has occasionally been reported although, in general, chlorhexidine is well tolerated and non-toxic when applied to skin or mucous membranes and is an important preoperative antiseptic.

3.4.2 Polyhexamethylene biguanides

The antimicrobial activity of chlorhexidine, a bis-biguanide, exceeds that of monomeric biguanides. This has stimulated the development of polymeric biguanides containing repeating biguanide groups linked by hexamethylene chains. One such compound is a commercially available heterodisperse mixture of polyhexamethylene biguanides (PHMB, polyhexanide) having the general formula shown in Fig. 17.4.

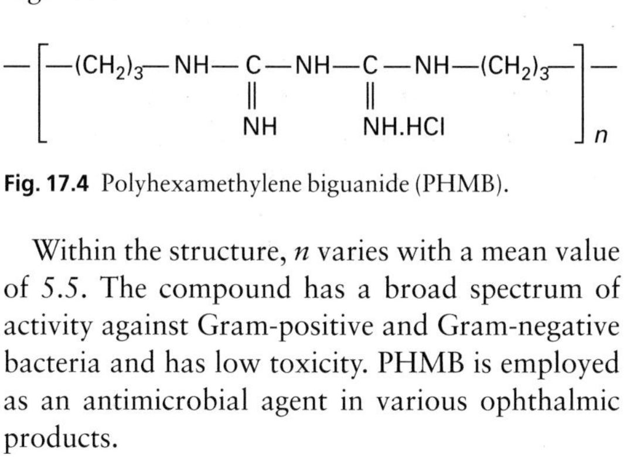

Fig. 17.4 Polyhexamethylene biguanide (PHMB).

Within the structure, *n* varies with a mean value of 5.5. The compound has a broad spectrum of activity against Gram-positive and Gram-negative bacteria and has low toxicity. PHMB is employed as an antimicrobial agent in various ophthalmic products.

3.5 Halogens

Chlorine and iodine have been used extensively since their introduction as disinfecting agents in the early 19th century. Preparations containing these halogens such as Dakin's solution and tincture of iodine were early inclusions in many pharmacopoeias and national formularies. More recent formulations of these elements have improved activity, stability and ease of use.

3.5.1 Chlorine

A large number of antimicrobially active chlorine compounds are commercially available, one of the most important being liquid chlorine. This is supplied as an amber liquid by compressing and cooling gaseous chlorine. The terms liquid and gaseous chlorine refer to elemental chlorine whereas the word 'chlorine' is normally used to signify a mixture of OCl^-, Cl_2, $HOCl$ and other active chlorine compounds in aqueous solution. The potency of chlorine disinfectants is usually expressed in terms of parts per million (ppm) or percentage of available chlorine (avCl).

3.5.2 Hypochlorites

Hypochlorites are the oldest and remain the most useful of the chlorine disinfectants, being readily available, inexpensive and compatible with most anionic and cationic surface-active agents. They exhibit a rapid kill against a wide spectrum of microorganisms including fungi and viruses. High levels of available chlorine will enable eradication of acid-fast bacilli and bacterial spores. To their disadvantage they are corrosive, suffer inactivation by organic matter and can become unstable. Hypochlorites are available as powders or liquids, most frequently as the sodium or potassium salts of hypochlorous acid (HOCl). Sodium hypochlorite exists in solution as follows:

$$NaOCl + H_2O \rightleftharpoons HOCl + NaOH$$

Undissociated hypochlorous acid is a strong oxidizing agent and its potent antimicrobial activity is dependent on pH as shown:

$$HOCl \rightleftharpoons H^+ + OCl^-$$

At low pH the existence of HOCl is favoured over OCl^- (hypochlorite ion). The relative microbiocidal effectiveness of these forms is of the order of 100:1. By lowering the pH of hypochlorite solutions the antimicrobial activity increases to an optimum at about pH 5; however, this is concurrent with a decrease in stability of the solutions. This problem may be alleviated by addition of NaOH (see above equation) in order to maintain a high pH during storage for stability. The absence of buffer allows the pH to be lowered sufficiently for activity on dilution to use-strength. It is preferable to prepare use-dilutions of hypochlorite on a daily basis.

3.5.3 *Organic chlorine compounds*

A number of organic chlorine, or chloramine, compounds are now available for disinfection and antisepsis. These are the *N*-chloro (= *N*-Cl) derivatives of, for example, sulphonamides giving compounds such as chloramine–T and dichloramine–T and halazone (Fig. 17.5), which may be used for the disinfection of contaminated drinking water.

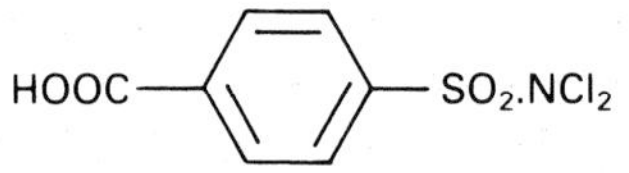

HOOC—⟨benzene ring⟩—SO$_2$.NCl$_2$

Fig. 17.5 Halazone.

A second group of compounds, formed by *N*-chloro derivatization of heterocyclic compounds containing a nitrogen in the ring, includes the sodium and potassium salts of dichloroisocyanuric acid (e.g. NaDCC). These are available in granule or tablet form and, in contrast to hypochlorite, are very stable on storage, if protected from moisture. In water they will give a known chlorine concentration. The antimicrobial activity of the compounds is similar to that of the hypochlorites when acidic conditions of use are maintained. It is, however, important to note that where inadequate ventilation exists, care must be taken not to apply the compound to acidic fluids or large spills of urine in view of the toxic effects of chlorine production. The Health and Safety Executive (HSE) has set the Occupational Exposure Standard (OES) short-term exposure limit at 1 ppm (see also section 2.5).

3.5.4 *Chloroform*

Chloroform (CHCl$_3$) has a narrow spectrum of activity. It has been used extensively as a preservative of pharmaceuticals since the last century, although more recently it has had limitations placed on its use. Marked reductions in concentration may occur through volatilization from products resulting in the possibility of microbial growth.

3.5.5 *Iodine*

Iodine has a wide spectrum of antimicrobial activity. Gram-negative and Gram-positive organisms, bacterial spores (on extended exposure), mycobacteria, fungi and viruses are all susceptible. The active agent is the elemental iodine molecule, I$_2$. As elemental iodine is only slightly soluble in water, iodide ions are required for aqueous solutions such as Aqueous Iodine Solution, BP 1988 (Lugol's Solution) containing 5% iodine in 10% potassium iodide solution. Iodine (2.5%) may also be dissolved in ethanol (90%) and potassium iodide (2.5%) solution to give Weak Iodine Solution, BP 1988 (Iodine Tincture).

The antimicrobial activity of iodine is less dependent than chlorine on temperature and pH, although alkaline pH should be avoided. Iodine is also less susceptible to inactivation by organic matter. Disadvantages in the use of iodine in skin antisepsis are staining of skin and fabrics coupled with possible sensitizing of skin and mucous membranes.

3.5.6 *Iodophors*

In the 1950s iodophors (iodo meaning iodine and phor meaning carrier) were developed to eliminate the disadvantages of iodine while retaining its antimicrobial activity. These allowed slow release of iodine on demand from the complex formed. Essentially, four generic compounds may be used as the carrier molecule or complexing agent. These give polyoxymer iodophors (i.e. with propylene or ethyene oxide polymers), cationic (quaternary ammonium) surfactant iodophors, non-ionic (ethoxylated) surfactant iodophors and polyvinylpyrrolidone iodophors (PVP-I or povidone-iodine). The non-ionic or cationic surface-active agents act as solubilizers and carriers, combining detergency with antimicrobial activity. The former type of surfactant especially, produces a stable, efficient formulation, the activity of which is further enhanced by the addition of phosphoric or citric acid to give a pH below 5 on use-dilution. The iodine is present in the form of micellar aggregates which disperse on dilution, especially below the critical micelle concentration (cmc) of the surfactant, to liberate free iodine.

When iodine and povidone are combined a chemical reaction takes place forming a complex between the two. Some of the iodine becomes organically linked to povidone, although the major portion of the complexed iodine is in the form of triiodide. Dilution of this iodophor results in a weakening of the iodine linkage to the carrier polymer with concomitant increases in elemental iodine in solution and antimicrobial activity.

The amount of free iodine the solution can generate is termed the 'available iodine'. This acts as a reservoir for active iodine, releasing it when required and therefore largely avoiding the harmful side-effects of high iodine concentration. Consequently, when used for antisepsis, iodophors should be allowed to remain on the skin for 2 minutes to obtain full advantage of the sustained-release iodine.

Cadexamer-I_2 is an iodophor similar to povidone-iodine. It is a 2-hydroxymethylene cross-linked (1–4) α-D-glucan carboxymethyl ether containing iodine. The compound is used especially for its absorbent and antiseptic properties in the management of leg ulcers and pressure sores where it is applied in the form of microbeads containing 0.9% iodine.

3.6 Heavy metals

Mercury and silver have long been known to have antibacterial properties and preparations of these metals were among the earliest used antiseptics; however, they have been replaced by less toxic compounds.

3.6.1 Mercurials

The organomercurial derivatives thiomersal and phenylmercuric nitrate or acetate (PMN or PMA) (Fig. 17.6) are bacteriostatic and are primarily employed as preservatives. Use of both compounds has declined considerably due to concerns about mercury toxicity and risk of hypersensitivity or local irritation. They are absorbed from solution by rubber closures and plastic containers to a significant extent.

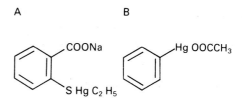

Fig. 17.6 Some organomercurials: A, thiomersal (sodium ethylmercurithiosalicylate); B, phenylmercuric acetate.

Thiomersal has been employed as a preservative for eye-drops and contact lens solutions. Its use as a preservative in vaccines is being phased out where possible because of suggestions that mercury in vaccines could be neurotoxic. The phenylmercuric salts (0.002%) have also been used for preservation of eye-drops but long-term use has led to keratopathy and they are not recommended for prolonged use.

3.7 Hydrogen peroxide and peroxygen compounds

Hydrogen peroxide and peracetic acid are high level disinfectants due to their production of the highly reactive hydroxyl radical. They have the added advantage that their decomposition products are non-toxic and biodegradable. The germicidal properties of hydrogen peroxide (H_2O_2) have been known for more than a century, but use of low concentrations of unstable solutions did little for its reputation. However, stabilized solutions are now available and due to its unusual properties and antimicrobial activity, hydrogen peroxide has a valuable role for specific applications. Its activity against the protozoan, *Acanthamoeba*, which can cause keratitis in contact lens wearers, has made it popular for disinfection of soft contact lenses. Concentrations of 3–6% are effective for general disinfection purposes. At high concentrations (up to 35%) and increased temperature hydrogen peroxide is sporicidal. Use has been made of this in vapour phase hydrogen peroxide decontamination of equipment and enclosed spaces.

Peracetic acid (CH_3COOOH) is the peroxide of acetic acid and is a more potent biocide than hydrogen peroxide, with excellent rapid biocidal activity against bacteria, including mycobacteria, fungi,

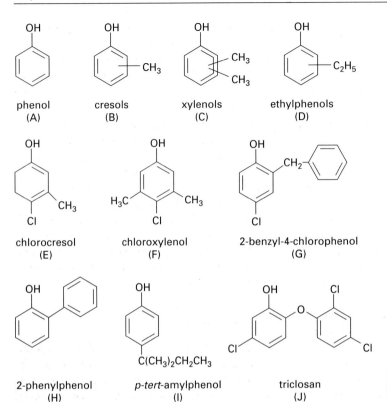

phenol
(A)

cresols
(B)

xylenols
(C)

ethylphenols
(D)

chlorocresol
(E)

chloroxylenol
(F)

2-benzyl-4-chlorophenol
(G)

2-phenylphenol
(H)

p-tert-amylphenol
(I)

triclosan
(J)

Fig 17.7 Structures of some common phenols possessing antimicrobial activity.

viruses and spores. It can be used in both the liquid and vapour phases and is active in the presence of organic matter. It is finding increasing use at concentrations of 0.2–0.35% as a chemosterilant of medical equipment such as flexible endoscopes. Its disadvantages are that it is corrosive to some metals. It is also highly irritant and must be used in an enclosed system. The combination of hydrogen peroxide and peracetic acid is synergistic and is marketed as a cold sterilant for dialysis machines.

3.8 Phenols

Phenols (Fig. 17.7) are widely used as disinfectants and preservatives. They have good antimicrobial activity and are rapidly bactericidal but generally are not sporicidal. Their activity is markedly diminished by dilution and is also reduced by organic matter. They are more active at acid pH. The main disadvantages of phenols are their caustic effect on skin and tissues and their systemic toxicity. The more highly substituted phenols are less toxic and can be used as preservatives and antiseptics; however, they are also less active than the simple phenolics, especially against Gram-negative organisms. To improve their poor aqueous solubility, phenolic disinfectants are often formulated with soaps, synthetic detergents, and/or solvents.

3.8.1 *Phenol (carbolic acid)*

Phenol (Fig. 17.7A) no longer plays any significant role as an antibacterial agent except as a preservative in some multi-dose parenteral products, e.g. vaccines. It is largely of historical interest, as it was used by Lister in the 1860s as a surgical antiseptic and has been a standard for comparison with other disinfectants in tests such as the Rideal Walker test.

3.8.2 Clear soluble fluids, black fluids and white fluids

Phenols obtained by distillation of coal or petroleum are known as the tar acids. These phenols are separated by fractional distillation according to their boiling point range into phenols, cresols, xylenols and high boiling point tar acids. As the boiling point increases bactericidal activity increases and tissue toxicity decreases, but there is increased inactivation by organic matter and decreased water solubility.

Clear soluble fluids are produced from cresols or xylenols. The preparation known as Lysol (Cresol and Soap Solution BP 1968) is a soap-solubilized formulation of cresol (Fig. 17.7B) that has been widely used as a general purpose disinfectant but has largely been superseded by less irritant phenolics. A higher boiling point fraction consisting of xylenols and ethylphenols (Fig. 17.7C and D) produces a more active, less corrosive product that retains activity in the presence of organic matter. A variety of proprietary products for general disinfection purposes are available with these phenols as active ingredients, and they are one of the most popular disinfectants for floor cleaning in hospitals. They possess rapid fungicidal and bactericidal activity, including mycobacteria.

Black fluids and white fluids are prepared by solubilizing the high boiling point tar acids. Black fluids are homogeneous solutions, which form an emulsion on dilution with water. White fluids are finely dispersed emulsions of tar acids, which on dilution with water produce more stable emulsions than do black fluids. Both types of fluid have good bactericidal activity. Preparations are very irritant and corrosive to skin, however, they are relatively inexpensive and are useful for household and general disinfection purposes. They must be used in adequate concentrations as activity is reduced by organic matter and is markedly affected by dilution.

3.8.3 Synthetic phenols

Many derivatives of phenol are now made by a synthetic process. A combination of alkyl or aryl substitution and halogenation of phenolic compounds has produced useful derivatives. Two of the most widely used chlorinated derivatives are *p*-chloro-*m*-cresol (chlorocresol, Fig. 17.7E) which is mostly employed as a preservative at a concentration of 0.1%, and *p*-chloro-*m*-xylenol (chloroxylenol, Fig. 17.7F) which is used for skin disinfection, although less than formerly. Chloroxylenol is sparingly soluble in water and must be solubilized, for example, in a suitable soap solution in conjunction with terpineol or pine oil. Its antimicrobial capacity is weak and is reduced by the presence of organic matter. Three other phenol derivatives common as active ingredients of general purpose disinfectant formulations, particularly in the USA, are: 2-benzyl-4-chlorophenol (Fig. 17.7G), 2-phenylphenol (Fig. 17.7H) and *p-tert*-amylphenol (Fig. 17.7I). A combination of amylphenol and phenylphenol is marketed as a sterilant.

3.8.4 Bisphenols

Bisphenols are composed of two phenolic groups connected by various linkages. Triclosan (Fig. 17.7J) is the most widely used. It is bacteriostatic at use-concentrations and has little anti-pseudomonal activity. It has been incorporated into medicated soaps, lotions and solutions and is also included in household products such as plastics and fabrics. There is concern about bacterial resistance developing to triclosan.

3.9 Surface-active agents

Surface-active agents or surfactants are classified as anionic, cationic, non-ionic or ampholytic according to the ionization of the hydrophilic group in the molecule. A hydrophobic, water-repellent group is also present. Within the various classes a range of detergent and disinfectant activity is found. The anionic and non-ionic surface-active agents, for example, have strong detergent properties but exhibit little or no antimicrobial activity. They can, however, render certain bacterial species more sensitive to some antimicrobial agents, possibly by altering the permeability of the outer envelope. Ampholytic or amphoteric agents can ionize to give anionic, cationic and zwitterionic (positively and negatively charged ions in the same molecule) activity. Consequently, they display both the detergent properties of the anionic surface-active agents and the antimicrobial activity of the cationic agents. They are used quite extensively in Europe for pre-surgical hand scrubbing, medical instrument disinfection and floor disinfection in hospitals.

Of the four classes of surface-active agents, however, the cationic compounds arguably play the most important role in an antimicrobial context.

3.9.1 Cationic surface-active agents

The cationic agents used for their antimicrobial activity all fall within the group known as the quaternary ammonium compounds that are variously described as QACs, quats or onium ions. These are organically substituted ammonium compounds as shown in Fig. 17.8A where the R substituents are alkyl or heterocyclic radicals to give compounds such as benzalkonium chloride (Fig. 17.8B), cetyltrimethylammonium bromide (cetrimide) (Fig. 17.8C) and cetylpyridinium chloride (Fig. 17.8D). Inspection of the structures of these compounds (Fig. 17.8B and C) indicates that a chain length in the range C_8 to C_{18} in at least one of the R substituents is a requirement for good antimicrobial activity. In the pyridinium compounds (Fig. 17.8D), three of the four covalent links may be satisfied by the nitrogen in a pyridine ring. Several 'generational' changes have arisen in the development of QACs. Compounds such as alkyldimethylbenzyl ammonium chloride, alkyldimethylethylbenzyl ammonium chloride and didecyldimethylammonium chloride are finding roles in disinfection where HIV and HBV are present. Polymeric quaternary ammonium salts such as polyquaternium 1 are finding increasing use as preservatives.

The QACs are most effective against microorganisms at neutral or slightly alkaline pH and become virtually inactive below pH 3.5. Not surprisingly, anionic agents greatly reduce the activity of these compounds. Incompatibilities have also been recorded with non-ionic agents, possibly due to the formation of micelles. The presence of organic matter such as serum, faeces and milk will also seriously affect activity.

QACs exhibit greatest activity against Gram-positive bacteria with a lethal effect observed using concentrations as low as 1:200 000. Gram-negative bacteria are more resistant, requiring a level of 1:30 000 or higher still if *Ps. aeruginosa* is present. Bacteriostasis is obtained at higher dilutions. A limited antifungal activity, more in the form of a static than a cidal effect, is exhibited. The QACs have not been shown to possess any useful sporicidal activity. This narrow spectrum of activity therefore limits the usefulness of the compounds, but as they are generally well tolerated and non-toxic when applied to skin and mucous membranes they have considerable use in treatment of wounds and abrasions and they are used as preservatives in certain preparations. Benzalkonium chloride and cetrimide are employed extensively in surgery, urology and gynaecology as aqueous and alcoholic solutions and as creams. In many instances they are used in conjunction with a biguanide disinfectant such as chlorhexidine. The detergent properties of the QACs also provide a useful activity, especially in hospitals, for general environmental sanitation.

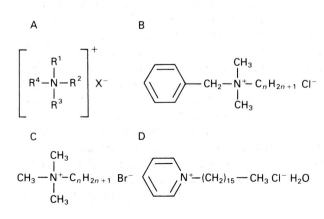

Fig 17.8 Quaternary ammonium compounds (QACs): A, general structure of QACs; B, benzalkonium chloride ($n = 8–18$); C, cetrimide ($n = 12–14$ or 16); D, cetylpyridinium chloride.

3.10 Other antimicrobials

The full range of chemicals that can be shown to have antimicrobial properties is beyond the scope of this chapter. The agents included in this section have limited use or are of historic interest.

3.10.1 Diamidines

The activity of diamidines is reduced by acid pH and in the presence of blood and serum. Propamidine and dibromopropamidine, as the isethionate salts, are the major diamidine derivatives employed as antimicrobial agents; propamidine in the form of eye-drops (0.1%) is used for amoebic infection and dibromopropamidine for topical treatment of minor infections.

3.10.2 Dyes

Crystal violet (Gentian violet), brilliant green and malachite green are triphenylmethane dyes widely used to stain bacteria for microscopic examination. They have bacteriostatic and fungistatic activity and have been applied topically for the treatment of infections. Due to concern about possible carcinogenicity, they are now rarely used.

The acridine dyes, acriflavine and aminacrine, have also been employed for skin disinfection and treatment of infected wounds or burns. They are slow acting and mainly bacteriostatic in effect, with no useful fungicidal or sporicidal activity. Acriflavine is a mixture of two components, proflavine and euflavine. Only euflavine has effective antimicrobial properties.

3.10.3 Quinoline derivatives

The quinoline derivatives of pharmaceutical interest are little used now. The antimicrobial activity of the derivatives is generally good against the Gram-positive bacteria although less so against Gram-negative species. The compound most frequently used in a pharmaceutical context is dequalinium chloride, a bisquaternary ammonium derivative of 4-aminoquinaldinium. It is formulated as a lozenge for the treatment of oropharyngeal infections.

3.11 Antimicrobial combinations and systems

As is apparent from the above information, there is no ideal disinfectant, antiseptic or preservative. All chemical agents have their limitations either in terms of their antimicrobial activity, resistance to organic matter, stability, incompatibility, irritancy, toxicity or corrosivity. To overcome the limitations of an individual agent, formulations consisting of combinations of agents are available. For example, ethanol and isopropanol have been combined with chlorhexidine, quaternary ammonium compounds, sodium hypochlorite and iodine to produce more active preparations. The combination of chlorhexidine and cetrimide is also considered to improve activity. Quaternary ammonium compounds and phenols have been combined with glutaraldehyde and formaldehyde so that the same effect can be achieved with lower, less irritant concentrations of the aldehydes. Some combinations are considered to be synergistic, e.g. hydrogen peroxide and peroxygen compounds. Care must be taken in deciding on disinfectant combinations, as the concentration exponents associated with each component of a disinfectant combination will have a considerable effect on the degree of activity.

Research into the resistance of microbial biofilms provides potential for improving elimination of this problematical microbial mode of growth. Bacteria often use a communication system, quorum sensing (QS), to regulate virulence factor production and the formation of biofilms. Chemicals that can block QS could be combined with disinfectants (or other antimicrobial agents) to provide effective elimination of biofilm infection. Increasing attention is also being focused on the incorporation of antimicrobial agents into materials that will form working surfaces or those of medical devices and implants. These 'bioactive' surfaces can be formed, for example, by incorporation of silver salts and alloys, biguanides and triclosan and have the ability to reduce infection arising from microbial adherence and biofilm formation.

Other means are available to potentiate the activity of disinfectants. Ultrasonic energy in combination with suitable disinfectants such as aldehydes and biguanides has been demonstrated to be useful in practice and ultraviolet radiation increases the activity of hydrogen peroxide. Superoxidized water provides an extremely active disinfectant with a mixture of oxidizing species produced from the electrolysis of saline. The main products are hypochlorous acid (144 mg/L) and free chlorine radicals. The antimicrobial activity is rapid against a wide range of microorganisms in the absence of organic matter.

4 Disinfection policies

The aim of a disinfection policy is to control the use of chemicals for disinfection and antisepsis and give guidelines on their use. The preceding descriptions within this chapter of the activities, advantages and disadvantages of the many disinfectants available allow considerable scope for choice and inclusion of agents in a policy to be applied to such areas as industrial plant, walls, ceilings, floors, air, cleaning equipment and laundries and to the extensive range of equipment in contact with hospital patients.

The control of microorganisms is of prime importance in hospital and industrial environments. Where pharmaceutical products (either sterile or non-sterile) are manufactured, contamination of the product may lead to its deterioration and to infection in the user. In hospital there is the additional consideration of patient care; therefore protection from nosocomial (hospital-acquired) infection and prevention of cross-infection must also be covered. Hospitals generally have a disinfection policy, although the degree of adherence to, and implementation of, the policy content can vary. A specialized Infection Control Committee comprising the pharmacist, the consultant medical microbiologist and senior nurse responsible for infection control should formulate a suitable policy. This core team may usefully be expanded to include, for example, a physician, a surgeon, nurse teachers and nurses from several clinical areas, the sterile services manager and the domestic superintendent. Purchasing may also be represented. This expanded committee will meet regularly to help with the implementation of the policy and reassess its efficiency. Reference to Tables 17.2–17.4 indicates the susceptibility of various microorganisms to the range of agents available and Table 17.5 presents examples of the range of formulations and uses. Although scope exists for choice of disinfectant in many of the areas covered by a policy, in certain instances specific recommendations are made as to the type, concentration and usage of disinfectant.

Categories of risk (to patients) may be assigned to equipment coming into contact with a patient, dictating the level of decontamination required and degree of concern. *High-risk* items have close contact with broken skin or mucous membrane or are those introduced into a sterile area of the body and should therefore be sterile. These include sterile instruments, gloves, catheters, syringes and needles. Liquid chemical disinfectants should only be used if heat or other methods of sterilization are unsuitable. *Intermediate-risk items* are in close contact with skin or mucous membranes and disinfection will normally be applied. Endoscopes, respiratory and anaesthetic equipment, wash bowls, bed-pans and similar items are included in this category. *Low-risk items* or areas include those detailed earlier such as walls, floors, etc., which are not in close contact with the patient. Cleaning is obviously important with disinfection being required, for example, in the event of contaminated spillage.

5 Further reading

Alvarado, C. J. & Reichelderfer, M. (2000) APIC guideline for infection prevention and control in flexible endoscopy. *Am J Infect Control,* 28, 138–155.

Ayliffe, G. A. J., Coates, D. & Hoffman, P. N. (1993) *Chemical Disinfection in Hospitals.* Public Health Laboratory Service, London.

British Medical Association (1989) *A Code of Practice for Sterilisation of Instruments and Control of Cross Infection.* BMA (Board of Science and Education), London.

British Standards Institution (1986) *Terms Relating to Disinfectants.* BS 5283: 1986 Glossary. Section one. British Standards Institution, London.

Block, S. S. (2001) *Disinfection, Sterilisation and Preservation,* 5th edn. Lippincott Williams & Wilkins, Philadelphia and London.

Coates, D. & Hutchinson, D. N. (1994) How to produce a hospital disinfection policy. *J Hosp Infect,* 26, 57–68.

Control of Substances Hazardous to Health (COSHH) Regulations (1999) (SI 437 1999) ISBN 0 11 082087 8.

Eggers, H. J. (1990) Experiments on antiviral activity of hand disinfectants. Some theoretical and practical considerations. *Zentralbl Bakteriol,* 273, 36–51.

Health and Safety Executive (1996) *Occupational Exposure Limits* EH40/96. Health and Safety Executive, Sheffield.

Holton, J., Nye, P. & McDonald, V. (1994) Efficacy of selected disinfectants against Mycobacteria and Cryptosporidia. *J Hosp Infect,* 27, 105–115.

Russell, A. D. (1990) Bacterial spores and chemical sporicidal agents. *Clin Microbiol Rev,* 3, 99–119.

Russell, A. D. (1996) Activity of biocides against mycobacteria. *J Appl Bacteriol,* 81, 87S-101S.

Russell, A. D., Hugo, W. B. & Ayliffe, G. A. J. (1999) In: *Principles and Practice of Disinfection, Preservation and Sterilisation,* 3rd edn. Blackwell Science, Oxford:.

Rutala, W.A. (1996) APIC guideline for selection and use of disinfectants. *Am J Infect Control,* 24, 313–342.

Scott, E. M., Gorman, S. P. & McGrath, S. J. (1986) An assessment of the fungicidal activity of antimicrobial agents used for hard-surface and skin disinfection. *J Clin Hosp Pharm,* 11, 199–205.

Sterilization, Disinfection and Cleaning of Medical Equipment: Guidance on Decontamination from the Microbiology Advisory Committee to Department of Health Medical Devices Directorate. Part 1 Principles (1993) HMSO.

Traore, O., Springthorpe, V .S. & Sattar, S. A. (2002) Testing chemical germicides against *Candida* species using quantitative carrier and fingerpad methods. *J Hosp Infect,* 50, 66–75.

van Bueren, J., Salman, H. & Cookson, B. D. (1995) The efficacy of thirteen chemical disinfectants against Human Immunodeficiency Virus (HIV). Medical Devices Agency Evaluation Report.

Chapter 18

Non-antibiotic antibacterial agents: mode of action and resistance

Stephen Denyer and A Denver Russell

1 Introduction

This group of drugs which comprises antiseptics, disinfectants and preservatives (often collectively termed biocides) have frequently been classified as non-specific protoplasmic poisons, and indeed such views are still sometimes expressed today. Such a broad generalization is, however, very far from the true position.

It is convenient to consider the modes of action in terms of the biocides' targets within the bacterial cell, and in the following pages various examples will be given; the targets to be considered are the cell wall, the cytoplasmic membrane and the cytoplasm. The range and complexity of the reactions involved will become apparent from this account and from Table 18.1 and Fig. 18.1, and it is worth emphasizing here that many of these substances exhibit concentration-dependent dual or even multiple roles. Much more detailed treatments of the subject will be found in the Further reading section at the end of this chapter. Experimental methods for determining the mode of action of an antimicrobial substance have been compiled (Denyer & Hugo, 1991).

For a chemical to exhibit antimicrobial activity it

Table 18.1 Cellular targets for non-antibiotic antibacterial drugs

Target or reaction attacked	Acridine dyes	Alcohols	Anilides (TCS, TCC)	Bronopol	Chlorhexidine	Copper II salts	Ethylene oxide	Formaldehyde	Glutaraldehyde	Hexachlorophane	Hydrogen peroxide	Hypochlorites, chlorine releasers	Iodine	Mercury II salts, mercurials organic	Phenols	β-Propiolactone	QACS	Silver salts	Sulphur dioxide, sulphites	Iso-thiazolones
1 Cell wall																				
2 Cytoplasmic membrane		+						+	+			+		+	+					
2.1 Action on membrane potentials			+																	
2.2 Action on membrane enzymes										+					+					
2.2.1 Electron transport chain						+				+										
2.2.2 Adenosine triphosphatase				+			+													
2.2.3 Enzymes with thiol groups							+		+		+	+	+	+		+		+	+	+
2.3 Action on general membrane permeability		+	+		+												+			
3 Cytoplasm																				
3.1 General coagulation					+++	++			++	+++				+++	++					
3.2 Ribosomes						+++								+	+++		+++	+++		
3.3 Nucleic acids	+										+									
3.4 Thiol groups				+		+	+		+		+	+	+	+		+		+		+
3.5 Amino groups							+	++	+			+	+			+			+	
4 High reactive compounds: multitarget reactors							+	+	+			+				+				

Crosses, indicating activity, which appear in several rows for a given compound, demonstrate the multiple actions for the compound concerned. This activity is nearly always concentration-dependent, and the number of crosses indicates the order of concentration at which the effect is elicited, i.e. +, elicited at low concentrations; +++, elicited at high concentrations.

When a cross appears in only one target row, this is the only known site of action of the drug.

QAC, quaternary ammonium compound.

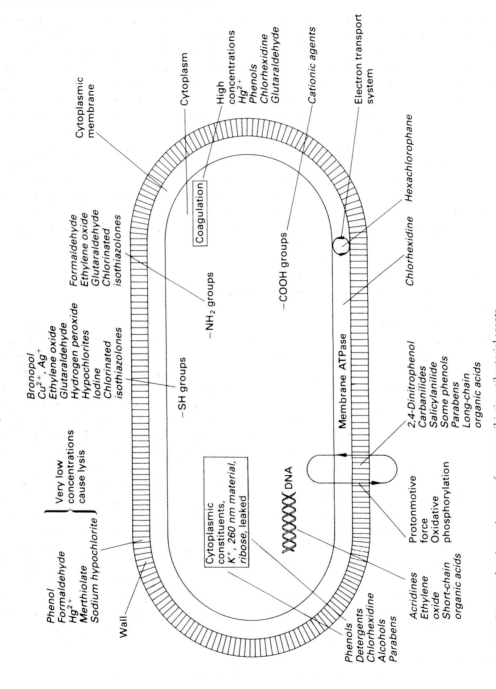

Fig. 18.1 Diagram showing main targets for non-antibiotic antibacterial agents.

usually has to undergo a sequence of events that begins with adsorption onto the cell surface. In the many cases where the chemical has an intracellular site of action, adsorption must be followed by passage through porin channels in Gram-negative cells (Chapter 3, section 2.2.1), diffusion across, or into, the lipid-rich cytoplasmic membrane, and finally, interaction with proteins, enzymes, nucleic acids or other targets within the cytoplasm. These processes are markedly influenced by the physicochemical characteristics of the biocide, e.g. ionization constant and lipid solubility, so the wide diversity of structures exhibited by biocide molecules (Chapter 17) complicates the prediction of antimicrobial potency and explanation of their mechanisms of action. Despite this, it is important to recognize that there is a basis upon which the mode of action might be deduced, because there are certain molecular features of biocides that are associated with activity against particular cellular targets.

Antimicrobial activity is often strongly influenced by the affinity of the biocide for structural or molecular components of the cell, and this, in turn, may depend upon the attraction of dissimilar charges or on hydrophobic interactions. Antimicrobial drugs whose active species is positively charged, e.g. quaternary ammonium compounds and chlorhexidine, display an affinity for the negative charges of sugar residues on the microbial cell surface or phosphate groups on the membrane(s); adsorption of these biocides, and thus their antimicrobial activity, is increased as the pH rises and the cell surface becomes more electronegative. Antimicrobial chemicals possessing a long alkyl chain on the other hand may integrate into the hydrophobic region of phospholipid molecules within the membrane and so cause membrane disruption and fatal permeability changes. Further examples of structure–activity relationships are afforded by the aldehydes, particularly glutaraldehyde, which is an electrophile that is able to react with molecules possessing thiol (SH) or amino groups, e.g. proteins. This reaction, too, increases with pH, so aldehydes are more active in alkaline conditions. Biocides containing heavy metal ions, e.g. silver or phenylmercury, also inactivate enzymes and structural proteins by virtue of interactions with thiol groups. A number of phenols and bisphenols incorporate a hydroxyl group that is capable of generating a labile proton, i.e. they are weak acids. A weakly acidic nature combined with significant lipid solubility are properties associated with uncoupling agents, i.e. those molecules that can disrupt the proton-motive force that is responsible for oxidative phosphorylation in the cell. It is thought that these molecules dissolve in the lipid bilayer of the membrane and act as proton conductors by virtue of their ionizability (section 3.1). This property, possessed by biocides like phenoxyethanol and fentichlor, results in the failure of many important energy-requiring processes in the cell, including the concentration and retention of sugars and amino acids.

2 Cell wall

This structure is the traditional target for a group of antibiotics which includes the penicillins (Chapter 10), but a little-noticed report which appeared in 1948 showed that low concentrations of disinfectant substances caused cell wall lysis such that a normally turbid suspension of bacteria became clear. It was thought that these low concentrations of disinfectant cause enzymes whose normal role is to synthesize the cell wall to reverse their role in some way and effect its disruption or lysis.

In the original report, the disinfectants (at the following percentages: formalin, 0.12; phenol, 0.32; mercuric chloride, 0.0008; sodium hypochlorite, 0.005 and merthiolate, 0.0004) caused lysis of *Escherichia coli*, streptococci and staphylococci.

Glutaraldehyde also owes part of its mode of action to its ability to react with, and provide irreversible cross-linking in, the cell wall. As a result, other cell functions are impaired. This phenomenon is especially found in Gram-positive cells.

3 Cytoplasmic membrane

Actions on the cytoplasmic membrane may be divided into three categories.
1 Action on membrane potentials.
2 Action on membrane enzymes.
3 Action on general membrane permeability.

3.1 Action on membrane potentials

Recent work has shown that bacteria, in common with chloroplasts and mitochondria, are able, through the membrane-bound electron transport chain aerobically, or the membrane-bound adenosine triphosphate (ATP) anaerobically, to maintain a gradient of electrical potential and pH such that the interior of the bacterial cell is negative and alkaline. This potential gradient and the electrical equivalent of the pH difference (1 pH unit = 58 mV at 37°C) give a potential difference across the membrane of 100–180 mV, with the inside negative. The membrane is impermeable to protons, whose extrusion creates the potential described.

These results may be expressed in the form of an equation, thus:

$$\Delta\rho = \Delta\psi - Z\Delta pH$$

where $\Delta\rho$ is the proton-motive force, $\Delta\psi$ the membrane electrical potential and ΔpH the transmembrane pH gradient, i.e. the pH difference between the inside and outside of the cytoplasmic membrane. Z is a factor converting pH units to millivolts so that all the units of the equation are the same, i.e. millivolts. Z is temperature-dependent and at 37°C has a value of 62.

This potential, or proton-motive force as it is also called, in turn drives a number of energy-requiring functions which include the synthesis of ATP, the coupling of oxidative processes to phosphorylation, a metabolic sequence called oxidative phosphorylation and the transport and concentration in the cell of metabolites such as sugars and amino acids. This, in a few simple words, is the basis of the chemiosmotic theory linking metabolism to energy-requiring processes.

Certain chemical substances have been known for many years to uncouple oxidation from phosphorylation and to inhibit active transport, and for this reason they are named uncoupling agents. They are believed to act by rendering the membrane permeable to protons, hence short-circuiting the potential gradient or proton-motive force.

Some examples of antibacterial agents which owe at least a part of their activity to this ability are tetrachlorosalicylanilide (TCS), tricarbanilide, trichlorocarbanilide (TCC), pentachlorophenol, di-(5-chloro-2-hydroxyphenyl) sulphide (fentichlor) and 2-phenoxyethanol.

3.2 Action on membrane enzymes

3.2.1 Electron transport chain

Hexachlorophane inhibits the electron transport chain in bacteria and thus will inhibit all metabolic activities in aerobic bacteria.

3.2.2 Adenosine triphosphatase

Chlorhexidine has been shown to inhibit the membrane ATPase and could thus inhibit anaerobic processes.

3.2.3 Enzymes with thiol groups

Mercuric chloride, other mercury-containing antibacterials and silver will inhibit enzymes in the membrane, and for that matter in the cytoplasm, which contain thiol, -SH, groups. A similar action is shown by 2-bromo-2-nitropropan-1,3-diol (bronopol) and *iso*-thiazolones. Under appropriate conditions the toxic action on cell thiol groups may be reversed by addition of an extrinsic thiol compound, e.g. cysteine or thioglycollic acid (see also Chapter 20). Particularly susceptible enzymes are the dehydrogenases involved in membrane-associated redox processes.

3.3 Action on general membrane permeability

This lesion was recognized early as being one effect of many disinfectant substances. The membrane, as well as providing a dynamic link between metabolism and transport, serves to maintain the pool of metabolites within it.

Treatment of bacterial cells with appropriate concentrations of such substances as cetrimide, chlorhexidine, phenol and hexylresorcinol causes a leakage of a group of characteristic chemical species. The potassium ion, being a small entity, is the first substance to appear when the cytoplasmic membrane is damaged. Amino acids, purines, pyrimidines and pentoses are examples of other substances which will leak from treated cells.

If the action of the drug is not prolonged or exerted in high concentration the damage may be reversible and leakage may only induce bacteriostasis.

3.3.1 Permeabilization

Drugs able to affect outer-membrane integrity have also been exploited as potentiators of antimicrobial agents (biocides, i.e. disinfectants, antiseptics and preservatives, and antibiotics) thereby helping these to penetrate the outer membrane of Gram-negative organisms and especially *Pseudomonas aeruginosa*.

Chelators, particularly ethylenediamine tetra-acetic acid (EDTA), have been used as potentiators of the action of chloroxylenol. Vaara has extensively reviewed the subject of permeabilization and Ayres, Furr and Russell have described a rapid method of evaluating the permeabilization of *Ps. aeruginosa* (see Further reading section).

4 Cytoplasm

Within the cytoplasm are a number of important subcellular particles, which include the ribosome and oxy- and deoxyribonucleic acids. Enzymes other than those in the membrane are also present in the cytoplasm.

Many early studies measured overall enzyme inhibition in bacterial cultures and a search was made for a peculiarly sensitive enzyme which might be identified as a target, interference with which would cause death. No such enzyme has been found.

4.1 General coagulation

High concentrations of disinfectants, e.g. chlorhexidine, phenol or mercury salts, will coagulate the cytoplasm and in fact it was this kind of reaction which gave rise to the epithet 'general protoplasmic poison', already referred to, providing an uncritical and dismissive definition of the mode of action of disinfectants. There is little doubt, however, that the disinfectants in use in the 1930s had just this effect when applied at high concentrations.

4.2 Ribosomes

These organelles, the sites of protein synthesis, are well-established targets for antibiotic action.

Both hydrogen peroxide and *p*-chloromercuribenzoate will dissociate the ribosome into its two constituent parts but whether this is a secondary reaction of the two chemicals is difficult to assess. There is no real evidence that the ribosome is a prime target for disinfectant substances.

4.3 Nucleic acids

Acridine dyes used as antiseptics, i.e. proflavine and acriflavine, will react specifically with nucleic acids, by fitting into the double helical structure of this unique molecule. In so doing they interfere with its function and can thereby cause cell death. There is evidence that a depletion of intracellular potassium caused by membrane damage can lead to the activation of latent ribonucleases and the consequent breakdown of RNA. Several biocides, including cetrimide and some phenols, are known to cause the release of nucleotides and nucleosides following an autolytic process. This is irreversible and has been proposed as an autocidal (suicide) process, committing the injured cell to death (Denyer & Stewart, 1998).

4.4 Thiol groups

Mention has been made of thiol groups in the cytoplasmic membrane as targets for certain antibacterial compounds. Thiol groups also occur in the cytoplasm and these groups will also serve as targets.

Bronopol, *iso*-thiazolones, chlorine, chlorine-releasing agents, hypochlorites and iodine will oxidize or react with thiol groups.

4.5 Amino groups

Formaldehyde, sulphur dioxide and glutaraldehyde react with amino groups. If these groups are essential for metabolic activity, cell death will follow reactions of this nature. Chlorinated *iso*-thiazolones as well as acting on –SH groups (section 4.4) can react with –NH$_2$ groups.

5 Highly reactive compounds: multitarget reactors

There are one or two chemical sterilants in use whose chemical reactivity is so high that they have a very wide spectrum of cell interactions and it is difficult to pinpoint the fatal reaction. In fact, it is safe to say that there is no single fatal reaction but that death results from the accumulated effects of many reactions; one or two specific reactions of compounds in this category have already been referred to.

β-Propiolactone is one example. It will alkylate amino, imino, hydroxyl and carboxyl groups, all of which occur in proteins, and react also with thiol and disulphide groups responsible for the secondary structure of proteins and the activity of some enzymes. Another example is ethylene oxide, which has a very similar range of chemical activity.

Sulphur dioxide, sulphites and bisulphites, used as preservatives in fruit juices, ciders and perrys are yet other examples.

6 Relative microbial responses to biocides

Different types of microbes show varying responses to biocides. This is demonstrated clearly in Table 18.2. Additionally, it must be noted that Gram-positive bacteria such as staphylococci and streptococci are generally more sensitive to biocides than are Gram-negative bacteria. Enterococci are frequently antibiotic-resistant, but are not necessarily more resistant to biocides than streptococci. Methicillin-resistant *Staphylococcus aureus* (MRSA) strains are rather more resistant to biocides, especially cationic ones, than methicillin-sensitive *Staph. aureus* (MSSA) strains. Among Gram-negative bacteria, the most marked resistance is shown by *Pseudomonas aeruginosa*, *Providencia stuartii* and *Proteus* species.

Mycobacteria are more resistant than other non-sporulating bacteria to a wide range of biocides. Examples of such organisms are *Mycobacterium tuberculosis*, the *M. avium intracellulare* (MAI) group and *M. chelonae* (*M. chelonei*). Of the bacteria, however, the most resistant of all to biocides are bacterial spores, e.g. *Bacillus subtilis*, *B. cereus*.

Moulds and yeasts show varying responses to biocides. Various types of protozoa are potentially pathogenic and inactivation by biocides may be problematic. Viral response to biocides depends upon the type and structure of the virus particle and on the nature of the biocide.

The most resistant of all infectious agents to chemical inactivation are the prions, which cause transmissible degenerative encephalopathies.

7 Bacterial resistance to biocides: general mechanisms

Bacterial resistance to biocides (Table 18.3) is usually considered as being of two types: (a) intrinsic (innate, natural), a natural property of an organism, or (b) acquired, either by chromosomal mutation or by the acquisition of plasmids or transposons. Intrinsic resistance to biocides is usually demonstrated by Gram-negative bacteria, mycobacteria and bacterial spores, whereas acquired resistance can result by mutation or, more frequently, by the acquisition of genetic elements, e.g. plasmid (or transposon)-mediated resistance to mercury compounds. Intrinsic resistance may also be exemplified by physiological (phenotypic) adaptation, a classical example of which is biofilm formation.

Table 18.2 Comparative responses of microorganisms to biocides

Type of microorganism	Biocide susceptibility or resistance
Bacteria	Non-sporing most susceptible, acid-fast bacteria intermediate, spores most resistant
Fungi	Fungal spores may be resistant
Viruses	Non-enveloped more resistant than enveloped
Parasites	Coccidia may be highly resistant
Prions	Usually highly resistant

Table 18.3 Intrinsic and acquired bacterial resistance to biocides

Distinguishing feature	Intrinsic resistance	Acquired resistance
General property	Natural property	Achieved by mutation or by acquisition of plasmid or transposon (Tn)
Mechanisms*		
(1) Alteration of biocide (enzymatic inactivation)	Chromosomally mediated, but not usually significant	Plasmid/Tn-mediated, e.g. mercurials
(2) Impaired uptake	Applies to several biocides	Less important
(3) Efflux	Not known	Cationic biocides and antibiotic-resistant staphylococci
Biofilm production	Phenotypic adaptation	Plasmid transfer may occur within biofilms
Pharmaceutical/clinical significance	High	Could be high in certain circumstances

* See Table 18.5 for additional information.

8 Intrinsic bacterial resistance

As already pointed out, staphylococci and strepto-cocci are generally more sensitive to biocides than Gram-negative bacteria; examples are provided in Table 18.4. On the other hand, mycobacteria and especially bacterial spores are much more resistant. A major reason for this variation in response is associated with the chemical composition and structure of the outer cell layers such that there is restricted uptake of a biocide. In consequence of this cellular impermeability, a reduced concentration of the antimicrobial compound is available at the target site(s) so that the cell may escape severe injury. Another, less frequently observed, mechanism is the presence of constitutive, biocide-degrading enzymes.

Intrinsic resistance may then be defined as a natural, chromosomally controlled property of a bacterial cell that enables it to circumvent the action of a biocide (see Table 18.3). A summary of intrinsic resistance mechanisms is provided in Table 18.5.

8.1 Gram-positive cocci

The cell wall of staphylococci is composed essentially of peptidoglycan and teichoic acids. Substances of high molecular weight can traverse the wall, a ready explanation for the sensitivity of these organisms to most biocides. However, the plasticity of the bacterial cell envelope is well known and the

Table 18.4 Sensitivity of microorganisms to chlorhexidine

Organism	Minimum inhibitory concentration *(µg/ml)
Gram-negative bacteria	
Pseudomonas aeruginosa	10–500
Proteus mirabilis	25–100
Burkholderia cepacia	5–100
Serratia marcescens	3–50
Salmonella typhimurium	14
Klebsiella aerogenes	1–12
Escherichia coli	1–5
Gram-positive bacteria	
Staphylococcus aureus	1–2
Enterococcus faecalis	1–3
Bacillus subtilis	1–3
Streptococcus mutans	0.1
Mycobacterium tuberculosis	0.7–6
Fungi	
Candida albicans	7–15
Trichophyton mentagrophytes	3
Penicillium notatum	200

* The minimum inhibitory concentration (MIC) is the lowest concentration of an antimicrobial agent that prevents growth. The lower the MIC value, the more active the agent.

growth rate and any growth-limiting nutrient will affect the physiological state of the cells. The thickness and degree of cross-linking of peptidoglycan may be modified and hence the sensitivity of the cells to antibacterial agents. Likewise 'fattened'

313

Table 18.5 Examples of intrinsic resistance mechanisms to biocides in bacteria

Type of resistance	Bacteria	Mechanism	Examples
Impermeability	Gram-negative	OM barrier	QACs, diamidines
	Mycobacteria	Waxy cell wall	QACs, chlorhexidine, organomercurials
	Bacterial spores	Spore coats and cortex	QACs, chlorhexidine, organomercurials, phenols
	Other Gram-positive	Phenotypic adaptation	Chlorhexidine
Enzymatic	Gram-negative	Chemical inactivation	Chlorhexidine

OM, outer membrane; QAC, quaternary ammonium compound.

cells of *Staph. aureus* which have been trained in the laboratory to contain much higher levels of cell wall lipid than normal cells, are less sensitive to higher phenols. Normally, staphylococci contain little or no cell wall lipid and consequently the lipid-enriched cells represent physiologically adapted cells that offer intrinsic resistance to certain biocidal agents.

8.2 Gram-negative bacteria

8.2.1 Enterobacteriaceae

8.2.1.1 Outer membrane as a permeability barrier
EDTA greatly enhances the permeability and sensitivity of the Enterobacteriaceae towards antimicrobial agents. By binding metal ions such as magnesium, which is essential for the stability of the outer membrane, EDTA releases 30–50% of the lipopolysaccharide (LPS) from the outer membrane together with some phospholipid and protein. The permeability barrier is effectively removed and the cells, which retain their viability, then become sensitive to large hydrophobic antibiotics such as fucidin and rifampicin against which they are normally resistant. This phenomenon extends to non-antibiotic agents such as the quaternary ammonium agents and esters of *p*-aminobenzoic acid (parabens; Chapter 17). More complete removal of the outer membrane and peptidoglycan with EDTA and lysozyme (a muramidase enzyme which degrades peptidoglycan) produces spheroplasts in Gram-negative bacteria. These osmotically fragile, but viable, cells are equivalent to protoplasts of Gram-positive bacteria, which are cells where the wall has been completely removed with lysozyme.

Both spheroplasts and protoplasts are equally sensitive to lysis by membrane-active agents such as quaternary ammonium compounds (QACs), phenols and chlorhexidine. This demonstrates that the difference in sensitivities of whole cells to these agents is not due to a difference in sensitivity of the target cytoplasmic membrane but in the different permeability properties of the overlying wall or envelope structures.

The outer membrane of Gram-negative bacteria plays an important role in limiting exposure of susceptible target sites to antibiotics and biocides. Thus, Gram-negative bacteria are usually less sensitive to many more antibacterial agents than Gram-positive organisms. This is particularly marked with inhibitors such as hexachlorophane, diamidines, QACs and some lipophilic acids.

The hydrated nature of amino acid residues lining the porin channels presents an energetically unfavourable barrier to the passage of hydrophobic molecules. In rough strains, the reduction in the amount of polysaccharide on the cell surface allows hydrophobic molecules to approach more closely the surface of the outer membrane and cross the outer membrane lipid bilayer by passive diffusion. This process is greatly facilitated in deep rough and heptose-less strains which have phospholipid molecules on the outer face of their outer membranes as well as on the inner face. The exposed areas of phospholipids favour the absorption and penetration of the hydrophobic agents.

Two pathways can be envisaged for penetration of antibacterial agents across the outer membrane:
1 hydrophilic, which is porin-mediated;
2 hydrophobic, involving diffusion.

This picture holds for all Gram-negative bacteria. It is especially important for the Enterobacteri-aceae which survive the antibacterial action of hydrophobic bile salts and fatty acids in the gut by the combined effects of the penetration barrier of their smooth LPS and the small size of their porin channels (which restricts passage of hydrophilic molecules to those of molecular weight < 650). By contrast, an organism like *Neisseria gonorrhoeae*, which does not produce an O-antigen polysaccha-ride on its LPS and is naturally rough, is very sensi-tive to hydrophobic molecules. Natural fatty acids help to defend the body against these organisms.

Cationic biocides which have strong surface-active properties and which attack the inner (cyto-plasmic) membrane, e.g. chlorhexidine and QACs, also damage the outer membrane and thus are be-lieved to mediate their own uptake into the cells. However, the QACs are considerably less active against wild-type than against deep rough strains of *Escherichia coli* and *Salmonella typhimurium*. It is clear, then, that the outer membrane must act as a permeability barrier against these compounds.

Studies with porin-deficient mutants of many Gram-negative species have confirmed that deter-gents do not use the porin channels to gain access to the cytoplasmic membrane. Porin-deficient strains in general show no difference in sensitivity to deter-gents compared with their parent strains, even though the permeability of their outer membrane to small hydrophilic molecules is reduced up to 100-fold. Other mutations affecting the stability of the outer membrane, such as loss of the lipoprotein which anchors it to the peptidoglycan, are asso-ciated with extreme sensitivity to membrane-active agents. Some mutants of *E. coli* are highly perme-able and sensitive to a wide range of antimicrobial agents, but have no major defect in envelope com-position. The explanation presumably lies in the way the individual components are organized in the envelope. As components are not covalently linked together, ionic interactions mediated by divalent metal ions play an important part in maintaining the integrity of the outer membrane.

Hospital isolates of *Serratia marcescens* may be highly resistant to chlorhexidine, hexachlorophane liquid soaps and detergent creams. The outer mem-brane probably determines this resistance to biocides.

Members of the genus *Proteus* are unusually re-sistant to high concentrations of chlorhexidine and other cationic biocides and are more resistant to EDTA than most other types of Gram-negative bac-teria. A less acidic type of LPS may be responsible for reduced binding of, and hence increased resis-tance to, cationic biocides. Decreased susceptibility to EDTA may result from the reduced divalent cation content of the *Proteus* outer membrane.

8.2.1.2 Efflux of biocides

Efflux is effectively the removal of an intracellular level of a biocide that would otherwise prove toxic to a bacterial cell. However, this has to be consid-ered in the context of the actual concentration of biocide used. Whilst low levels of a biocide may be pumped out of a cell, at higher concentrations a competition would ensue between the damage in-flicted on that cell and an efflux pump attempting to remove the toxic element. Under such circum-stances, inactivation of the organism would occur rather than removal of the biocide.

Efflux may be both an intrinsic and acquired resistance mechanism.

8.2.2 Pseudomonads

Pseudomonas aeruginosa is notorious for its ability to survive in the environment, particularly in moist conditions. It is a dangerous contaminant of medi-cines, surgical equipment, clothing and dressings, with the ability to cause serious infections in immunocompromised patients. The intrinsic resistance of Gram-negative bacteria is especially apparent with *Ps. aeruginosa*; many disinfectants and preservatives possess insufficient activity against it to be of any use. Added to the problem of natural resistance to antimicrobials is the organ-ism's extensive repertoire of phenotypic variation.

The basis of the greater resistance of *Ps. aerugi-nosa* compared with other Gram-negative bacteria (see Table 18.4) is probably due, at least in part, to the properties of the envelope because when this is removed, the resulting spheroplasts are just as sen-sitive as those of other organisms. The outer mem-brane is not significantly different from that of other organisms in terms of overall composition with the same components (LPS, proteins, phospholipid and peptidoglycan) being present. However, one difference is the number of phosphate groups present in the lipid A region of the LPS. This is significantly higher in *Ps. aeruginosa* than in members of the Enterobacteriaceae and might account for the unusual sensitivity of the organism to EDTA. The high phosphate content means that the outer membrane is unusually dependent upon divalent metal ions for stability; their removal by EDTA therefore has a dramatic effect upon cell wall integrity. Magnesium-depleted cells of *Ps. aeruginosa* are extremely resistant to EDTA. Presumably the lower magnesium content of the cell envelope reflects a decreased phosphorylation of lipid A. Other effects follow from magnesium depletion, including complex changes in lipid composition and increased production of an outer-membrane protein known as H1, which is believed to replace magnesium ions in binding together LPS molecules on the cell surface.

Biocide efflux must also be considered in the pseudomonads. For example, one mechanism of resistance of *Ps. aeruginosa* to the bisphenol triclosan involves an active efflux pump.

Burkholderia (formerly *Pseudomonas*) *cepacia* is intrinsically resistant to a number of biocides, notably benzalkonium chloride and chlorhexidine. Again, the outer membrane is likely to act as a permeability barrier. By contrast, *Ps. stutzeri* (an organism implicated in eye infections caused by some cosmetic products) is invariably intrinsically sensitive to a range of biocides, including QACs and chlorhexidine. This organism contains less wall muramic acid than other pseudomonads but it is unclear as to whether this could be a contributory factor in its enhanced biocide susceptibility.

8.3 Mycobacteria

Mycobacteria consist of a fairly diverse group of acid-fast bacteria. The best-known members are *M. tuberculosis* and *M. leprae*, the causative agents of tuberculosis and leprosy, respectively. Other mycobacteria can also cause serious infection, e.g. members of the MAI group, and there are many opportunistic species.

Mycobacteria show a high level of resistance to inactivation by biguanides (e.g. chlorhexidine), QACs and organomercurials. Phenols may or may not be mycobactericidal. Alkaline glutaraldehyde exerts a lethal effect but more slowly than against other non-sporulating bacteria, but MAI is more resistant than *M. tuberculosis*. Recently, glutaraldehyde-resistant *M. chelonae* strains have been isolated from endoscope washers. These strains remain sensitive to a new disinfectant used in endoscopy, the aromatic dialdehyde *ortho*-phthalaldehyde.

The mycobacterial cell wall is highly hydrophobic, with a mycoylarabinogalactanpeptidoglycan skeleton composed of two covalently linked polymers, an arabinagalactan mycolate (mycolic acid, D-arabinose and D-galactose) and a peptidoglycan containing *N*-glycomuramic acid instead of *N*-acetylmuramic acid. The mycolic acids have an important role to play in reducing cell wall permeability to hydrophilic molecules. However, porins are present which are similar to those found in *Ps. aeruginosa* cell envelopes so that only low molecular weight hydrophilic substances can enter the cell via this route.

Overall, the mechanisms involved in the role of the mycobacterial cell wall as a permeability barrier are poorly understood and it is not known why MAI and *M. chelonae*, in particular, are more resistant than other species of mycobacteria.

8.4 Bacterial spores

Bacterial spores of the genera *Bacillus* and *Clostridium* are invariably the most resistant of all types of bacteria to biocides. Many biocides, e.g. biguanides and QACs, will kill (or at low concentrations be bacteriostatic to) non-sporulating bacteria but not bacterial spores. Other biocides such as alkaline glutaraldehyde are sporicidal, although higher concentrations for longer contact periods may be necessary than for a bactericidal effect.

8.4.1 Spore structure

A typical bacterial spore has several components (Chapter 3, see Fig. 3.7). The germ cell (protoplast or core) and germ cell wall are surrounded by the cortex, external to which are the inner and outer spore coats. An exosporium is present in some spores but may surround just one spore coat. The protoplast is the location of RNA, DNA, dipicolinic acid (DPA) and most of the calcium, potassium, manganese and phosphorus present in the spore. Also present are substantial amounts of low molecular weight basic proteins, the small acid-soluble spore proteins (SASPs, see below) which are rapidly degraded during germination. The cortex consists largely of peptidoglycan, some 45–60% of the muramic acid residues not having either a peptide or an N-acetyl substituent but instead forming an internal amide known as muramic lactam. The cortical membrane (germ cell wall, primordial cell wall) is a dense inner layer of the cortex that develops into the cell wall of the emergent cell when the cortex is degraded during germination. Two membranes, the inner and outer forespore membranes, surround the forespore during germination. The inner forespore membrane eventually becomes the cytoplasmic membrane of the germinating spore, whereas the outer forespore membrane persists in the spore integuments.

The spore coats make up a major portion of the spore, consisting mainly of protein with smaller amounts of complex carbohydrates and lipid and possibly large amounts of phosphorus. The outer spore coat contains the alkali-resistant protein fraction and is associated with the presence of disulphide-rich bonds. The alkali-soluble fraction is found in the inner spore coats and consists predominantly of acidic polypeptides which can be dissociated to their unit components by treatment with sodium dodecyl sulphate.

8.4.2 Spore development (sporulation) and resistance

Response to a biocide depends upon the cellular stage of development. Sporulation, a process in which a bacterial spore develops from a vegetative cell, involves seven stages (I–VII; Chapter 3); of these, stages IV–VII (cortex and coat development) are the most important in relation to the development of biocide resistance. Resistance to biocidal agents develops during sporulation and may be an early, intermediate or late/very late event. For example, resistance to chlorhexidine occurs at an intermediate stage, at about the same time as heat

resistance, whereas decreasing susceptibility to glutaraldehyde is a very late event.

8.4.3 Mature spores and resistance

Spore coatless forms, produced by treatment of spores under alkaline conditions with UDS (urea plus dithiothreitol plus sodium lauryl sulphate), have been of value in estimating the role of the coats in limiting access of biocides to their target sites. However, this treatment removes a certain amount of spore cortex also. The amount of cortex remaining can be further reduced by subsequent use of lysozyme. The spore coats have an undoubted role to play in conferring resistance of spores to biocides. The cortex also acts as a barrier to some extent.

SASPs, comprising about 10–20% of the protein in the dormant spore, exist in two forms (α/β and γ) and are degraded during germination. They are essential for expression of spore resistance to ultraviolet radiation and also appear to be involved in resistance to some biocides, e.g. hydrogen peroxide. Spores (α^-/β^-) deficient in α/β-type SASPs are much more peroxide-sensitive than are wild-type (normal) spores. It has been proposed that in wild-type spores DNA is saturated with α/β-type SASPs and is thus protected from free radical damage.

8.4.4 Germination, outgrowth and susceptibility

During germination and/or outgrowth, cells regain their sensitivity to antibacterial agents. Some inhibitors act at the germination stage (e.g. phenolics, parabens), whereas others such as chlorhexidine and the QACs do not affect germination but inhibit outgrowth. Glutaraldehyde, at low concentrations, is an effective inhibitor of both stages. During germination, several degradative changes occur in the spore, e.g. loss of dry weight, decrease in optical density, loss of dipicolinic acid, increase in stainability, increase in oxygen consumption, whereas biosynthetic processes (RNA, DNA, protein, cell wall syntheses) become apparent during outgrowth.

Table 18.6 Examples of acquired resistance mechanisms to biocides in bacteria

Type of resistance	Bacteria	Mechanism	Examples
Enzymatic	Gram-positive*	Plasmid/Tn-encoded inactivation	Mercury compounds
	Gram-negative		Mercury compounds, formaldehyde
Impaired uptake	Gram-negative	Plasmid-encoded porin modification	QACs
Efflux	Gram-positive*	Plasmid-encoded expulsion from cells	QACs
			Chlorhexidine?

QAC, quaternary ammonium compound.
* Non-mycobacterial, non-sporing bacteria.

8.5 Physiological (phenotypic) adaptation to intrinsic resistance

Bacteria grown under different conditions may show wide response to biocides. For example, fattened cells of Staph. aureus obtained by repeated subculturing in glycerol-containing media are more resistant to benzylpenicillin and higher phenols.

Both nutrient limitation and reduced growth rates may alter the sensitivity of bacteria to biocides. These changes in susceptibility can be considered as the expression of intrinsic resistance brought about by exposure to environmental conditions. These aspects assume greater importance when organisms existing as biofilms are considered. The association of microorganisms with solid surfaces leads to the generation of biofilms, which may be considered as consortia of bacteria organized within an extensive exopolysaccharide polymer (glycocalyx). The physiology of bacteria existing at different parts of biofilm is affected because the cells experience different nutrient conditions. Growth rates are likely to be reduced within the depths of a biofilm, one reason being the growth-limiting concentrations of essential nutrients that are available. Consequently, the sessile organisms present differ phenotypically from the planktonic-type cells found in liquid cultures. Frequently, bacteria within a biofilm are less sensitive to a biocide than planktonic cells.

Another reason for this decreased susceptibility is the prevention of access of a biocide to the underlying cells. The glycocalyx, as well as the rate of growth of the biofilm microcolony in relation to the diffusion rate of the biocide across the biofilm, can affect susceptibility. A possible third mechanism involves the increased production of degradative enzymes by attached cells, but the importance of this has yet to be determined. Quorum sensing between bacteria appears to be an important factor. In addition, it has recently been claimed that persisters are responsible for the high resistance of biofilm cells to both biocides and antibiotics.

The non-random distribution of bacteria in biofilms has important implications for industry (biofouling, corrosion) and in medical practice (use of indwelling devices, which might become infected when within the human body, thereby making treatment more difficult).

9 Acquired bacterial resistance to biocides

Acquired resistance to biocides results from genetic changes in a cell and arises either by mutation or by the acquisition of genetic material (plasmids, transposons) from another cell (Table 18.6).

9.1 Resistance acquired by mutation

Acquired, non-plasmid-encoded resistance to biocides can result when bacteria are exposed to gradually increasing concentrations of a biocide. Examples are provided by highly QAC-resistant Serratia marcescens, and chlorhexidine-resistant Pr. mirabilis, Ps. aeruginosa and Ser. marcescens. However, in view of the multiple target sites associated with biocide action, it is unlikely that mutation plays a key role in resistance.

9.2 Plasmid-encoded resistance

9.2.1 Resistance to cations and anions

Among the Enterobacteriaceae, plasmids may carry genes specifying resistance to antibiotics and in some instances to mercury, organomercury and other cations and some anions. Mercury resistance is inducible and is not the result of training or tolerance. Transposon (Tn)*501*, conferring mercury resistance, has been widely studied. Plasmids conferring resistance to mercury are of two types:

1 'narrow-spectrum', conferring resistance to Hg(II) and to a few specified organomercurials;
2 'broad-spectrum', encoding resistance to those in (1) plus other organomercury compounds.

There is enzymatic reduction of mercury to Hg metal and its vaporization in narrow-spectrum resistance, and enzymatic hydrolysis followed by vaporization in broad-spectrum. Plasmid-encoded resistance to other metallic ions has also been described but, apart from silver, is probably of little clinical relevance.

Plasmid-mediated resistance to silver salts is of particular importance in the hospital environment, because silver nitrate and silver sulphadiazine may be used topically for preventing infections in severe burns. It may have increased relevance in the future arising from the use of silver-coated connectors in catheter systems. Silver reduction is not a primary resistance mechanism as sensitive and resistant cells can equally convert Ag^+ to metallic silver. Plasmid-mediated resistance to silver salts is, in fact, difficult to demonstrate, but where it has been shown to occur, decreased accumulation rather than silver reduction is believed to be the mechanism involved.

9.2.2 Resistance to other biocides

Plasmid-mediated resistance to other biocides has not been widely studied and the results to date may be somewhat conflicting. Plasmid-encoded resistance to formaldehyde has been described in *Ser. marcescens*, presumably due to aldehyde degradation. There is evidence that some plasmids are responsible for producing surface changes in cells and that the response depends not only on the plasmid but also on the host cell. Gram-negative bacteria showing high resistance to QACs and chlorhexidine as well as to antibiotics have been isolated but it has not been possible to establish a linked association of resistance in these organisms.

MRSA strains are a frequent problem in hospital infection, such strains often showing multiple antibiotic resistance. Furthermore, increased resistance to some cationic biocides (chlorhexidine, QACs, diamidines and the now little used crystal violet and acridines) and to another cationic agent, ethidium bromide, is found in MRSA strains carrying genes encoding gentamicin resistance. At least three determinants have been identified as being responsible for low-level biocide resistance in clinical isolates of *Staph. aureus*: *qacA*, which encodes resistance to QACs, acridines, ethidium bromide and low-level resistance to chlorhexidine; *qacB*, which is similar but specifies resistance to the intercalating dyes and QACs; and the genetically unrelated *qacC* which specifies resistance to QACs and low-level resistance to ethidium bromide. Other *qac* genes have since been identified.

Evidence has been presented for the expulsion (efflux) of acridines, ethidium bromide, crystal violet, QACs, diamidines and chlorhexidine. Recombinant *Staph. aureus* plasmids transferred into *E. coli* cells are responsible for conferring resistance in the latter organisms to these agents. Multidrug resistance to antibiotics and cationic biocides has also been described in coagulase-negative staphylococci (*Staph. epidermidis*) mediated by multidrug export genes *qacA* and *qacC*.

The clinical relevance of biocide resistance in antibiotic-resistant staphylococci is, however, unclear. It has been claimed that the resistance of these organisms to cationic-type biocides confers a selective advantage, i.e. survival, when such disinfectants are employed clinically. However, it is important to note that the in-use concentrations are generally several times higher than those to which the organisms are resistant.

10 Sensitivity and resistance of fungi

10.1 General comments

Surprisingly little is known about the resistance of yeasts, fungi and fungal spores to disinfectants and preservatives. They are a major source of potential contamination in pharmaceutical product preparation and aseptic processing as they abound in the environment. It is, however, possible to make some general observations:

- moulds are often, but not invariably, more resistant than yeasts, e.g. to chlorhexidine and organomercurials;
- fungicidal concentrations are often much higher than those needed to inhibit growth, and inactivation may be comparatively slow;
- biocides are often considerably less active against yeasts and moulds than against non-sporulating bacteria.

For example, *Candida albicans* and (especially) *Aspergillus niger* are much more resistant to a variety of biocides than Gram-positive and Gram-negative bacteria.

10.2 Mechanisms of fungal resistance

By analogy with bacteria, two basic mechanisms of fungal resistance to biocides can be envisaged:

1 *Intrinsic (natural, innate) resistance.* In one form of intrinsic resistance, the fungal cell wall (see Chapter 4) is considered to present a barrier to exclude or, more likely, to reduce the penetration by, biocide molecules. The evidence to date is sketchy but the available information tentatively links cell wall glucan, wall thickness and consequent relative porosity to the sensitivity of *Saccharomyces cerevisiae* to chlorhexidine.

Another type of intrinsic resistance is shown by organisms that are capable of producing constitutive enzymes which degrade biocide molecules. Heavy metal activity is reduced by some strains of *Sacch. cerevisiae* which produce hydrogen sulphide; this combines with heavy metals (e.g. copper, mercury) to form insoluble sulphides thereby rendering the organisms more tolerant than non-enzyme-producing counterparts. Inactivation of other fungitoxic agents has also been described, e.g. the role of formaldehyde dehydrogenase in resistance to formaldehyde and the degradation of potassium sorbate by a *Penicillium* species. Degradation by fungi of biocides such as chlorhexidine, QACs and other aldehydes does not appear to have been reported.

2 *Acquired resistance.* There is no evidence linking the presence of plasmids in fungal cells and the ability of the organisms to acquire resistance to fungicidal or fungistatic agents. The development of resistance to antiseptic-type agents has not been widely studied, but acquired resistance to organic acids has been demonstrated, presumably by mutation, although efflux might also be involved.

11 Sensitivity and resistance of protozoa

Several distinct types of protozoa (e.g. *Giardia*, *Cryptosporidium*, *Naegleria*, *Entamoeba* and *Acanthamoeba*) are potentially pathogenic and may be acquired from water. A resistant cyst stage is included in their life cycle, the trophozoite form being sensitive to biocides. Little is known about mechanisms of inactivation by chemical agents and there appear to have been few significant studies linking excystment and encystment with the development of sensitivity and resistance, respectively.

From the evidence currently available, it is likely that the cyst cell wall acts in some way as a permeability barrier, thereby conferring intrinsic resistance to the cyst form.

12 Sensitivity and resistance of viruses

An important hypothesis was put forward in the USA by Klein and Deforest in 1963 and modified in 1983. Essentially the original concept was based on whether viruses could be classified as: 'lipophilic', i.e. those, such as herpes simplex virus, which possessed a lipid envelope; or 'hydrophilic', e.g. poliovirus, which did not contain a lipid envelope.

In the later (1983) modification, three groups were considered (Fig. 18.2):

1 lipid-enveloped viruses, which were inactivated by lipophilic biocides;

2 non-lipid picornaviruses (pico = very small, e.g. polio and Coxsackie viruses, all of which are RNA viruses);

3 other, larger, non-lipid viruses, e.g. adenoviruses.

Viruses in groups 2 and 3 are much more resistant to biocides.

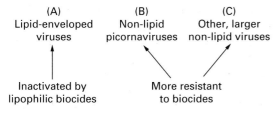

Fig. 18.2 Viral responses to biocides.

Although many papers have been published on the virucidal (viricidal) activity of biocides there is little information available about the uptake of biocides and their penetration into viruses of different types, or of their interaction with viral protein and nucleic acid.

13 Activity of biocides against prions

Prions are the simplest known infectious agents because they appear to consist largely, or exclusively, of protein, and contain no detectable nucleic acid; this distinguishes them from viruses and viroids (Chapter 1). A prion protein is a naturally occurring material that arises in mammalian brains and nervous tissue and is coded by a gene located on chromosome 20 in humans. The protein may exist in two forms: the natural, harmless form, which is thought to comprise four α-helices; this may undergo a conformational change to the infectious and β-sheet form. The process is autocatalytic, so that β-sheet molecules can cause the normal ones to convert to the infectious form and cease their normal function, ultimately with fatal consequences. These conformational changes cause degeneration of nervous tissue which, under the microscope, exhibits a sponge-like appearance. As a result, prion diseases are termed transmissible spongiform (or degenerative) encephalopathies and are exemplified primarily by scrapie in sheep, bovine spongiform encephalopathy (BSE) in cattle and Creutzfeldt–Jakob disease (CJD) in humans.

Prions are of particular significance in a pharmaceutical context because of the need to decontaminate surgical or other hospital equipment that has been in contact with diseased tissue. Prion proteins are very stable and resist proteolytic enzymes, heat,

ionizing radiation and the action of most biocides. Agents that have proved to be largely, or in some cases totally, ineffective, include chloroform, ethanol, phenol, iodophors, hydrogen peroxide, formaldehyde and ethylene oxide. Glutaraldehyde possesses some useful activity, but the most reliable means of inactivating prions that have been identified to date are 1 hour's exposure to either 1 M sodium hydroxide or a solution of sodium hypochlorite containing 20 000 ppm of free chlorine.

14 Pharmaceutical and medical relevance

The inherent variability in biocidal sensitivity of microorganisms has several important practical implications. For example, the population of bacteria making up the normal flora contaminating the working surfaces, floor, air or water supply in an environment such as a hospital pharmacy will probably contain a very low number of naturally resistant organisms. These might be resistant to the agent used as a disinfectant because they have acquired additional genetic information or lost, by mutation, genes involved in controlling the expression of other genes. In the absence of the antimicrobial agent, the resistant strains would have no competitive advantage over the sensitive strains, and in fact they might grow more slowly and would not predominate in the population. Under the selective pressure introduced by continual use of one kind of disinfectant, resistant strains would predominate as the sensitive strains are eliminated. Eventually the entire population would be resistant to the disinfectant and a serious contamination hazard would arise. This fact is of significance in the design of suitable hospital disinfection policies.

Tuberculosis is on the increase in developed countries such as the USA and UK; furthermore, MAI may be associated with AIDS sufferers. Hospital-acquired opportunist mycobacteria may cause disseminated infection and also lung infections, endocarditis and pericarditis. Transmission of mycobacterial infection by endoscopy is rare, despite a marked increase in the use of flexible fibreoptic endoscopes, but bronchoscopy is probably the greatest hazard for the transmission of *M. tuberculosis* and other mycobacteria. Thus, biocides used for bronchoscope disinfection must be chosen carefully to ensure that such transmission does not occur.

15 Further reading

Ayres, H., Furr, J. R. & Russell, A. D. (1993) A rapid method of evaluating permeabilizing activity against *Pseudomonas aeruginosa*. *Lett Appl Microbiol*, **17**, 149–187.

Collier, P .J., Ramsey, A J., Austin, P. & Gilbert, P. (1991) Uptake and distribution of some isothiazolone biocides in *Escherichia coli* and *Schizosaccharomyces pombe* NCYC 1354. *Int J Pharm*, **66**, 201–206 [and preceding two papers].

Denyer, S .P. & Hugo, W. B. (1991) *Mechanisms of Action of Chemical Biocides: their Study and Exploitation.* Society for Applied Bacteriology Technical Series No. 27. Blackwell Scientific Publications, Oxford.

Denyer, S. P. & Stewart, G. S. A. B. (1998) Mechanisms of action of disinfectants. *Int Biodeter Biodegrad*, **41**, 261–268.

Fraise, A., Lambert, P. & Maillard, J-Y. (2004) Russell, Hugo & Ayliffe's *Principles and Practice of Disinfection, Preservation and Sterilization,* 4th edn. Blackwell Science, Oxford.

Fuller, S. J., Denyer, S. P., Hugo, W.B ., Pemberton, D., Woodcock, P. M. & Buckley, A. J. (1985) The mode of action of 1,2-benzisothiazolin-3 one on *Staphylococcus aureus. Lett Appl Microbiol*, **1**, 13–15.

Garland, A. J. M. (1999) A review of BSE and its inactivation. *Eur J Parenteral Sci*, **4**, 85–92.

Hugo, W. B. (1967) The mode of action of antiseptics. *J Appl Bacteriol*, **30**, 17–50.

Hugo, W. B. (1976a) Survival of microbes exposed to chemical stress. In: *The Survival of Vegetative Microbes* (eds T.R.G. Gray & J.R. Postgate), pp. 383–413. 26th Symposium of the Society for General Microbiology. Cambridge University Press, Cambridge.

Hugo, W. B. (1976b) The inactivation of vegetative bacteria by chemicals. In: *The Inactivation of Vegetative Bacteria* (eds FA. Skinner & W.B. Hugo), pp. 1–11. Symposium of the Society of Applied Bacteriology. Academic Press, London.

Hugo, W. B. (1980) The mode of action of antiseptics. In: *Wirkungmechanisma von Antiseptica* (eds H. Wigert & W. Weufen), pp. 39–77. VEB Verlag, Berlin.

Hugo, W. B. (1992) Disinfection mechanisms. In: *Principles and Practice of Disinfection, Preservation and Sterilization* (eds A.D. Russell, W.B. Hugo & G.A.J. Ayliffe), 2nd edn, pp. 187–210. Blackwell Scientific Publications, Oxford.

Hugo, W. B. (1971) *The Inhibition and Destruction of the Microbial Cell.* Academic Press, London.

Klein, M. & Deforest, A. (1983) Principles of viral inactivation. In: *Disinfection, Sterilization and Preservation* (ed. S.S. Block), 3rd edn, pp. 422–434. Lea & Febiger, Philadelphia.

Nikaido, H. & Vaara, M. (1985) Molecular basis of bacterial outer membrane permeability. *Microbiol Rev*, **49**, 1–32.

Nikaido, H., Kim, S.-H. & Rosenberg, E. Y. (1993) Physical organization of lipids in the cell wall of *Mycobacterium chelonae. Mol Microbiol*, **8**, 1025–1030.

Russell, A. D. (1999) Bacterial resistance to disinfectants: present knowledge and future problems. *J Hosp Infect*, **43** (Suppl), S57–S68.

Russell, A. D. (2002) Introduction of biocides into clinical practice and the impact on antibiotic resistance. *J Appl Microbiol Symp Suppl.*

Russell, A. D. & Chopra, I. (1996) *Understanding Antibacterial Action and Resistance,* 2nd edn. Ellis Horwood, Chichester.

Russell, A. D. & Day, M. J. (1996) Antibiotic and biocide resistance in bacteria. *Microbios*, **85**, 45–65.

Russell, A. D. & Furr, J. R. (1996) Biocides: mechanisms of antifungal action and fungal resistance. *Sci Progr*, **79**, 27–48.

Russell, A. D. & Hugo, W. B. (1994) Antimicrobial activity and action of silver. In: *Progress in Medicinal Chemistry* (eds G.P. Ellis & D.K. Luscombe), vol. 39, pp. 351–370. Elsevier, Amsterdam.

Russell, A. D. & Russell, N. J. (1995) Biocides: activity, action and resistance. In: *Fifty Years of Antimicrobials: Past Perspectives and Future Trends* (eds P.A. Hunter, G.K. Derby & N.J. Russell), 53rd Symposium of the Society for General Microbiology, pp. 327–365. Cambridge University Press, Cambridge.

Setlow, P. (1994) Mechanisms which contribute to the long-term survival of spores of *Bacillus* species. *J Appl Bact Symp Suppl*, **76**, 49S–60S.

Stickler, D. J. & King, J. B. (1999) Intrinsic resistance to non-antibiotic antibacterial agents. In: *Principles and Practice of Disinfection, Preservation and Sterilisation* (eds A.D. Russell, W.B. Hugo & G.A.J. Ayliffe), 3rd edn. Blackwell Science, Oxford.

Taylor, D. M. (1999) Inactivation of unconventional agents of the transmissible degenerative encephalopathies. In: *Principles and Practice of Disinfection, Preservation and Sterilization* (eds A.D. Russell, W.B. Hugo & G.A.J. Ayliffe), 3rd edn. Blackwell Science, Oxford.

Vaara, M. (1992) Agents that increase the permeability of the outer membrane. *Microbiol Rev*, **56**, 395–411.

Chapter 19
Sterile pharmaceutical products

James Ford

1 Introduction

Parenteral drug delivery systems and many medicinal products, such as dressings and sutures, must be sterile to avoid the possibilities of microbial degradation or infection occurring as a result of their use. Sterility is also important for any material or instrument likely to contact broken skin or internal organs. Although pathogenic bacteria, fungi or viruses pose the most obvious danger to a patient, it should be also realized that microorganisms usually regarded as non-pathogenic and which inadvertently gain access to body cavities in sufficient numbers may cause a severe, possibly fatal infection. Consequently, injections, ophthalmic preparations, irrigation fluids, dialysis solutions, sutures and ligatures, implants, certain surgical dressings, as well as instruments necessary for their use or administration, must be presented in a sterile condition.

Whilst there is always a chance of an idiosyncratic reaction between a medicine and a patient caused by sensitivity, allergic reaction or unwanted side-effects, for sterile products there is the added requirement that they must be free of viable microorganisms. This consequently means the product should be manufactured in a manner that reduces to the lowest likelihood the risk of microbial contamination. Thus a sterile product should not contain viable bacteria, yeasts or fungi, nor other microorganisms such as rickettsiae, mycoplasmas or protozoa and viruses. The absence of prion particles is also desirable but difficult to demonstrate (see Chapter 2). Sterilization processes concentrate on the destruction or removal of microorganisms. Each process is designed to remove the most problematic microorganism (i.e. the smallest bacteria in filtration or the most heat-resistant bacterial spores in heat sterilization processes) on the basis that, once a sterilization process has been chosen, elimination of the most problematic species will have led to the elimination of all less resistant microorganisms.

The principles behind the sterilization processes are described in Chapter 20. The choice of method is determined largely by the ability of the formulation and container to withstand the physical stresses applied during the sterilization process. All products intended for sterilization should be manufactured under clean conditions and therefore will be of low microbial content (bioburden) prior to sterilization. Under these conditions, the sterilization process will not be overtaxed and will generally be within the safety limits needed to provide the required level of sterility assurance (Chapter 20). The next section emphasizes parenteral products, but the practices described apply to many other types of sterile product.

2 Types of sterile product

The most obviously recognized sterile pharmaceutical preparations are injections. These vary from very small volume antigenic products to large volume, total parenteral nutrition products. Other sterile products include ophthalmic preparations, creams and dusting powders. This section describes their formulation and packaging and the constraints imposed by sterilization on stability, formulation and packaging of some of the more common sterile products.

2.1 Injections

Injections may be aqueous solutions, oily solutions (because of poor aqueous solubility or the necessity for a prolongation of drug activity), aqueous suspensions or oily suspensions. They may be aseptically produced or terminally sterilized in their final containers. Those drugs that are unstable in solution may be presented as a freeze-dried (lyophilized) powder. The choice of final packaging should not determine the method of sterilization.

2.1.1 Formulation philosophy

An injection must be manufactured under conditions that result in a product containing the minimum possible levels of particles and pyrogenic substances. Its formulation and packaging must maintain physical and chemical stability throughout the production processes, the intended shelf-life and during administration. To achieve this, excipients such as buffers and anti-oxidants may be required to ensure chemical stability, and solubilizers, such as propylene glycol or polysorbates, may be necessary for drugs with poor aqueous solubility to maintain the drug in solution. Table 19.1 lists some chemical constituents of common injections and ophthalmic preparations.

Many injections are formulated as aqueous solutions, with Water for Injections as the vehicle. Their formulation depends upon several factors including the aqueous solubility of the active ingredient, the dose, its thermal stability, the route of administration, and whether the product is to be offered as a multiple-dose product (i.e. with doses removed on different occasions) or as a single-dose form (as the term suggests, only one dose per container). Most injections are prepared as a single-dose form but this is mandatory for certain routes, e.g. spinal injections where the intrathecal route is used, and large volume intravenous infusions. Multiple-dose

Table 19.1 Some examples of excipients used in formulations and reasons for their inclusion

Product	Excipients	Reason for inclusion
Diazepam Injection	Ethanol	Co-solvent
	Propylene glycol	Co-solvent
Insulin (Humalin®) Isophane Injection (Eli-Lilly)	m-Cresol	Preservative
	Glycerol	Tonicity modifier
	Phenol	Preservative
	Protamine sulphate	Forms insulin complex
	Dibasic sodium phosphate	Buffer
	Zinc oxide	Adjusts zinc content
	Hydrochloric acid	pH adjustment
	Sodium hydroxide	pH adjustment
Promethazine Hydrochloride Injection USP	Disodium edetate	Chelating agent
	Sodium metabisulphite	Anti-oxidant
	Phenol	Preservative
	Sodium acetate	Buffer
	Acetic acid	Buffer
Minims Chloramphenicol Eye Drops	Borax	Buffer
	Boric acid	Buffer
Minims Prednisolone Sodium Phosphate Eye Drops	Disodium edetate	Chelating agent
	Sodium chloride	Tonicity adjustment
	Sodium dihydrogen phosphate	Buffer
	Sodium hydroxide	pH adjustment

injections may require the inclusion of a suitable preservative to prevent contamination following the removal of each dose. Injections used for several routes, including the intrathecal and intracardiac routes, must not contain a preservative because of potential long-term damage to the patient.

Some types of injections must be isotonic with blood serum. This applies particularly to large volume intravenous infusions if at all possible; hypotonic solutions cause lysis of red blood corpuscles and thus must not be used for this purpose. Conversely, hypertonic solutions can be employed; these induce shrinkage, but not lysis, of red cells, which recover their shape later. Intraspinal injections must also be isotonic to reduce pain at the site of injection; so should intramuscular and subcutaneous injections. Adjustment to isotonicity can be determined from either the depression of freezing point or from sodium chloride equivalents. The depression of the freezing point depends on the number of dissolved particles (molecules or ions) present in a solution. The following equation:

$$W = (0.52 - a)/b$$

where W is the percentage (w/v) of adjusting substance, a is the freezing point of unadjusted solution and b is the depression of the freezing point of water induced by 1% w/v of adjusting substance, allows the determination of how much adjusting substance is required to produce isotonicity with blood plasma.

Alternatively the sodium chloride equivalent, which is produced by dividing the value for the depression of freezing point produced by a solution of the substance by the corresponding value of a solution of sodium chloride of the same strength, may be used. Fuller details of each method may be found in the *Pharmaceutical Codex* (1993).

2.1.2 Intravenous infusions

These consist of large volume injections or drips (500 ml or more) that are infused at various rates (50–500 ml/h) into the venous system. They are generally sterilized in an autoclave. Examples include isotonic solutions of sodium chloride or glucose that are used to maintain fluid and electrolyte balance, for replacement of extracellular body fluids (e.g. after surgery or prolonged periods of fluid loss), as a supplementary energy source as 1 litre of 5% w/v glucose yields 714 kJ of energy or as a vehicle for drugs. Other important examples are blood products, which are collected and processed in sterile containers, and plasma substitutes, e.g. dextrans and degraded gelatin. Dextrans are glucose polymers in which the glucose monomers are joined by 1,6 alpha links; they are produced by certain bacteria of the genus *Leuconostoc*, e.g. *Leuconostoc mesenteroides*.

2.1.2.1 Intravenous additives

A common hospital practice is to add drugs to infusions immediately before administration. Regularly used additives include potassium chloride, lignocaine, heparin, certain vitamins and antibiotics. Potentially this can be a hazardous practice. For instance, the drug may precipitate in the infusion fluid because of the pH (e.g. amphotericin) or the presence of calcium salts (e.g. thiopentone). The drug may degrade rapidly (e.g. ampicillin in 5% w/v glucose). Multiple additions may lead to precipitation of one or both of the drugs or to accelerated degradation. Finally drug loss may occur because of sorption by the container. For instance, insulin is adsorbed by glass or by PVC; glyceryl trinitrite and diazepam are absorbed by PVC. Apart from these problems, if the addition is not carried out under strict aseptic conditions the fluid can become contaminated with microorganisms during the procedure. Thus any addition should be made in a laminar-flow work-station or isolator, and the fluid should, ideally, be administered within 24 hours of preparation.

Another approach to the problem of providing an intravenous drug additive service is to add the drug to a small volume (50–100 ml) infusion in a collapsible plastic container and store the preparation at −20°C in a freezer. The infusion can be removed when required and thawed rapidly in a microwave oven. Many antibiotics are stable for several months when stored in minibags at −20°C and are unaffected by the thawing process. Other antibiotics, e.g. ampicillin, degrade even when frozen.

2.1.2.2 Total parenteral nutrition

Total parenteral nutrition (TPN) is the use of mixtures of amino acids, vitamins, electrolytes, trace elements and an energy source (glucose and fat) in the long-term feeding of patients who are unconscious or unable to take food. All or most of the ingredients to feed a patient for 1 day are combined aseptically in one large (3-litre capacity) collapsible plastic bag, the contents of which are infused over a 12–24-hour period. Transfer of amino acid, glucose and electrolyte infusions, and the addition of vitamins and trace elements must be carried out with great care under aseptic conditions to avoid microbial contamination. These solutions often provide good growth conditions for bacteria and moulds. Fats are administered as oil-in-water emulsions comprising small droplets of a suitable vegetable oil (e.g. soyabean) emulsified with egg lecithin and sterilized by autoclaving. In many cases, the fat emulsion is added to the 3-litre bag. Thus TPN fluids are complex mixtures and a multitude of potential interactions, both chemical and physicochemical, may occur between their individual components resulting in decomposition, creaming, precipitation or even the formation of toxic by-products. Trace elements, calcium, vitamins and lipids are particularly prone to affecting the stability.

Although many vitamins may be administered as a single dose at various time intervals, many of the patient's requirements will be found in what is basically an emulsion formulation, prepared aseptically and thus with no terminal sterilization. The product usually contains both essential and non-essential amino acids rather than fully formed protein and energy is provided at a ratio of 0.6–1.1 MJ per gram of protein nitrogen. A mixture of carbohydrate (glucose) and fat (as an emulsion) provides the energy. Electrolytes, trace elements and vitamins are included as required. Thus the TPN fluid is prepared to suit the individual patient's needs. The fact that the product contains so many ingredients makes TPN fluids extremely difficult to prepare, and once vitamins are added, their chemical instability reduces the shelf-life. During preparation, TPN fluids are compounded from individual solutions or emulsions. Generally, the bulk of the final volume is derived from glucose solutions, amino acid solutions and fat emulsions; small volume solutions are added to these before filling. During compounding electrolytes are added to the amino acid solutions and phosphate salts to the dextrose (glucose) solutions, which are then mixed and the lipid emulsions added. This order of mixing is adopted because the pH of glucose solutions decreases due to degradation during their sterilization and addition of emulsions to this low pH solution might cause emulsion instability. The mixing of the amino acids with the glucose solutions provides a vehicle with some degree of buffering capacity. Calcium might precipitate as the phosphate if its salts were to be added directly to the phospholipid emulsion. Vitamins are added to the lipid emulsion or to the bag immediately before use.

A number of other difficulties may be encountered. Polyunsaturated acids are subject to hydrolysis. Any residual air might cause oxidation of labile vitamins, e.g. vitamin C. Lipids (the fat emulsions and fat-soluble vitamins formulated as an emulsion) may extract plasticizer from a plastic container, especially if the bag is based on PVC. Any electrolytes may compromise emulsion stability by altering the electrochemistry around the dispersed oil droplets thus allowing the droplets to move closer to each other (due to a disruption of the Stern layer) and coalesce; a less noticeable problem would be changes in the globule size. Additionally, the plastic bag might absorb the oil-soluble vitamins and care has to be taken in the selection of the container to avoid moisture loss. As a final example of the complex nature of TPN fluids, amino acids may undergo the Maillard reaction with glucose, resulting in discoloration.

2.1.3 Small volume injections

This category comprises single-dose injections, usually of 1–2 ml but as high as 50 ml, dispensed in borosilicate glass ampoules, plastic (polyethylene or polypropylene) ampoules or, rarely, multiple-dose glass vials of 5–25 ml capacity stoppered with a rubber closure through which a hypodermic needle can be inserted, e.g. insulins, vaccines. The closure is designed to reseal after withdrawal of the needle. It is unwise to include too many doses in a multiple-dose container because of the risk of microbial contamination during repeated use. Preservatives must be added to injections in multiple-dose containers to prevent contamination during withdrawal of successive doses. However, preservatives may not be used in injections in which the total volume to be injected at one time exceeds 15 ml. This may occur if the solubility of a drug is such that a therapeutic dose can only be achieved in this volume of solvent. There is also an absolute prohibition on the inclusion of preservatives in intra-arterial, intracardiac, intrathecal or subarachnoid, intracisternal and peridural injections, and in various ophthalmic injections.

2.1.3.1 Small volume oily injections

Certain small volume injections are available where the drug is dissolved in a viscous oil because it is insoluble in water and therefore a non-aqueous solvent is used. In addition, drugs in non-aqueous solvents provide a depot effect, e.g. for hormones. The intramuscular route of injection must be used. The vehicle may be a metabolizable fixed oil such as arachis oil or sesame oil (but not a mineral oil) or an ester, such as ethyl oleate, which is also capable of being metabolized. The latter is less viscous and therefore easier to administer, but the depot effect is of shorter duration. The drug is normally dissolved in the oil, filtered under pressure and distributed into ampoules. After sealing, the ampoules are sterilized by dry heat. A preservative is probably ineffective in such a medium and therefore offers very little protection against contamination in a multiple-dose oily injection.

2.1.4 Freeze-dried products

In brief, freeze-drying (lyophilization) consists of preparing the drug solution (with buffers and cryoprotectants), filtering through a bacteria-proof filter, dispensing into containers, removing water in a freeze-drier, then capping and closing the containers. In the future it is probable that many biotechnology products will be freeze-dried

Freeze-drying is an aseptic process whereby water is removed from a frozen product mainly by sublimation, i.e. by the conversion of ice directly into the vapour state without the intermediary of liquid water. It is a batch process, of relatively long duration, and is used frequently for drugs of poor stability. Drugs are reconstituted into solution immediately prior to injection. The process consists of three stages:
- Freezing, which slows down degradation and solidifies the product.
- Primary drying whereby energy is provided to the system and a vacuum applied to expedite the removal of moisture at sub-ambient temperatures.
- Secondary drying, whereby the product is heated to remove the last traces (2%) of water.

A number of characteristics of the formulation control the behaviour of the product during the lyophilization cycle. These include the glass transition temperature and the collapse temperature. The maintenance of sterility and retention of the appropriate Sterility Assurance Level (SAL) is implicit in the freeze-drier design (Murgatroyd, 2001). Although membrane-filtered sterile solutions may be used to fill containers to be placed into the freeze-drier, other measures to maintain sterility are also employed. These include using steam sterilization of the drier; gaseous sterilization has not been widely adopted. The temperature of shelves is regulated using a circulating fluid such as dimethylsiloxane oil. Electronics and computerization have led to the accumulation of better data for validation. Stoppering systems allow the successful sealing of the containers and gas entering the drier may be filtered to effect sterilization.

2.1.5 Packaging, closures and blow-fill technology

The packaging and closures must prevent vehicle, excipient or drug loss during sterilization and storage. Additionally, ingress of microorganisms must be prevented. The packaging must not contribute any significant amounts of extractable chemicals to the contents, e.g. vulcanizing agents from rubbers or plasticizers from polyvinylchloride (PVC) infusion containers.

2.1.5.1 Glass containers

Single-dose injections are usually packed in glass ampoules containing 1, 2 or 5 ml of product. To ensure removal of the correct dose-volume by syringe and needle, it is necessary to add an appropriate overage to the ampoule. Thus a 1-ml ampoule will actually contain 1.1 ml of product and a 2-ml ampoule should contain 2.15 ml of product.

Many injectables are sealed with a rubber closure held on by an aluminium screw-cap or crimp-on ring. The rubber should be non-fragmenting, not release soluble extractives, and be sufficiently soft and pliable to seal around the needle inserted immediately prior to use. Although bottles are sterilized by autoclaving, it is still possible for the infusions in glass bottles to become contaminated with microorganisms before use through the seal. For instance, during the final part of the autoclave cycle, bottles may be spray-cooled with water to hasten the cooling process. However, if there is a poor fit between bottle lip and rubber plug (a skirted inset type is used) it is possible for the spray-cooling water to spread by capillary movement between bottle thread and screw-cap and even to enter the bottle contents. Failure may also result from any imperfection of the bottle or plug. Microorganisms may gain access to the product within the containers during storage if hairline cracks (due to bad handling or rough treatment) are present which permit fluid seepage. Finally, contamination may occur during use if poor aseptic techniques are applied when setting up the infusion, via an ineffective air inlet (which allows replacement of the infused fluid with air in glass bottles) or when changing the giving set or bottle.

Three types of glass are suitable for use in the manufacture of containers for injectable preparations. These are a neutral borosilicate glass, a sulphated soda glass and a soft, moderately hydrolytic resistant glass. The glasses are classified on their hydrolytic resistance. The choice for a container depends on the properties of the solution they are used to package. The advantages of glasses as container materials include their chemical resistance, the fact that they do not absorb or leach organic materials, their impermeability to water vapour and other gases, their transparency, their ability to form rigid strong stable containers which resist puncture, their ability to hold a vacuum and their overall stability to moist heat or dry heat sterilization. However, glass containers may break and crack during the sterilization process, they are attacked by alkaline solutions (and so may be a problem with, for example, sodium citrate bladder irrigation), they are heavy and require venting during administration of their contents.

2.1.5.2 Closures

Closures are composed of a polymer and include curing agents, activators, anti-oxidants, plasticizers, fillers and pigments within their formulae. They have to be selected with the drug product in mind to avoid chemical incompatibility and possible reaction with the ingredients in the product formulation. 'Sorption of the preservative from multiple-dose formulations has frequently been a problem and therefore closures may require saturation with the ingredients in the product prior to packaging.

Closures should be flexible to conform to the shape of the vial, resilient so as to reseal after each needle puncture, tough so that low fragmentation levels occur when punctured, non-thermoplastic so that the heat sterilization process is tolerated and chemically compatible with the drug formulation. Early closures were sulphur-based, and easily cured with accelerators to speed up the curing rate. Unfortunately, a high degree of water-extractable by-products could be taken up by the product that they were intended to protect. Consequently they have been replaced by modern polymer formulations with low extract curatives. Bromobutyl and chlorobutyl rubbers show superior performance although special polymers, e.g. nitrile rubbers, are used for mineral oil products. Problems of incompatibility may be overcome by film bonding a fluorocarbon barrier film to the surfaces of the closures.

2.1.5.3 Plastic containers

Most infusions are now packed in plastic containers. The plastic material should be pliable, thermo-resistant, transparent and non-toxic. The plastics may contain anti-oxidants, stabilizers, lubricants, plasticizers, fillers and colorants. Suitable materials are polyvinylchloride (PVC) (which may present a problem with moisture loss) and polyethylene. The former is transparent and very pliable, allowing the pack to collapse as the contents are withdrawn (consequently no air inlet is required). These packs are also amenable to the inclusion of ports into the bag, allowing greater safety during use. Such ports may be protected by sterile overseals.

Two problems arise: (i) the possibility of toxic extractives, e.g. diethyl phthalate, from the plastic entering the fluid if poor quality PVC is used and (ii) moisture permeability leading to loss of water if the packs are not protected by a water impermeable outer wrap. Bags of high-quality polyethylene are readily moulded (although separate ports cannot be included), translucent and free from potential toxic extractives. Again, these packs normally collapse readily during infusion. An important advantage of all plastic packs is that the containers are hermetically sealed prior to autoclaving and therefore spray-cooling water cannot enter the pack unless there is seal failure, an easily detected occurrence. However, autoclaving of plastic bags is more complex than that of bottled fluids because a steam/air mixture is necessary to prevent bursting of the bags when heated (air ballasting); adequate mixing of the steam and air is therefore required to prevent layering of gases inside the chamber.

2.1.5.4 Blow-fill technology

Blow-fill technology is an aseptic process whereby the container is formed from thermoplastic granules, filled with sterile solution and sealed, all within one automatic operation. The bulk solution should have a low bioburden and is delivered to the machine through a filling system that has been previously sanitized and steam sterilized *in situ*. Concern has been expressed that the machine itself may generate particles. The plastic granules are composed usually of polyethylene, polypropylene or one of their copolymers and are heat extruded at ~200°C into a tube. The two halves of a mould close around this tube and seal the base. The required quantity of sterile fluid is filled into the container, which is then sealed. Products packed in this way include intravenous solutions, and small volume parenteral, ophthalmic and nebulizer solutions. The technique offers lower costs than conventional packaging.

2.1.5.5 Cartridges and ready-to-use syringes

Small volume injections may also be packaged in cartridges or directly into disposable syringes. The latter are immediately available for use but have a high cost of production and their fixed content may lead to waste of material that remains uninjected after single use. Cartridges are lower cost and may be fitted into injection pens; many insulin products are produced in this manner because of their low waste and ease of use, their not requiring the patient to draw a dose volume into a separate syringe. Cartridges have a plunger stopper at one end of a cylindrical glass body containing the product for injection, and the other end is sealed with a rubber-lined crimp cap. Processing steps include preparing the bulk sterile solution for injection, washing and siliconizing the plunger stoppers, caps and glass cartridges, inserting the plunger stopper, filling and closing. The product is then sterilized, but care has to be taken that the internal pressures that develop during the autoclave cycle do not force the cartridge plunger out of the cartridge.

2.1.6 Quality control of ampoules and infusion containers

2.1.6.1 Particulate contamination

Because of the possible clinical consequences (such as granuloma of the lung) of injecting solid particles into the bloodstream, the number of particles present in injections and other solutions used in body cavities must be restricted. The *British Pharmacopoeia* (2002) states that injectable preparations which are solutions 'when examined under suitable conditions of visibility are clear and practically free from particles'. It also sets limits for sub-visible particles in injections based on the principle of light blockage. Not more than 100 particles per ml greater than 5 μm and not more than 50 per ml greater than 10 μm should be generally obtained. The *British Pharmacopoeia* (2002) describes a microscopic method for determination of the particulate contamination of injections and intravenous infusions. The counting methods should estimate extraneous particles, but not bubbles, that are unin-

tentionally present in the solutions. If the method provides a means for identifying and detecting the particles, insight may be gained into their possible origin. Filtration and observation using light microscopy have clear advantages including simplicity and allowing the operator to visualize the particles.

All parenterally injected solutions should be checked for particulate contamination but the above procedure is clearly impractical as a bulk screening exercise. Those products contaminated with particulate matter should be rejected. In practice, all products may be tested individually by humans against split white/black screens and/or under polarized light for obvious particulate contamination and again there is a method described in pharmacopoeias based on the split screen technique. Nowadays optical control equipment can take over this arduous and boring employment.

2.1.6.2 Integrity of seals

The integrity of sealing of ampoules should be assessed on an individual basis. Two techniques are available that depend on dye ingress under vacuum or electronic means. With dye intrusion, the ampoules are submerged in a dye solution and under an applied vacuum. Any container that has cracks in its structure or is not sealed will admit the dye when the vacuum is reduced. On washing, badly sealed ampoules will be coloured. This technique underestimates the problem of bad sealing. In the alternative technique, high frequency spark testing, the presence of a leak causes a change in a high frequency electrical signal placed across the ampoule. The method is limited to aqueous products with a high conductivity. It is a very sensitive technique and detects weak seals not detected by the dye test. In reality, both tests should be used in parallel.

2.2 Non-injectable sterile fluids

There are many other types of solution in a sterile form for use particularly in hospitals.

2.2.1 Non-injectable water

This is sterile water, not necessarily of injectable water standards, which is used widely during surgical procedures for wound irrigation, moistening of tissues, washing of surgeons' gloves and instruments during use and, when warmed, as a haemostat. Isotonic saline may also be used. Topical water (as it is often called) is prepared in 500-ml and 1-litre polyethylene or polypropylene containers with a wide neck and tear-off cap to allow for ease of pouring.

2.2.2 Urological (bladder) irrigation solutions

These are used for rinsing of the urinary tract to aid tissue integrity and cleanliness during or after surgery. Either water or glycine solution is used, the latter eliminating the risk of intravascular haemolysis when electrosurgical instruments are used. These are sterile solutions produced in collapsible or semi-rigid plastic containers of up to 3-litre capacity.

2.2.3 Peritoneal dialysis and haemodialysis solutions

Peritoneal dialysis solutions are admitted into the peritoneal cavity as a means of removing accumulated waste or toxic products following renal failure or poisoning. They contain electrolytes and glucose (1.4–7% w/v) to provide a solution equivalent to potassium-free extracellular fluid; lactate or acetate is added as a source of bicarbonate ions. Slightly hypertonic solutions are usually employed to avoid increasing the water content of the intravascular compartment. A more hypertonic solution containing a higher glucose concentration is used to achieve a more rapid removal of water. In fact, the peritoneal cavity behaves as if it were separated from the body organs by a semi-permeable membrane. Warm peritoneal solution (up to 5 litres) is perfused into the cavity for 30–90 minutes and then drained out completely. This procedure can then be repeated as often as required. As the procedure requires larger volumes, these fluids are commonly packed in 2.5-litre containers. It is not uncommon to add drugs (for instance potassium chloride or heparin) to the fluid prior to use.

Haemodialysis is the process of circulating a patient's blood through a machine via tubing composed of a semi-permeable material such that waste products permeate into the dialysing fluid and the blood then returns to the patient. Haemodialysis solutions need not be sterile but must be free from heavy bacterial contamination.

2.2.4 Inhaler solutions

In cases of severe asthmatic attacks, bronchodilators and steroids for direct delivery to the lungs may be needed in large doses. This is achieved by direct inhalation via a nebulizer device; this converts a liquid into a mist or fine spray. The drug is diluted in small volumes of Water for Injections before loading into the reservoir of the machine. This vehicle must be sterile and preservative-free and is therefore prepared as a terminally sterilized unit dose in polyethylene nebules.

2.3 Ophthalmic preparations

2.3.1 Design philosophy

Medication intended for instillation on to the surface of the eye is formulated in aqueous solution as eye-drops or lotion or in an oily base as an ointment. Because of the possibility of eye infection occurring, particularly after abrasion or damage to the corneal surface, all ophthalmic preparations must be sterile. As there is a very poor blood supply to the anterior chamber, defence against microbial invasion is minimal; furthermore it appears to provide a particularly good environment for growth of bacteria. As well as being sterile, eye products should also be relatively free from particles that might cause damage to the cornea. However, unlike aqueous injections the recommended vehicle is purified water because the presence of pyrogens is not clinically significant.

Another type of sterile ophthalmic product is the contact lens solution. However, unlike the other types this is not used for medication purposes but merely as wetting, cleaning and soaking conditions for contact lenses.

2.3.2 Eye-drops

Some typical excipients for eye-drops are given in Table 19.1. Eye-drops are presented for use in (i) sterile single-dose plastic sachets (often termed Minims®) containing 0.3–0.5 ml of liquid, (ii) multiple-dose amber fluted eye-dropper bottles including the rubber teat as part of the closed container or supplied separately or (iii) plastic bottles with integral dropper. A breakable seal indicates that the dropper or cap has not been removed prior to initial use. Although a standard design of bottle is used in hospitals, many proprietary products are manufactured in plastic bottles designed to improve safety and care of use. The maximum volume in each container is limited to 10 ml. Because of the likelihood of microbial contamination of eye-dropper bottles during use (arising from repeated opening or contact of the dropper with infected eye tissue or the hands of the patient), it is essential to protect the product with a preservative. Eye-drops for surgical theatre use should be supplied in single-dose containers.

Examples of preservatives are phenylmercuric nitrate or acetate (0.002% w/v), chlorhexidine acetate (0.01% w/v), thiomersal (0.01% w/v) and benzalkonium chloride (0.01% w/v). Chlorocresol is too toxic to the corneal epithelium, but 8-hydroxyquinoline and thiomersal may be used in specific instances. The principal consideration in relation to antimicrobial properties is the activity of the bactericide against *Pseudomonas aeruginosa*, a major source of serious nosocomial eye infections. Although benzalkonium chloride is probably the most active of the recommended preservatives, it cannot always be used because of its incompatibility with many compounds commonly used to treat eye diseases, nor should it be used to preserve eye-drops containing anaesthetics. As benzalkonium chloride reacts with natural rubbers, silicone or butyl rubber teats should be substituted and products should not be stored for more than 3 months after manufacture because silicone rubber is permeable to water vapour. As with all rubber components, the rubber teat should be pre-equilibrated with the preservative before use. Thermostable eye-drops and lotions are sterilized at 121°C for 15 minutes. For thermolabile drugs, filtration sterilization followed by aseptic filling into sterile containers is necessary. Eye-drops in plastic bottles are prepared aseptically.

In order to lessen the risk of eye-drops becoming heavily contaminated, either by repeated inoculation or by the growth of resistant organisms in the solution, use is restricted, after the container is first opened, to 1 month. This is usually reduced to 7 days for hospital ward use on one eye of a single patient. The period is shorter in the hospital environment because of the greater danger of contamination by potential pathogens, particularly pseudomonads.

2.3.3 Eye lotions

Eye lotions are isotonic solutions used for washing or bathing the eyes. They are sterilized by autoclaving in relatively large volume containers (100 ml or greater) of coloured fluted glass with a rubber closure and screw-cap, or packed in plastic containers with a screw-cap or tear-off seal. They may contain a preservative if intended for intermittent domiciliary use for up to 7 days. If intended for first aid or similar purposes, however, no bactericide is included and any remaining solution is discarded after 24 hours.

2.3.4 Eye ointments

Eye ointments are prepared in a semi-solid base (e.g. Simple Eye Ointment BP, which consists of yellow soft paraffin [8 parts], liquid paraffin [1 part] and wool fat [1 part]). The base is filtered when molten to remove particles and sterilized at 160°C for 2 hours. The drug is incorporated prior to sterilization if heat-stable, or added aseptically to the sterile base. Finally the product is aseptically packed in clear sterile aluminium or plastic tubes. As the product contains virtually no water the danger of bacteria proliferating in the ointment is negligible.

2.3.5 Contact lens solutions

Most contact lenses are worn for optical reasons as an alternative to spectacles. Contact lenses are of two types, namely hard lenses that are hydrophobic, and soft lenses, which may be either hydrophilic or hydrophobic. The surfaces of lenses must be wetted before use and wetting solutions are used for this purpose. Hard, and more especially, soft lenses become heavily contaminated with protein material during use and therefore must be cleaned before disinfection. Contact lenses are potential sources of eye infection and, consequently, microorganisms should be removed before the lens is again inserted into the eye. Lenses must also be clean and easily wettable by lachrymal secretions. Contact lens solutions are thus sterile solutions of the various types described below. Apart from achieving their stated functions, either singly or in combination, all solutions must be non-irritating and must protect against microbial contamination during use and storage.

2.3.5.1 *Wetting solutions*

These are used to hydrate the surfaces of hard lenses after disinfection. As they must also cope with chance contamination, they must contain a preservative as well as a wetting agent. They may be isotonic with lachrymal secretions and be formulated to a pH of about 7.2 for compatibility with normal tears.

2.3.5.2 *Cleaning solutions*

These are responsible for the removal of ocular debris and protein deposits, and contain a cleaning agent that consists of a surfactant and/or an enzyme product. As they must also cope with chance contamination, they contain a preservative, are isotonic and have a pH of about 7.2.

2.3.5.3 *Soaking solutions*

These are solutions for disinfection of lenses but also maintain the lenses in a hydrated state. The antimicrobial agents used for disinfecting hard lenses are those used in eye-drops (benzalkonium, chlorhexidine, phenylmercuric acetate or nitrate, thiomersal and chlorbutol). Ethylene diamine tetra-acetic acid (EDTA) is usually present as a synergist. Benzalkonium chloride and chlorbutol are strongly bound to hydrophilic soft contact lenses and therefore cannot be used in storage solutions for these; chlorhexidine and thiomersal are usually employed. It must be added that the concentrations of all preservatives used in contact lens solutions are lower than those employed in eye-drops, to minimize irritancy. Hydrogen peroxide is becoming commonly used but must be inactivated before the

lenses are inserted onto the eyes. Finally, heat may be utilized as an alternative method to disinfect soft contact lenses, especially the hydrophilic types. Lenses are boiled in isotonic saline.

2.4 Dressings

Dressings and surgical materials are used widely in medicine, both as a means of protecting and providing comfort for wounds and for many associated activities such as cleaning and swabbing. They may or may not be used on areas of broken skin. If there is a potential danger of infection arising from the use of a dressing then it must be sterile. For instance, sterile dressings must be used on all open wounds, both surgical and traumatic, on burns and during and after catheterization at a site of injection. It is also important to appreciate that sterile dressings must be packaged in such a way that they can be applied to the wound aseptically.

Dressings are described in the *British Pharmacopoeia* (2002). Methods for their sterilization include autoclaving, dry heat, ethylene oxide and ionizing radiation. Any other effective method may be used. The choice is governed principally by the stability of the dressing constituents to the stress applied and the nature of their components. Most celluloses and synthetic fibres withstand autoclaving, but there are exceptions. For instance, boric acid tenderizes cellulose fibres during autoclaving, and dressings containing waxes cannot be sterilized by moist heat. Certain constituents are also adversely affected on exposure to large doses of gamma-radiation. Examples of dressings that are required to be sterile are listed in Table 19.2, together with other dressings and materials that may be sterilized when required.

A very important aspect of dressings production is packaging. The packaging material must allow correct sterilization conditions (e.g. permeation of moisture or ethylene oxide), retain the dressing in a sterile condition and allow for its removal without contamination prior to use. All dressings intended for aseptic handling and application must be double wrapped. For steam sterilization they may be individually wrapped in fabric, paper or nylon and sterilized in metal drums, cardboard boxes or bleached Kraft paper. The choice of method also determines

Table 19.2 Uses of surgical dressings and methods of sterilization

Dressing	Uses	Method of sterilization
Required to be sterile		
Chlorhexidine gauze dressing	Medicated open wound dressing, burns, grafts	Any combination of dry heat, gamma-radiation and ethylene oxide
Framycetin gauze dressing	Medicated open wound dressing, burns, grafts	
Knitted viscose primary dressing	Ulcerative and granulating wounds	
Paraffin gauze dressing	Burns, scalds and grafts	
Perforated film absorbent dressing	Postoperative wounds	
Polyurethane foam dressing	Burns, ulcers, grafts, granulating wounds	
Semi-permeable adhesive dressing	Adhesive dressing for open wounds, i.v. sites, stoma care, etc.	
Sodium fusidate gauze dressing	Medicated open wound dressing, burns, grafts	
May be sterile for use in certain circumstances		
Absorbent cotton wool	Swabbing, cleaning, medication application	Any method
Elastic adhesive dressing	Protective wound dressings	Ethylene oxide or gamma-radiation
Plastic wound dressings	Protective dressing (permeable or occlusive)	Ethylene oxide or gamma-radiation
Absorbent cotton gauze	Absorbent wound dressing	Any method
Gauze pads	Swabbing, dressing, wound packing	Any method
Absorbent viscose wadding	Wound cleaning, swabbing, skin antiseptic	Any method

the design of the autoclave cycle. Providing that adequate steam penetration is assured dressings may be sterilized in downward displacement autoclaves which rely on displacement of air by steam. However, high pre-vacuum autoclaves in which virtually all the air is removed before the admission of steam are much more commonly employed. This method ensures rapid heating up of dressings, reduces the time needed to achieve sterilization (e.g. 134°C for 4 minutes) and shortens the overall sterilization cycle.

A recent development is the use of spray-on dressings. A convenient type is an acrylic polymer dissolved in ethyl acetate and packed as an aerosol. This should be self-sterilizing. The film after application is able to maintain the sterility of a clean wound for up to 2 weeks. However, they can only be used on clean, relatively dry wounds.

2.5 Implants

Implants are small, sterile cylinders of drug, inserted beneath the skin or into muscle tissue to provide slow absorption and prolonged action therapy. This is principally based on the fact that such drugs, invariably hormones, are almost insoluble in water and yet the implant provides a rate of dissolution sufficient for a therapeutic effect. Implants are manufactured from the pure drug made into tablet form by compression or fusion. No other ingredient can be included because this may be insoluble or toxic, or most importantly may influence the rate of drug release. Copolymers such as polylactic acid/polyglycolic acid may be used as the implant matrix to provide a controlled rate of drug delivery.

Compression of sterile drugs must be conducted under aseptic conditions using sterile machine parts and materials. After manufacture, the outer surface of the implant is sterilized by immersion in 0.002% w/v phenylmercuric nitrate at 75°C for 12 hours. After the surface has been dried, each implant is placed aseptically into a sterile glass vial with a cotton-wool plug at both ends. This prevents damage and reduces the risk of glass specules, formed when the vial is opened, adhering to the implant. This compression process is not ideal and fusion processes may be used provided that the drug is heat-stable. The pure drug is melted at 5–10°C above its melting temperature and poured into moulds. The interior of the implant will be automatically sterilized by this process if the melting temperature is high enough. It is also possible to dry heat sterilize the implant after packaging provided that the melting temperature is above 160°C. Clearly, it is easier to manufacture sterile implants by fusion as the process does not require pre-sterilized ingredients or aseptic processing. The implant hardness is also very convenient.

2.6 Absorbable haemostats

The reduction of blood loss during or after surgical procedures where suturing or ligature is either impractical or impossible can often be accomplished by the use of sterile, absorbable haemostats. These consist of a soft pad of solid material packed around and over the wound that can be left *in situ* and absorbed by body tissues over a period of time, usually up to 6 weeks. The principal mechanism of action of these is their ability to encourage platelet fracture because of their fibrous or rough surfaces, and to act as a matrix for complete blood clotting. Four products commonly used are: oxidized cellulose, absorbable gelatin sponge, human fibrin foam and calcium alginate.

2.6.1 Oxidized cellulose

This consists of cellulose material that has been partially oxidized. White gauze is the most common form, although lint is also used. It can be absorbed by the body in 2–7 weeks, depending on the size. Its action is based principally on a mechanical effect and it is used in the dry state. As it inactivates thrombin, its activity cannot be enhanced by thrombin incorporation.

2.6.2 Absorbable gelatin foam

This insoluble foam is produced by whisking warm gelatin solution to form a uniform foam, which is then dried. It can be cut into suitable shapes, packed in metal or paper containers and sterilized by dry heat (150°C for 1 hour). Moist heat destroys the physical properties of the material. Immediately before use, it can be moistened with normal saline containing thrombin. It behaves as a mechanical

haemostat providing the framework on which blood clotting can occur.

2.6.3 Human fibrin foam

This is a dry sponge of human fibrin prepared by clotting a foam of human fibrinogen solution with human thrombin. It is then freeze-dried, cut into shapes and sterilized by dry heat at 130°C for 3 hours. Before use it is saturated with thrombin solution. Blood coagulation occurs in contact with the thrombin in the interstices of the foam.

2.6.4 Calcium alginate

This is composed of the sodium and calcium salts of alginic acid formed into a powder of fibrous material and sterilized by autoclaving. It aids clotting by forming a sodium-calcium alginate complex in contact with tissue fluids acting principally as a mechanical haemostat. It is relatively slowly absorbed and some residues may occasionally remain in the tissues.

2.7 Surgical ligatures and sutures

The use of strands of material to tie off blood or other vessels (ligature) and to stitch wounds (suture) is an essential part of surgery. Both absorbable and non-absorbable materials are available for this purpose.

2.7.1 Sterilized surgical catgut

This consists of absorbable strands of collagen derived from mammalian tissue, particularly the intestine of sheep. Because of its source, it is particularly prone to bacterial contamination, and even anaerobic spores may be found in such material. Therefore sterilization is a particularly difficult process. As collagen is converted to gelatin when exposed to moist heat, autoclaving cannot be used. The official method is to pack the 'plain' catgut strands (up to 350 cm in length) on a metal spindle in a glass or other suitable container with a tubing fluid, the purpose of which is to maintain both flexibility and tensile strength after sterilization. Probably the most suitable method is to expose the material to gamma-radiation. There is minimal loss of tensile strength and the container can be over-wrapped prior to sterilization to provide a sterile container surface for opening aseptically. The alternative method involves placing the coiled suture immersed in a tubing fluid (commonly 95% ethyl alcohol with or without 0.002% w/v phenylmercuric nitrate) and storing for sufficient time to ensure sterilization. The outer surface of the vial must be sterilized before opening to avoid contamination of the suture when removed. Therefore the vial is immersed in 1% w/v formaldehyde in ethanol before use. It cannot be heated. A non official method of sterilization is to immerse the catgut in a non-aqueous solvent (naphthalene or toluene) and heat at 160°C for 2 hours. The catgut becomes hard and brittle during the process, and is aseptically transferred to an aqueous tubing fluid to restore its flexibility and tensile strength.

Catgut is packed in single threads up to 350 cm in length of various thicknesses related to tensile strength in single-use glass or plastic containers that cannot be resealed after use. Any remaining material should be discarded. Hardened catgut is prepared by treating strands with certain agents to prolong resistance to digestion. If hardened with chromium compounds, the material is known as chromicized catgut.

2.7.2 Non-absorbable types

Sutures and ligatures are also made from many materials not absorbed by the body tissues. These consist of uniform strands of metal or organic material that will not cause any tissue reactions and are capable of being sterilized. Depending on the physical stability of each material, they are preferably sterilized by autoclaving or gamma-radiation. They are packed in single-dose sachets, either dry or surrounded by a preserving fluid with or without a bactericide. The different materials are described in the *British Pharmacopoeia* (2002); they include linen (adversely affected by gamma-rays), nylon (either monofilament or plaited), silk and polypropylene.

2.8 Instruments and equipment

The method chosen for sterilization of instruments

(see Table 19.3) depends on the nature of the components and the design of the item. The wide range of instruments that may be required in a sterile condition includes syringes (glass or plastic disposable), needles, giving sets, metal surgical instruments (e.g. scalpels, scissors, forceps), rubber gloves, catheters, etc. Relatively complicated equipment such as pressure transducers, pacemakers, kidney dialysis equipment, incubators and aerosol machine parts may also be sterilized. Artificial joints could also be included in the vast range of items required in modern medical practice in a sterile condition. The choice of method depends largely on the physical stability of the items and the appropriate technique in particular situations. For instance, incubators necessitate a chemical method of sterilization. On the other hand, even delicate instruments like pressure transducers are now available that can withstand autoclaving.

3 Sterilization considerations

Sterilization processes are discussed in detail in Chapter 20. However, it is axiomatic that whatever method is chosen, the process should not cause damage to the product. By reference mostly to moist heat sterilization processes (the reader should remember that there are parallel approaches to other methods of sterilization) this section illustrates the factors that must be considered in the design of a sterilization process.

The simplest method of sterilization, for an aqueous product, is to expose it to the standard moist heat sterilization conditions, i.e. holding the product at 121°C for 15 minutes, a process termed overkill. These conditions are quite severe and therefore milder conditions might be considered, i.e. a lower holding temperature than 121°C, or a shorter holding period than 15 minutes for a product prone to degradation. The minimum holding period for moist heat sterilization might be considered to be 8 minutes at 121°C. However, in reality a slightly shorter holding period may be satisfactory if the lethality of the whole autoclave cycle (including heat up and cooling phases) is calculated using F_0 values (Chapter 20) and shown to afford the requisite sterility assurance level. F_0 values ≥ 8 minutes

Table 19.3 Methods* commonly used to sterilize or disinfect equipment

Equipment	Method of treatment	Sterilization or disinfection	Preferred method	Comments
Syringes (glass)	Dry heat	Sterilization	Dry heat using assembled syringes	Autoclave not recommended; difficulty with steam penetration unless plungers and barrels sterilized separately
Syringes (glass), dismantled	Moist heat	Sterilization		
Syringes (disposable)	Gamma-radiation	Sterilization	Gamma-radiation	Possibility of 'crazing' of syringes after ethylene oxide
	Ethylene oxide			
Needles (all metal)	Dry heat	Sterilization	Dry heat	
Needles (disposable)	Gamma-radiation	Sterilization	Gamma-radiation	
	Ethylene oxide			
Metal instruments (including scalpels)	Autoclave	Sterilization	Dry heat	Cutting edges should be protected from mechanical damage during the process
	Dry heat			
Disposable instruments	Gamma-radiation	Sterilization	Gamma-radiation	
	Ethylene oxide			
Rubber gloves	Autoclave	Sterilization	Gamma-radiation	If autoclave used, care should be taken with drying at end of process. Little oxidative degradation when high vacuum autoclave used
	Gamma-radiation			
	Ethylene oxide			
Administration (giving) sets	Gamma-radiation	Sterilization	Gamma-radiation	
	Ethylene oxide			
Respirator parts	Moist heat (autoclave)	Sterilization	Sterilization by dry heat where possible	Chemicals not recommended; may be microbiologically ineffective, may present hazard to patient safety by compromising the safety devices on the machine
	Moist heat (low temperature steam, or hot water at 80°C)	Disinfection		
Dialysis machines	Chemical	Disinfection	Formalin	Ethylene oxide not recommended in NHS for practical reasons
Fragile heat-sensitive equipment	Ethylene oxide	Sterilization	Ethylene oxide under expert supervision	
	Chemical	Disinfection		

* 1. Disposable equipment should not be re-sterilized or re-used. 2. Ethylene oxide is a difficult process to control and the Department of Health discourages its use in hospitals. 3. Low temperature steam with formaldehyde is of value in the sterilization/disinfection of some heat-sensitive materials. 4. Chemical agents, e.g. gluteraldehyde, hypochlorite.

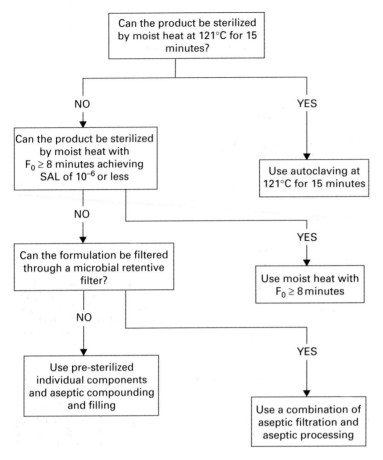

Fig. 19.1 Decision tree for sterilization choices for aqueous products (from CPMP/QWP/054/98).

are normally considered satisfactory. Use of lower temperatures and times gives an autoclave process partly based on the initial bioburden and partly on the known stability of the product.

3.1 Decision trees

Where it is not possible to sterilize a product in its final container by terminal heat sterilization at 121°C for 15 minutes, decisions have to be made to use an alternative method. The options include filtration in combination with aseptic processing, but readers should note that aseptic processing by itself is not a method of sterilization, rather of preventing contamination of the product whilst it is manufactured from individually sterilized components.

The European Agency for the Evaluation of Medicinal Products in 2000 produced an Annex for Guidance on Development Pharmaceuticals (CPMP/QWP/155/96) showing decision trees for the selection of sterilization methods. The tree for the sterilization choices for aqueous products is shown in Fig. 19.1. The initial premise is that if the products may be sterilized at 121°C for 15 minutes, that process should be used. The next alternative is that if the product is stable when an $F_0 \geq 8$ minutes can be used, then the reduced moist heat process should be undertaken. If heat processes are unsuitable (an $F_0 < 8$ minutes will not guarantee sterility), then filtration through a microbial filter should be chosen as the process to render the product sterile. If that process cannot be utilized then pre-sterilizing of stable components and aseptic compounding and filling must be considered. The described methods generally show decreasing levels of sterility assurance on moving down the tree. It is imperative

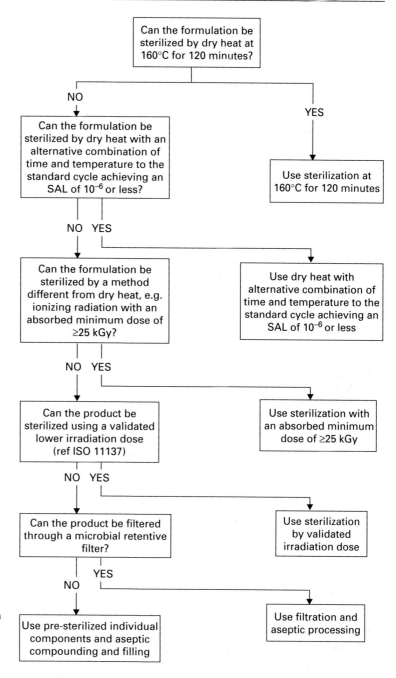

Fig. 19.2 Decision tree for sterilization choices for non-aqueous liquid, semi-solid or dry powder products (from CPMP/QWP/054/98).

therefore to remember that the highest level of sterility assurance is achieved in conjunction with the lowest pre-sterilization bioburden. The use of inappropriate heat-labile packaging material cannot by itself be the reason for the use of aseptic pro-

cessing and any manufacturer should use the best sterilization method achievable for a given formulation before selecting the packaging material. The manufacture of biotechnology products, which are typically heat-labile peptides, proteins or nucleic acids, will provide a challenge to sterility as their overall stability dictates their positioning near the bottom of the decision tree. They may require sterilization by sub-micron (< 0.1 μm) filtration and filling and finishing using aseptic processes. The overall SAL for terminally sterilized products should be $< 10^{-6}$ and for aseptically produced products is $< 10^{-3}$.

Figure 19.2 gives the decision tree for sterilization choices for non-aqueous liquid, semi-solid or dry powder products. Intermediary decisions, based on radiation and not found with aqueous products, may be seen in the tree.

3.2 Problems of drug stability

Certain issues of product instability may be resolved by formulation or careful selection of vehicle. Aminophylline injection, for example, is a solution of the drug in Water for Injections free from carbon dioxide, as the presence of this gas causes precipitation of the active. Similarly, promethazine injection is a solution of the active in Water for Injections free from dissolved air as the presence of oxygen would cause promethazine oxidation. Removal of these gases can be accomplished by prior boiling; additionally the product may be packed under an atmosphere of nitrogen to eliminate oxygen from the head space in the ampoule.

Formulations may be further stabilized by the inclusion of inactive ingredients with specific functions. Although the *British Pharmacopoeia* (2002) describes chloramphenicol eye-drops as a sterile solution of chloramphenicol in purified water, normally the system is buffered for stability with a boric acid/sodium borate buffer (see Table 19.1). Sodium metabisulphite may be found in many products as an anti-oxidant to prevent degradation of the active, examples being promethazine injection and adrenaline injection. The presence of antimicrobial preservatives may be found in multiple-dose products, to prevent microbial growth following contamination during use. Many of these formulation considerations relate to stability of the product during storage but an understanding of thermostability is required for the selection of the appropriate sterilization process.

The choice of sterilization method depends on the thermostability of the active ingredient. Moist heat sterilization can only be applied to drugs that are heat-stable in aqueous solution and are not subject to hydrolysis. Where aqueous solutions are so unstable that chemical stabilization is impossible, consideration should be given to sterilization of the drug itself by dry heat processes (160°C for 2 hours or its equivalent at higher temperatures) in its final container and dissolution immediately before use by the addition of sterile Water for Injections BP. For drugs which are both thermolabile and unstable in aqueous solution, a sterile solution of the drug may be freeze-dried in its final container and is again reconstituted as above just before use. Examples include many antibiotics and Hyaluronidase Injection BP.

4 Quality control and quality assurance of sterile products

It is not the aim of this section to review the entirety of quality control of sterile products or of the chemical assays and requirements of drugs and excipients prior to formulation. Therefore only those techniques with importance either to microbiology or the confirmation of sterility of the final product are introduced.

4.1 Bioburden

It should be obvious from previous sections that a successful sterilization process is dependent on a product having a low pre-sterilization bioburden. This will also be true of the individual ingredients, which must have low levels of microbial contamination or else there is a danger that the contaminants will find their way into the final product or be a source of pyrogens (see section 4.4). Sterilization should be considered as the removal of the bioburden.

Underestimating the level of microbial contamination prior to the terminal sterilization process will lead to a miscalculation of the sterilization dose requirements to achieve the desired sterility assurance level. The bioburden must be maintained within certain limits to justify the chosen sterilization process. When a higher number of organisms or more resistant microorganisms are encountered during manufacture of batches than was determined during the initial validation, those batches must be assumed not to be sterile. The bioburden is an estimate of the total viable count of microorganisms present pre-sterilization, and a knowledge of the resistance characteristics of these organisms is often an integral part of the sterility assurance calculation. To build some degree of safety into the sterilization process the sterilization conditions should be set to destroy all the bioburden by assuming that ALL the contaminating microorganisms are the most resistant of the species identified in that bioburden. Sterility assurance, as implied in the schemes shown in Figs 19.1 and 19.2 can only be achieved with a low bioburden and fully validated, correctly functioning sterilizers.

4.2 The test for sterility

The broad basis of the test for sterility is that it examines samples of the final product for the presence of microorganisms. Theoretically, the test for sterility should be applied to all products that are designated as sterile. However, the test does not examine all samples in a batch, its results can only be considered valid if all items in a batch are treated similarly (*British Pharmacopoeia*, 2002). Clearly for products which are terminally sterilized this might seem a reasonable assumption but only if there is uniform heat distribution in an autoclave or hot air oven or uniform delivery of a radiation dose. With aseptically produced products there are dangers because not all items in a batch may have been treated similarly. A successful test only shows that no microbial contamination was found in the samples examined under the test conditions. Extension of the result to a whole batch requires the assurance that every unit in the batch was manufactured in such a manner that it would also have passed the test with a high degree of probability. This highlights the weakness of the test for sterility and why the controls of sterilization processes are very important and probably of greater assurance in confirming the sterility of a batch. The test, however, remains one of few analytical methods that examine a product for sterility; the practical aspects of sterility tests are considered in Chapter 20 and the limitations of sterility testing have been discussed by Brown & Gilbert (1977).

4.3 Parametric release

As there are significant limitations with the test for sterility, many authorities place considerable reliance on the validation and reliable performance of sterilizers and their sterilization cycles. Parametric release takes this reliance a step further by allowing batches of terminally sterilized products to be released without being subjected to the test for sterility. The sterilization cycle will be validated to have a sterility assurance level of 10^{-6} or less as the minimum safety factor. Validation studies would include heat distribution, heat penetration, bioburden, container closure and cycle lethality studies. For a product to be subject to parametric release, pre-sterilization bioburden testing on each batch would be completed, and the comparative resistance of isolated spore-formers checked. Each cycle would include the use of chemical or biological indicators. It is hoped that these actions will provide a significantly higher level of assurance of sterility than provided by the test for sterility. In practice this requires confirmation that each part of the manufacturing process has been satisfactorily completed, the initial pre-sterilization bioburden is within agreed limits, that the controls for the sterilizing cycle were satisfactory and that the correct time cycles were achieved. In practice parametric release should only be used when experience has been gained on a reliably controlled and adequately validated process and where a relationship has been proved between end-product testing and in-process monitoring.

Clearly reproducibility, regular monitoring and documentation are required. However, parametric release would imply abandoning the sterility test, an option that many manufacturers have not yet adopted, possibly because of the fear of litigation based on the premise that any sterile product would, if tested, have passed the test for sterility.

4.4 Pyrogens

The discovery that aqueous solutions may lead to an increase in body temperature when injected into a patient dates back to the 19th century. The agents responsible for this fever were termed 'pyrogens'. In theory a pyrogen is any substance that, when injected into a mammal, elicits a rise in body temperature, and substances produced by some Gram-positive bacteria, mycobacteria, fungi and also viruses conform to this definition. The most common pyrogens, however, and those of major significance to the pharmaceutical industry, are produced by Gram-negative bacteria and are termed endotoxins; they are lipopolysaccharides (LPS) found in the cell walls. The presence of pyrogens in aqueous solutions was first demonstrated by injection into rabbits whose body temperature was recorded. More sensitive methods have since been developed, mostly based on the discovery that a fraction of the horseshoe crab blood reacts with LPS as a clotting agent.

Two pharmacopoeial limit tests exist. That for pyrogens uses rabbits to assess pharmacological activity and therefore the presence of pyrogens of all kinds. The test for bacterial endotoxins uses lysed amoebocytes (blood cells) of the horseshoe crab and is therefore termed the *Limulus* amoebocyte lysate (LAL) test. This may be extended to many drug and device products and clearly will be developed in the future to assess the presence of endotoxins in biotechnology products.

4.4.1 Physiological effects of pyrogens

The most characteristic effect following injection of pyrogens into humans is a rise of body temperature but it is only one of a number of dose-dependent diverse effects. Pyrogens elevate the circulating levels of inflammatory cytokines, which may be followed by fever, blood coagulation, hypotension, lymphopenia, neutrophilia, elevated levels of plasma cortisol and acute phase proteins. Low doses of pyrogens induce asymptomatic inflammatory reactions. Moderate doses induce fever and changes in plasma composition. Injection of high pyrogenic doses results in shock, characterized by cardiovascular dysfunction, vasodilation, vasoconstriction, endothelium dysfunction and multiple organ dysfunction or failure and death.

4.4.2 Characteristics of bacterial endotoxin

The release of LPS from bacteria takes place after death and lysis. Many Gram-negative bacteria, e.g. *Escherichia coli* and *Proteus*, *Pseudomonas*, *Enterobacter* and *Klebsiella* species produce pyrogenic LPS which is composed of two main parts: a hydrophilic polysaccharide chain with antigenic regions, and a hydrophobic lipid group termed lipid A which is responsible for many of the biological activities. The molecular size of the polysaccharide chain is very variable, and consequently the molecular weight of the LPS may vary from 5000 to 25 000 to several million Daltons. LPS is unusually thermostable and insensitive to pH changes. Molecules are able to withstand 120°C for over 3 hours. Extremes of pH are required for rapid destruction of the LPS.

4.4.3 Sources

The sources of pyrogens in parenteral products include: water used at the end stages of the purification and crystallization of the drug or excipients, water used during processing; packaging components; and the chemicals, raw materials or equipment used in the preparation of the product. The presence of endotoxins on devices may be attributed to water in the manufacturing process, the washing of components such as filter media to be used for the manufacture of filters, or the washing/rinsing of tubing or other plastic devices prior to their sterilization. Additionally, if the drug is biologically produced, incomplete removal of the microorganisms during purification can result in high endotoxin levels.

4.4.4 Measurement of pyrogens

Pyrogens are generally assessed using rabbits which are stored in carefully controlled conditions and whose temperature is monitored before the administration of the test product. The *British Pharmacopoeia* (2002) describes a test initially based on three rabbits; the number is progressively increased if the product fails at any one of four stages (Table 19.4). Samples of the product under test are injected into the marginal ear vein at a dose no greater than

Table 19.4 Increases of temperature used to determine outcome of pyrogen tests

Number of rabbits	Material passes if summed response does not exceed	Material fails if summed response exceeds
3	1.15°C	2.65°C
6	2.80°C	4.30°C
9	4.45°C	5.95°C
12	6.60°C	6.60°C

10 ml/kg. The animals are monitored for the 3-hour period immediately after injection, at 30-minute intervals. The test assumes that the maximum rise in temperature will be detected in this 3-hour period immediately after injection. Table 19.4 describes the criteria for pass or fail as the number of rabbits used increases to the maximum of 12.

A number of limitations of the rabbit pyrogen test are recognized. Repeated use of animals leads to endotoxin tolerance. There is low reactivity to the endotoxin produced by certain species, e.g. *Legionella*. There is also variability in control results when identical standardized endotoxin preparations are used, which is probably related to factors affecting the rabbits such as seasonal variation, inter-laboratory factors, rabbit species variations and other biological variation. Care must be taken in testing radiopharmaceuticals, and certain drugs may, themselves, elicit a rise in temperature on administration. The test is therefore inadequate for radiopharmaceuticals, cancer chemotherapeutic agents, hypnotics and narcotics, vitamins, steroids and some antibiotics. The presence of pyrogens may be hidden by the pharmacological activity of the product's components. Finally the rabbit test is insufficiently sensitive to detect endotoxin in intrathecal products where only low levels of pyrogens are acceptable.

4.4.5 Measurement of bacterial endotoxins

The LAL test is considerably more sensitive than the pyrogen test. As mentioned above, although the *Legionella* endotoxin is not very pyrogenic to rabbits it is easily detected by the LAL test. It has been estimated that there is a 1000-fold difference in sensitivity between the two tests but the LAL test only detects endotoxins of Gram-negative bacteria and not all pyrogens. However, the LAL test may be used for radiopharmaceuticals.

LAL test reagent comes from the American horseshoe crab *Limulus polyphemus*. The endotoxin-induced coagulation of its blood is based on an enzyme-mediated interaction of LAL with endotoxins. The reagents are obtained from the blood of freshly captured horseshoe crabs whose amoebocytes are concentrated, washed and lysed with endotoxin-free water. The LAL is separated from the remaining cellular debris and its activity optimized using metallic cations, pH adjustment and additives and then freeze-dried. Certain preparations interfere with the interaction between LAL and endotoxin. Chemical inhibitors may cause chelation of the divalent cations necessary for the reaction, protein denaturation or inappropriate pH changes. Physical inhibition may result from adsorption of endotoxin or be caused by viscosity of the product. Even the type of glassware may affect the test. Siliconized glassware or plastic can inhibit gel-clot formation, or prevent accurate spectrophotometric readings of the reaction end-point.

The samples of products are incubated with *Limulus* amoebocyte lysate at 37°C. If endotoxins are present a solid gel forms, indicating the presence of endotoxins. The *British Pharmacopoeia* (2002) describes six separate methodologies for the test for endotoxin. These are (A) gel-clot limit test; (B) gel-clot: semi quantitative; (C) turbidimetric kinetic method; (D) chromogenic kinetic method; (E) chromogenic end-point method; and (F) turbidimetric end-point method. There are checks for interfering factors. Any validated method may be used, but the gel-clot method is the referee test in the case of dispute. Coloured products cannot be tested by turbidimetric and chromogenic methods, as precipitate formation may be mistaken for a positive response.

Kinetic LAL methods are claimed to increase the efficiency of large-scale testing, probably important when validation of depyrogenation cycles or preparation of components for aseptic processing are required. For all procedures, test validation must be conducted to rule out interference, which may be either inhibition or enhancement. Depyrogenated glassware must be used throughout.

The gel-clot method is most commonly used. The test is conducted by adding the LAL reagent to an equal volume of test solution, agitating and storing at 37°C for 1 hour when the end-point is determined by inversion of the tubes. If a solid clot remains intact the product is considered to contain endotoxins. Chromogenic methods utilize colorimetry but do not depend on the clottable protein. A synthetic substrate is used that contains an amino acid sequence similar to that of coagulogen, the clottable protein. The activated proclotting enzyme cleaves a p-nitroanilide chromophore from the synthetic substrate and the colour produced is proportional to the amount of endotoxin. The turbidimetric LAL method is based on the fact that an increase in endotoxin concentration will cause a proportional increase in turbidity caused by the precipitation of the clottable protein, coagulogen. The optical density is read spectrophotometrically either at a fixed time or constantly for kinetic assays as turbidity develops. The kinetic methods depend on the relationship between the logarithm of the response and the logarithm of the endotoxin concentration. The end-point methods relate endotoxin levels to the quantity of chromophore released or the amount of precipitation.

4.4.6 Endotoxins in parenteral pharmaceuticals

The limits for endotoxin are based on the dose of the product. Put simply, the endotoxin limit, EL, which represents the maximum amount of endotoxin that is allowed in a specific dose, is inversely related to the dose of the drug; it may be assessed from the following equation (*United States Pharmacopoeia*, 2002):

$$EL = K/M$$

where K is the threshold human pyrogenic dose of endotoxin per kg body weight and M is the maximum human dose of the product in kg body weight that would be administered in a single 1-hour period. M recognizes that the pharmacological effects of endotoxin are dose-dependent. The endotoxin limit is the level at which a product is adjudged pyrogenic or non-pyrogenic. Gel-clot reagent sensitivities are generally in the range 0.015–0.5 EU/ml. As examples of endotoxin limits, the *United States Pharmacopoeia* (2002) states limits of " 0.5 EU/ml for Dextrose Infusion, " 5 EU/mg promethazine in Promethazine Injection USP, " 10 EU/mg of mitomycin in Mitomycin for Injection USP and " 24 EU/mg warfarin sodium in Warfarin Sodium for Injection. The *British Pharmacopoeia* (2002) has a limit of 0.25 IU/ml in Glucose Intravenous Infusion; this value is similar for many BP intravenous infusions. As another example insulin should contain " 10 IU/mg of endotoxin. The endotoxin limit for drugs gaining access to the CSF is reduced to 0.2 EU/kg because the intrathecal route is the most toxic route for endotoxins.

4.4.7 Depyrogenation and the production of apyrogenic products

Pyrogens and endotoxins are difficult to remove from products once present and it is easier to keep components relatively endotoxin-free rather than to remove it from the final product. Rinsing or dilution is one way of eliminating pyrogenic activity provided that the rinsing fluid is apyrogenic. Closures and vials should be washed with pyrogen-free water before sterilization. Pyrogens in vials or glass components may be destroyed by dry heat sterilization at high temperatures. A recommended condition for depyrogenation of glassware and equipment is heating at 250°C for 45 minutes. Pyrogens are also destroyed at 650°C in 1 minute or at 180°C in 4 hours. The *British Pharmacopoeia* (2002) states that dry heat at temperatures > 220°C may be used for the depyrogenation of glassware. These processes equate to incineration, although removal by washing, also termed dilution, may be used. Filtration, irradiation or ethylene oxide treatment have limited value in reducing pyrogen or endotoxin loads.

The removal of pyrogens from Water for Injections may be effected by distillation or reverse osmosis. Distillation is the most reliable method for removing endotoxin. Care has to be taken to avoid splashing in the still as pyrogens have been carried over in droplets. Another source of endotoxins is the Water for Injection system. Generally circulating hot water at temperatures above 75°C provides an environment that is not conducive to microbial growth and thus the formation of endotoxin. Circulating water at approximately 60°C causes some concern as some Gram-negative organisms, e.g. *Legionella pneumophilia*, will survive and grow at 57°C. The water-producing systems may be sanitized by circulating water at 75–80°C.

Pyrogen-free water can be produced using an ultrafiltration membrane with a nominal molecular weight limit that is low enough to ensure the removal of endotoxins under all conditions. Hollow fibre polysulphone membranes can be sanitized with sodium hydroxide, which efficiently destroys pyrogens. A nominal molecular weight limit of 5000 Da should efficiently remove endotoxins. However, many endotoxin-producing microorganisms multiply in ambient temperature Water for Injection systems, especially reverse osmosis (RO) systems. Reverse osmosis filters are not absolute and may be used in series in order to manufacture pyrogen-free water.

5 Acknowledgement

The contribution of Professor Mike Allwood, who wrote the chapter on sterile products in previous editions of this book, is gratefully acknowledged. The European Agency for the Evaluation of Medicinal Products is acknowledged for permission to use Figs 19.1 and 19.2.

6 Further reading

Annex for Guidance on Development Pharmaceuticals (CPMP/QWP/155/96). EMEA The European Agency for the Evaluation of Medicinal Products (2000).

British Pharmacopoeia Commission (2002) *British Pharmacopoeia*. The Stationery Office, London.

Brown, M.R.W. & Gilbert, P. (1977) Increasing the probability of sterility of medicinal products. *J Pharm Pharmacol*, 29, 517–523.

Cooper, J.F. (2001) The bacterial endotoxins test: past, present and future. *Eur J Parenteral Sci*, 6, 89–93.

Guerret, J. & Murano, R.A. (2002) The unique challenges of manufacturing parenteral nutrition products. *Eur J Parenteral Sci*, 7, 127–130.

ISO 11137 Sterilization of health care products — Requirements for validation and routine control — Radiation sterilization (1995).

Murgatroyd, K. (2001) Freeze drying — a review. *Eur J Parenteral Sci*, 6, 21–25.

Pharmaceutical Codex (1994) London: The Pharmaceutical Press.

United States Pharmacopoeia (2002) US Pharmacopoeial Convention, Rockville, MD.

Chapter 20
Sterilization procedures and sterility assurance

Stephen Denyer and Norman Hodges

1 Introduction

Sterilization is an essential stage in the processing of any product destined for parenteral administration, or for contact with broken skin, mucosal surfaces, or internal organs, where the threat of infection exists. In addition, the sterilization of microbiological materials, soiled dressings and other contaminated items is necessary to minimize the health hazard associated with these articles.

Sterilization processes involve the application of a biocidal agent or physical microbial removal process to a product or preparation with the object of killing or removing all microorganisms. These processes may involve elevated temperature, reactive gas, irradiation or filtration through a microorganism-proof filter. The success of the process depends upon a suitable choice of treatment conditions, e.g. temperature and duration of exposure. It must be remembered, however, that with all articles to be sterilized there is a potential risk of product damage, which for a pharmaceutical preparation may result in reduced therapeutic efficacy, stability or patient acceptability. Thus, there is a need to achieve a balance between the maximum acceptable risk of failing to achieve sterility and the maximum level of product damage that is acceptable. This is best determined from a knowledge of the properties of the sterilizing agent, the properties of the product to be sterilized and the nature of the likely contaminants. A suitable sterilization process may then be selected to ensure maximum microbial kill/removal with minimum product deterioration.

2 Sensitivity of microorganisms

The general pattern of resistance of microorganisms to biocidal sterilization processes is independent of the type of agent employed (heat, radiation or gas), with vegetative forms of bacteria and fungi, along with the larger viruses, showing a greater sensitivity to sterilization processes than small viruses and bacterial or fungal spores. The choice of suitable reference organisms for testing the efficiency of sterilization processes (see section 12.3) is therefore made from the most durable bacterial spores; these are usually represented *by Bacillus stearothermophilus* for moist heat, certain strains of *B. subtilis* for dry heat and gaseous sterilization, and *B. pumilus* for ionizing radiation.

Ideally, when considering the level of treatment necessary to achieve sterility a knowledge of the type and total number of microorganisms present in a product, together with their likely response to the proposed treatment, is necessary. Without this information, however, it is usually assumed that organisms within the load are no more resistant than the reference spores or than specific resistant product isolates. In the latter case, it must be remembered that resistance may be altered or lost entirely by laboratory subculture and the resistance characteristics of the maintained strain must be regularly checked.

A sterilization process may thus be developed without a full microbiological background to the product, instead being based on the ability to deal with a 'worst case' condition. This is indeed the situation for official sterilization methods, which must be capable of general application, and modern pharmacopoeial recommendations are derived from a careful analysis of experimental data on bacterial spore survival following treatments with heat, ionizing radiation or gas.

However, the infectious agents responsible for spongiform encephalopathies such as bovine spongiform encephalopathy (BSE) and Creutzfeldt–Jakob disease (CJD) exhibit exceptional degrees of resistance to all known lethal agents. Recent work has even cast doubts on the adequacy of the process of 18-minute exposure to steam at 134–138°C which has been officially recommended for the destruction of these agents (and which far exceeds the lethal treatment required to achieve adequate destruction of bacterial spores).

2.1 Survivor curves

When exposed to a killing process, populations of microorganisms generally lose their viability in an exponential fashion, independent of the initial number of organisms. This can be represented graphically with a 'survivor curve' drawn from a plot of the logarithm of the fraction of survivors against the exposure time or dose (Fig. 20.1). Of the typical curves obtained, all have a linear portion which may be continuous (plot A), or may be modified by an initial shoulder (B) or by a reduced rate of kill at low survivor levels (C). Furthermore, a short activation phase, representing an initial increase in viable count, may be seen during the heat treatment of certain bacterial spores. Survivor curves have been employed principally in the examination of heat sterilization methods, but can equally well be applied to any biocidal process.

2.2 Expressions of resistance

2.2.1 D-*value*

The resistance of an organism to a sterilizing agent can be described by means of the D-value. For heat and radiation treatments, respectively, this is defined as the time taken at a fixed temperature or the radiation dose required to achieve a 90% reduction in viable cells (i.e. a 1 log cycle reduction in survivors; Fig. 20.2A). The calculation of the D-value assumes a linear type A survivor curve (Fig. 20.1), and must be corrected to allow for any deviation from linearity with type B or C curves. Some typical D-values for resistant bacterial spores are given in Table 20.1.

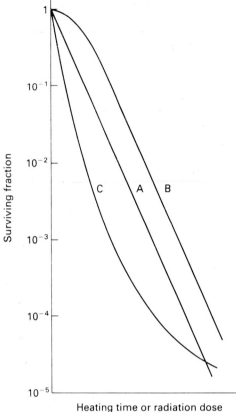

Fig. 20.1 Typical survivor curves for bacterial spores exposed to moist heat or gamma-radiation.

2.2.2 Z-value

For heat treatment, a D-value only refers to the resistance of a microorganism at a particular temperature. In order to assess the influence of temperature changes on thermal resistance a relationship between temperature and log D-value can be developed, leading to the expression of a z-value, which represents the increase in temperature needed to reduce the D-value of an organism by 90% (i.e. 1 log cycle reduction; Fig. 20.2B). For bacterial spores used as biological indicators for moist heat (*B. stearothermophilus*) and dry heat (*B. subtilis*) sterilization processes, mean z-values are given as 10°C and 22°C, respectively. The z-value is not truly independent of temperature but may be considered essentially constant over the temperature ranges used in heat sterilization processes.

2.3 Sterility assurance

The term 'sterile', in a microbiological context, means no surviving organisms whatsoever. Thus, there are no degrees of sterility; an item is either sterile or it is not, and so there are no levels of contamination which may be considered negligible or insignificant and therefore acceptable. From the survivor curves presented, it can be seen that the

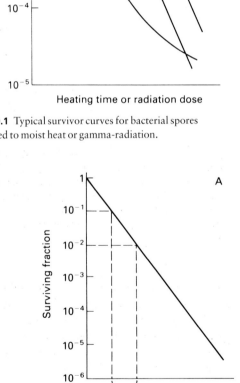

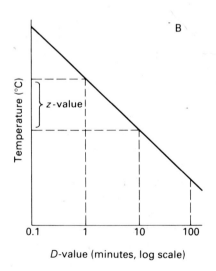

Fig. 20.2 Calculation of: (A) D-value; (B) z-value.

Table 20.1 Inactivation factors (IF) for selected sterilization protocols and their corresponding biological indicator (BI) organisms

Sterilization protocol	BI organism	D-value	Log IF
Moist heat (121°C for 15 minutes)	*B. stearothermophilus*	1.5 min	10
Dry heat (160°C for 2 hours)	*B. subtilis* var. *niger*	Max. 10 min	Min. 12
Irradiation (25 kGy; 2.5 Mrad)	*B. pumilus*	3 kGy (0.3 Mrad)	8.3

elimination of viable microorganisms from a product is a time-dependent process, and will be influenced by the rate and duration of biocidal action and the initial microbial contamination level. It is also evident from Fig. 20.2A that true sterility, represented by zero survivors, can only be achieved after an infinite exposure period or radiation dose. Clearly, then, it is illogical to claim, or expect, that a sterilization procedure will guarantee sterility. Thus, the likelihood of a product being produced free of microorganisms is best expressed in terms of the probability of an organism surviving the treatment process, a possibility not entertained in the absolute term 'sterile'. From this approach has arisen the concept of sterility assurance or a microbial safety index which gives a numerical value to the probability of a single surviving organism remaining to contaminate a processed product. For pharmaceutical products, the most frequently applied standard is that the probability, post-sterilization, of a non-sterile unit is ″1 in 1 million units processed (i.e. ″10^{-6}). The sterilization protocol necessary to achieve this with any given organism of known D-value can be established from the inactivation factor (IF) which may be defined as:

$$IF = 10^{t/D}$$

where t is the contact time (for a heat or gaseous sterilization process) or dose (for ionizing radiation) and D is the D-value appropriate to the process employed.

Thus, for an initial burden of 10^2 spores an inactivation factor of 10^8 will be needed to give the required sterility assurance of 10^{-6} (Fig. 20.3). The sterilization process will therefore need to produce sufficient lethality to achieve an 8 log cycle reduction in viable organisms; this will require exposure of the product to eight times the D-value of the reference organism ($8D$). In practice, it is generally

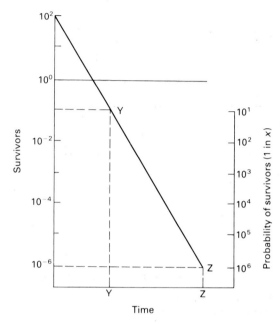

Fig. 20.3 Sterility assurance. At Y, there is (literally) 10^{-1} bacterium in one bottle, i.e. in 10 loads of single containers, there would be one chance in 10 that one load would be positive. Likewise, at Z, there is (literally) 10^{-6} bacterium in one bottle, i.e. in 1 million (10^6) loads of single containers, there is one chance in 1 million that one load would be positive.

assumed that the contaminant will have the same resistance as the test spores unless full microbiological data are available to indicate otherwise. The inactivation factors associated with certain sterilization protocols and their biological indicator organisms are given in Table 20.1.

3 Sterilization methods

A sterilization process should always be considered

a compromise between achieving good antimicrobial activity and maintaining product stability. It must, therefore, be validated against a suitable test organism and its efficacy continually monitored during use. Even so, a limit will exist as to the type and size of microbial challenge that can be handled by the process without significant loss of sterility assurance. Thus, sterilization must not be seen as a 'catch-all' or as an alternative to good manufacturing practices but must be considered as only the final stage in a programme of microbiological control. The *European Pharmacopoeia* (2002) recognizes five methods for the sterilization of pharmaceutical products. These are: (i) steam sterilization (heating in an autoclave); (ii) dry heat; (iii) ionizing radiation; (iv) gas sterilization; and (v) filtration. In addition, other approaches involving steam and formaldehyde and ultraviolet (UV) light have evolved for use in certain situations. For each method, the possible permutations of exposure conditions are numerous, but experience and product stability requirements have generally served to limit this choice. Nevertheless, it should be remembered that even the recommended methods and regimens do not necessarily demonstrate equivalent biocidal potential (see Table 20.1), but simply offer alternative strategies for application to a wide variety of product types. Thus, each should be validated in their application to demonstrate that the minimum required level of sterility assurance can be achieved (sections 2.3 and 9).

In the following sections, factors governing the successful use of these sterilizing methods will be covered and their application to pharmaceutical and medical products considered. Methods for monitoring the efficacy of these processes are discussed in section 12.

4 Heat sterilization

Heat is the most reliable and widely used means of sterilization, affording its antimicrobial activity through destruction of enzymes and other essential cell constituents. These lethal events proceed most rapidly in a fully hydrated state, thus requiring a lower heat input (temperature and time) under conditions of high humidity where denaturation and hydrolysis reactions predominate, rather than in the dry state where oxidative changes take place. This method of sterilization is limited to thermostable products, but can be applied to both moisture-sensitive and moisture-resistant items for which dry (160–180°C) and moist (121–134°C) heat sterilization procedures are respectively used. Where thermal degradation of a product might possibly occur, it can usually be minimized by selecting the higher temperature range, as the shorter exposure times employed generally result in a lower fractional degradation.

4.1 Sterilization processes

In any heat sterilization process, the articles to be treated must first be raised to sterilization temperature and this involves a heating-up stage. In the traditional approach, timing for the process (the holding time) then begins. It has been recognized, however, that during both the heating-up and cooling-down stages of a sterilization cycle

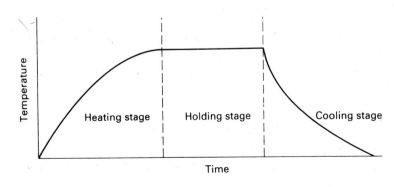

Fig. 20.4 Typical temperature profile of a heat sterilization process.

(Fig. 20.4), the product is held at an elevated temperature and these stages may thus contribute to the overall biocidal potential of the process.

A method has been devised to convert all the temperature–time combinations occurring during the heating, sterilizing and cooling stages of a moist heat (steam) sterilization cycle to the equivalent time at 121°C. This involves following the temperature profile of a load, integrating the heat input (as a measure of lethality), and converting it to the equivalent time at the standard temperature of 121°C. Using this approach, the overall lethality of any process can be deduced and is defined as the *F*-value; this expresses heat treatment at any temperature as equal to that of a certain number of minutes at 121°C. In other words, if a moist heat sterilization process has an *F*-value of *x*, then it has the same lethal effect on a given organism as heating at 121°C for *x* minutes, irrespective of the actual temperature employed or of any fluctuations in the heating process due to heating and cooling stages. The *F*-value of a process will vary according to the moist heat resistance of the reference organism; when the reference spore is that of *B. stearothermophilus* with a *z*-value of 10°C, then the *F*-value is known as the F_0-value.

A relationship between *F*- and *D*-values, leading to an assessment of the probable number of survivors in a load following heat treatment, can be established from the following equation:

$$F = D(\log N_0 - \log N)$$

in which *D* is the *D*-value at 121°C, and N_0 and *N* represent, respectively, the initial and final number of viable cells per unit volume.

The *F*-concept has evolved from the food industry and principally relates to the sterilization of articles by moist heat. Because it permits calculation of the extent to which the heating and cooling phases contribute to the overall killing effect of the autoclaving cycle, the *F*-concept enables a sterilization process to be individually developed for a particular product. This means that adequate sterility assurance can be achieved in autoclaving cycles in which the traditional pharmacopoeial recommendation of 15 minutes at 121°C is not achieved. The holding time may be reduced below 15 minutes if there is a substantial killing effect during the heating and cooling phases, and an adequate cycle can be achieved even if the 'target' temperature of 121°C is not reached. Thus, *F*-values offer both a means by which alternative sterilizing cycles can be compared in terms of their microbial killing efficiency, and a mechanism by which overprocessing of marginally thermolabile products can be reduced without compromising sterility assurance. The *European Pharmacopoeia* (2002) emphasizes that when a steam sterilization cycle is designed on the basis of F_0 data, it may be necessary to perform continuous and rigorous microbiological monitoring during routine manufacturing in order consistently to achieve an acceptable sterility assurance level.

F_0 values may be calculated either from the 'area under the curve' of a plot of autoclave temperature against time constructed using special chart paper on which the temperature scale is modified to take into account the progressively greater lethality of higher temperatures, or by use of the equation below:

$$F_0 = \Delta t \Sigma 10^{(T-121)/z}$$

where Δt = time interval between temperature measurements; T = product temperature at time t; z is (assumed to be) 10°C.

Thus, if temperatures were being recorded from a thermocouple at 1.00-minute intervals then Δt = 1.00, and a temperature of, for example, 115°C maintained for 1 minute would give an F_0 value of 1 minute $\times 10^{(115-121)/10}$ which is equal to 0.25 minutes. In practice, such calculations could easily be performed on the data from several thermocouples within an autoclave using computer-driven software, and, in a manufacturing situation, these would be part of the batch records. Such a calculation facility is offered as an optional extra by most autoclave manufacturers.

Application of the *F*-value concept has been largely restricted to steam sterilization processes although there is a less frequently employed, but direct parallel in dry heat sterilization (see section 4.3).

4.2 Moist heat sterilization

Moist heat has been recognized as an efficient biocidal agent from the early days of bacteriology, when it was principally developed for the sterilization of culture media. It now finds widespread application in the processing of many thermostable products and devices. In the pharmaceutical and medical sphere it is used in the sterilization of dressings, sheets, surgical and diagnostic equipment, containers and closures, and aqueous injections, ophthalmic preparations and irrigation fluids, in addition to the processing of soiled and contaminated items (Chapter 19).

Sterilization by moist heat usually involves the use of steam at temperatures in the range 121–134°C, and while alternative strategies are available for the processing of products unstable at these high temperatures, they rarely offer the same degree of sterility assurance and should be avoided if at all possible. The elevated temperatures generally associated with moist heat sterilization methods can only be achieved by the generation of steam under pressure.

By far the most commonly employed standard temperature/time cycles for bottled fluids and porous loads (e.g. surgical dressings) are 121°C for 15 minutes and 134°C for 3 minutes, respectively. Not only do high temperature-short time cycles often result in lower fractional degradation, they also afford the advantage of achieving higher levels of sterility assurance due to greater inactivation factors (Table 20.2). The 115°C for 30 minute cycle was considered an acceptable alternative to 121°C for 15 minutes prior to the publication of the 1988 *British Pharmacopoeia*, but it is no longer considered sufficient to give the desired sterility assurance levels for products which may contain significant concentrations of thermophilic spores.

4.2.1 Steam as a sterilizing agent

To act as an efficient sterilizing agent, steam should be able to provide moisture and heat efficiently to the article to be sterilized. This is most effectively done using saturated steam, which is steam in thermal equilibrium with the water from which it is derived, i.e. steam on the phase boundary (Fig. 20.5). Under these circumstances, contact with a cooler surface causes condensation and contraction, drawing in fresh steam and leading to the immediate release of the latent heat, which represents approximately 80% of the total heat energy. In this way, heat and moisture are imparted rapidly to

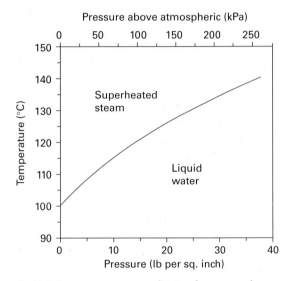

Fig. 20.5 Pressure–temperature diagram for water at the phase boundary.

Table 20.2 Pressure-temperature relationships and antimicrobial efficacies of alternative steam sterilization cycles

| Temperature (°C) | Holding time (minutes) | Steam pressure | | Inactivation factor* (decimal reductions) |
		(kPa)	(psi)	
115	30	69	10	5
121	15	103	15	10
126	10	138	20	21
134	3	207	30	40

* Calculated for a spore suspension having a D_{121} of 1.5 minutes and a z value of 10°C.

articles being sterilized and dry porous loads are quickly penetrated by the steam.

Steam for sterilization can either be generated within the sterilizer, as with portable bench or 'instrument and utensil' sterilizers, in which case it is constantly in contact with water and is known as 'wet' steam, or can be supplied under pressure (350–400 kPa) from a separate boiler as 'dry' saturated steam with no entrained water droplets. The killing potential of 'wet' steam is the same as that of 'dry' saturated steam at the same temperature, but it is more likely to soak a porous load, creating physical difficulties for further steam penetration. Thus, major industrial and hospital sterilizers are usually supplied with 'dry' saturated steam and attention is paid to the removal of entrained water droplets within the supply line to prevent introduction of a water 'fog' into the sterilizer.

If the temperature of 'dry' saturated steam is increased, then, in the absence of entrained moisture, the relative humidity or degree of saturation is reduced and the steam becomes superheated (Fig. 20.5). During sterilization this can arise in a number of ways, for example by overheating the steam-jacket (see section 4.2.2), by using too dry a steam supply, by excessive pressure reduction during passage of steam from the boiler to the sterilizer chamber, and by evolution of heat of hydration when steaming overdried cotton fabrics. Superheated steam behaves in the same manner as hot air as condensation and release of latent heat will not occur unless the steam is cooled to the phase boundary temperature. Thus, it proves to be an inefficient sterilizing agent and, although a small degree of transient superheating can be tolerated, a maximum acceptable level of 5°C superheat is set, i.e. the temperature of the steam is never greater than 5°C above the phase boundary temperature at that pressure.

The relationship between temperature and pressure holds true only in the presence of pure steam; adulteration with air contributes to a partial pressure but not to the temperature of the steam. Thus, in the presence of air the temperature achieved will reflect the contribution made by the steam and will be lower than that normally attributed to the total pressure recorded. Addition of further steam will raise the temperature but residual air surrounding

articles may delay heat penetration or, if a large amount of air is present, it may collect at the bottom of the sterilizer, completely altering the temperature profile of the sterilizer chamber. It is for these reasons that efficient air removal is a major aim in the design and operation of a boiler-fed steam sterilizer.

4.2.2 Sterilizer design and operation

Steam sterilizers, or autoclaves as they are also known, are stainless steel vessels designed to withstand the steam pressures employed in sterilization. They can be: (i) 'portable' sterilizers, where they generally have internal electric heaters to produce steam and are used for small pilot or laboratory-scale sterilization and for the treatment of instruments and utensils; or (ii) large-scale sterilizers for routine hospital or industrial use, operating on 'dry' saturated steam from a separate boiler (Fig. 20.6). Because of their widespread use within pharmacy this latter type will be considered in greatest detail.

There are two main types of large sterilizers, those designed for use with porous loads (i.e. dressings) and generally operated at a minimum temperature of 134°C, and those designed as bottled fluid sterilizers employing a minimum temperature of 121°C. The stages of operation are common to both and can be summarized as air removal and steam admission, heating-up and exposure, and drying or cooling. Many modifications of design exist and in this section only general features will be considered. Fuller treatments of sterilizer design and operation can be found in *Health Technical Memorandum 2010* (1994).

General design features. Steam sterilizers are constructed with either cylindrical or rectangular chambers, with preferred capacities ranging from 400 to 800 litres. They can be sealed by either a single door or by doors at both ends (to allow through-passage of processed materials; see Chapter 21). During sterilization the doors are held closed by a locking mechanism which prevents opening when the chamber is under pressure and until the chamber has cooled to a pre-set temperature, typically 80°C.

In the larger sterilizers the chamber may be surrounded by a steam-jacket which can be used to

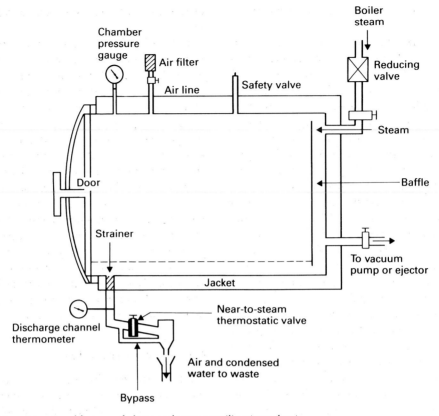

Fig. 20.6 Main constructional features of a large-scale steam sterilizer (autoclave).

heat the autoclave chamber and promote a more uniform temperature throughout the load. The same jacket can also be filled with water at the end of the cycle to facilitate cooling and thus reduce the overall cycle time. The chamber floor slopes towards a discharge channel through which air and condensate can be removed. Temperature is monitored within the opening of the discharge channel and by thermocouples in dummy packages; jacket and chamber pressures are followed using pressure gauges. In hospitals and industry, it is common practice to operate sterilizers on an automatic cycle, each stage of operation being controlled by a timer responding to temperature- or pressure-sensing devices.

The stages of operation are as follows.

1 *Air removal and steam admission.* Air can be removed from steam sterilizers either by downward displacement with steam, evacuation or a combina-tion of the two. In the downward displacement sterilizer, the heavier cool air is forced out of the discharge channel by incoming hot steam. This has the benefit of warming the load during air removal, which aids the heating-up process. It finds widest application in the sterilization of bottled fluids where bottle breakage may occur under the combined stresses of evacuation and high temperature. For more air-retentive loads (i.e. dressings), how-ever, this technique of air removal is unsatisfactory and mechanical evacuation of the air is essential before admission of the steam. This can either be to an extremely high level (e.g. 2.5 kPa) or can involve a period of pulsed evacuation and steam ad-mission, the latter approach improving air extrac-tion from dressings packs. After evacuation, steam penetration into the load is very rapid and heating-up is almost instantaneous. It is axiomatic that packaging and loading of articles within a sterilizer be so organized as to facilitate air removal.

During the sterilization process, small pockets of entrained air may still be released, especially from packages, and this air must be removed. This is achieved with a near-to-steam thermostatic valve incorporated in the discharge channel. The valve operates on the principle of an expandable bellows containing a volatile liquid which vaporizes at the temperature of saturated steam thereby closing the valve, and condenses on the passage of a cooler air-steam mixture, thus reopening the valve and discharging the air. Condensate generated during the sterilization process can also be removed by this device. Small quantities of air will not, however, lower the temperature sufficiently to operate the valve and so a continual slight flow of steam is maintained through a bypass around the device in order to flush away residual air.

It is common practice to package sterile fluids, especially intravenous fluids, in flexible plastic containers. During sterilization these can develop a considerable internal pressure in the airspace above the fluid and it is therefore necessary to maintain a proportion of air within the sterilizing chamber to produce sufficient overpressure to prevent these containers from bursting (air ballasting). In sterilizers modified or designed to process this type of product, air removal is therefore unnecessary but special attention must be paid to the prevention of air 'layering' within the chamber. This is overcome by the inclusion of a fan or through a continuous spray of hot water within the chamber to mix the air and steam. Air ballasting can also be employed to prevent bottle breakage.

2 *Heating-up and exposure.* When the sterilizer reaches its operating temperature and pressure the sterilization stage begins. The duration of exposure may include a heating-up time in addition to the holding time and this will normally be established using thermocouples in dummy articles.

3 *Drying or cooling.* Dressings packs and other porous loads may become dampened during the sterilization process and must be dried before removal from the chamber. This is achieved by steam exhaust and application of a vacuum, often assisted by heat from the steam-filled jacket if fitted. After drying, atmospheric pressure within the chamber is restored by admission of sterile filtered air.

For bottled fluids the final stage of the sterilization process is cooling, and this needs to be achieved as rapidly as possible to minimize thermal degradation of the product and to reduce processing time. In modem sterilizers, this is achieved by circulating water in the jacket that surrounds the chamber or by spray-cooling with retained condensate delivered to the surface of the load by nozzles fitted into the roof of the sterilizer chamber. This is often accompanied by the introduction of filtered, compressed air to minimize container breakage due to high internal pressures (air ballasting). Containers must not be removed from the sterilizer until the internal pressure has dropped to a safe level, usually indicated by a temperature of <80°C. Occasionally, spray-cooling water may be a source of bacterial contamination and its microbiological quality must be carefully monitored.

4.3 Dry heat sterilization

The lethal effects of dry heat on microorganisms are due largely to oxidative processes which are less effective than the hydrolytic damage which results from exposure to steam. Thus, dry heat sterilization usually employs higher temperatures in the range 160–180°C and requires exposure times of up to 2 hours depending upon the temperature employed.

Again, bacterial spores are much more resistant than vegetative cells and their recorded resistance varies markedly depending upon their degree of dryness. In many early studies on dry heat resistance of spores their water content was not adequately controlled, so conflicting data arose regarding the exposure conditions necessary to achieve effective sterilization. This was partly responsible for variations in recommended exposure temperatures and times in different pharmacopoeias.

Dry heat application is generally restricted to glassware and metal surgical instruments (where its good penetrability and non-corrosive nature are of benefit), non-aqueous thermostable liquids and thermostable powders (see Chapter 19). In practice, the range of materials that are actually subjected to dry heat sterilization is quite limited, and consists largely of items used in hospitals. The major industrial application is in the sterilization of glass bottles which are to be filled aseptically, and here the attraction of the process is that it not only achieves an adequate sterility assurance level, but that it may also destroy bacterial endotoxins (products of Gram-negative bacteria, also known as pyrogens, that cause fever when injected into the body). These are difficult to eliminate by other means. For the purposes of depyrogenation of glass, temperatures of approximately 250°C are used.

The *F*-value concept that was developed for steam sterilization processes has an equivalent in dry heat sterilization although its application has been limited. The F_H designation describes the lethality of a dry heat process in terms of the equivalent number of minutes exposure at 170°C, and in this case a *z*-value of 20°C has been found empirically to be appropriate for calculation purposes; this contrasts with the value of 10°C which is typically employed to describe moist heat resistance.

4.3.1 Sterilizer design

Dry heat sterilization is usually carried out in a hot air oven which comprises an insulated polished stainless steel chamber, with a usual capacity of up to 250 litres, surrounded by an outer case containing electric heaters located in positions to prevent cool spots developing inside the chamber. A fan is fitted to the rear of the oven to provide circulating air, thus ensuring more rapid equilibration of temperature. Shelves within the chamber are perforated to allow good airflow. Thermocouples can be used to monitor the temperature of both the oven air and articles contained within. A fixed temperature sensor connected to a chart recorder provides a permanent record of the sterilization cycle. Appropriate door-locking controls should be incorporated to prevent interruption of a sterilization cycle once begun.

Recent sterilizer developments have led to the use of dry heat sterilizing tunnels where heat transfer is achieved by infrared irradiation or by forced convection in filtered laminar airflow tunnels. Items to be sterilized are placed on a conveyer belt and pass through a high temperature zone (250–300+ °C) over a period of several minutes.

4.3.2 Sterilizer operation

Articles to be sterilized must be wrapped or enclosed in containers of sufficient strength and integrity to provide good post-sterilization protection against contamination. Suitable materials are paper, cardboard tubes or aluminium containers. Container shape and design must be such that heat penetration is encouraged in order to shorten the heating-up stage; this can be achieved by using narrow containers with dull non-reflecting surfaces. In a hot-air oven, heat is delivered to articles principally by radiation and convection; thus, they must be carefully arranged within the chamber to avoid obscuring centrally placed articles from wall radiation or impending air flow. The temperature variation within the chamber should not exceed ±5°C of the recorded temperature. Heating-up times, which may be as long as 4 hours for articles with poor heat-conducting properties, can be reduced by preheating the oven before loading. Following sterilization, the chamber temperature is usually allowed to fall to around 40°C before removal of sterilized articles; this can be accelerated by the use of forced cooling with filtered air.

5 Gaseous sterilization

The chemically reactive gases ethylene oxide $(CH_2)_2O$ and formaldehyde (methanal, H.CHO) possess broad-spectrum biocidal activity, and have found application in the sterilization of re-usable surgical instruments, certain medical, diagnostic and electrical equipment, and the surface sterilization of powders. Sterilization processes using ethylene oxide sterilization are far more commonly used on an international basis than those employing formaldehyde.

Ethylene oxide treatment can also be considered as an alternative to radiation sterilization in the commercial production of disposable medical devices (Chapter 19). These techniques do not, however, offer the same degree of sterility assurance as heat methods and are generally reserved for temperature-sensitive items.

The mechanism of antimicrobial action of the two gases is assumed to be through alkylation of sulphydryl, amino, hydroxyl and carboxyl groups on proteins and imino groups of nucleic acids. At the concentrations employed in sterilization protocols, type A survivor curves (section 2.1, Fig. 20.1) are produced, the lethality of these gases increasing in a non-uniform manner with increasing concentration, exposure temperature and humidity. For this reason, sterilization protocols have generally been established by an empirical approach using a standard product load containing suitable biological indicator test strips (section 12.3). Concentration ranges (given as weight of gas per unit chamber volume) are usually in the order of 800–1200 mg/L for ethylene oxide and 15–100 mg/L for formaldehyde, with operating temperatures in the region of 45–63°C and 70–75°C, respectively. Even at the higher concentrations and temperatures, the sterilization processes are lengthy and therefore unsuitable for the re-sterilization of high-turnover articles. Further delays occur because of the need to remove toxic residues of the gases before release of the items for use. In addition, because recovery of survivors in sterility tests is more protracted with gaseous sterilization methods than with other processes, an extended quarantine period may also be required.

As alkylating agents, both gases are potentially mutagenic and carcinogenic (as is the ethylene chlorohydrin that results from ethylene oxide reaction with chlorine); they also produce symptoms of acute toxicity including irritation of the skin, conjunctiva and nasal mucosa. Consequently, strict control of their atmospheric concentrations is necessary and safe working protocols are required to protect personnel. Formaldehyde can normally be detected by smell at concentrations lower than those permitted in the atmosphere, whereas this is not true for ethylene oxide. Table 20.3 summarizes the comparative advantages afforded by ethylene oxide and low temperature steam formaldehyde (LTSF) processes.

5.1 Ethylene oxide

Ethylene oxide gas is highly explosive in mixtures of >3.6% v/v in air; in order to reduce this explosion hazard it is usually supplied for sterilization purposes as a 10% mix with carbon dioxide, or as an

Table 20.3 Relative merits of ethylene oxide and low-temperature steam formaldehyde (LTSF) processes

Advantages of ethylene oxide over LTSF	Advantages of LTSF over ethylene oxide
Wider international regulatory acceptance	Less hazardous because formaldehyde is not flammable and is more readily detected by smell
Better gas penetration into plastics and rubber	
	Cycle times may be shorter
Relatively slow to form solid polymers (with the potential to block pipes, etc.)	The gas is obtained readily from aqueous solution (formalin) which is a more convenient source than gas in cylinders
With long exposure times it is possible to sterilize at ambient temperatures	
Very low incidence of product deterioration	

8.6% mixture with HFC 124 (2-chloro-1,1,1,2 tetrafluoroethane), which has replaced fluorinated hydrocarbons (freons). Alternatively, pure ethylene oxide gas can be used below atmospheric pressure in sterilizer chambers from which all air has been removed.

The efficacy of ethylene oxide treatment depends upon achieving a suitable concentration in each article and this is assisted greatly by the good penetrating powers of the gas, which diffuses readily into many packaging materials including rubber, plastics, fabric and paper. This is not without its drawbacks, however, as the level of ethylene oxide in a sterilizer will decrease due to absorption during the process and the treated articles must undergo a desorption stage to remove toxic residues. Desorption can be allowed to occur naturally on open shelves, in which case complete desorption may take many days, e.g. for materials like PVC, or it may be encouraged by special forced aeration cabinets where flowing, heated air assists gas removal, reducing desorption times to between 2 and 24 hours.

Organisms are more resistant to ethylene oxide treatment in a dried state, as are those protected from the gas by inclusion in crystalline or dried organic deposits. Thus, a further condition to be satisfied in ethylene oxide sterilization is attainment of a minimum level of moisture in the immediate product environment. This requires a sterilizer humidity of 30–70% and frequently a preconditioning of the load at relative humidities of >50%.

5.1.1 Sterilizer design and operation

An ethylene oxide sterilizer consists of a leak-proof and explosion-proof steel chamber, normally of 100–300-litre capacity, which can be surrounded by a hot-water jacket to provide a uniform chamber temperature. Successful operation of the sterilizer requires removal of air from the chamber by evacuation, humidification and conditioning of the load by passage of subatmospheric pressure steam followed by a further evacuation period and the admission of preheated vaporized ethylene oxide from external pressurized canisters or single-charge cartridges. Forced gas circulation is often employed to minimize variations in conditions throughout the sterilizer chamber. Packaging materials must be air-, steam- and gas-permeable to permit suitable conditions for sterilization to be achieved within individual articles in the load. Absorption of ethylene oxide by the load is compensated for by the introduction of excess gas at the beginning or by the addition of more gas as the pressure drops during the sterilization process. The same may also be true for moisture absorption, which is compensated for by supplementary addition of water to maintain appropriate relative humidity.

After treatment, the gases are evacuated either directly to the outside atmosphere or through a special exhaust system. Filtered, sterile air is then admitted either for a repeat of the vacuum/air cycle or for air purging until the chamber is opened. In this way, safe removal of the ethylene oxide is achieved, reducing the toxic hazard to the operator. Sterilized articles are removed directly from the chamber and arranged for desorption. The operation of an ethylene oxide sterilizer should be monitored and controlled automatically. A typical operating cycle for pure ethylene oxide gas is given in Fig. 20.7.

5.2 Formaldehyde

Formaldehyde gas for use in sterilization is produced by heating formalin (37% w/v aqueous solution of formaldehyde) to a temperature of 70–75°C with steam, leading to the process known as LTSF. Formaldehyde has a similar toxicity to ethylene oxide and although absorption to materials appears to be lower, similar desorption routines are recommended. A major disadvantage of formaldehyde is low penetrating power and this limits the packaging materials that can be employed to principally paper and cotton fabric.

5.2.1 Sterilizer design and operation

An LTSF sterilizer is designed to operate with subatmospheric pressure steam. Air is removed by evacuation and steam is admitted to the chamber to allow heating of the load and to assist in air removal. The sterilization period starts with the release of formaldehyde by vaporization from formalin (in a vaporizer with a steam-jacket) and continues through either a simple holding stage or through a series of pulsed evacuations and steam and formaldehyde admission cycles. The chamber temperature is maintained by a thermostatically controlled water-jacket, and steam and condensate are removed via a drain channel and an evacuated condenser. At the end of the treatment period formaldehyde vapour is expelled by steam flushing and the load is dried by alternating stages of evacuation and admission of sterile, filtered air. A typical pulsed cycle of operation is shown in Fig. 20.8.

6 Radiation sterilization

Several types of radiation find a sterilizing application in the manufacture of pharmaceutical and medical products, principal among which are accelerated electrons (particulate radiation), gamma-rays and UV light (both electromagnetic radiations). The major target for these radiations is believed to be microbial DNA, with damage occur-

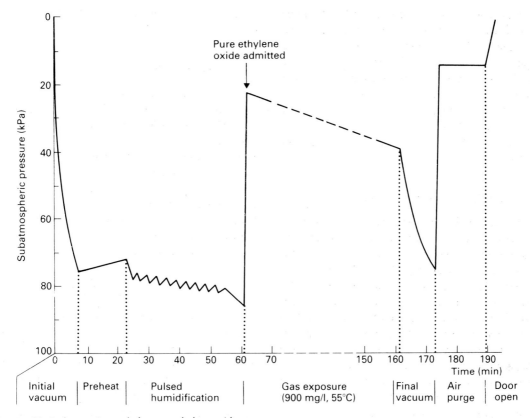

Fig. 20.7 Typical operating cycle for pure ethylene oxide gas.

ring as a consequence of ionization and free radical production (gamma-rays and electrons) or excitation (UV light). This latter process is less damaging and less lethal than ionization, and so UV irradiation is not as efficient a sterilization method as electron or gamma-irradiation. As mentioned earlier (section 2), vegetative bacteria generally prove to be the most sensitive to irradiation (with notable exceptions, e.g. *Deinococcus* (*Micrococcus*) *radiodurans*), followed by moulds and yeasts, with bacterial spores and viruses as the most resistant (except in the case of UV light where mould spores prove to be most resistant). The extent of DNA damage required to produce cell death can vary and this, together with the ability to carry out effective repair, probably determines the resistance of the organism to radiation. With ionizing radiations (gamma-ray and accelerated electrons), microbial resistance decreases with the presence of moisture

or dissolved oxygen (as a result of increased free radical production) and also with elevated temperatures.

Radiation sterilization with high energy gamma-rays or accelerated electrons has proved to be a useful method for the industrial sterilization of heat-sensitive products. However, undesirable changes can occur in irradiated preparations, especially those in aqueous solution where radiolysis of water contributes to the damaging processes. In addition, certain glass or plastic (e.g. polypropylene, PTFE) materials used for packaging or for medical devices can also suffer damage. Thus, radiation sterilization is generally applied to articles in the dried state; these include surgical instruments, sutures, prostheses, unit-dose ointments, plastic syringes and dry pharmaceutical products (Chapter 19). With these radiations, destruction of a microbial population follows the classic survivor curves

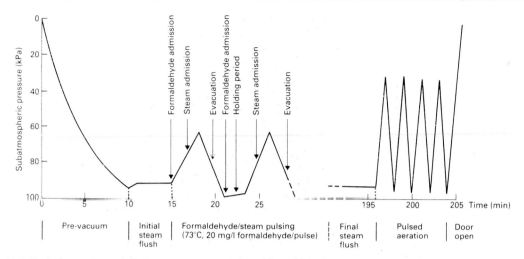

Fig. 20.8 Typical operating cycle for low-temperature steam and formaldehyde treatment.

(see Fig. 20.1) and a *D*-value, given as a radiation dose, can be established for standard bacterial spores (e.g. *Bacillus pumilus*) permitting a suitable sterilizing dose to be calculated. In the UK it is usual to apply a dose of 25 kGy (2.5 Mrad) for pharmaceutical and medical products, although lower doses are employed in the USA and Canada.

UV light, with its much lower energy, causes less damage to microbial DNA. This, coupled with its poor penetrability of normal packaging materials, renders UV light unsuitable for sterilization of pharmaceutical dosage forms. It does find applications, however, in the sterilization of air, for the surface sterilization of aseptic work areas, and for the treatment of manufacturing-grade water.

6.1 Sterilizer design and operation

6.1.1 Gamma-ray sterilizers

Gamma-rays for sterilization are usually derived from a cobalt-60 (^{60}Co) source (caesium-137 may also be used), with a half-life of 5.25 years, which on disintegration emits radiation at two energy levels of 1.33 and 1.17 MeV. The isotope is held as pellets packed in metal rods, each rod carefully arranged within the source and containing up to 20 kCi (740×10^{12} Bq) of activity; these rods are replaced or re-arranged as the activity of the source either drops or becomes unevenly distributed. A typical ^{60}Co installation may contain up to 1 MCi (3.7×10^{16} Bq) of activity. For safety reasons, this source is housed within a reinforced concrete building with walls some 2 m thick, and it is only raised from a sunken water-filled tank when required for use. Control devices operate to ensure that the source is raised only when the chamber is locked and that it is immediately lowered if a malfunction occurs. Articles being sterilized are passed through the irradiation chamber on a conveyor belt or monorail system and move around the raised source, the rate of passage regulating the dose absorbed (Fig. 20.9).

Radiation monitors are continually employed to detect any radiation leakage during operation or source storage, and to confirm a return to satisfactory background levels within the sterilization chamber following operation. The dose delivered is dependent upon source strength and exposure period, with dwell times typically up to 20 hours. The difference in radiation susceptibilities of microbial cells and humans may be gauged from the fact that a lethal human dose would be delivered by an exposure of seconds or minutes.

6.1.2 Electron accelerators

Two types of electron accelerator machine exist, the electrostatic accelerator and the microwave linear

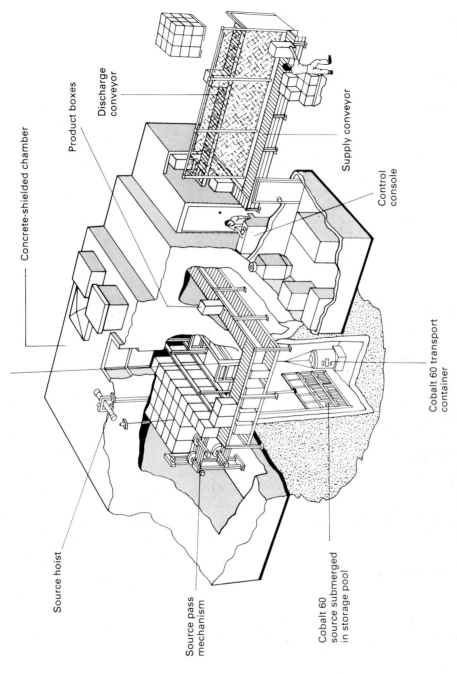

Concrete-shielded chamber

Product boxes

Discharge conveyor

Supply conveyor

Control console

Source hoist

Source pass mechanism

Cobalt 60 source submerged in storage pool

Cobalt 60 transport container

Fig. 20.9 Diagram of a typical cobalt-60 irradiation plant.

accelerator, producing electrons with maximum energies of 5 MeV and 10 MeV, respectively. Although higher energies would achieve better penetration into the product, there is a risk of induced radiation and so they are not used. In the first, a high energy electron beam is generated by accelerating electrons from a hot filament down an evacuated tube under high potential difference, while in the second, additional energy is imparted to this beam in a pulsed manner by a synchronized travelling microwave. Articles for treatment are generally limited to small packs and are arranged on a horizontal conveyor belt, usually for irradiation from one side but sometimes from both. The sterilizing dose is delivered more rapidly in an electron accelerator than in a ^{60}Co plant, with exposure times for sterilization usually amounting to only a few seconds or minutes. Varying extents of shielding, depending upon the size of the accelerator, are necessary to protect operators from X-rays generated by the bremsstrahlung effect.

6.1.3 Ultraviolet irradiation

The optimum wavelength for UV sterilization is around 260 nm. A suitable source for UV light in this region is a mercury lamp giving peak emission levels at 254 nm. These sources are generally wall- or ceiling-mounted for air disinfection, or fixed to vessels for water treatment. Operators present in an irradiated room should wear appropriate protective clothing and eye shields.

7 Filtration sterilization

The process of filtration is unique among sterilization techniques in that it removes, rather than destroys, microorganisms. Further, it is capable of preventing the passage of both viable and non-viable particles and can thus be used for both the clarification and sterilization of liquids and gases. The principal application of sterilizing-grade filters is the treatment of heat-sensitive injections and ophthalmic solutions, biological products and air and other gases for supply to aseptic areas (see Chapters 19 and 21).

They may also be required in industrial applications where they become part of venting systems on fermenters, centrifuges, autoclaves and freeze-driers. Certain types of filter (membrane filters) also have an important role in sterility testing, where they can be employed to trap and concentrate contaminating organisms from solutions under test. These filters are then placed in a liquid nutrient medium and incubated to encourage growth and turbidity (section 13.1).

The major mechanisms of filtration are sieving, adsorption and trapping within the matrix of the filter material. Of these, only sieving can be regarded as absolute as it ensures the exclusion of all particles above a defined size. It is generally accepted that synthetic membrane filters, derived from cellulose esters or other polymeric materials, approximate most closely to sieve filters; while fibrous pads, sintered glass and sintered ceramic products can be regarded as depth filters relying principally on mechanisms of adsorption and entrapment. Some of the characteristics of filter media are summarized in Table 20.4. The potential hazard of microbial multiplication within a depth filter and subsequent contamination of the filtrate (microbial grow-through) should be recognized.

7.2 Filtration sterilization of liquids

In order to compare favourably with other methods

Table 20.4 Some characteristics of membrane and depth filters

Characteristic	Membrane	Depth
Absolute retention of microorganisms greater than rated pore size	+	−
Rapid rate of filtration	+	−
High dirt-handling capacity	−	+
Grow-through of micro-organisms	Unlikely	+
Shedding of filter components	−	+
Fluid retention	−	+
Solute adsorption	−	+
Good chemical stability	Variable (depends on membrane)	+
Good sterilization characteristics	+	+

+, applicable; −, not applicable.

of sterilization the microorganism removal efficiency of filters employed in the processing of liquids must be high. For this reason, membrane filters of 0.2–0.22 µm nominal pore diameter are chiefly used, while sintered filters are used only in restricted circumstances, i.e. for the processing of corrosive liquids, viscous fluids or organic solvents. It may be tempting to assume that the pore size is the major determinant of filtration efficiency and two filters of 0.2 µm pore diameter from different manufacturers will behave similarly. This is not so because, in addition to the sieving effect, trapping within the filter matrix, adsorption and charge effects all contribute significantly towards the removal of particles. Consequently, the depth of the membrane, its charge and the tortuosity of the channels are all factors which can make the performance of one filter far superior to that of another. The major criterion by which filters should be compared, therefore, is their titre reduction values, i.e. the ratio of the number of organisms challenging a filter under defined conditions to the number penetrating it. In all cases, the filter medium employed must be sterilizable, ideally by steam treatment; in the case of membrane filters this may be for once-only use, or, in the case of larger industrial filters, a small fixed number of re-sterilizations; sintered filters may be re-sterilized many times. Filtration sterilization is an aseptic process and careful monitoring of filter integrity is necessary as well as final product sterility testing (section 13).

Membrane filters, in the form of discs, can be assembled into pressure-operated filter holders for syringe mounting and in-line use or vacuum filtration tower devices. Filtration under pressure is generally considered most suitable, as filling at high flow rates directly into the final containers is possible without problems of foaming, solvent evaporation or air leaks. To increase the filtration area, and hence process volumes, several filter discs can be used in parallel in multiple-plate filtration systems or, alternatively, membrane filters can be fabricated into plain or pleated cylinders and installed in cartridges. Membrane filters are often used in combination with a coarse-grade fibreglass depth prefilter to improve their dirt-handling capacity.

7.2 Filtration sterilization of gases

The principal application for filtration sterilization of gases is in the provision of sterile air to aseptic manufacturing suites, hospital isolation units and some operating theatres. Filters employed generally consist of pleated sheets of glass microfibres separated and supported by corrugated sheets of Kraft paper or aluminium; these are employed in ducts, wall or ceiling panels, overhead canopies, or laminar airflow cabinets (Chapter 21). These high-efficiency particulate air (HEPA) filters can remove up to 99.997% of particles >0.3 µm in diameter and thus are acting as depth filters. In practice their microorganism removal efficiency is rather better as the majority of bacteria are found associated with dust particles and only the larger fungal spores are found in the free state. Air is forced through HEPA filters by blower fans, and prefilters are used to remove larger particles to extend the lifetime of the HEPA filter. The operational efficiency and integrity of a HEPA filter can be monitored by pressure differential and airflow rate measurements, and dioctylphthalate smoke particle penetration tests.

Other applications of filters include sterilization of venting or displacement air in tissue and microbiological culture (carbon filters and hydrophobic membrane filters); decontamination of air in mechanical ventilators (glass fibre filters); treatment of exhausted air from microbiological safety cabinets (HEPA filters); and the clarification and sterilization of medical gases (glass wool depth filters and hydrophobic membrane filters).

8 New sterilization technologies

Heat is the means of terminal sterilization that is preferred by the regulatory authorities because of its relative simplicity and the high sterility assurance that it affords. However, a significant number of traditional pharmaceutical products and many recently developed biotechnology products are damaged by heat, as are many polymer-based medical devices and surgical implants; for such products alternative sterilization processes must be adopted. Whilst radiation is a viable option for many dry materials, radiation-induced damage is common in aqueous drug solutions, and gaseous methods are also inappropriate for liquids. Aseptic manufacture from individually sterilized ingredients is a suitable solution to the problem of making sterile thermolabile products, but it affords a lower degree of sterility assurance than steam sterilization and is both time-consuming and expensive. For these reasons alternative sterilization strategies have been developed in recent years, and although they are not currently in widespread use, it is likely that some will be further refined and become much more widespread in the 21st century. Two processes that have progressed to the stage of commercial exploitation are those employing high intensity light and low temperature plasma. It must be stressed, however, that whilst the need to develop alternative strategies for the terminal sterilization of protein- or nucleic acid-containing biotechnology products is one of the stimuli for the investigation of new methods in general, these particular processes are unsuitable for such products.

8.1 High-intensity light

UV light has long been known to have the potential to kill all types of microorganisms, but its penetrating power is so poor that it has found practical application only in the decontamination of air (e.g. in laminar-flow workstations and operating theatres), shallow layers of water and surfaces. UV light does not penetrate metal at all, nor glass to any useful degree, but it will penetrate those polymers that do not contain unsaturated bonds or aromatic groups (e.g. polyethylene and polypropylene — but not polystyrene, polycarbonate or polyvinyl chloride). High intensity light sterilization is based upon the generation of short flashes of broad wavelength light from a xenon lamp that has an intensity almost 100 000 times that of the sun; approximately 25% of the flash is UV light. The procedure has been applied to the sterilization of water and studied as a means of terminal sterilization for injectables in UV-transmitting plastic ampoules in a blow-fill-seal operation. Although pulsed light is unlikely to be useful for coloured solutions or those that contain solutes with a high UV absorbance, it is likely that the procedure will be readily applicable not only to

water but to some simple solutions of organic molecules, e.g. dextrose-saline injection.

8.2 Low temperature plasma

Plasma is a gas or vapour that has been subjected to an electrical or magnetic field which causes a substantial proportion of the molecules to become ionized. It is thus composed of a cloud of neutral species, ions and electrons in which the numbers of positive and negatively charged particles are equal. Plasmas may be generated from many substances but those from chlorine, glutaraldehyde and hydrogen peroxide have been shown to possess the greatest antimicrobial activity.

Low temperature plasma is a method of sterilization that is applicable to most of the items and materials for which ethylene oxide is used, i.e. principally medical devices rather than drugs; it cannot be used to sterilize liquids, powders and certain fabrics. Commercial plasma sterilizers, which have been available since the early 1990s, typically consist of a sterilization chamber of about 75 litres; this is evacuated, then filled with hydrogen peroxide vapour which is subsequently converted to a plasma by application of an electric field. An alternative commercial plasma sterilizer utilizes alternating cycles of peracetic acid vapour and a plasma containing oxygen, hydrogen and an inert carrier gas. The cycle times are typically from 60 to 90 minutes and the operating temperatures are <50°C. Major benefits of plasma sterilization include: elimination of the requirement to remove toxic gases at the end of the cycle (in contrast to ethylene oxide and LTSF processes); there is no requirement for the treated device to be aired to remove residual gas and there is no significant corrosion or reduction in sharpness of exposed surgical instruments.

9 Sterilization control and sterility assurance

A product to be labelled 'sterile' must be free of viable microorganisms. To achieve this, the product, or its ingredients, must undergo a sterilization process of sufficient microbiocidal capacity to ensure a minimum level of sterility assurance. It is essential that the required conditions for sterilization be achieved and maintained through every operation of the sterilizer.

Historically, the quality control of sterile products consisted largely, or in some cases, even exclusively, of a sterility test, to which the product was subjected at the end of the manufacturing process. However, a growing awareness of the limitations of sterility tests in terms of their ability to detect low concentrations of microorganisms has resulted in a shift in emphasis from a crucial dependence on end-testing to a situation in which the conferment of the status 'sterile' results from the attainment of satisfactory quality standards throughout the whole manufacturing process. In other words, the quality is 'assured' by a combination of process monitoring and performance criteria; these may be considered under four headings:

- Bioburden determinations (section 10)
- Environmental monitoring (section 11)
- Validation and in-process monitoring of sterilization procedures (section 12)
- Sterility testing (section 13).

In well-understood and well-characterized sterilization processes (e.g. heat and irradiation), where physical measurements may be accurately made, sterility can be assured by ensuring that the manufacturing process as a whole conforms to the established protocols for the first three of the above headings. In this case the process has satisfied the required parameters thereby permitting parametric release (i.e. release based upon process data) of the product without recourse to a sterility test (see Chapter 19).

10 Bioburden determinations

The term 'bioburden' is used to describe the concentration of microorganisms in a material; this may be either a total number of organisms per millilitre or per gram, regardless of type, or a breakdown into such categories as aerobic bacteria or yeasts and moulds. Bioburden determinations are normally undertaken by the supplier of the raw material, whose responsibility it is to ensure that the material supplied conforms to the agreed specification, but they may also be checked by the recipient. The

maximum permitted concentrations of contaminants may be those specified in various pharmacopoeias or the levels established by the manufacturer during product development.

The level of sterility assurance that is achieved in a terminally sterilized product is dependent upon the design of the sterilization process itself and upon the bioburden immediately prior to sterilization (see Chapters 15, 19 and 21). However, the adoption of high standards for the quality of the raw materials is not, in itself, a strategy that will ensure that the product has an acceptably low bioburden immediately prior to sterilization. It is necessary also to ensure that the opportunities for microbial contamination during manufacture are restricted (see below), and that those organisms that are present initially do not normally find themselves in conditions conducive to growth. It is for these reasons that manufacturing processes are designed to utilize adverse temperatures, extreme pH values and organic solvent exposures in order to prevent an increase in the microbial load. For example, water is the most common, and potentially the most significant, source of contamination in the manufactured product, and maintenance of water at elevated temperatures is commonly employed as a means of limiting the growth of organisms such as *Pseudomonas* spp., which can proliferate during storage, even in distilled or deionized water. Precautions such as these ensure that chemically synthesized raw materials have bioburdens that are generally much lower than those found in 'natural' products of animal, vegetable or mineral origin.

11 Environmental monitoring

The levels of microbial contamination in the manufacturing areas (Chapter 21) are monitored on a regular basis to confirm that the numbers do not exceed specified limits. The concentrations of bacteria and of yeasts/moulds in the atmosphere may be determined either by use of 'settle plates' (Petri dishes of suitable media exposed for fixed periods, on which the colonies are counted after incubation) or by use of air samplers which cause a known volume of air to be passed over an agar surface. Similarly, the contamination on surfaces, including manufacturing equipment, may be measured using swabs or contact plates (also known as Rodac — replicate organism detection and counting — plates) which are specially designed Petri dishes slightly overfilled with agar, which, when set, projects very slightly above the plastic wall of the dish. This permits the plate to be inverted onto or against any solid surface, thereby allowing transfer of organisms from the surface onto the agar.

Less commonly, environmental monitoring can extend also to the operators in the manufacturing area whose clothing, e.g. gloves or face masks, may be sampled in order to estimate the levels and types of organisms that may arise as product contaminants from those sources.

12 Validation and in-process monitoring of sterilization procedures

There are several definitions of 'validation' but, in simple terms, the word means demonstrating that a process will consistently produce the results that it is intended to. Thus, with respect to sterile products, validation would be necessary for each of the individual aspects of the manufacturing process, e.g. environmental monitoring, raw materials quality assessment, the sterilization process itself and the sterility testing procedure. Of these, it is the sterilization process that is likely to be subject to the most detailed and complex validation procedures, and these will be used to exemplify the factors to be considered. A typical validation procedure for a steam sterilization process is likely to incorporate most, or all, of the following features:

• The calibration and testing of all the physical instruments used to monitor the process, e.g. thermocouples, pressure gauges and timers.
• Production of evidence that the steam is of the desired quality (e.g. that the chamber temperature is that expected for pure steam at the measured pressure).
• The conduct of leak tests and steam penetration tests using both an empty chamber and a chamber filled with the product to be sterilized in the intended load conformation.
• The use of biological indicators either alone or in combination with bioburden organisms to demonstrate that the sterilization cycle is capable of producing an acceptable level of sterility assurance under 'worst case' conditions.
• The production of data to demonstrate repeatability of the above (typically for three runs).
• Comprehensive documentation of all of these aspects.

There are different approaches to the demonstration of adequate sterility assurance in steam sterilization depending upon the thermostability and knowledge of the pre-sterilization bioburden. Where the product is known to be stable, an overkill approach may be adopted in which biological indicators (section 12.3) containing 10^6 test organisms are inactivated in half the proposed exposure time (thus achieving a 12 log reduction and a sterility assurance level of 10^{-6} in the full exposure period). For a marginally thermostable product the cycle could be validated on the basis of measurements of the worst case bioburden level and the heat resistance of the bioburden organisms; such an approach would necessitate rigorous control of the bioburden during routine manufacturing. In the UK, biological indicators are used primarily in validation rather than routine monitoring of heat sterilization processes, although their use in routine manufacturing may be required in other countries. Chemical indicators of sterilization (section 12.2) are more convenient to use than biological indicators, but as they provide no direct measure of the efficacy of the process in terms of microbial killing they are considered to be less useful. Physical measurements of temperature, pressure, time, relative humidity, etc. are of such fundamental importance to the assurance of sterility that records of these parameters are retained for each batch of sterilized product.

12.1 Physical indicators

In heat sterilization processes, a temperature record chart is made of each sterilization cycle with both dry and moist heat (i.e. autoclave) sterilizers; this chart forms part of the batch documentation and is compared against a master temperature record (MTR). It is recommended that the temperature be taken at the coolest part of the loaded sterilizer. Further information on heat distribution and penetration within a sterilizer can be gained by the use of thermocouples placed at selected sites in the chamber or inserted directly into test packs or bottles. For gaseous sterilization procedures, elevated temperatures are monitored for each sterilization cycle by temperature probes, and routine leak tests are performed to ensure gas-tight seals. Pressure and humidity measurements are recorded. Gas concentration is measured independently of pressure rise, often by reference to weight of gas used. In radiation sterilization, a plastic (often perspex) dosimeter which gradually darkens in proportion to the radiation absorbed gives an accurate measure of the radiation dose and is considered to be the best technique currently available for following the radiosterilization process.

Sterilizing filters are subject to a bubble point pressure test, which is a technique employed for determining the pore size of filters, and may also be used to check the integrity of certain types of filter device (membrane and sintered glass; section 7) immediately after use. The principle of the test is that the wetted filter, in its assembled unit, is subjected to an increasing air or nitrogen gas pressure differential. The pressure difference recorded when the first bubble of gas breaks away from the filter is related to the maximum pore size. When the gas pressure is further increased slowly, there is a general eruption of bubbles over the entire surface. The pressure difference here is related to the mean pore size. A pressure differential below the expected value would signify a damaged or faulty filter. A modification to this test for membrane filters involves measuring the diffusion of gas through a wetted filter at pressures below the bubble point pressure (diffusion rate test); a faster diffusion rate than expected would again indicate a loss of filter integrity. In addition, a filter is considered ineffective when an unusually rapid rate of filtration occurs.

Efficiency testing of HEPA filters used for the supply of sterile air to aseptic workplaces (Chapter 21) is normally achieved by the generation upstream of dioctylphthalate (DOP) or sodium chloride particles of known dimension followed by detection in downstream filtered air. Retention efficiency is recorded as the percentage of particles removed under defined test conditions. Microbiological tests are not normally performed.

12.2 Chemical indicators

Chemical monitoring of a sterilization process is based on the ability of heat, steam, sterilant gases and ionizing radiation to alter the chemical and/or physical characteristics of a variety of chemical substances. Ideally, this change should take place only when satisfactory conditions for sterilization prevail, thus confirming that the sterilization cycle has been successfully completed. In practice, however, the ideal indicator response is not always achieved and so a necessary distinction is made between (i) those chemical indicators which integrate several sterilization parameters (i.e. temperature, time and saturated steam) and closely approach the ideal; and (ii) those which measure only one parameter and consequently can only be used to distinguish processed from unprocessed articles. Thus, indicators which rely on the melting of a chemical substance show that the temperature has been attained but not necessarily maintained.

Chemical indicators generally undergo melting or colour changes (some examples are given in Fig. 20.10), the relationship of this change to the sterilization process being influenced by the design of the test device (Table 20.5). It must be remembered, however, that the changes recorded do not necessarily correspond to microbiological sterility and consequently the devices should never be employed as sole indicators in a sterilization process. Nevertheless, when included in strategically placed containers or packages, chemical indicators are valuable monitors of the conditions prevailing at the coolest or most inaccessible parts of a sterilizer.

12.3 Biological indicators

Biological indicators (BIs) for use in thermal, chemical or radiation sterilization processes consist of standardized bacterial spore preparations which are usually in the form either of suspensions in water or culture medium or of spores dried on paper, aluminium or plastic carriers. As with chemical indicators, they are usually placed in dummy packs located at strategic sites in the sterilizer. Alternatively, for gaseous sterilization these may also be placed within a tubular helix (Line-Pickerill) device. After the sterilization process, the aqueous

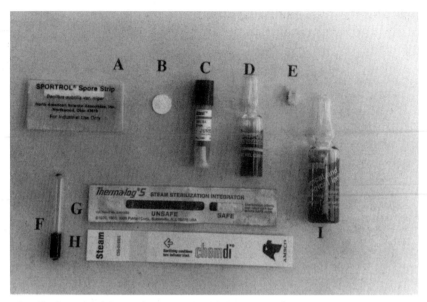

Fig. 20.10 Examples of biological and chemical indicators used for monitoring sterilization processes. (A and B) A spore strip (in a glassine envelope) and a spore disc, respectively; the spores are dried onto absorbent paper or fabric. (C) Attest™ indicator comprising a plastic vial containing a spore strip together with a sealed glass ampoule of culture medium; the ampoule is crushed after exposure and the medium immerses the strip. (D) Chemspor™ indicator in which bacterial spores are suspended in culture medium; the horizontal band on the ampoule also darkens on autoclaving to enable steam-exposed and non-exposed ampoules to be distinguished. (E) Plastic carrier with dried *Bacillus stearothermophilus* spores designed for monitoring low-temperature steam and formaldehyde cycles. (F) Browne's tube™; the liquid within the tube changes colour on heat exposure. (G) Thermalog™ strip in which a blue dye progresses from left to right during heat exposure. (H) Chemdi™ displays colour change in arrowed section of the strip after heating. (I) Chemspor™ which is a combined chemical and biological indicator; the ampoule contains a spore suspension in culture medium together with a second, smaller ampoule which contains a chemical indicator.

suspensions or spores on carriers are aseptically transferred to an appropriate nutrient medium, which is then incubated and periodically examined for signs of growth. Spores of *Bacillus stearothermophilus* in sealed ampoules of culture medium are used for steam sterilization monitoring, and these may be incubated directly at 55°C; this eliminates the need for an aseptic transfer. Aseptic transfers are also avoided by the use of self-contained units where the spore strip and nutrient medium are present in the same device ready for mixing after use.

The bacterial species to be used in a BI must be selected carefully, as it must be non-pathogenic and should possess above-average resistance to the particular sterilization process. Resistance is adjudged from the spore destruction curve obtained upon exposure to the sterilization process; recommended BI spores and their decimal reduction times (*D*-values;

section 2.2.1) are shown in Table 20.6. Great care must be taken in the preparation and storage of BIs to ensure a standardized response to sterilization processes. Indeed, while certainly offering the most direct method of monitoring sterilization processes, it should be realized that BIs may be less reliable monitors than physical methods and are not recommended for routine use, except in the case of gaseous sterilization.

One of the long-standing criticisms of BIs is that the incubation period required in order to confirm a satisfactory sterilization process imposes an undesirable delay on the release of the product. This problem has been overcome, with respect to steam sterilization at least, by the use of a detection system in which a spore enzyme, α-glucosidase (reflective of spore viability), converts a non-fluorescent substrate into a fluorescent product in as little as 1 hour.

Table 20.5 Examples of chemical indicators for monitoring sterilization processes

Sterilization method	Principle	Device	Parameter(s) monitored
Heat Autoclaving or dry heat	Temperature-sensitive coloured solution	Sealed tubes partly filled with a solution which changes colour at elevated temperatures; rate of colour change is proportional to temperature, e.g. Browne's tubes	Temperature, time
Dry heat only	Temperature-sensitive chemical	Usually a temperature-sensitive white wax concealing a black marked or printed (paper) surface; at a predetermined temperature the wax rapidly melts exposing the background mark(s)	Temperature
Heating in an autoclave only	Steam-sensitive chemical	Usually an organic chemical in a printing ink base impregnated into a carrier material. A combination of moisture and heat produces a darkening of the ink, e.g. autoclave tape. Devices of this sort can be used within dressings packs to confirm adequate removal of air and penetration of saturated steam (Bowie–Dick test)	Saturated steam
	Capillary principle (Thermalog S)	Consists of a blue dye in a waxy pellet, the melting-point of which is depressed in the presence of saturated steam. At autoclaving temperatures, and in the continued presence of steam, the pellet melts and travels along a paper wick forming a blue band the length of which is dependent upon both exposure time and temperature	Temperature, saturated steam, time
Gaseous sterilization Ethylene oxide (EO)	Reactive chemical	Indicator paper impregnated with a reactive chemical which undergoes a distinct colour change on reaction with EO in the presence of heat and moisture. With some devices rate of colour development varies with temperature and EO concentration	Gas concentration, temperature, time (selected devices); NB a minimum relative humidity (rh) is required for device to function
	Capillary principle (Thermalog G)	Based on the same 'migration along wick' principle as Thermalog S. Optimum response in a cycle of 600 mg/L EO, temperature 54°C, rh 40–80%. Lower EO levels and/or temperature will slow response time	Gas concentration, temperature, time (selected cycles)
Low temperature steam and formaldehyde	Reactive chemical	Indicator paper impregnated with a formaldehyde-, steam- and temperature-sensitive reactive chemical which changes colour during the sterilization process	Gas concentration, temperature, time (selected cycles)
Radiation sterilization	Radiochromic chemical	Plastic devices impregnated with radiosensitive chemicals which undergo colour changes at relatively low radiation doses	Only indicate exposure to radiation
	Dosimeter device	Acidified ferric ammonium sulphate or ceric sulphate solutions respond to irradiation by dose-related changes in their optical density	Accurately measure radiation doses

Table 20.6 Biological indicators recommended by the EP (2002) for monitoring sterilization processes

Sterilization process	Species	Inoculum size	D-value
Steam sterilization (121°C)	*Bacillus stearothermophilus*	$>5 \times 10^5$	>1.5 min
Dry heat (160°C)	*Bacillus subtilis* var *niger*	$>1 \times 10^5$	5–10 min
Hydrogen peroxide and peracetic acid	*Bacillus stearothermophilus*	$>5 \times 10^5$	–
Ethylene oxide (EtOx)	*Bacillus subtilis* var *niger*	$>5 \times 10^5$	>2.5 min at 54°C, 60% relative humidity and 600 mg/L EtOx
Formaldehyde	*Bacillus subtilis* var *niger*	$>5 \times 10^5$	–
Ionizing radiation	*Bacillus pumilus*	$>1 \times 10^7$	1.9 kGy

Filtration sterilization requires a different approach from biological monitoring, the test effectively measuring the ability of a filter to produce a sterile filtrate from a culture of a suitable organism. For this purpose, *Serratia marcescens*, a small Gram-negative rod-shaped bacterium (minimum dimension 0.5 μm), has been used for filters of 0.45 μm pore size, and a more rigorous test involving *Brevundimonas diminuta* (formerly *Pseudomonas diminuta*) having a minimum dimension of 0.3 μm is applied to filters of 0.22 μm pore size. The latter filters are defined as those capable of completely removing *Brev. diminuta* from suspension. In this test, using this organism, a realistic inoculum level must be adopted, as the probability of bacteria appearing in the filtrate rises as the number of *Brev. diminuta* cells in the test challenge increases; a standardized inoculum size of 10^7 cells cm^{-2} is normally employed. The extent of the passage of this organism through membrane filters is enhanced by increasing the filtration pressure. Thus, successful sterile filtration depends markedly on the challenge conditions. Such tests are used as part of the filter manufacturer's characterization and quality assurance process, and a user's initial validation procedure. They are not employed as a test of filter performance in use.

13 Sterility testing

A sterility test is essentially a test which assesses whether a sterilized pharmaceutical or medical product is free from contaminating microorganisms by incubation of either the whole or a part of that product with a nutrient medium. It thus becomes a destructive test and is of questionable suitability for testing large, expensive or delicate products or equipment. Furthermore, by its very nature such a test is a statistical process in which part of a batch is randomly sampled and the chance of the batch being passed for use then depends on the sample passing the sterility test. (Random sampling should be applied to products that have been processed and filled aseptically. With products sterilized in their final containers, samples should be taken from the potentially coolest or least sterilant-accessible part of the load.)

A further limitation is that which is inherent in a procedure intended to demonstrate a negative. A sterility test is intended to demonstrate that no viable organisms are present, but failure to detect them could simply be a consequence of the use of unsuitable media or inappropriate cultural conditions. To be certain that no organisms are present it would be necessary to use a universal culture medium suitable for the growth of any possible contaminant and to incubate the sample under an infinite variety of conditions. Clearly, no such medium or combination of media are available and, in practice, only media capable of supporting non-fastidious bacteria, yeasts and moulds are employed. Furthermore, in pharmacopoeial tests, no attempt is made to detect viruses, which on a size basis, are the organisms most likely to pass through a sterilizing filter. Nevertheless, the sterility test does have an important application in monitoring the microbiological quality of filter-sterilized, aseptically filled products and does offer a final check on terminally sterilized articles. In the UK, test procedures laid down by the *European Pharmacopoeia* must be followed; this provides details of the sample sizes to be adopted in particular cases. The principles of these tests are discussed below.

13.1 Methods

There are three alternative methods available when conducting sterility tests.

1 The direct inoculation procedure involves introducing test samples directly into nutrient media. The *European Pharmacopoeia* (2002) recommends two media: (i) fluid mercaptoacetate medium (also known as fluid thioglycollate medium), which contains glucose and sodium mercaptoacetate (sodium thioglycollate) and is particularly suitable for the cultivation of anaerobic organisms (incubation temperature 30–35°C); and (ii) soyabean casein digest medium (also known as tryptone soya broth), which will support the growth of both aerobic bacteria (incubation temperature 30–35°C) and fungi (incubation temperature 20–25°C). Other media may be used provided that they can be shown to be suitable alternatives. Limits are placed upon the ratio of the weight or volume of added sample relative to the volume of culture medium so as to avoid reducing the nutrient properties of the medium or creating unfavourably high osmotic pressures within it.

2 Membrane filtration is the technique recommended by most pharmacopoeias and, consequently, the method by which the great majority of products are examined. It involves filtration of fluids through a sterile membrane filter (pore size ″0.45 μm); any microorganism present being retained on the surface of the filter. After washing *in situ*, the filter is divided aseptically and portions are transferred to suitable culture media which are then incubated at the appropriate temperature for the required period of time. Water-soluble solids can be dissolved in a suitable diluent and processed in this way and oil-soluble products may be dissolved in a suitable solvent, e.g. isopropyl myristate.

3 A sensitive method for detecting low levels of contamination in intravenous infusion fluids involves the addition of a concentrated culture medium to the fluid in its original container, such that the resultant mixture is equivalent to single strength culture medium. In this way, sampling of the entire volume is achieved.

With the techniques discussed above, the media employed should previously have been assessed for nutritive (growth-supporting) properties and a lack of toxicity using specified organisms. It must be remembered that any survivors of a sterilization process may be damaged and thus must be given the best possible conditions for growth.

As a precaution against accidental contamination, product testing must be carried out under conditions of strict asepsis using, for example, a laminar airflow cabinet to provide a suitable environment (Chapter 21).

The *European Pharmacopoeia* (2002) indicates that it is necessary to conduct control tests that confirm the adequacy of the facilities by sampling of air and surfaces and carrying out tests using samples 'known' to be sterile (negative controls). In reality, this means samples that have been subjected to a very reliable sterilization process, e.g. radiation, or samples that have been subjected to a sterilization procedure more than once. In order to minimize the risk of introducing contaminants from the surroundings or from the operator during the test itself, isolators are often employed which physically separate the operator from the materials under test. These are designed on the same principle as a glove box, but on a much larger and more sophisticated scale, so the operator works inside a sterile cubicle but is separated from the atmosphere within it by a flexible moulded covering (rather like a space suit) which is an integral part of the cubicle base (Fig. 20.11).

13.2 Antimicrobial agents

Where an antimicrobial agent comprises the product or forms part of the product, for example as a preservative, its activity must be nullified in some way during sterility testing so that an inhibitory action in preventing the growth of any contaminating microorganisms is overcome. This is achieved by the following methods.

13.2.1 Specific inactivation

An appropriate inactivating (neutralizing) agent (Table 20.7) is incorporated into the culture media. The inactivating agent must be non-toxic to microorganisms, as must any product resulting

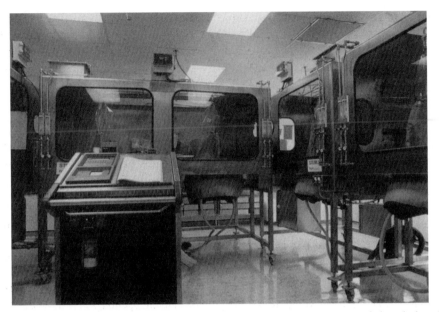

Fig. 20.11 Isolators used for sterility testing. The operator works within the hood which is suspended inside the cubicle; the hydrogen peroxide generator which is used to sterilize the isolators is shown in the left foreground. (Courtesy of GlaxoSmithKline.)

from an interaction of the inactivator and the antimicrobial agent.

Although Table 20.7 lists only benzylpenicillin and ampicillin as being inactivated by β-lactamase (from *B. cereus*), other β-lactams may also be hydrolysed by β-lactamases. Other antibiotic-inactivating enzymes are also known (Chapter 13) and have been considered as possible inactivating agents, e.g. chloramphenicol acetyltransferase (inactivates chloramphenicol) and enzymes that modify aminoglycoside antibiotics.

13.2.2 Dilution

The antimicrobial agent is diluted in the culture medium to a level at which it ceases to have any activity, for example phenols, cresols and alcohols (see Chapter 11). This method applies to substances with a high dilution coefficient, η.

13.2.3 Membrane filtration

This method has traditionally been used to overcome the activity of antibiotics for which there

Table 20.7 Inactivating agents*

Inhibitory agents	Inactivating agents
Phenols, cresols	None (dilution)
Alcohols	None (dilution)
Parabens	Dilution and Tween
Mercury compounds	-SH compounds
Quaternary ammonium compounds	Lecithin + Lubrol W; Lecithin + Tween (Letheen)
Benzylpenicillin† ⎫ Ampicillin ⎬	β-Lactamase from *Bacillus cereus*
Other antibiotics†	None (membrane filtration)
Sulphonamides	p-Aminobenzoic acid

* Neutralizing agents.
† See text.

are no inactivating agents, although it could be extended to cover other products if necessary, e.g. those containing preservatives for which no specific or effective inactivators are available. Basically, a solution of the product is filtered through a hydrophobic-edged membrane filter that will retain any contaminating microorganisms. The membrane is washed *in situ* to remove any traces of antibiotic adhering to the membrane and is then transferred to appropriate culture media.

13.3 Positive controls

It is essential to show that microorganisms will actually grow under the conditions of the test. For this reason positive controls have to be carried out; in these, the ability of small numbers of suitable microorganisms to grow in media in the presence of the sample is assessed. The microorganism used for positive control tests with a product containing or comprising an antimicrobial agent must, if at all possible, be sensitive to that agent, so that growth of the organism indicates a satisfactory inactivation, dilution or removal of the agent. The *European Pharmacopoeia* suggests the use of designated strains of *Staphylococcus aureus*, *Bacillus subtilis* and *Pseudomonas aeruginosa* as appropriate aerobic organisms, *Clostridium sporogenes* as an anaerobe and *Candida albicans* or *Aspergillus niger* as fungi.

In practice, a positive control (medium with added test sample) and a negative control (medium without it) are inoculated simultaneously, and the rate and extent of growth arising in each should be similar. However, the negative control without the test sample, is, in effect, exactly the same as the growth promotion control that is also described in the test procedure, so, for the organisms concerned, it is not necessary to do both.

All the controls may be conducted either before, or in parallel with, the test itself, providing that the same batches of media are used for both. If the controls are carried out in parallel with the tests and one of the controls gives an unexpected result, the test for sterility may be declared invalid, and, when the problem is resolved, the test may be repeated.

13.4 Specific cases

Specific details of the sterility testing of parenteral products, ophthalmic and other non-injectable preparations, catgut and surgical sutures will be found in the *European Pharmacopoeia*. These procedures cannot conveniently be applied to items like surgical dressings and medical devices because they

are too big. In such cases the most convenient approach is to immerse the whole object in culture medium in a sterile flexible bag, but care must be taken to ensure that the liquid penetrates to all parts and surfaces of the material.

13.5 Sampling

A sterility test attempts to infer the state (sterile or non-sterile) of a batch from the results of an examination of part of a batch, and is thus a statistical operation. Suppose that p represents the proportion of infected containers in a batch and q the proportion of non-infected containers. Then, $p + q = 1$ or $q = 1 - p$.

Suppose also that a sample of two items is taken from a large batch containing 10% infected containers. The probability of a single item taken at random being infected is $p = 0.1$ (10% = 0.1), whereas the probability of such an item being non-infected is given by $q = 1 - p = 0.9$. The probability of both items being infected is $p^2 = 0.01$, and of both items being non-infected, $q^2 = (1 - p)^2 = 0.81$. The probability of obtaining one infected item and one non-infected item is $1 - (0.01 + 0.81) = 0.18 = 2pq$.

In a sterility test involving a sample size of n containers, the probability p of obtaining n consecutive 'steriles' is given by $q^n = (1 - p)^n$. Values for various levels of p (i.e. proportion of infected containers in a batch) with a constant sample size are given in Table 20.8, which shows that the test cannot detect low levels of contamination. Similarly, if different sample sizes are employed (based also upon $(1 - p)^n$) it can be shown that as the sample size increases, the probability of the batch being passed as sterile decreases.

It can be seen from the above that a sterility test can only show that a proportion of the products in a batch is sterile. Thus, the correct conclusion to be drawn from a satisfactory test result is that the batch has passed the sterility test not that the batch is sterile.

13.6 Re-tests

Under certain circumstances a sterility test may be repeated, but the only justification for repeating the test is unequivocal evidence that the first test was

Table 20.8 Sampling in sterility testing

	Infected items in batch (%)					
	0.1	1	5	10	20	50
p	0.001	0.01	0.05	0.1	0.2	0.5
q	0.999	0.99	0.95	0.9	0.8	0.5
Probability *P**, of drawing 20† consecutive sterile items:	0.98	0.82	0.36	0.12	0.012	<0.00001

* Calculated from $P = (1 - p)^{20} = q^{20}$.
† 20 is the sample size required by the EP for batches of >500 items.

invalid; a re-test cannot be viewed as a second opportunity for the batch to pass when it has failed the first time. Circumstances that may justify a re-test would include, for example, failure of the air filtration system in the testing facility which might have permitted airborne contaminants to enter the product or media during testing, non-sterility of the media used for testing, or evidence that contamination arose during testing from the operating personnel or a source other than the sample under test.

14 The role of sterility testing

The techniques discussed in this chapter comprise an attempt to achieve, as far as possible, the continuous monitoring of a particular sterilization process. The sterility test on its own provides no guarantee as to the sterility of a batch; however, it is an additional check and, as it will detect gross failure, continued compliance with the test does give confidence as to the efficacy of a sterilization or aseptic process. Failure to carry out a sterility test, despite the major criticism of its inability to detect other than gross contamination, may have important legal and moral consequences.

15 Acknowledgements

The assistance of the following is gratefully acknowledged: F.J. Ley, Isotron plc, Swindon (for discussions and permission to reproduce Fig. 20.9); M.S. Copson, Albert Browne Ltd, Leicester (for discussions and permission to reproduce Fig. 20.6). GlaxoSmithKline plc for permission to use Fig. 20.11.

16 Appendix

Examples of typical conditions employed in the sterilization of pharmaceutical and medical products.

Sterilization method	Conditions
Moist heat (autoclaving)	121°C for 15 min
	134°C for 3 min
Dry heat	160°C for 120 min
	170°C for 60 min
	180°C for 30 min
Ethylene oxide	Gas concentration:
	800–1200 mg/L
	45–63°C
	30–70% relative humidity
	1–4 hours sterilizing time
Low-temperature steam and formaldehyde	Gas concentration:
	15–100 mg/L
	Steam admission to 73°C
	40–180 min sterilizing time depending on type of process
Irradiation Gamma-rays or accelerated electrons	25 kGy (2.5 Mrad) dose
Filtration	≤0.22 μm pore size, sterile membrane filter

17 Further reading

Baird, R. M. & Bloomfield, S. F. (1996) *Microbial Quality Assurance in Cosmetics, Toiletries and Non-sterile Pharmaceuticals*. Taylor & Francis, London.

Baird, R. M., Hodges, N. A. & Denyer, S.P. (2000) *Handbook of Microbiological Quality Control: Pharmaceuticals and Medical Devices*. Taylor & Francis, London.

Block, S. S. (2001) *Disinfection, Sterilization and Preservation*, 5th edn. Lippincott Williams and Wilkins, Philadelphia.

European Agency for the Evaluation of Medicinal Products (2000) *Decision trees for the selection of sterilization methods*. Annex to Note for Guidance on Development of Pharmaceutics. Committee for Proprietary Medicinal Products, London. CPMP/QWP/054/98 Corr.

European Pharmacopoeia, 4th edn (2002) Council of Europe, Strasbourg.

Fraise, A. P., Lambert, P. A. & Mailland, J.-Y. (2004) *Principles and Practice of Disinfection, Preservation and Sterilization*, 5th edn. Blackwell Scientific Publications, Oxford.

Gilbert, P. & Allison, D. (1996) Redefining the 'sterility' of sterile products. *Eur J Parenteral Sci*, 1, 19–23.

Health Technical Memorandum (1994) *Sterilisers*. HTM 2010. Department of Health, London.

Medicines Control Agency (2002) *Rules and Guidance for Pharmaceutical Manufacturers and Distributors*. The Stationery Office, London.

Parenteral Society (2001) Microbiology Special Issue. *Eur J Parenteral Sci*, 6(4).

Prince, R. (2001) *Microbiology in Pharmaceutical Manufacturing*. Davis Horwood International Publishing, Godalming, UK.

Soper, C. J. & Davies, D. J. G. (1990) Principles of sterilization. In: *Guide to Microbiological Control in Pharmaceuticals* (eds S.P. Denyer & R.M. Baird), pp. 157–181. Ellis Horwood, Chichester.

Chapter 21
Factory and hospital hygiene

Robert Jones

1 Introduction

There are many definitions of *quality* (see Sharp, 2000). For the purpose of pharmaceutical products the term *quality* is usually taken to mean *fitness for purpose*. Not only must the product have the desired therapeutic properties; it must also be safe for administration by the route intended. Some products such as injections must be sterile, while others such as oral drugs need not be sterile, but must be free from pathogens that can be contracted via the oral route (*British Pharmacopoeia*, 2003, Appendix XVI D). A great deal more space in the literature is dedicated to quality of sterile products, but this reflects the *additional* quality assurance required compared with that for non-sterile products (Sharp, 2000).

Manufacturing is carried out in both industry and hospitals. In the latter, batches tend to be much smaller, sometimes only one item, and the products are stored for much less time, usually less than 24 hours (Beaney, 2001).

The difficulty in demonstrating quality is that the tests carried out are designed to detect its absence. For example, the test for sterility (Chapter 20) involves taking samples at random and testing for microorganisms. The absence of microorganisms only allows an estimate of the statistical *probability* that the batch is sterile. Therefore it is important that a product be manufactured in a suitable environment by a procedure that minimizes the possibility of contamination occurring. At the end of this process the tests can be performed as an *additional* measure.

The UK Orange Guide (Rules and Guidance for Pharmaceutical Manufacturers and Distributors, 2002) emphasizes the fundamental point that the manufacture of sterile products:

> must strictly follow carefully established and validated methods of preparation and procedure. Sole reliance for sterility or other quality aspects must not be placed on any terminal process or finished product test.

This chapter summarizes measures for the control, during manufacture, of one important feature of product quality, the level of microbial contamination. It is designed to complement and be read in conjunction with Chapters 15, 16, 17, 19, 20 and 23.

1.1 Definitions

Several terms used in industrial and hospital production must be defined to enable the reader to follow this chapter. These definitions are given in sections 1.1.1 to 1.1.5. The inter-relationship between quality assurance, good manufacturing practice, quality control and in-process control is shown in Fig. 21.1.

1.1.1 Manufacture

Manufacture is the complete cycle of production of a medical product. This cycle includes the acquisition of all raw materials, their processing into a final product, and its subsequent packaging and distribution.

1.1.2 Quality assurance (QA)

This term refers to the sum total of the arrange-ments made to ensure that the final product is of the quality required for its intended purpose. It consists of good manufacturing practice plus factors such as original product design and development.

1.1.3 Good manufacturing practice (GMP)

Good manufacturing practice (GMP) comprises that part of quality assurance that is aimed at ensuring the product is consistently manufactured to a quality appropriate for its intended use. GMP requires that: (i) the manufacturing process is fully defined before it is commenced; and (ii) the necessary facilities are provided. In practice, this means that:
- personnel must be adequately trained
- suitable premises and equipment employed
- correct materials used
- approved procedures adopted
- suitable storage and transport facilities available
- appropriate records made.

1.1.4 Quality control (QC)

Quality control refers to the part of GMP that ensures that (i) at each stage of manufacture the necessary tests are conducted; and (ii) the product is not released until it has passed these tests. An example is the test for pyrogens applied to sterile pharmaceutical products (Chapter 19).

1.1.5 In-process control

This comprises any test on a product, the environment or the equipment that is made during the manufacturing process. An example of this is testing that an autoclave is functioning correctly (Gardner & Peel, 1998).

2 Control of microbial contamination during manufacture: general aspects

A pharmaceutical product may become contaminated by a number of means and at several points during manufacture. There are several ways in which this risk can be minimized. Any such measures require an understanding of the risks involved (Chapters 15 and 16).

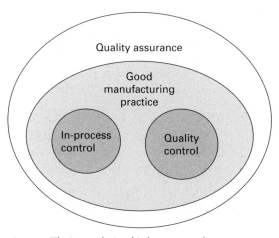

Fig. 21.1 The inter-relationship between quality assurance, good manufacturing practice, quality control and in-process control.

2.1 Hazard analysis of critical control points (HACCP)

Hazard analysis of critical control points (HACCP) has been widely used in the food industry and is becoming more commonly used in the pharmaceutical industry (Jahnke, 1997). HACCP is a tool for evaluating steps in a manufacturing process. It provides a structured thought process for GMP. The seven steps involved are:

1 Analysis and identification of the potential risk (hazard) represented by each step in the process.
2 Determination of the critical control points (CCP) where it is necessary to control the hazards.
3 Definition of the limits within which each critical parameter should be controlled.
4 Establishment (and validation) of in-process control methods and tests to be used to determine, for each critical control point, whether or not the potential hazard is maintained within the defined limits.
5 Establishment of corrective measures designed to correct any out of control situation at each and every CCP.
6 Confirmation that the HACCP regime (and hence the manufacturing process adopted) is functioning as intended.
7 Documentation of the entire system, in terms of both HACCP steps to be followed, and of the results obtained.

2.2 Environmental cleanliness and hygiene

Microorganisms may be transferred to a product from working surfaces, fixtures and equipment. Pooled stagnant water is a frequent source of contamination. Thus it is essential that all working areas are kept clean, dry and tidy. Any cracks where microorganisms may accumulate must be eliminated. All walls, floors and ceilings should be easy to clean. This requires impervious and washable surfaces, free from open joints or ledges. Coving should be used at junctions between walls and floors or ceilings. All services such as pipes, light fittings and ventilation points should be sited so that inaccessible recesses are avoided. A rigorous disinfection policy must be in place (Chapter 17). All equipment must be easy to dismantle and clean and should be inspected for cleanliness before use.

Fall-out of dust- and droplet-borne microorganisms from the atmosphere is an obvious route for contamination. Therefore 'clean' air (section 3.1.4) is a prerequisite during manufacturing processes and the spread of dust during manufacture or packaging must be avoided. Microorganisms may thrive in certain liquid preparations and creams and lotions (Chapters 15 and 16), so the manufacture of such products should, as far as possible, be in a closed system; this serves a dual purpose as it also prevents evaporative loss.

Personnel are another source of potential contamination. High standards of personal hygiene are essential. Operatives should be free from communicable disease and open lesions on the exposed body surfaces. To ensure high standards of personal cleanliness, adequate hand-washing facilities and protective garments, including headgear and gloves, must be provided. Staff should be trained in the principles of GMP and in the practice (and theory) of the tasks assigned. Staff employed in the manufacture of sterile products should also receive basic training in microbiology.

2.3 Quality of starting materials

Raw materials, including water supplies, are an important source of microorganisms in the manufacturing area and can lead to contamination of both the environment and final product. Materials of natural origin, plant or animal, are usually associated with an extensive microbial flora and require careful storage to prevent growth of the organisms and spoilage of the material. If stable, natural products with a high microbial count may be sterilized. Staff handling raw materials must be given adequate training to prevent cross-contamination.

The many grades of water used in pharmaceutical manufacturing are discussed in Chapter 15. Water for manufacturing may be potable mains water, water purified by ion exchange, reverse osmosis or distillation, or Water for Injection. Water used for parenteral products must be apyrogenic and is usually produced in a specially designed still. Although pyrogens are not volatile, some are carried over mechanically into the distillate with the entrainment (spray), so a spray trap, consisting of a series of baffles, is fitted to the distilling flask to prevent spray and pyrogens from entering the condenser tubes. Water prepared in this way can be used immediately for the preparation of injections, provided they are sterilized within 4 hours of water collection. Alternatively, the water can be kept for longer periods at a temperature above 65°C (usually 80°C) to prevent bacterial growth with consequent pyrogen production. Ultraviolet radiation may be useful in reducing bacterial count but must not be regarded as a sterilizing agent (Chapter 20).

2.4 Process design

The manufacturing process must be fully defined and capable of providing, with the facilities available, a product that is microbiologically acceptable and conforms to specifications. The process must be fully evaluated before starting to ensure that it is suitable for routine production operations. Processes and procedures must also be subject to frequent reappraisal and should be re-evaluated when any significant changes are made in the equipment or materials used.

2.5 Quality control and documentation

The lower the microbiological count of the starting materials, the more readily the quality of the product can be controlled. Microbiological standards should be set for all raw materials as well as microbial limits for in-process samples and the final product. Microbiological quality assurance also covers the validation of cleaning and disinfectant solutions and the monitoring of the production environment by microbial counts. This monitoring should be carried out while normal production operations are in progress. In addition, sterile manufacture requires extra safeguards. Operators must be adequately trained and their aseptic technique monitored both by observation and microbial testing. Air filter and sterility efficiency must also be evaluated (Chapter 20). The final tests that are usually conducted on the finished product are those for pyrogens (endotoxin test, Chapter 19) and sterility (Chapter 20).

Documentation is a vital part of quality assurance. Details of starting materials, packaging materials, and intermediate, bulk and finished products should be recorded, so that the history of each batch may be traced. Distribution records must be kept. This information is of paramount importance in the event that a defective batch has to be recalled.

2.6 Packaging, storage and transport

Packaging serves a number of functions: it keeps the contents in, it should keep contaminants out and it is labelled to permit identification of its contents. The product is contained within primary packaging. In industry these packages are then placed inside secondary packaging for storage and transport. This secondary packaging may take the form of cartons, boxes, trays or shrink-wrapping. Consideration must be given to both the fabrics of the packaging and its cleaning (Chapter 15) and also the actual process of packaging. Where terminal sterilization is carried out, the packaging must be suitable for the process. Packaging of aseptically processed products into a sterile container (section 3) must be carried out in grade A environment (Table 21.1). A discussion of packaging beyond the scope of this chapter is given by Sharp (2000).

3 Manufacture of sterile products

The various types of sterile product are described in Chapter 19, and methods available for terminal sterilization in Chapter 20. For production purposes an important distinction exists between sterile products which have been terminally sterilized (Fig. 21.2a) and those which are not. Terminal sterilization involves the product being sealed in its container and then sterilized, usually by heat, but ionizing radiation or, less commonly, ethylene oxide may be employed. Such a product must be produced in a clean area (sections 3.1.1–3.1.8). A product that cannot be terminally sterilized is prepared aseptically (Fig. 21.2b) from previously sterilized materials or by sterile filtration and then filled into sterile containers. Strict aseptic conditions are required throughout (sections 3.2.1–3.2.4).

Vaccines, consisting of dead microorganisms, microbial extracts or inactivated viruses (see Chap-

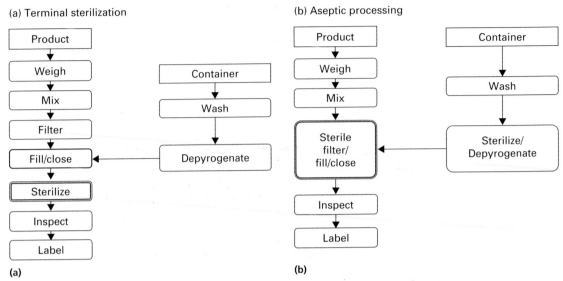

Fig. 21.2 A comparison of (a) terminal sterilization and (b) aseptic processing in sterile manufacturing.

ter 23) may be filled in the same premises as other sterile medicinal products. The completeness of inactivation (or killing or removal of live organisms) must be proved before processing. Separate premises are needed for the filling of live or attenuated vaccines and for the preparation of other products derived from live organisms. Non-sterile products and sterile products must not be processed in the same area.

3.1 Clean and aseptic areas: general requirements

3.1.1 *Design of premises*

Sterile production should be carried out in a purpose-built unit separated from other manufacturing areas and thoroughfares. The unit should be designed to encourage separation of each stage of production but should ensure a safe and organized workflow. A plan of such a facility is shown in Fig. 21.3. Sterilized products held in quarantine pending sterility test results (Chapter 20) must be kept separate from those awaiting sterilization.

3.1.2 *Internal surfaces, fittings and floors*

Particulate, as well as microbial, contamination must be prevented. To this end all surfaces must have smooth, impervious surfaces which will: (i) prevent accumulation of dust or other particulate matter; and (ii) permit easy, repeated cleaning and disinfection. Smooth rounded coving should be used where the wall meets the floor and the ceiling.

Suitable flooring may be provided by welded sheets of polyvinyl chloride (PVC); cracks and open joints that might harbour dirt and microorganisms must be avoided. The preferred surfaces for walls are plastic, epoxy-coated plaster, plastic fibreglass or glass reinforced polyester. Often the final finish for the floor, wall and ceiling is achieved using continuous welded PVC sheeting. False ceilings should be adequately sealed to prevent contamination from the space above. Use should be made of well-sealed glass panels, especially in dividing walls, to ensure good visibility and allow satisfactory supervision. Doors and windows should be flush with the walls. Windows should not be openable.

Internal fittings such as cupboards, drawers and shelves should be kept to a minimum. They must be sited where they do not interfere with the laminar flow of the filtered air supply. Stainless steel or laminated plastic are the preferred materials for such fittings. Stainless steel trolleys may be used to transport equipment and materials within the clean and

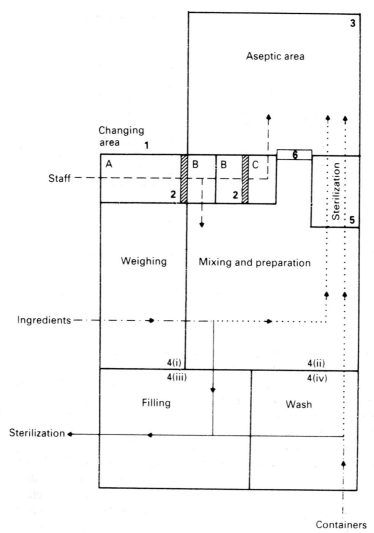

Fig. 21.3 Example of a diagrammatic representation of the layout and workflow of a sterile products manufacturing unit. **1,** the changing area in this example is built on the black (A)–grey (B)–white (C) principle; passage into the clean area is through A and B (see section 3.1.6) whereas entry to the aseptic area is first through A and B followed by C (see section 3.2.2). **2,** Dividing step-over sill. **3,** For details of aseptic area requirements, see text; a laminar airflow work station would be included in this area. **4i–4iv,** These areas are clean areas. In filling rooms for terminally sterilized products, care should be exercised to protect containers from airborne contamination. The final rinse point (i.e. where the containers are finally washed) should be sited as near as possible to the filling point. **5,** Articles which are to be transferred directly to the aseptic area from elsewhere must be sterilized by passage through a double-ended sterilizer. Solutions manufactured in the clean area may be brought into the aseptic area through a sterilizing-grade membrane filter. **6,** Double-doored hatchway through which presterilized articles may be passed into the aseptic area (see section 3.2.3). Note: inspection, holding and final packaging areas have been omitted. Direction of workflow: ——▸——, for terminally sterilized products; · · ·▸· · ·, for aseptically prepared products; —·▸·—, shared stages of preparation.

aseptic areas but must remain confined to their respective units. Equipment must be designed so that it may be easily cleaned and sterilized or disinfected.

3.1.3 Services

Clean and aseptic areas must be adequately illuminated; lights are best housed in translucent panels set in a false ceiling. Electrical switches and sockets must be flush with the wall. When required, gases should be pumped in from outside the unit. Pipes and ducts, if they must be brought into the clean area, must be sealed through the walls. Additionally, in order to prevent dust accumulation, they must be boxed in or readily cleanable. Alternatively they may be sited above false ceilings.

Sinks should be of stainless steel with no overflow, and water must be of at least potable quality. Wherever possible, drains should be avoided. If installed they must be fitted with effective, readily cleanable traps and with air breaks to prevent backflow. Any floor channels should be open, shallow and cleanable and connected to drains outside the area. They should be monitored microbiologically.

Sinks and drains should be excluded from aseptic areas except where radiopharmaceuticals are being processed when sinks are a requirement.

3.1.4 Air supply

Areas for sterile manufacture are classified according to the required characteristics of the environment. Each operation requires an appropriate level of microbial and particulate cleanliness; four grades (Table 21.1) are specified in *Rules and Guidance for Pharmaceutical Manufacturers and Distributors* (2002). The air supplied to the manufacturing environment substantially influences environmental quality.

Filtered air (Chapter 15) is used to achieve the necessary standards; this should be maintained at positive pressure throughout a clean or aseptic area, with the highest pressure in the most critical rooms (aseptic or clean filling rooms) and a progressive reduction through the preparation and changing rooms (Fig. 21.4); a minimum pressure differential of 10–15 Pa is normally required between each class of room. A minimum of 20 changes of air per hour is usual in clean and aseptic rooms. The air inlet points should be situated in or near the ceiling, with

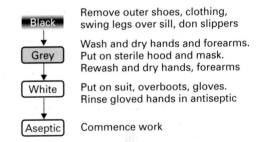

Fig. 21.4 Entry into aseptic area.

Table 21.1 Environmental grades and typical manufacturing operations

| Environmental grade | Typical operations | | Area designation in Fig. 21.3 |
	Aseptically prepared products	Terminally sterilized products (TSP)	
A	Aseptic preparation and filling in a protective work unit	Filling of products at particular microbiological risk	3
B	Background environment to grade A preparation areas	Background environment to grade A preparation areas	3
C	Preparation of solutions to be filtered	Preparation of 'at risk' solutions Filling of products	4ii 4ii
D	Handling of components after washing	Preparation of solutions and components for subsequent filling	4iv (aseptic) 4ii (TSP)

Table 21.2 Basic operating standards for the manufacture of sterile products

| Environmental grade | Operating standards* | | Recommended limit of viable airborne microorganisms (cfu/m³) |
| | Maximum permitted number of airborne particles/m³ equal to or above specified size | | |
	0.5 µm	5 µm	
A	3 500	0	<1
B	350 000	2 000	10
C	3 500 000	20 000	100
D	ND	ND	200

ND, not defined.

* Particulate burdens for the manufacturing environment 'at rest' are more rigorous for grades B, C and D.

the final filters placed as close as possible to the point of input to the room.

The greatest risk of contamination of a product comes from its immediate environment. Additional protection is needed in both the filling area of the clean room and in the aseptic suite. This can be provided by a workstation supplied with a unidirectional flow of filtered sterile air. This is known as a laminar flow cabinet. Displacement of air may be vertical or horizontal with a minimum homogeneous airflow of 0.45 m/s at the working position. Consequently airborne contamination is not added to the workspace and any generated by manipulations is swept away by the laminar air currents. A fuller description of high efficiency particulate air (HEPA) filters in laminar flow cabinets is given by Gardner and Peel (1998).

The efficacy of the filters through which the air is passed should be monitored at predetermined intervals. Air quality may be monitored by volumetric air sampler or settle plate. Table 21.2 describes the maximum concentrations of non-viable particles and viable airborne microorganisms permitted in the four grades of air.

3.1.5 Clothing

Clothing worn in the clean area must be of non-shedding fibres; terylene is a suitable fabric. Airborne contamination, both microbial and particulate, is reduced when trouser suits, close-fitting at the neck, wrists and ankles, are worn. Clean suits should be provided once a day, but fresh headwear, overshoes and powder-free gloves are necessary for each working session. Special laundering facilities are desirable. Additional requirements for aseptic rooms are discussed in section 3.2.1.

3.1.6 Changing facilities

Entry to a clean or aseptic area should be through a changing room fitted with interlocking doors; this acts as an airlock to prevent influx of air from outside. This route is for personnel only, not for the transfer of materials and equipment. Staff entering the changing room should already be clad in the standard factory or hospital protective clothing.

For entry into a clean area, passage through the changing room should be from a 'black' to a 'grey' area, via a dividing step-over sill (Fig. 21.4). Movement through these areas and finally into the clean room is permitted only when observing a strict protocol, whereby outer garments are removed in the 'black' area and clean room trouser-suits donned in the 'grey' area. After hand-washing in a sink fitted with elbow- or foot-operated taps the operator may enter the clean room.

The changing procedure for entry to an aseptic area is described in section 3.2.2.

3.1.7 Cleaning and disinfection

A strict disinfection policy is necessary if microbial contamination is to be kept to a minimum. Cleaning agents used include alkaline detergents and ionic and non-ionic surfactants. A wide range of chemical disinfectants is available (Chapter 17). Clear soluble phenolics are commonly used for interior services and fittings. Disinfectants for working surfaces are alcohols (70% ethanol or isopropanol) or, less commonly, chlorine-base agents such as hypochlorites. Skin may be disinfected with cationic detergents such as cetrimide or chlorhexidine, usually formulated with 70% alcohol to avoid the need for rinsing. Gloved hands may be disinfected with these detergents (so offering residual activity) or 70% alcohol alone. Rotation of different disinfectants reduces the risk of the emergence of resistant strains. In-use dilutions must not be stored unless sterilized. Disinfectants and detergents for use in grade A/B areas must be sterile prior to use.

As mentioned in section 3.1.2, smooth polished surfaces are most readily cleaned. Floors and horizontal surfaces should be cleaned and disinfected daily, walls and ceilings as often as required, but the interval should not exceed 1 month. Regular microbiological monitoring should be carried out to determine the efficacy of disinfection procedures. Records must be kept and immediate remedial action taken should normal levels for that area be exceeded.

3.1.8 Operation

The number of persons involved in sterile manufacture should be kept to a minimum to avoid the inevitable turbulence and shedding of particles and organisms associated with the operatives (Chapter 15). All operations should be undertaken in a controlled and methodical manner as excessive activity may increase this turbulence and shedding.

Containers made from fibrous materials such as paper, cardboard and sacking are generally heavily contaminated (especially with moulds and bacterial spores) and should not be taken into clean areas. Ingredients that must be brought into clean areas must first be transferred to suitable metal or plastic containers.

Containers and closures for terminally sterilized products must be thoroughly cleaned before use and should undergo a final washing and rinsing process in apyrogenic distilled water (which has been passed through a bacteria-proof membrane filter) immediately prior to filling. Containers and closures for use in aseptic manufacture must, in addition, be sterilized after washing and rinsing in preparation for aseptic filling (Fig. 21.2).

3.2 Aseptic areas: additional requirements

Additional requirements for aseptic areas, over and above those discussed in sections 3.1.1–3.1.8, are discussed below.

3.2.1 Clothing

Clothing requirements in addition to those in section 3.1.5 are necessary for aseptic areas. The operative is a potential source of microorganisms and it is imperative that steps are taken to prevent this contamination. The operative must wear sterile protective headwear, totally enclosing hair and beard, powder-free rubber or plastic gloves, a non-fibre-shedding facemask (to prevent the release of droplets) and footwear. A suitable garment is a one- or two-piece trouser-suit. An example of such clothing is shown in Fig. 21.5. Fresh sterile clothing should be provided each time a person enters an aseptic area.

3.2.2 Entry to aseptic areas

Entry to an aseptic suite is usually through a 'black-grey-white' changing procedure (Fig. 21.4), where white represents the highest level of cleanliness. Movement from 'black' to 'white' is via two changing rooms, the 'grey' area also serving as an entry to the clean room (Figs 21.3 and 21.4 and section 3.1.6).

3.2.3 Equipment and operation

Any articles entering the aseptic area must be sterilized. In order to achieve this, articles should be transferred via a double-ended sterilizer (i.e. with a door at each end). If they are not to be discharged

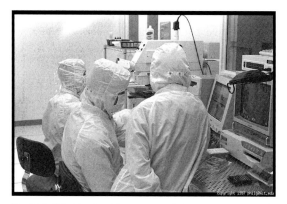

Fig. 21.5 Working in a clean room (photo courtesy http://philip.greenspun.com).

directly to the aseptic area, they should be (i) double-wrapped before sterilization; (ii) transferred immediately after sterilizing into a clean environment until required; (iii) transferred from this clean environment via a double-doored hatch (where the outer wrapping is removed) to the aseptic area (where the inner wrapper is removed at the workbench). Hatches and sterilizers must be designed so that only one door may be opened at any one time. Solutions manufactured in the clean room may be brought into the aseptic area through a sterile 0.22-μm membrane filter.

Workbenches, including laminar flow units, and equipment, should be disinfected immediately before and after each work session. Equipment must be of the simplest design possible for the operation being performed.

Aseptic manipulations must be carried out in the grade A air of a laminar flow cabinet. Speed, accuracy and economy of movement are essential features of good aseptic technique. It is therefore essential that workers are well trained and motivated and familiar with the task in hand. Observation and microbiological monitoring of the operator and of the environment are very important. Air quality is measured using settle plates or slit samplers, work surfaces by taking swabs or by use of contact plates (Chapter 20).

Under no circumstances must living microorganisms, including those used for vaccine preparation (Chapter 23) and for biological monitoring, be introduced into the aseptic area.

3.2.4 *Isolator and blow/fill/seal technology*

All aseptic packaging should be carried out in a grade A environment with a grade B background (Table 21.1). Advances in technology now permit the production of self-contained workstations, or isolators, which incorporate many of the design principles of clean rooms and laminar flow cabinets. The isolator (see Fig. 20.11) protects both the product from contamination by the operator and the operator from any hazardous materials. Direct interaction between the operator and the product is minimized by providing a grade A laminar flow of air with a positive pressure, the internal space being accessed by means of a glove/sleeve system. A grade D background (Table 21.1) is considered adequate for such operations.

Blow/fill/seal units are purpose-built pieces of equipment, which carry out these three steps in a continuous process within a controlled environment. Containers, which are formed from thermoplastic granules, are blown to form the correct shape, filled and heat-sealed. These units are fitted with a grade A air shower and operated in a grade C environment for aseptic manufacture and a grade D background for products which are to be terminally sterilized.

4 Guide to Good Pharmaceutical Manufacturing Practice

Between 1971 and 1983 the essential features of GMP were covered in the UK by three editions of the *Guide to Good Pharmaceutical Manufacturing Practice*, frequently referred to as 'The Orange Guide'. This guide was prepared by the UK Medicines Inspectorate in consultation with industrial, hospital, professional and other interested parties. The principles of this national guide were subsequently assimilated into the EC *Guide to Good Manufacturing Practice for Medicinal Products* in 1989 and are now published as *Rules and Guidance for Pharmaceutical Manufacturers and Distributors* (2002) by the Medicines Control Agency, Department of Health. Two important recent publications from the Pharmaceutical Press are *Quality in the Manufacture of Medicines and Other*

Health Care Products (Sharp, 2000) and *Quality Assurance of Aseptic Preparation Services* (Beaney, 2001), which discusses manufacturing in hospitals.

Compliance with GMP is one of the major factors considered by the Licensing Authority when examining an application for a licence to manufacture under the Medicines Act (1968). Similar codes exist in the USA and other countries.

5 Conclusions

Quality assurance is not just a process; it is a way of thinking. All staff should be well trained and motivated and be working to a common goal: the production of a pharmaceutical product of a quality that is safe for the patient. The procedures should not be seen as a chore or burden to make work more difficult, but essential steps in the production of a safe, satisfactory product. Self-inspection and external audit of procedures are important processes in maintaining standards of cleanliness. Even after manufacture and distribution it is vital that the products are used properly, especially multi-use containers that are subject to potential in-use contamination.

The manufacture of non-sterile products requires that certain standards of cleanliness, personal hygiene, production methods and storage must be met. Many such products are for oral and topical use and one might wonder why such stringent parameters need be in place. However, there have been controlled hospital studies and case reports associating these products with nosocomial (hospital-acquired) infection (Chapter 16). Furthermore, methods of controlling pathogens also control spoilage organisms (Chapter 16), which could cause the industry considerable expense. Spoilage organisms can alter the aesthetic qualities (such as smell, taste, appearance), physical properties (pH, viscosity) and efficacy of the product, in addition to producing toxins.

Greater stringency is required for terminally sterilized products. Such environmental and process controls might seem overzealous, but it is better to minimize risk at all stages rather than to rely on final product testing (section 1). The lower the bioburden the easier it is to achieve the required sterility assurance level in the terminal sterilization process (Chapter 20). It is also important to exclude pyrogens and particulate matter that would not be removed by sterilization.

Where products are processed aseptically even higher standards of cleanliness are necessary. The importance of the knowledge and commitment of the operatives cannot be overemphasized, both in hospital and industry. A majority of reported incidents of defective products have been traced to human rather than technological error.

6 Further reading

Baird, R. M., Hodges N. A. & Denyer S. P. (2000) *Handbook of Microbiological Quality Control: Pharmaceuticals and Medical Devices.* Taylor & Francis, London.

Beaney, A. M. (2001) *Quality Assurance of Aseptic Preparation Services*, 3rd edn. Pharmaceutical Press, London.

British Pharmacopoeia (2003) HMSO, London.

Denyer, S. & Baird, R. (1990) *Guide to Microbiological Control in Pharmaceuticals.* Ellis Horwood, Chichester.

Gardner, J. F. & Peel, M. M. (1998) *Sterilization, Disinfection and Infection Control*, 3rd edn. Churchill Livingstone, Melbourne.

Jahnke, M. (1997) Use of the HACCP concept for the risk analysis of pharmaceutical manufacturing processes. *Eur J Parenter Sci*, **2**, 113–117.

Lund, W. (1994) *The Pharmaceutical Codex*, 12th edn. Pharmaceutical Press, London.

Rules and Guidance for Pharmaceutical Manufacturers and Distributors (2002) HMSO, London.

Sharp, J. (2000) *Quality in the Manufacture of Medicines and Other Health Care Products.* Pharmaceutical Press, London.

[There are two relevant computer-aided learning (CAL) packages produced by CoAcS (www.coacs.com): *Good Manufacturing Practice* and *Pharmaceutical Microbiology Tutorial*.]

Chapter 22
Manufacture of antibiotics

Sally Varian

1 Introduction

Industrial manufacture of most antibiotics is based on the large scale production of microorganisms which convert raw materials into antibiotics. This process is commonly referred to as a fermentation. Other much longer-established fermentation processes include wine and beer making. Strictly speaking, fermentations are biological processes occurring in the absence of air (oxygen). However, the term is now commonly applied to any large-scale cultivation of microorganisms, whether aerobic (with oxygen) or anaerobic (without oxygen).

Following production by fermentation, antibiotics are recovered, concentrated and purified by a series of downstream processing stages. For semisynthetic antibiotics there will then be chemical conversion stages to produce the bulk antibiotic or active pharmaceutical ingredient (API). The bulk antibiotic (API) is formulated into the required dosage form: tablets, vials for injection, solutions, ointments and so on. Stages up to bulk API are commonly termed primary manufacture; stages from API to formulated product are termed secondary manufacture.

2 Background

Benzylpenicillin (penicillin G, originally just 'penicillin') is the first antibiotic to have been manufactured in bulk. It is still universally prescribed and is also used as input material for some semisynthetic antibiotics (Chapter 10). Developments associated with the penicillin fermentation process have been a significant factor in the development of modern biotechnology and therefore it is an appropriate example to illustrate key aspects of manufacture.

Despite the ever-increasing use of complex instrumentation, the application of feedback control techniques and the use of computers, the science of antibiotic fermentation is still imperfectly developed. Processes are difficult to optimize and no two apparently 'identical' batches will ever be entirely the same. This is because living cell populations change both quantitatively and qualitatively throughout the production cycle and small changes in control parameters, such as a fluctuation in air pressure or a power dip, can potentially impact a batch and the effect may vary dependent upon the age of the batch. Also there tends to be significant batch to batch variation in the complex nutrients commonly used in the fermentations.

No single product can exemplify all the important features of antibiotic manufacture. Benzylpenicillin is a β-lactam. Brief accounts are given of the manufacture of two other β-lactams, penicillin V (phenoxymethylpenicillin) and cephalosporin C, to illustrate further key points. However, important as the β-lactams are, they are but one of many families of antibiotics (Chapter 10). Furthermore, most industrial microorganisms used to make β-lactams are fungi; this is atypical of antibiotics as a whole where bacteria, particularly *Streptomyces* spp., predominate. Chapter 10 and some of the further reading at the end of this chapter provide the broad perspective, including information on those antibiotics made by total or partial chemical synthesis.

All the examples are of batched fermentations, i.e. of processes where sterile medium in a vessel is inoculated, the broth fermented for a defined period (usually hours or days), the tank emptied and the broth extracted by downstream processing to yield the antibiotic. During the fermentation, nutrients, antifoam agents and air are supplied, the pH is controlled and exhaust gases are removed. After emptying, the tank is cleaned and prepared for a new batch ('turned round'). In continuous fermentations, sterile medium is added to the fermentation with a balancing withdrawal of broth for product extraction. This has a number of advantages providing the system can be run without contamination. One advantage is long fermentation runs of many weeks, hence greater productivity per vessel due to fewer turn rounds. In continuous culture the growth rate can be held at an optimum value for product fermentation. It is therefore suitable for products whose synthesis is proportional to cell density, but is not generally an economical process for antibiotic production where synthesis is not associated with growth and there are additional concerns about strain degeneration.

3 The production of benzylpenicillin

3.1 The organism

The original organism for the production of penicillin, *Penicillium notatum*, was isolated by Flem-ing in 1926 as a chance contaminant. By 1940, Florey and Chain produced purified penicillin and its tremendous curative potential became apparent. However, the liquid surface culture techniques necessary for the cultivation of this obligate aerobe were lengthy, labour-intensive and prone to contamination. The isolation of a higher-yielding organism, *P. chrysogenum*, from an infected Cantaloupe melon obtained in a market in Peoria, Illinois, USA, was the key advance. This organism could be grown in deep fermentations in sealed tanks under stirred and aerated conditions, in vessels as large as $250\,\text{m}^3$, and thus started the antibiotic manufacturing industry.

From this one ancestral fungus penicillin manufacturers evolved production strains by what became classic strain selection procedures. Large numbers of isolates were screened to identify higher-yielding variants, generally after some type of mutagenic treatment. This cycle of mutation and selection was repeated many times. The selected variants can produce over 20 g/l of culture compared with the 2 mg/l produced by the 'wild' strain, especially when fermented on media under particular control conditions developed in parallel with the strains.

However, there comes a time when sequential improvements in penicillin productivity obtained by these standard strain improvement techniques (physical and chemical mutagenesis in conjunction with a variety of selection techniques that apply pressure for high-yielding variants) become subject to rate-limiting returns. At first, it is easy to double the 'titre' with each campaign; later in the genealogy even a 5% improvement would be regarded as excellent.

Recent developments may well prove to have transformed this situation. Tremendous progress has been made since the mid-1980s both in the isolation and manipulation of the biosynthetic genes in this pathway and in the related routes to the cephalosporins (via the cephalosporin C-producing fungus *Acremonium chrysogenum*) and the cephamycins (via the cephamycin C-producing bacterium *Streptomyces clavuligerus*). Antibiotic manufacturers can now apply recombinant DNA technology to the industrial strains of filamentous microorganisms used to produce β-lactams and there are real prospects of making genetic changes that will very significantly increase productivity. These are discussed further, later in this chapter. There is plenty of scope for improvement, because the best current industrial strains and processes convert little more than 10% of all elemental carbon into penicillin.

Production strains are stored in a dormant form by an appropriate culture preservation technique. Thus, a spore suspension may be mixed with a sterile, finely divided, inert support and desiccated. Alternatively, spore suspensions or vegetative cells can be lyophilized or stored in liquid nitrogen biostats.

All laboratory operations are carried out in laminar flow cabinets in rooms in which filtered air is maintained at a slight positive pressure relative to their outer environment. Operators wear sterilized clothing and work aseptically. Antibiotic fermentations are, of strict necessity, pure culture aseptic processes, without foreign growth, i.e. contamination by other microorganisms.

3.2 Inoculum preparation

The aim is to develop for the production stage fermenter a pure inoculum in sufficient volume and in the fast-growing (logarithmic) phase so that a high population density is quickly established. Figure 22.1 shows a typical route by which the inoculum is produced. The time taken for each seed stage is measured in days and decreases as the sequence progresses. The final inoculum to the production stage is generally 1–10% of the total volume of the fermenter. If the fermenter is under-inoculated there may be an extended lag before growth starts and the fermentation period will be prolonged. This is both uneconomic and may result in degenerative growth

which affects performance, quality and hence also cost.

The inoculum stage media are designed to provide the organism with all the nutrients required for that stage. Adequate oxygen is provided in the form of sterile air and the temperature is controlled at the desired level. Principal criteria for transfer to the next stage in the progression are freedom from foreign growth and growth to a pre-determined cell density.

Typical of fungi, the organism grows as branching filaments (hyphae) and by the time that the culture has progressed to the production stage it is very viscous.

3.3 The fermenter

A typical fermenter is a closed, vertical, cylindrical, stainless steel vessel with convexly dished ends and of 25–250 m^3 capacity. Its height is usually two to three times its diameter. Figure 22.2 shows such a vessel diagrammatically, and Fig. 22.3 gives a view inside an actual vessel.

3.3.1 Oxygen supply

The penicillin fermentation needs large quantities of dissolved oxygen, which is supplied as filter-sterilized air from a compressor. Oxygen is critical to aerobic processes and its supply is a crucial aspect of fermenter design and batch control. As oxygen is poorly soluble in water, steps are taken to assist its passage into the liquid phase and from aqueous solution into the cell, the latter being particularly problematic in viscous broths. One option is to introduce air into the bottom of the vessel via a ring 'sparger' with multiple small holes rather than through a single large orifice. This breaks the air

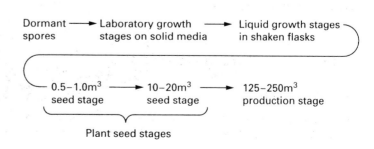

Fig. 22.1 Stages in the preparation of inoculum for the benzylpenicillin fermentation.

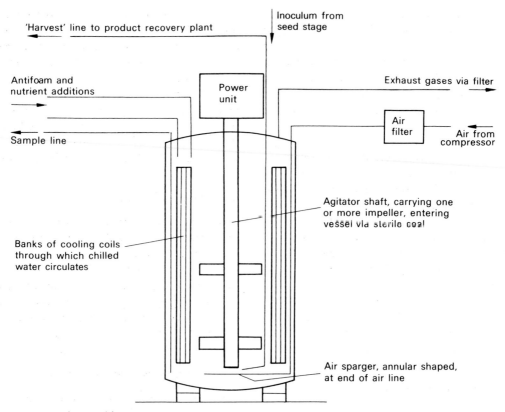

Fig. 22.2 Diagram of a typical fermenter.

Inoculum from
seed stage

'Harvest' line to product recovery plant

Antifoam and
nutrient additions

Power
unit

Exhaust gases via filter

Air
filter

Air from
compressor

Sample line

Agitator shaft, carrying one
or more impeller, entering
vessel via sterile seal

Banks of cooling coils
through which chilled
water circulates

Air sparger, annular shaped,
at end of air line

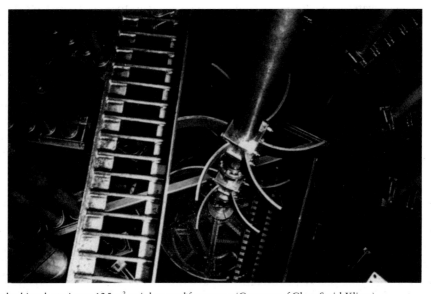

Fig. 22.3 View looking down into a 125 m^3 stainless steel fermenter. (Courtesy of GlaxoSmithKline.)

flow into smaller bubbles which have a greater surface area to volume ratio and hence greater oxygen transfer. These bubbles lose oxygen as they rise up the tank and, at the same time, carbon dioxide diffuses into them. The vessel is kept under a positive head pressure which promotes the dissolution of oxygen and in addition reduces the chances of contamination.

Impellers and baffles assist the transfer of oxygen as well as helping to achieve the correct blend of shear and of bulk circulation from the power supplied, and generally promoting mixing of cells and nutrients. Impellers are mounted on a rotating vertical stirrer shaft which is mechanically driven by a powerful electric motor. This is a major expense as very large amounts of energy are consumed. Baffles located at the vessel perimeter further increase turbulence.

There has been considerable research into novel, energetically more efficient methods of aeration, and the next generation of fermenters may include some that are radically different in design.

3.3.2 Temperature control

The production of benzylpenicillin is very sensitive to temperature. A lot of metabolic heat is generated and the fermentation temperature has to be reduced by controlled cooling. This heat transfer is achieved by circulating chilled water through banks of pipes inside the vessel (which also serve as baffles) or through external 'limpet' coils on the jacket of the vessel. These coils consist of continuous lengths of pipe welded in a shallow spiral round the vessel. This cooling water system is also used to cool batched medium which has been sterilized in the vessel prior to its inoculation.

3.3.3 Defoaming agents and instrumentation

Microbial cultures may foam when they are subjected to vigorous mechanical stirring and aeration. If this foaming is not controlled, culture is lost by entrainment in the exhaust gases and so there are systems, often automatic, for detecting incipient foaming, for temporarily applying backpressure to contain the culture within the vessel and for the aseptic addition of defoaming agents.

Instrumentation is also fitted to provide a continuous display of important variables such as temperature and pH, the power used by the electric motor, airflow, dissolved oxygen and exhaust gas analysis. Manual or computer feedback control can be based either directly on the signals provided by the probes and sensors or on derived data calculated from those signals, such as the respiratory coefficient or the rate of change of pH. Analysis of exhaust gases can provide valuable physiological information.

3.3.4 Media additions

Not all the nutrients required during fermentation are initially provided in the culture medium. Some are sterilized separately by batch or continuous sterilization and then added whilst the fermentation is in progress, usually via automatic systems that allow a preset programme of continuous or discrete aseptic additions. This type of fermentation is called fed batch.

3.3.5 Transfer and sampling systems

Aseptic systems are used to transfer the inoculum to the vessel, to allow the removal of routine samples during fermentation, for early harvesting of aliquots when the vessel becomes full as a consequence of the media additions and to transfer the final contents to the extraction plant when fermentation is complete. Asepsis is assured by engineering design and by steam, which must reach all parts of the vessels and associated pipework. Any pockets of air or rough surfaces that steam does not penetrate could act as reservoirs for foreign growth.

Sampling is essential to monitor the amount of growth, the running levels of key nutrients and the penicillin concentration. It is necessary also to check that there has been no contamination by unwanted microorganisms.

3.4 Control of the fermentation

If growth in the fermenter proceeds unchecked at the rate prevailing in the seed stages, the culture would become very dense and the available aeration would no longer be sufficient to maintain penicillin production. Should oxygen availability fall below a critical level, benzylpenicillin biosynthesis is greatly reduced although culture growth continues. Accordingly, conditions are so adjusted that fast growth is achieved only until the cell population has reached the maximum density that the vessel can support. Further net growth is constrained by deliberately limiting the supply of a key nutrient (in practice, a sugar). The cells can then be stimulated to an 'overproduction' of benzylpenicillin while restricting the amount of growth and a stable, highly productive cell population can be sustained.

3.4.1 Batched medium

The medium initially batched into the fermenter is a complex one but designed only to support the desired amount of early growth. The principal nitrogen source is corn steep liquor (CSL), a by-product of the maize starch-producing industry. This material was originally found to be specifically useful for the penicillin fermentation, but it is recognized as valuable in many fungal antibiotic media. Apart from its primary purpose in supplying cheap and readily available nitrogen, CSL also contains a useful range of carbon compounds, such as acids and sugars, together with inorganic ions and growth factors—in short, it is virtually a complete growth medium in itself. However, like some of the fed nutrients, CSL is a complex nutrient, not chemically defined, derived from natural products and with significant batch-to-batch variation. It is therefore one of the reasons why no two fermentations are ever absolutely identical. In recent years a number of manufacturers have moved from using these relatively cheap but chemically undefined complex nutrients to defined media, thus reducing variability in their fermentation processes.

The batched medium contains subsidiary nitrogen sources and additional essential nutrients such as calcium (added in the form of chalk to counter the natural acidity of the CSL), magnesium, sulphate, phosphate, potassium and trace metals. The medium is sterilized with steam at or above 120°C either in the fermenter itself or in ancillary plant, which may be worked continuously.

3.4.2 Fed nutrients

The sterile medium is stirred and aerated and its pH and temperature are adjusted to the appropriate values. It is then inoculated and the growth phase begins. The initial carbon source is sufficient in quantity to maintain early growth but not sufficient to provide the energy that penicillin production and maintenance of the cell population need during the rest of the fermentation. Carbon for these subsequent stages is 'fed' continuously in such a way as to limit net growth. Either sucrose or glucose is used, possibly as cheaper, impure forms, such as molasses or starch hydrolysate. As the concentration of residual sugar in the broth is too low to measure, the rate of feeding has to be learned by experience and modified on the basis of systematic observation. An alternative way of attaining carbon limitation without the complication of a carefully monitored carbon feed rate is to supply all the carbohydrate at the outset as lactose. The rate-limiting hydrolysis of lactose to hexose is then relied upon to give a steady, slow feed of assimilable carbohydrate. Originally, all benzylpenicillin was manufactured using lactose in this way and some manufacturers still prefer this technique. Calcium, magnesium, phosphate and trace metals added initially are usually sufficient to last throughout the fermentation, but the microorganisms need further supplies of nitrogen and sulphur to balance the carbon feed. Fed nitrogen is often supplied as ammonia gas. The word 'balance' is used quite deliberately; the whole system is a balanced one. Thus, the carbon and nitrogen feeds not only satisfy the organisms' requirements for these elements in the correct molar ratio, they also maintain an adequate reserve of ammonium ion and contribute to pH control, the carbon metabolism being acidogenic and balanced by the alkalinity of the ammonia. Sulphate is usually supplied in combination with the sugar feed and, by obtaining the correct ratio, there is a balanced presentation of sulphate with an adequate pool of intermediates.

The growth phase passes rapidly into the antibiotic-production phase. The optimum pH and temperature for growth are not those for penicillin production and there may be changes in the control of these parameters. The only other event that marks the onset of the production phase is the addition of phenylacetic acid (PAA) by continuous feed.

All feeds are sterilized before they are metered in to the fermenter. Contaminants resistant to the antibiotic rarely find their way into the fermenter, but when they do their effects are so damaging that prevention is of paramount importance. Any foreign growth has the potential to disrupt the fermentation process with both quality and financial implications. For example, a resistant β-lactamase-producing, fast-growing bacterial contaminant can destroy the penicillin already made, as well as consuming nutrients intended for the fungus, causing loss of pH control and interfering with the subsequent extraction process. Hence the key requirement in both design and operation of all stages of the fermentation is that aseptic operations be maintained with growth of the process microorganism but no unwanted foreign growth by contaminating microorganisms.

3.4.3 Stimulation by PAA

Phenylacetic acid (PAA) supplies the side-chain of benzylpenicillin (see also Chapter 10); without PAA, the organisms synthesize only small quantities of this penicillin. Indeed, it was the chance presence of phenylacetyl compounds in CSL (formed by phenylalanine in the grain by the natural bacterial flora during processing) that caused it to be established in early experiments as the best of the cheap complex nitrogen sources and led to the use of PAA. Not only does PAA stimulate benzylpenicillin biosynthesis but it also suppresses the formation of other (unwanted) penicillins. High levels of PAA are, however, toxic and PAA is also expensive. The feed is controlled to supply an adequate standing level of PAA without approaching the toxic limit; the feed is reduced just before the end of the process so that the amount of unused (irrecoverable) precursor in the final culture is not excessive.

3.4.4 Termination

When to stop a fermentation is a very complex decision and several factors have to be taken into account. Quite often a manufacturer will find it appropriate to harvest shortly after the first signs of a faltering in the efficiency of conversion of the most costly raw material into antibiotic.

3.5 Extraction

3.5.1 Removal of cells

At harvest, the benzylpenicillin is in solution extracellularly, together with a range of other metabolites and medium constituents. The first step in downstream processing is to separate the cells from the liquid broth by techniques such as filtration, ultrafiltration or centrifugation. This stage is carried out under conditions that avoid contamination with β-lactamase-producing microorganisms which could lead to serious or total loss of product.

3.5.2 Isolation of benzylpenicillin

The next stage is to isolate the benzylpenicillin. Solvent extraction is the generally accepted process although other methods are available, including ion-exchange chromatography and precipitation. In aqueous solution at pH 2–2.5, there is a high partition coefficient in favour of certain organic solvents such as amyl acetate, butyl acetate and methyl isobutyl ketone. The extraction has to be carried out quickly, as benzylpenicillin is very unstable at these low pH values. The penicillin is then extracted back into an aqueous buffer at pH 7.5, the partition coefficient now being strongly in favour of the aqueous phase. The solvent is recovered by distillation for re-use. The benzylpenicillin is then crystallized, blended and dried. The downstream processing stages are designed not only to recover the antibiotic but also to ensure that it is of the appropriated potency and purity and that this is achieved by cost-effective processes.

3.5.3 Further processing

Benzylpenicillin is produced as various salts according to its intended use, whether as an input to semisynthetic β-lactam antibiotics manufacture or for clinical use in its own right. The treatment of the crude penicillin extract varies according to the objective but involves formation of an appropriate salt, usually followed by treatment to remove pyrogens, and by sterilization. This last is usually achieved by filtration but pure metal salts of benzylpenicillin can be safely sterilized by dry heat if desired.

For parenteral use, the antibiotic is packed in sterile vials as a freeze-dried power (reconstituted before use) or suspension. For oral use it is prepared in any of the standard presentations, such as film-coated tablets. Searching tests are carried out on a significant number of random samples of the finished product to ensure that it satisfies the stringent quality control requirements for potency, purity, freedom from pyrogens and sterility.

4 The production of penicillin V

By the addition of different acyl donors to the medium, different penicillins can be biologically synthesized. For example, penicillin V is made by a similar process to benzylpenicillin, but with phenoxyacetic acid as the precursor instead of PAA. In the biosynthetic pathway, the α-aminoadipyl side-chain of isopenicillin N is replaced by a phenoxyacetyl group.

The microorganism is again *P. chrysogenum*. A manufacturer may use the same mutant strain to make both products or may have different mutants for the two penicillins. Parallel situations of a single organism producing more than one natural product occur with other types of antibiotics; for example strains of *Streptomyces aureofaciens* are used for both chlortetracycline and demethylchlortetracycline fermentations.

Like benzylpenicillin, penicillin V is still used in its own right, but can also be used as a starting material for the manufacture of semisynthetic penicillins which cannot be made by direct fermentation.

5 The production of cephalosporin C

It is possible to convert penicillin V or benzylpenicillin to a cephalosporin by chemical ring expansion. The first-generation cephalosporin cephalexin, for example, can be made in this way. Most cephalosporins used in clinical practice, however, are semi-synthetics produced from the fermentation product cephalosporin C.

The ancestral strain of *Acremonium chrysogenum* (at that time called *Cephalosporium acremonium*) was isolated on the Sardinian coast in 1945 following an observation that the local sewage outlet into the sea cleared at a quite remarkable rate. Developments were slow because the activity was associated with a number of different types of compound. Cephalosporin C was first isolated in 1952, but it was a further decade before clinically useful semi-synthetic cephalosporins became available.

The biosynthetic route to cephalosporin C is identical to that of the penicillins as far as isopenicillin N. The further route to cephalosporin C is shown below. Note the branch into a third series of β-lactam drugs, the cephamycins (see Chapter 10).

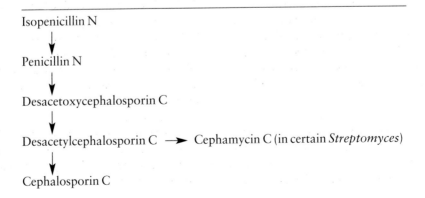

Isopenicillin N
↓
Penicillin N
↓
Desacetoxycephalosporin C
↓
Desacetylcephalosporin C ⟶ Cephamycin C (in certain *Streptomyces*)
↓
Cephalosporin C

The similarities in the routes to the three classes of antibiotics have facilitated progress in the understanding of the underlying molecular genetics. Most of the genes coding for the relevant enzymes have been isolated. Modern DNA techniques are being targeted at rate-limiting biosynthetic steps. Amplification of gene copy numbers, improving gene expression efficiencies, transferring genes to bacterial host organisms and manipulation of pathways of antibiotic synthesis all have potential in strain development. However, in the production of antibiotics, economic benefits from the application of recombinant DNA technology have thus far been limited.

Manufacturing processes for cephalosporin C and benzylpenicillin are broadly similar. In common with many other antibiotic fermentations, no specific precursor feed is necessary for cephalosporin C. There is sufficient acetyl group substrate available from the organism's metabolic pool for the terminal acetyltransferase reaction.

The product is extracted from the culture fluid by adsorption onto carbon or resins rather than by solvent. This illustrates an important general point that antibiotic manufacturing processes differ from one another much more in their product recovery stages than in their fermentation stages. Figure 22.4 illustrates a typical production route for inoculum to bulk antibiotic.

6 Good manufacturing practice (GMP)

All stages of antibiotic manufacture from fermentation through to finished product are governed by the code of good manufacturing practice (GMP), of which quality control is one aspect. GMP requires that 'there should be a comprehensive system, so designed, documented, implemented and controlled, and so furnished with personnel, equipment and other resources as to provide assurance that products will consistently be of a quality appropriate to their intended use'.

Quality control is concerned with testing the quality of the product by a combination of in-process and final product testing. However, that a product meets specification does not necessarily mean that it is suitable for use. GMP is about ensuring that quality is built in to all stages of the manufacturing process. Basic GMP requirements outlined in the Medicines Control Agency Rules and Guidance (the "Orange Guide") are as follows:

1 All manufacturing processes should be clearly defined and be capable of consistently producing material of the required quality and complying with specification.

2 Critical steps of manufacturing processes and significant changes to processes should be validated.

3 All necessary facilities for GMP should be provided including:

(a) appropriately qualified and trained personnel;
(b) adequate premises and space;
(c) suitable equipment and services;
(d) correct materials, containers and labels;
(e) approved procedures and instructions; and
(f) suitable storage and transport.

4 Instructions and procedures are written in an instructional form in clear and unambiguous language, specifically applicable to the facilities provided.

5 Operators are trained to carry out procedures correctly.

6 Records are to be made during manufacture which demonstrate that all the steps required by the defined procedures have been taken and that the quantity and quality of the product was as expected. Any significant deviations are to be fully recorded and investigated.

7 Records of manufacture and distribution, which enable the complete history of a batch to be traced, are retained in a comprehensible and accessible form.

8 The distribution (wholesaling) of the products minimizes any risk to quality.

9 A system is available to recall any batch of product, from sale or supply.

10 All complaints are examined, the cause of quality defects investigated and appropriate measures taken in respect of the defective products and to prevent recurrence.

Failure to comply with current GMP may result in a number of sanctions from the regulatory authorities, up to and including recall of product from the marketplace and withdrawal of manufacturing

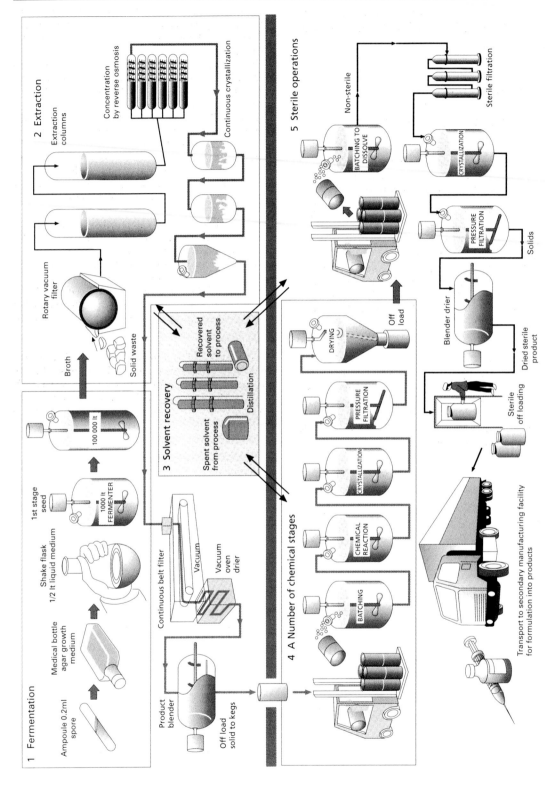

Fig. 22.4 Typical production route for cephalosporins.

1 Fermentation

Ampoule 0.2ml spore

Medical bottle agar growth medium

Shake flask 1/2 lt liquid medium

1st stage seed

1000 lt FERMENTER

100 000 lt

2 Extraction

Extraction columns

Concentration by reverse osmosis

Continuous crystallization

Rotary vacuum filter

Broth

Solid waste

3 Solvent recovery

Recovered solvent to process

Spent solvent from process

Distillation

Continuous belt filter

Vacuum

Vacuum oven drier

Product blender

Off load solid to kegs

4 A Number of chemical stages

BATCHING

CHEMICAL REACTION

CRYSTALLIZATION

PRESSURE FILTRATION

DRYING

Off load

5 Sterile operations

Non-sterile

BATCHING TO DISSOLVE

Sterile filtration

CRYSTALLIZATION

PRESSURE FILTRATION

Solids

Blender drier

Dried sterile product

Sterile off loading

Transport to secondary manufacturing facility for formulation into products and marketing licences. Thus appropriate standards for the manufacture of antibiotics are monitored and maintained.

7 Further reading

Bu'Lock, J. D., Nisbet, L. J. & Winstanley, D. J. (eds) (1983) *Bioactive Microbial Products*, Vol. II, *Development and Production*. Academic Press, London.

Calam, C. T. (1987) *Process Development in Antibiotic Fermentations*, Cambridge Studies in Biotechnology, 4 (eds Sir James Baddiley, N. H. Carery, J. F. Davidson, I. J. Higgins & W. G. Potter). Cambridge University Press, Cambridge.

Finch, R. G. (1996) Antibacterial chemotherapy: principles of use. *Medicine*, **24**, 24–26.

Greenwood, D. (1995) *Antimicrobial Chemotherapy*, 3rd edn. Oxford University Press, Oxford.

Hugo, W. B. & Mol, H. (1972) Antibiotics and chemotherapeutic agents. In: *Materials and Technology* (eds L. W. Codd, K. Dijkoff, J. H. Fearon, C. J. vanOss, H. G. Roeberson & E. G. Stanford). Longman & de Bussy, London.

Lambert, H. P., O'Grady, F., Greenwood, D. & Finch, R. G. (1996) *Antibiotic and Chemotherapy*, 7th edn. Churchill Livingstone, Edinburgh.

Mandell, G. L., Douglas, R. G. & Bennett, J. E. (eds) (1995) *Principles and Practice of Infectious Diseases*, 4th edn. John Wiley, New York.

Medicines Control Agency (2002) *Rules and Guidance for Pharmaceutical Manufacturers and Distributors*. Her Majesty's Stationery Office, London.

Peberdy, J. F. (ed.) (1987) *Penicillin and Acremonium*, Biotechnology Handbooks, 1 (series eds T. Atkinson & R. F. Sherwood). Plenum Press, New York. (See, in particular, Chapters 2 and 5.)

Office for Official Publications of the European Community (2002) *The Rules Governing Medicinal Products in the European Community*, Vol. IV, *Guide to Good Manufacturing Practice for the Manufacture of Medicinal Products*.

Queener, S. W. (1990) Molecular biology of penicillin and cephalosporin biosynthesis. *Antimicrobial Agents and Chemotherapy*, **34**, 943–948.

Rohm, H. J., Reed, G., Puhler, A. & Stadler, P. (eds) (1993) *Biotechnology*, Vol. III, *Bioprocessing*. VCH, New York.

Smith, J. E. (1985) *Biotechnology Principles*. Aspects of Microbiology Series No 11. Van Nostrand Reinhold, Workinham.

Stowell, J. D., Bailey, P. J. & Winstanley, D. J. (eds) (1986) *Bioactive Microbial Products*, Vol. III, *Downstream Processing*. Academic Press, London.

Van Damme, E. J. (1984) *Biotechnology of Industrial Antibiotics*. Marcel Dekker, New York.

Verrall, M. S. (ed.) (1985) *Discovery and Isolation of Microbial Products*. Society of Chemical Industry Series in Biological Chemistry and Biotechnology. Ellis Horwood, Chichester.

A good source of articles on individual antibiotics, groups of antibiotics, fermentation plant and related topics is the series *Progress in Industrial Microbiology* edited originally by D. J. D. Hockenhull and published by Heywood Books, London. These articles normally carry extensive references to the original literature.

Chapter 23
The manufacture and quality control of immunological products

Michael Corbel

1 Introduction

Immunological products comprise a group of pharmaceutical preparations with diverse origins but with a common pharmacological purpose: the modification of the immune status of the recipient, either to provide immunity to infectious disease, or in the case of *in vivo* diagnostics, to provoke an indication of immune status. The immunological products that are currently available are of the following types: vaccines; *in vivo* diagnostics; immune sera; human immunoglobulins; monoclonal antibodies; and antibody targeted therapeutics and diagnostics.

Vaccines are by far the most important immunological products. They have enabled the control or eradication of numerous infectious diseases affecting humans and their domesticated animals. For example, the systematic application of smallpox vaccine, deployed under the aegis of the World Health Organization, achieved the eradication of one of the most devastating infections. Diphtheria, tetanus, whooping cough, poliomyelitis, measles and rubella vaccines have been applied worldwide through national or UNICEF-sponsored health-care programmes and have virtually eliminated these diseases in those countries in which there have been the resources and the will to deploy them effectively. Vaccines that provide protection against many other infections are available for use in appropriate circumstances. Some, such as hepatitis B, *Haemophilus influenzae* b (Hib) and new conjugate vaccines against meningococci and pneumococci, have received fairly limited application but have the potential to make a huge impact on morbidity and mortality throughout the world.

The range of disorders that may be prevented or treated by vaccines has enlarged considerably beyond infectious diseases. Vaccines are undergoing evaluation for several other purposes including: therapy of cancer; prevention of allergies; desensitization of allergic patients; fertility control; and treatment of addictions.

In vivo diagnostics such as tuberculins, mallein, histoplasmin, coccidioidin and brucellin, are used to demonstrate an immune response, and hence previous exposure, to specific pathogens as an aid to diagnosis. Others, such as the Schick test (diphtheria) toxin are used to detect the presence of protective immunity. Because of their limitations, the trend has been to phase out these preparations, and tuberculins (as purified protein derivative, PPD) are now by far the most important of this group.

Immune sera, which were once very widely used in the prophylaxis and treatment of many infections, have more limited use today. Vaccines and antibiotics have superseded some and lack of proven therapeutic benefit has caused others to be relegated to immunological history. However, some still play an important role in the management of specific conditions. Thus, diphtheria and botulinum antitoxins prepared in horses remain the only specific treatments for diphtheria and botulism respectively. Equine tetanus antitoxin is still used as an effective prophylactic in some parts of the world, although largely replaced by human tetanus immunoglobulin in developed countries. Similarly, antivenins prepared in horses, sheep, goats or other animals against the venoms of snakes, spiders, scorpions and marine invertebrates still provide the only effective treatment for venomous bites and stings and are important therapeutic agents in some parts of the world.

Human immunoglobulins have important but limited uses, for example in the prophylaxis of hepatitis A, hepatitis B, tetanus and varicella zoster. Additional specific immunoglobulins against diphtheria and botulism toxins are under development and vaccinia immunoglobulin may be reintroduced. Monoclonal antibodies to bacterial endotoxin, to cytokines involved in the pathogenesis of septic shock and to specific infectious agents have been developed and evaluated clinically but have yet to enter into general use. Immune sera and human immunoglobulins depend for their protective effects on their content of antibodies derived, in the case of immune sera, from immunized animals and, in the case of immunoglobulins, from humans who have been immunized or who have high antibody titres as a consequence of prior infection. The form of immunity conferred is known as passive immunity and is achieved immediately but is limited in its duration to the time that protective levels of antibodies remain in the circulation (see also Chapter 9).

Vaccines achieve their protective effects by stimulating the immune system of the recipient to produce T cells or antibodies that impede the attachment of infectious agents, promote their destruction or neutralize their toxins. This form of protection, known as active immunity, develops in the course of days and in the case of many vaccines develops adequately only after two or three doses of vaccine have been given at intervals of days or weeks. Once established, this immunity can last for years but it may need to be reinforced by 'booster' doses of vaccine given at relatively long intervals. The immunogenicity of some vaccines can be improved by formulating them with adjuvants. The latter are a heterogeneous collection of substances which enhance the immune response. Aluminium hydroxide gel (hydrated aluminium oxide) and aluminium phosphate are the only ones in general use in human vaccines. A much wider range of substances including oily emulsions, saponin, immune-stimulating complexes (ISCOMS), monophosphoryl lipid A and others are used in veterinary vaccines and some are under investigation for use in human vaccines.

Different types of infectious agent require preferential mobilization of different arms of the immune response. For example, toxigenic bacterial infections require the production of toxin neutralizing antibodies, intracellular bacterial infections such as tuberculosis require cell-mediated responses involving cytotoxic T lymphocytes and activated macrophages, whereas many viral infections will require neutralizing antibody and cytotoxic T-cell responses for effective protection. Achieving the appropriate response can be difficult and in the past has had to be approached empirically. This is why most successful viral vaccines have been based on live attenuated strains, which simulate natural infection. Non-living vaccines have been effective against many bacterial infections but markedly less so against those requiring cell-mediated responses. The development of more selective vaccine adjuvants and delivery systems promises to put the future process of vaccine design on a more rational basis.

A property common to vaccines, immune sera and human immunoglobulins is their high specificity of action. Each provides immunity to only one infection. Where it is necessary to protect against more than one type of agent, monospecific preparations can be combined. For example, botulism antitoxin usually covers types A, B and E; meningococcal polysaccharide vaccine may cover groups A, C, W_{125} and Y; pneumococcal polysaccharide vaccine usually covers 23 serotypes. Heterologous preparations may also be combined as in measles/mumps/rubella and diphtheria/tetanus/pertussis vaccines. With the increasing number of vaccines for infants and young children, the trend is to produce more complex combinations such as diphtheria/tetanus/pertussis/hepatitis B/inactivated polio/Hib vaccine, to minimize the number of injections. The possible additive or interactive effects of the various components on the immune system have raised concerns about the safety of such combinations. While some evidence of reduced responses to certain components has been obtained, there is little to support suggestions of serious adverse effects from current combinations.

In addition to the three main types of immunological products that are widely available, more specialized preparations include: synthetic peptide immune response modifiers such as those used to block T-cell responses in multiple sclerosis; labelled monoclonal antibodies for cancer therapy or diagnosis; and hybrid toxins containing a bacterial or plant toxin subunit attached to an antibody or human cell receptor-binding protein, and also intended mainly for cancer therapy. These have rather limited applications and for the most part, are designed to suppress or exploit the specificity of immune responses rather than to stimulate them.

Principles of immunity are discussed in Chapter 8, whereas Chapter 9 describes a vaccination and immunization programme.

2 Vaccines

The vaccines currently used for the prevention of in-

fectious diseases of humans are all derived, directly or indirectly, from pathogenic microorganisms. The basis of vaccine manufacture thus consists of procedures which produce from infectious agents, their components or their products, immunogenic preparations that are devoid of pathogenic properties but which, nonetheless, can still induce a protective response in their recipients. The methods that are used in vaccine manufacture are constrained by technical limitations, costs, problems of delivery to the recipient/patient, by regulatory issues and, most of all, by the biological properties of the pathogens from which vaccines are derived. Those vaccines currently in use in conventional immunization programmes are of several readily distinguishable types.

Live vaccines. These are preparations of live bacteria, viruses or other agents which, when administered by an appropriate route, cause subclinical or mild infections. In the course of such an infection the components of the microorganisms in the vaccine evoke an immune response which provides protection against the more serious natural disease. Live vaccines have a long history, dating from the development of smallpox vaccine. Initially, material from mild cases of smallpox was used for inoculation. This process of 'variolation' was hazardous and could produce fatalities and secondary smallpox cases. A much safer alternative was introduced in 1796 by the Gloucestershire physician, Edward Jenner, following observations made by Benjamin Jesty, a local farmer, that an attack of the mild condition known as 'cowpox' protected milkmaids from smallpox during epidemics of this dreaded disease. For many years the cowpox vaccine was propagated by serial transfer from person to person and at some point evolved into a distinctive virus, vaccinia, with some features of both cowpox and smallpox viruses. Vaccinia was eventually used to eradicate smallpox. Its significance was that it could stimulate a high degree of immunity to smallpox while producing only a localized infection in the recipient.

The natural occurrence of cross-protective organisms of low pathogenicity seems to be a rare event and attenuated strains have usually had to be selected by laboratory manipulation. Thus the bacille Calmette-Guérin (BCG) strain of *Mycobacterium bovis* used to protect against human tuberculosis caused by the related species *M. tuberculosis*, was produced by many sequential subcultures on ox bile medium. This process resulted in deletion of many genes present in virulent *M. bovis*, including some essential for pathogenicity. Similarly, treatment of a virulent strain of *Salmonella typhi* with nitrosoguanidine, which produced multiple mutations, gave rise to the live attenuated typhoid vaccine strain Ty21a. More recently developed attenuated strains of *S. typhi* and *Vibrio cholerae* have been selected by directed mutagenesis processes which can produce defined mutations in specific genes.

Perhaps surprisingly, all of the most successful attenuated viral vaccine strains in current use were produced by empirical methods long before the genetic basis of pathogenesis by the specific pathogen was understood. Thus, attenuated strains of polio virus for use as a live, oral vaccine (Sabin) were selected by growth of viruses isolated from human cases under cultural conditions that did not permit replication of neuropathogenic virus. Comparable procedures were used to select the attenuated virus strains that are currently used in live measles, mumps, rubella and yellow fever vaccines.

Now, attenuated strains of pathogens can be selected by deliberate selective modification of genes responsible for encoding factors determining pathogenesis, such as toxins or immunomodulators, or metabolites essential for *in vivo* growth. Live vaccine strains can also be genetically modified by incorporating genes that encode protective antigens for other infectious agents. Several of these are under evaluation at present although none is yet in general use.

Killed vaccines. Killed vaccines are suspensions of bacteria, viruses or other pathogenic agents, that have been killed by heat or by disinfectants such as phenol, ethanol or formaldehyde. Killed microorganisms obviously cannot replicate and cause an infection and so it is necessary for each dose of a killed vaccine to contain sufficient antigenic material to stimulate a protective immune response. Killed vaccines therefore usually have to be relatively concentrated suspensions. Even so, such preparations are often rather poorly protective, possibly because of partial destruction of protective antigens during the killing process or inadequate expression

of these during *in vitro* culture. At the same time, because they contain all components of the microorganism they can be somewhat toxic. It is thus often necessary to divide the total amount of vaccine that is needed to induce protection into several doses that are given at intervals of a few days or weeks. Such a course of vaccination takes advantage of the enhanced 'secondary' response that occurs when a vaccine is administered to an individual person whose immune system has been sensitized by a previous dose of the same vaccine. The best known killed vaccines are whooping cough (pertussis), typhoid, cholera, plague, inactivated polio vaccine (Salk type) and rabies vaccine. The trend now is for these rather crude preparations to be phased out and replaced by better-defined subunit vaccines containing only relevant protective antigens, e.g. acellular pertussis and typhoid Vi polysaccharide vaccines.

Toxoid vaccines. Toxoid vaccines are preparations derived from the toxins that are secreted by certain species of bacteria. In the manufacture of such vaccines, the toxin is separated from the bacteria and treated chemically to eliminate toxicity without eliminating immunogenicity, a process termed 'toxoiding'.

A variety of reagents have been used for toxoiding, but by far the most widely employed and generally successful has been formaldehyde.

The treated toxins are sometimes referred to as formol toxoids. Toxoid vaccines are very effective in the prevention of those diseases such as diphtheria, tetanus, botulism and clostridial infections of farm animals, in which the infecting bacteria produce disease through the toxic effects of secreted proteins which enzymically modify essential cellular components. Many of the clostridial toxins are lytic enzymes. Detoxification is also required for the pertussis toxin component of acellular pertussis vaccines.

Anthrax adsorbed vaccine is not toxoided but relies on the use of cultural conditions that favour production of the protective antigen (binding and internalization factor) rather than the lethal factor (protease) and oedema factor (adenyl cyclase) components of the toxin. Selective adsorption to aluminium hydroxide or phosphate also slows release of residual toxin.

Bacterial cell component vaccines. Rather than

use whole cells, which may contain undesirable and potentially reactogenic components such as lipopolysaccharide endotoxins, a more precise strategy is to prepare vaccines from purified protective components. These are of two main types, proteins and capsular polysaccharides. Often more than one component may be needed to ensure protection against the full range of prevalent serotypes. The potential advantage of such vaccines is that they evoke an immune response only to the component, or components, in the vaccine and thus induce a response that is more specific and effective. At the same time, the amount of unnecessary material in the vaccine is reduced and with it the likelihood of adverse reaction. Vaccines that have been based on one or more capsular polysaccharides include: *Haemophilus influenzae* type b vaccine; the *Neisseria meningitidis* ACWY vaccines; the 23-valent pneumococcal polysaccharide vaccine; and the typhoid Vi vaccine. These have the disadvantage that they are T-cell-independent antigens and thus do not evoke immunological memory, or effective protective responses in the very young. This problem can be overcome by chemically coupling the polysaccharides to T-cell-dependent protein carriers.

The pertussis vaccine is another example where, traditionally, whole bacterial cells have been used, but recent developments have led to an acellular pertussis vaccine that may contain detoxified toxin, either alone or combined with several other bacterial antigens.

Conjugate vaccines. The performance of certain types of antigen that give weak or inappropriate immune responses can often be improved by chemically conjugating them to more immunogenic carriers. Among others, polysaccharide–protein, peptide–protein, protein–protein, lipid–protein and alkaloid–protein conjugate vaccines may be prepared in this way. These have a wide range of applications, including prevention of infection, tumour therapy, fertility control and treatment of addictions. This approach has been very successful against infections caused by bacteria that produce polysaccharide capsules. The latter are T-independent antigens and induce weak responses without immunological memory. They are particularly ineffective in the very young.

Viral subunit vaccines. Three viral subunit vaccines are widely available, two influenza vaccines and a hepatitis B vaccine. The influenza vaccines are prepared by treating intact influenza virus particles from embryonated hens' eggs infected with influenza virus with a surface-active agent such as a non-ionic detergent. This disrupts the virus particles, releasing the virus subunits. The two that are required in the vaccine, haemagglutinin and neuraminidase, can be recovered and concentrated by centrifugation methods. The hepatitis B vaccine was, at one time, prepared from hepatitis B surface antigen (HbsAg) obtained from the blood of carriers of hepatitis B virus. This very constrained source of antigen has been replaced by production in yeast or mammalian cells that have been genetically engineered to express HbsAg during fermentation.

For further information see Ada (1994), Ellis (1999), Mizrahi (1990), Pastoret *et al.* (1997), Perlmann & Wigzell (1999), Plotkin & Mortimer (2003) and Powell & Newman (1995) (Further reading section).

2.1 The seed lot system

The starting point for the production of all microbial vaccines is the isolation of the appropriate infectious agent. Such isolates have usually been derived from human infections and in some cases have yielded strains suitable for vaccine production very readily; in other instances a great deal of manipulation and selection in the laboratory have been needed before a suitable strain has been obtained. For example, bacterial strains may need to be selected for high toxin yield or production of abundant capsular polysaccharide; viral strains may need to be selected for stable attenuation.

Once a suitable strain is available, the practice is to grow, often from a single viable unit, a substantial culture which is distributed in small amounts in a large number of ampoules and then stored at −70°C or below, or freeze-dried. This is the original seed lot. From this seed lot, one or more ampoules are used to generate the working seed from which a limited number of batches of vaccine are generated. These are first examined exhaustively in the laboratory and then, if found to be satisfactory, tested for safety and efficacy in clinical trials. Satisfactory results in the clinical trials validate the seed lot as the material from which batches of vaccine for routine use can subsequently be produced.

It is important that the full history of the seed is known, including the nature of the culture media used to propagate the strain since isolation. If at all possible, media prepared from animal products should be avoided. If this is not practicable, media components must be from sources certified free of transmissible spongiform encephalopathy (TSE) agents.

2.2 Production of the bacteria and the cellular components of bacterial vaccines

The bacteria and cellular components needed for the manufacture of most bacterial vaccines are prepared in laboratory media by well-established fermentation methods. The end-product of the fermentation, the harvest, is processed to provide a concentrated and purified bulk lot of vaccine component that may be conveniently stored for long periods or even sold to other manufacturers prior to further processing. It is important that the materials, equipment, facilities and working practices are of a standard acceptable for the manufacture of pharmaceutical products. The requirements for this are defined as Good Manufacturing Practice (GMP). Guidelines on the basic requirements have been published by the World Health Organization (Anon, 1999a,b).

2.3 Fermentation

The production of a bacterial vaccine batch begins with the resuscitation of the bacterial seed contained in an ampoule of the seed lot stored at −70°C or below, or freeze-dried. The resuscitated bacteria are first cultivated through one or more passages in pre-production media. Then, when the bacteria have multiplied sufficiently, they are used to inoculate a batch of production medium. Again, all media used must be from sources certified free of TSEs. Wherever possible, medium components of animal origin, especially human and ruminant, should be avoided.

The production medium is usually contained in a large fermenter, the contents of which are continuously stirred. Usually the pH and the oxidation-reduction potential of the medium are monitored and adjusted throughout the growth period in a manner intended to produce the greatest bacterial yield (see also Chapter 22 for details of fermenter design and operation). In the case of rapidly growing bacteria the maximum yield is obtained after about a day but in the case of bacteria that grow slowly the maximum yield may not be reached before 2 weeks. At the end of the growth period the contents of the fermenter, which are known as the harvest, are ready for the next stage in the production of the vaccine

2.3.1 Processing of bacterial harvests

The harvest is a very complex mixture of bacterial cells, metabolic products and exhausted medium. In the case of a live attenuated vaccine it should be innocuous, and all that is necessary is for the bacteria to be separated and resuspended under aseptic conditions in an appropriate diluent, possibly for freeze-drying. In a vaccine made from a virulent strain of pathogen the harvest may be intensely dangerous and great care is necessary in the subsequent processing. Adequate containment will be required and for class 3 pathogens such as *Salmonella typhi* or *Yersinia pestis* or bulk production of bacterial toxins, dedicated facilities that will provide complete protection for the operators and the environment are essential.

• *Killing.* The process by which the live bacteria in the culture are rendered non-viable and harmless. Heat and disinfectants are usually employed. Heat and/or formalin or thiomersal are used to kill the cells of *Bordetella pertussis* used to make whole cell pertussis vaccines. Phenol was used to kill the *Vibrio cholerae* and the *Sal. typhi* cells used in the now obsolete whole cell cholera and typhoid vaccines.

• *Separation.* The process by which the bacterial cells are separated from the culture fluid and soluble products. Centrifugation using either a batch or continuous flow process, or ultrafiltration, is commonly used. Precipitation of the cells by reducing the pH has been used as an alternative. In the case of vaccines prepared from cells, the supernatant fluid is discarded and the cells are resuspended in a saline diluent; where vaccines are made from a constituent of the fluid, the cells are discarded.

- *Fractionation.* This is the process by which components are extracted from bacterial cells or from the medium in which the bacteria are grown and obtained in a purified form. The polysaccharide antigens of *Neisseria meningitidis* are usually separated from the bacterial cells by treatment with hexadecyltrimethylammonium bromide followed by extraction with calcium chloride and selective precipitation with ethanol. Those of *Streptococcus pneumoniae* are usually extracted with sodium deoxycholate, deproteinized and then fractionally precipitated with ethanol. The purity of an extracted material may be improved by resolubilization in a suitable solvent and re-precipitation. These procedures are often supplemented with filtration through membranes or ultrafilters with specific molecular size cut-off points. After purification, a component may be freeze-dried, stored indefinitely at low temperature and, as required, incorporated into a vaccine in precisely weighed amount at the blending stage.
- *Detoxification.* The process by which bacterial toxins are converted to harmless toxoids. Formaldehyde is used to detoxify the toxins of *Corynebacterium diphtheriae*, *Clostridium botulinum* and *Cl. tetani*. The detoxification may be performed either on the whole culture in the fermenter or on the purified toxin after fractionation. Traditionally the former approach has been adopted, as it is much safer for the operator. However, the latter gives a purer product. The pertussis toxin used in acellular vaccines may be detoxified with formaldehyde, glutaraldehyde, or both, hydrogen peroxide or tetranitromethane. In the case of genetically detoxified pertussis toxin, a treatment with a low concentration of formaldehyde is still performed to stabilize the protein.
- *Further processing.* This may include physical or chemical treatments to modify the product. For example polysaccharides may be further fractionated to produce material of a narrow molecular size specification. They may then be activated and conjugated to carrier proteins to produce glyco-conjugate vaccines. Further purification may then be required to eliminate unwanted reactants and by-products. These processes must be done under conditions that minimize extraneous microbial contamination. If sterility is not achievable then strict bioburden limits are imposed.
- *Adsorption.* The adsorption of the components of a vaccine on to a mineral adjuvant. The mineral adjuvants, or carriers, most often used are aluminium hydroxide and aluminium phosphate; rarely calcium phosphate. Their effect is to increase the immunogenicity and decrease the toxicity, local and systemic, of a vaccine. Diphtheria vaccine, tetanus vaccine, diphtheria/tetanus vaccine and diphtheria/tetanus/pertussis (whole cell or acellular) vaccine, are generally prepared as adsorbed vaccines.
- *Conjugation.* The linking of a vaccine component that induces an inadequate immune response, with a vaccine component that induces a good immune response. For example, the immunogenicity for infants of the capsular polysaccharide of *H. influenzae* type b is greatly enhanced by the conjugation of the polysaccharide with diphtheria or tetanus toxoid, or with the outer-membrane protein of *Neisseria meningitidis*.

2.4 Production of the viruses and the components of viral vaccines

Viruses replicate only in living cells, so the first viral vaccines were necessarily made in animals: smallpox vaccine in the dermis of calves and sheep; and rabies vaccines in the spinal cords of rabbits and brains of mice. Such methods are no longer used in advanced vaccine production; the only intact animal hosts that are still used are embryonated hens' eggs. Almost all the virus that is needed for viral vaccine production is obtained from cell cultures infected with virus of the appropriate strain.

2.4.1 Growth of viruses

Embryonated hens' eggs are still the most convenient hosts for growth of the viruses that are needed for influenza and yellow fever vaccines. Influenza viruses accumulate in high titre in the allantoic fluid of the eggs and yellow fever virus accumulates in the nervous system of the embryos. It is important to use eggs from disease-free flocks and emphasis is placed on screening the latter for various avian viruses. The allantoic fluid or embryos must be harvested under conditions that minimize extraneous microbial contamination.

Where cell cultures are used for virus production, they must be of known origin, obtained from validated sources and shown to be free of extraneous agents. The media used in their production should not contain components of human or animal origin, unless the latter are from TSE-free sources.

2.4.2 *Processing of viral harvests*

The processing of the virus-containing material from infected embryonated eggs may take one or other of several forms. In the case of influenza vaccines the allantoic fluid is centrifuged to provide a concentrated and partially purified suspension of virus. This concentrate is treated with organic solvent or detergent to split the virus into its components when split virion or surface antigen vaccines are prepared. The chick embryos used in the production of yellow fever vaccine are homogenized in sterile water to provide a virus-containing pulp. Centrifugation then precipitates most of the embryonic debris and leaves much of the yellow fever virus in an aqueous suspension.

Cell cultures provide infected fluids that contain little debris and can generally be satisfactorily clarified by filtration. Because most viral vaccines made from cell cultures consist of live attenuated virus, there is no inactivation stage in their manufacture. There are, however, two important exceptions: inactivated poliomyelitis virus vaccine is inactivated with dilute formaldehyde or β-propiolactone and rabies vaccine is inactivated with β-propiolactone. The preparation of these inactivated vaccines also involves a concentration stage — by adsorption and elution of the virus in the case of poliomyelitis vaccine and by ultrafiltration in the case of rabies vaccine. When processing is complete the bulk materials may be stored until needed for blending into final vaccine. Because of the lability of many viruses, however, it is necessary to store most purified materials at temperatures of −70°C.

2.5 Blending

Blending is the process in which the various components of a vaccine are mixed to form a final bulk. It is undertaken in a large, closed vessel fitted with a stirrer and ports for the addition of constituents and withdrawal of the final blend. When bacterial vaccines are blended, the active constituents usually need to be greatly diluted and the vessel is first charged with the diluents, usually containing a preservative. Thiomersal has been widely used in the past but is now being phased out and replaced by phenoxy ethanol or alternatives. A single-component final bulk is made by adding bacterial suspension, bacterial component or concentrated toxoid in such quantity that it is at the required concentration in the final product. A multiple-component final bulk of a combined vaccine is made by adding each required component in sequence. When viral vaccines are blended, the need to maintain adequate antigenicity or infectivity may preclude dilution, and tissue culture fluids, or concentrates made from them, are often used undiluted or, in the case of multi-component vaccines, merely diluted one with another. After thorough mixing, a final bulk may be divided into a number of moderate sized volumes to facilitate handling.

2.6 Filling and drying

As vaccine is required to meet orders, bulk vaccine is distributed into single-dose ampoules or into multi-dose vials as necessary. Vaccines that are filled as liquids are sealed and capped in their containers, whereas vaccines that are provided as dried preparations are freeze-dried before sealing.

The single-component bacterial vaccines are listed in Table 23.1. For each vaccine, notes are provided of the basic material from which the vaccine is made, the salient production processes and tests for potency and for safety. The multi-component vaccines that are made by blending together two or more of the single-component vaccines are required to meet the potency and safety requirements for each of the single components that they contain. The best known of the combined bacterial vaccines is the adsorbed diphtheria, tetanus and pertussis vaccine (DTPer/Vac/Ads) that is used to immunize infants, and the adsorbed diphtheria and tetanus vaccine (DT/Vac/Ads) that is used to reinforce the immunity of school entrants. The trend is to

Table 23.1 Bacterial vaccines used for the prevention of infectious disease in humans

Vaccine	Source material	Processing	Potency assay	Safety tests
Anthrax*	Medium from cultures of *B. anthracis*	**1** Separation of protective antigen from medium **2** Adsorption	3 + 3 quantal assay in guinea-pigs using challenge with *B. anthracis*	Exclusion of live *B. anthracis* and of anthrax toxin
BCG*	Cultures of live BCG cells in liquid or on solid media	**1** Bacteria centrifuged from medium **2** Resuspension in stabilizer **3** Freeze-drying	Viable count; induction of sensitivity to tuberculin in guinea-pigs	Exclusion of virulent mycobacteria; excessive dermal reactivity
Diphtheria (adsorbed)*	Cultures of *C. diphtheriae* in liquid medium	**1** Separation and concentration of toxin **2** Conversion of toxin to toxoid **3** Adsorption of toxoid to adjuvant	3 + 3 quantal assay in guinea-pigs using intradermal challenge with diphtheria toxin	Inoculation of guinea-pigs to exclude untoxoided toxin
Haemophilus influenzae type b*	Cultures of *H. influenzae* type b	**1** Separation of capsular polysaccharide **2** Conjugation with a protein	Estimation of capsular polysaccharide content and molecular size	Absence of unreacted intermediates. Endotoxin assay
Neisseria meningitidis types A and C†	Cultures of *N. meningitidis* of serotypes A and C	**1** Precipitation with hexadecyl-trimethyammonium bromide **2** Solubilization and purification **3** Blending **4** Freeze-drying	Estimation of capsular polysaccharide content and molecular size	
Pneumococcal polysaccharide	Cultures of 23 serotypes of *Strep. pneumoniae*	**1** Precipitation of extracted polysaccharides with ethanol **2** Blending into polyvalent vaccine	Physico-chemical estimation of polysaccharides	
Tetanus (adsorbed)*	Cultures of *Cl. tetani* in liquid medium	**1** Conversion of toxin to toxoid **2** Separation and purification of toxoid **3** Adsorption to adjuvant	3 + 3 quantal assay in mice using subcutaneous challenge with tetanus toxin	Inoculation of guinea-pigs to exclude presence of untoxoided toxin
Typhoid† whole cell	Cultures of *Sal. typhi* grown in liquid media	**1** Killing with heat or phenol **2** Separation and resuspension of bacteria in saline	Induction of antibodies in rabbits	Exclusion of live *Sal. typhi*
Typhoid Vi capsular polysaccharide antigen	Cultures of *Sal. typhi* grown in liquid medium	Extraction of capsular antigen	Estimation of capsular antigen and molecular size	Endotoxin assay

Table 23.1 *Continued*

Vaccine	Source material	Processing	Potency assay	Safety tests
Typhoid live vaccine†	Cultures of *Sal. typhi* Strain Ty21A	Encapsulation	Estimation of content of live bacteria	Absence of live enteric pathogens
Whooping cough (pertussis) whole cell*	Cultures of *Bord. pertussis* grown in liquid or on solid media	**1** Harvest **2** Killing with formalin **3** Resuspension	3 + 3 quantal assay in mice using intracerebral challenge with live *Bord. pertussis*	Estimation of bacteria to limit content to 20×10^9 per human dose; weight gain test in mice to exclude excess toxicity
Whooping cough (pertussis) (acellular)†	Cultures of *Bord. pertussis*	**1** Harvest **2** Extraction, detoxification and blending of cell components	Immunogenicity assay	Specific toxin and endotoxin assays

* Vaccines used in conventional immunization schedules.

† Vaccines used to provide additional protection when circumstances indicate a need.

Diphtheria and pertussis vaccines are seldom used as single-component vaccines but as components of diphtheria/tetanus vaccines and diphtheria/tetanus/pertussis vaccines. Combined diphtheria/tetanus/pertussis/Hib and diphtheria/tetanus/pertussis/Hep B vaccines with or without inactivated polio vaccine are available.

Bacterial vaccines of restricted availability include anthrax, botulism, plague, Q fever, typhus and tularaemia vaccines.

produce more complex combinations, and hepta- or octavalent preparations are now available.

The single-component viral vaccines are listed in Table 23.2 with notes similar to those provided with the bacterial vaccines. The only combined viral vaccine that is widely used is the measles, mumps and rubella vaccine (MMR Vac). In a sense however, both the inactivated (Salk) poliovaccine (Pol/Vac (inactivated)) and the live (Sabin) polio-vaccine (Pol/Vac (oral) are combined vaccines in that they are both mixtures of virus of each of the three serotypes of poliovirus. Influenza vaccines, too, are combined vaccines in that they usually contain components from several virus strains, usually from two strains of influenza A and one strain of influenza B.

2.7 Quality control

The quality control of vaccines is intended to provide assurances of both the probable efficacy and the safety of every batch of every product. It is executed in three ways:

- in-process control;
- final product control; and
- a requirement that for each product the starting materials, intermediates, final product and processing methods are consistent.

The results of all quality control tests must be recorded in detail and authorized by a Qualified Person as, in those countries in which the manufacture of vaccines is regulated by law, they are part of the evidence on which control authorities judge the acceptability or otherwise of each batch of each preparation.

2.7.1 In-process control

In-process quality control is the control exercised over starting materials and intermediates. Its importance stems from the opportunities that it provides for the examination of a product at the stages in its manufacture at which testing is most likely to provide the most meaningful information. The WHO recommendations and national authorities stipulate many in-process controls but

Table 23.2 Viral vaccines used for the prevention of infectious diseases in humans

Vaccine	Source material	Processing	Potency assay	Safety tests
Hepatitis A†	Human diploid cells infected with hepatitis A virus	**1** Separation of virus from cells **2** Inactivation with formaldehyde **3** Adsorption to $Al(OH)_3$ gel	Assay of antigen content by ELISA	Inoculation of cell cultures to exclude presence of live virus
Hepatitis B†	Yeast cells genetically modified to express surface antigen	**1** Separation of HbsAg from yeast cells **2** Adsorption to $Al(OH)_3$ gel	Immunogenicity assay or HbsAg assay by ELISA	Test for presence of yeast DNA
Influenza (split virion)†	Allantoic fluid from embryonated hens' eggs infected with influenza viruses A and B	**1** Harvest of viruses **2** Disruption with surface active agent or solvent **3** Blending of components of different serotypes	Assay of haemagglutinin content by single radial diffusion	Inoculation of embryonated hens' eggs to exclude live virus
Influenza (surface antigen)†	Allantoic fluid from embryonated hens' eggs infected with influenza viruses A and B	**1** Inactivation and disruption **2** Separation of haemagglutinin and neuraminidase **3** Blending of haemagglutinins and neuraminidase of different serotypes	Assay of haemagglutinin content by single radial diffusion	Inoculation of embryonated hens' eggs to exclude live virus
Measles*	Chick embryo cell cultures infected with attenuated measles virus	**1** Clarification **2** Freeze-drying	Infectivity titration in cell cultures	Tests to exclude presence of extraneous viruses
Mumps*	Chick embryo cell cultures infected with attenuated mumps virus	**1** Clarification **2** Freeze-drying	Infectivity titration in cell cultures	Tests to exclude presence of extraneous viruses
Poliomyelitis (inactivated)	Human diploid cell cultures infected with each of the three serotypes of poliovirus	**1** Clarification **2** Inactivation with formaldehyde **3** Concentration **4** Blending of virus of each serotype	Estimation of D antigen content	Inoculation of cell cultures and monkey spinal cords to exclude live virus
Poliomyelitis (live or oral)* (Sabin type)	Cell cultures infected with attenuated poliovirus of each of the three serotypes	**1** Clarification **2** Blending with beta-propiolactone	Infectivity titration in cell cultures	Neurovirulence test in monkeys
Rubella* (German measles)	Human diploid cell cultures infected with rabies virus	**1** Clarification **2** Blending with stabilizer **3** Freeze-drying	Infectivity titration in cell cultures	Tests to exclude presence of extraneous viruses

Table 23.2 *Continued*

Vaccine	Source material	Processing	Potency assay	Safety tests
Varicella†	Human diploid cell cultures infected with attenuated varicella virus	**1** Clarification **2** Freeze-drying	Infectivity titration in cell cultures	Tests to exclude presence of extraneous viruses
Yellow fever†	Aqueous homogenate of chick embryos infected with attenuated yellow fever virus 17D	**1** Centrifugation to remove cell debris **2** Freeze-drying	Infectivity titration in cell cultures by plaque assay	Tests to exclude extraneous viruses

* Vaccines used in conventional immunization programmes.

† Vaccines used to provide additional protection when circumstances indicate a need.

Measles, mumps and rubella vaccines are generally administered in the form of a combined measles/mumps/rubella vaccine (MMR vaccine).

Viral vaccines of restricted availability include Congo Crimean haemorrhagic fever vaccine, dengue fever vaccine, Japanese encephalitis B vaccine, smallpox vaccine, tick-borne encephalitis vaccine and Venezuelan encephalitis vaccine.

ELISA, enzyme-linked immunosorbent assay.

manufacturers often perform tests in excess of those stipulated, especially sterility tests (Chapter 20) as, by so doing, they obtain assurance that production is proceeding normally and that the final product is likely to be satisfactory. Numerous examples of in-process control exist for various types of vaccine but three demonstrate the principle.

The quality control of both diphtheria and tetanus vaccines requires that the products are tested for the presence of free toxin, that is for specific toxicity due to inadequate detoxification with formaldehyde, at the final product stage. By this stage, however, the toxoid concentrates used in the preparation of the vaccines have been much diluted and, as the volume of vaccine that can be inoculated into the test animals (guinea-pigs) is limited, the tests are relatively insensitive. In-process control, however, provides for tests on the undiluted concentrates and thus increases the sensitivity of the method at least 100-fold.

An example from virus vaccine manufacture is the titration, prior to inactivation, of the infectivity of the pools of live poliovirus used to make inactivated poliomyelitis vaccine. Adequate infectivity of the virus from the tissue cultures is an indicator of the adequate virus content of the starting material

and, as infectivity is destroyed in the inactivation process, there is no possibility of performing such an estimation after formolization.

A more general example from virus vaccine production is the rigorous examination of tissue cultures to exclude contamination with infectious agents from the source animal or, in the cases of human diploid cells or cells from continuous cell lines, to detect cells with abnormal characteristics. Monkey kidney cell cultures are tested for simian herpes B virus, simian virus 40, mycoplasma and tubercle bacilli. Cultures of human diploid cells and continuous line cells are subjected to detailed karyological examination (examination of chromosomes by microscopy) to ensure that the cells have not undergone any changes likely to impair the quality of a vaccine or lead to undesirable side-effects.

2.7.2 Final product control

2.7.2.1 Assays

Vaccines containing killed microorganisms or their products are generally tested for potency in assays in which the amount of the vaccine that is required to protect animals from a defined challenge dose of the appropriate pathogen, or its product, is compared with the amount of a standard vaccine that is required to provide the same protection. The usual format of the test is the 3 + 3 dose quantal assay that is used to estimate the potency of whole cell pertussis vaccine (*British Pharmacopoeia*, 2003). Three logarithmic serial doses of the test vaccine and three logarithmic serial doses of the standard vaccine are made and each is used to inoculate a group of 16 mice. In the case of both the test vaccine and the standard, the middle dose is chosen on the basis of experience, so that it is sufficient to induce a protective response in about 50% of the animals to which it is given. Each lower dose may then be expected to protect < 50% of the mice to which it is given and each higher dose to protect > 50% of the animals. Fourteen days later all of the mice are inoculated ('challenged') with virulent *Bordetella pertussis* and, after a further 14 days, the number of mice surviving in each of the six groups is counted. The number of survivors in each group is used to calculate the potency of the test vaccine relative to the potency of the standard vaccine by the statistical method of probit analysis (Finney, 1971). The potency of the test vaccine may be expressed as a percentage of the potency of the standard vaccine. However, as the standard vaccine will have an assigned potency in International Units (IU), it is more usual to express the potency of the test vaccine in similar units. Tests similar to that used to estimate the potency of pertussis vaccine are prescribed for the potency determinations of diphtheria vaccine and tetanus vaccines. In these cases the respective bacterial toxins are used as the challenge material (*British Pharmacopoeia*, 2003).

Vaccines containing live microorganisms are generally tested for potency by determining their content of viable particles. In the case of the most widely used live bacterial vaccine, BCG vaccine, dilutions of vaccine are prepared in a medium which inhibits clumping of cells, and fixed volumes are dropped on to solid media capable of supporting mycobacterial growth. After a fortnight the colonies generated by the drops are counted and the live count of the undiluted vaccine is calculated. The potency of live viral vaccines is estimated in much the same way except that a substrate of living cells is used. Dilutions of vaccine are inoculated on to tissue culture monolayers in Petri dishes or in plastic trays, and the infective particle count of the vaccine is calculated from the infectivity of the dilutions as indicated by plaque formation, cytopathic effect, haemadsorption or other effect and the dilution factor involved.

2.7.2.2 Safety tests

Because many vaccines are derived from basic materials of intense pathogenicity — the lethal dose of tetanus toxin for a mouse is estimated to be $3 \times 10^{-5}\,\mu g$ — safety testing is of paramount importance. Effective testing provides a guarantee of the safety of each batch of every product and most vaccines in the final container must pass one or more safety tests as prescribed in a pharmacopoeial monograph. This generality does not absolve a manufacturer from the need to perform 'in-process' tests as required, but it is relaxed for those preparations that have a final formulation that makes safety tests on the final product either impractical or meaningless.

Bacterial vaccines are regulated by relatively simple safety tests. Those vaccines composed of killed bacteria or bacterial products must be shown to be completely free from the living microorganisms used in the production process. Inoculation of appropriate bacteriological media with the final product provides an assurance that all organisms have been killed. Those vaccines prepared from toxins, for example, diphtheria and tetanus toxoids, require in addition, a test system capable of revealing inadequately detoxified toxins; this can be done by inoculation of guinea-pigs, which are exquisitely sensitive to both diphtheria and tetanus toxins. A test for sensitization of mice to the lethal effects of histamine is used to detect active pertussis toxin in pertussis vaccines. The trend is to replace *in vivo* assays by cell culture methods where possible. Inoculation of guinea-pigs is also used to exclude the presence of abnormally virulent organisms in BCG vaccine. Molecular genetic methods, such as nucleic acid amplification to probe for genes specific to virulent strains, are now available but not yet in routine use for vaccine testing.

Viral vaccines can present problems of safety testing far more complex than those experienced with most bacterial vaccines. With killed viral vaccines the potential hazards are those due to incomplete virus inactivation and the consequent presence of residual live virus in the preparation. The tests used to detect such live virus consist of the inoculation of susceptible tissue cultures and of susceptible animals. The cultures are examined for cytopathic effects, and the animals for symptoms of disease and histological evidence of infection at autopsy. This test is of particular importance in inactivated poliomyelitis vaccines, the vaccine being injected intraspinally into monkeys. At autopsy, sections of brain and spinal cord are examined microscopically for the histological lesions indicative of proliferating poliovirus.

With attenuated viral vaccines the potential hazards are those associated with reversion of the virus during production to a degree of virulence capable of causing disease in recipients. To a large extent this possibility is controlled by very careful selection of a stable seed but, especially with live attenuated poliomyelitis vaccine, it is usual to compare the neurovirulence of the vaccine with that of a vaccine known to be safe in field use. The technique involves the intraspinal inoculation of monkeys with both the reference vaccine and the test vaccine followed by comparison of the neurological lesions and symptoms, if any, that are caused. If the vaccine causes abnormalities in excess of those caused by the reference it fails the test. A modification of this test which uses transgenic mice instead of monkeys is now available. An *in vitro* method (MAPREC test) which relies on detecting RNA sequences specific to virulent virus has also been developed.

2.7.2.3 Tests of general application

In addition to the tests designed to estimate the potency and to exclude the hazards peculiar to each vaccine there are a number of tests of more general application. These relatively simple tests are as follows.

1 *Sterility.* In general, vaccines are required to be sterile. The exceptions to this requirement are smallpox vaccine made from the dermis of animals and bacterial vaccines such as BCG, Ty21A and tularaemia vaccine, which consist of living but attenuated strains. These have a bioburden limit which defines the number of permissible microorganisms but excludes pathogens. WHO recommendations and pharmacopoeial monographs stipulate, for vaccine batches of different size, the numbers of containers that must be tested and found to be sterile. The preferred method of sterility testing is membrane filtration, as this technique permits the testing of large volumes without dilution of the test media. The test system must be capable of detecting aerobic and anaerobic bacteria and fungi (see Chapter 20).

2 *Freedom from abnormal or general toxicity.* The purpose of this simple test is to exclude the presence in a final container of a highly toxic contaminant. Five mice of 17–22 g and two guinea-pigs of 250–350 g are inoculated with one human dose or 1.0 ml, whichever is less, of the test preparation. All must survive for 7 days without signs of illness. Current pharmacopoeial monographs usually do not require this test if another *in vivo* test has been performed on the product.

3 *Pyrogenicity or endotoxin content.* The pyrogenicity of a specified dose of product when administered to rabbits can be assayed by a standard pharmacopoeial method but the trend is to replace this with an *in vitro* assay for endotoxin (Chapter 19). The capacity of the product to induce gelation of *Limulus polyphemus* amoebocyte lysate is determined against a reference endotoxin preparation and the result is expressed as IU of endotoxin.

4 *Presence of aluminium and calcium.* The quantity of aluminium in vaccines containing aluminium hydroxide or aluminium phosphate as an adjuvant is limited to 1.25 mg per dose and it is usually estimated compleximetrically. The quantity of calcium is limited to 1.3 mg per dose and is usually estimated by atomic absorption spectrometry.

5 *Free formaldehyde.* Inactivation of bacterial toxins with formaldehyde may lead to the presence of small amounts of free formaldehyde in the final product. The concentration, as estimated by colour development with acetylacetone, must not exceed 0.02%.

6 *Phenol concentration.* When phenol is used to preserve a vaccine its concentration must not exceed 0.25% w/v or, in the case of some vaccines, 0.5% w/v. Phenol is usually estimated by the colour reaction with amino-phenazone and hexacyanoferrate.

3 *In-vivo* diagnostics

3.1 Preparation

The most widely used of these are the tuberculins employed to detect sensitization by mycobacterial proteins and hence the possible presence of infection. These are prepared by growing approved strains of *Mycobacterium tuberculosis* (or *M. bovis* or *M. avium* in preparations intended for veterinary use) in a protein-free medium for several weeks. The culture is then steamed for a prolonged period to kill surviving bacteria and to facilitate release of tuberculo-proteins from the cells. The culture supernate is recovered by centrifugation and further concentrated by evaporation and sterile filtered to make a product known as Old Tuberculin. The crude material may then be standardized against a reference preparation by titration in the skin of guinea-pigs sensitized to *M. tuberculosis*. In practice, further purification is usually performed by precipitation with trichloracetic acid or other protein precipitant to produce Purified Protein Derivative, which is standardized. Concentrated preparations containing 100 000 IU per ml are used to formulate working strengths such as 1000, 100 or 10 IU per ml. These have to be diluted in a medium containing a Tween surfactant to reduce adsorption to glass. The concentrated material can be used for intradermal testing by a multi-prong device such as the Heaf or Tine method.

3.2 Quality control

Apart from standardization of potency, which also serves as an identity test, the material must be checked for sterility and for the absence of viable mycobacteria. Because of their slow growth the latter may not be detected by conventional sterility tests and it is usual to perform check tests by guinea-pig inoculation, or by prolonged culture on Lowenstein-Jensen medium. The product is also checked for absence of reactogenicity in unsensitized guinea-pigs and if required by the regulatory authority, for abnormal toxicity.

Analogous intradermal test reagents such as mallein, histoplasmin and coccidioidin, are produced by similar methods. Their use has declined however, as they, like the tuberculin test, measure exposure and sensitization to the antigens of the agent but not necessarily active infection.

4 Immune sera

4.1 Preparation

Immune sera are preparations derived from the blood of animals, usually horses, but mules, donkeys, sheep or goats are also used. The animals must be in good health, free of infections and from sources free of TSEs, and kept under veterinary supervision. To prepare an immune serum, horses or other animals are injected with a sequence of spaced doses of an antigen until a trial blood sample shows that the injections have induced a high titre of antibody to the injected antigen. An adjuvant may be used if required. A large volume of blood is then removed by venepuncture and collected into a vessel containing sufficient citrate solution to prevent clotting. The blood cells are allowed to settle and the supernatant plasma is drawn off. Alternatively, the blood can be mechanically defibrinated. The crude plasma can be sterilized by filtration and dispensed for use, but it is preferable to fractionate it to separate the immune globulin. This is done by fractional precipitation of the plasma by the addition of ammonium sulphate. The globulin fraction is recovered and treated with pepsin to yield a refined immune product containing the Fab fragment. This refined globulin contains no more than a trace of the albumin that was present in the plasma. It is less antigenic, has a longer half-life in the circulation and is less likely to provoke anaphylaxis or serum sickness than whole serum or crude globulin (Harms, 1948). The antibody content of the refined product is determined, the product is diluted to the required concentration and transferred into ampoules. Two or more monovalent immune sera may be blended together to provide a multivalent immune serum.

4.2 Quality control

The quality of immune sera is controlled by potency tests and by conventional tests for safety and sterility. The potency tests have a common design in that, in the case of all immune sera, the potency is estimated by comparing the amount of the product that is required to neutralize an effect of a homologous toxin with the amount of a standard preparation that is required to achieve the same effect. Serial dilutions of the immune serum and of a standard preparation are made and to each is added a constant amount of the homologous antigen. Each mixture is then inoculated into a group of animals, usually guinea-pigs or mice, and the dilutions of the immune serum and of the standard, which neutralize the effects of toxin, are noted. As the potencies of the standard preparations are expressed in IU, the potencies of the immune sera are determined in corresponding units per millilitre (*British Pharmacopoeia*, 2003). The quality of globulin fractions is usually monitored by gel electrophoresis to detect contaminating proteins and uncleaved immunoglobulin and by size exclusion high performance liquid chromatography to detect aggregates.

Table 23.3 lists the immune sera for which there is currently a demand, or a potential need, and indicates their required potencies and the salient features of the potency assay methods.

5 Human immunoglobulins

5.1 Source material

Human immunoglobulins are preparations of the immunoglobulins, principally immunoglobulin G

(IgG) subclasses, that are present in human blood. They are derived from the plasma of donated blood and from plasma obtained by plasmapheresis. Normal immunoglobulin, that is immunoglobulin that has relatively low titres of antibodies representative of those present in the population at large, is prepared from pools of plasma obtained from not fewer than a thousand individuals. Specific immunoglobulins, that is immunoglobulins with a high titre of a particular antibody, are usually prepared from smaller pools of plasma obtained from individuals who have suffered recent infections or who have undergone recent immunization and who thus have a high titre of a particular antibody. Each contribution of plasma to a pool is tested for the presence of hepatitis B surface antigen (HbsAg), for antibodies to human immunodeficiency viruses 1 and 2 (HIV 1 and 2) and for antibodies to hepatitis C virus in order to identify, and to exclude from a pool, any plasma capable of transmitting infection from donor to recipient. Donors who have been resident for 6 months or more in areas endemic for transmissible spongiform bovine encephalopathy, which currently includes the UK, are also excluded.

5.2 Fractionation

The immunoglobulins are obtained from the plasma pools by fractionation methods that are based on ethanol precipitation in the cold with rigorous control of protein concentration, pH and ionic strength (Cohn *et al.*, 1946). The variation of

Table 23.3 Immune sera used in the prevention or treatment of infections in humans

Immunoserum	Potency assay method	Potency requirement
Botulinum antitoxin	Neutralization of the lethal effects of botulinum toxins A, B and E in mice	500 IU/ml type A 500 IU/ml type B 50 IU/ml type E
Diphtheria antitoxin	Neutralization of the erythrogenic effect of diphtheria toxin in the skin of guinea-pigs	1000 IU/ml if prepared in other species
Tetanus antitoxin	Neutralization of the paralytic effect of tetanus toxin in mice	1000 IU/ml for prophylaxis 3000 IU/ml for treatment

In each of the assays of potency the amount of the immune serum and the amount of a corresponding standard antitoxin that are required to neutralize the effects of a defined dose of the corresponding toxin are determined. The two determined amounts and the assigned unitage of the standard antitoxin are then used to calculate the potency of the immune serum in International Units (IU).

Table 23.4 Immunoglobulins used in the prevention and treatment of infections in humans

Immunoglobulins	Potency assay method	Potency requirement
Normal	Neutralization tests in cell cultures or in animals	Measurable amounts of one bacterial antibody and of one viral antibody for which there are international standards
Hepatitis B	Radioimmunoassay or enzyme immunoassay	Not less than 100 IU/ml
Measles	Neutralization of the infectivity of measles virus for cell cultures	Not less than 50 IU/ml
Rabies	Neutralization of the infectivity of rabies virus for mice	Not less than 150 IU/ml
Tetanus	Neutralization of the paralytic effect of tetanus toxin in mice	Not less than 50 IU/ml
Varicella/zoster	ELISA in parallel with a standard varicella-zoster immunoglobulin	Not less than 100 IU/ml

In each of the assays of potency the amount of the immunoglobulin and the amount of a corresponding standard preparation that are required to neutralize the infectivity or other biological activity of a defined amount of virus or to neutralize a defined amount of a bacterial toxin are determined. The two determined amounts and the assigned unitage of the standard preparation are then used to calculate the potency of the immunoglobulins in International Units (IU). ELISA, enzyme-linked immunosorbent assay.

Kistler & Nitschmann (1962) is widely used. Some of the fractionation steps may contribute to the safety of immunoglobulins by inactivating or removing contaminating viruses that have not been detected by tests on the blood donations. The immunoglobulins may be presented either as a freeze-dried or a liquid preparation at a concentration that is 10–20 times that in plasma. Glycine may be added as a stabilizer and thiomersal as a preservative.

5.3 Quality control

The quality control of immunoglobulins includes potency tests and conventional tests for safety and sterility. The potency tests consist of toxin or virus neutralization tests that parallel those used for the potency assay of immune sera, except that for in-process control of some immunoglobulins wider use is made of *in vitro* assays. In addition to the safety and sterility tests, total protein is determined by nitrogen estimations, the protein composition by sodium dodecyl sulphate-polyacrylamide gel electrophoresis and molecular size by high performance liquid chromatography. The presence of immunoglobulins derived from species other than humans is excluded by precipitin tests. Table 23.4

lists six human immunoglobulins and their requisite potencies and indicates the methods by which the potencies are determined.

6 Further reading

Ada, G. L. (1994) *Strategies in Vaccine Design*. RG Landes, Austin.

Anon (1999a) *A WHO Guide to Good Manufacturing Practice (GMP) Requirements. Part 1. Standard Operating Procedures and Master Formulae*. WHO/VSQ/97.01. World Health Organization, Geneva.

Anon (1999b) *A WHO Guide to Good Manufacturing Practice (GMP) Requirements. Part 2. Validation*. WHO/VSQ/97.02. World Health Organization, Geneva.

British Medical Association and Pharmaceutical Press (2002) *The British National Formulary*. BMA, London. [This publication contains a useful section on immunological products. New editions appear at intervals.]

British Pharmacopoeia (2003) The Stationery Office, London.

Cohn, E. J., Strong, L. E., Hughes, W. L., Hulford, D. J., Ashworth, J. N., Melin, M. & Taylor, H. I. (1946) Preparation and properties of serum proteins IV. *J Am Chem Soc*, **68**, 459–475.

Ellis, R. W. (1999) *Combination Vaccines. Development, Clinical Research and Approval*. Humana Press, Totowa, NJ.

Finney, D. J. (1971) *Probit Analysis*. Cambridge University Press, London.

Harms, A. J. (1948) The purification of antitoxic plasmas by enzyme treatment and heat denaturation. *Biochem J, 42*, 340–347.

Kistler, P. & Nitschmann, H. S. (1962) Large scale production of human plasma fractions. *Vox Sang, 7*, 414–424.

Mizrahi, A. (1990) Bacterial vaccines. *Advances in Biotechnological Processes 15*. Wiley-Liss, New York.

Pastoret, P., Blancou, J., Vannier, P. & Verschueren, C. (1997) *Veterinary Vaccinology*. Elsevier, Amsterdam.

Perlmann, P. & Wigzell, H. (1999) *Vaccines. Handbook of Experimental Pharmacology*, Vol 133. Springer, Berlin.

Plotkin, S. A. & Mortimer, E. A. (2003) *Vaccines*, 3rd edn. WB Saunders, Philadelphia.

Powell, M. F. & Newman, M. J. (1995) *Vaccine Design. The Subunit and Adjuvant Approach*. Plenum Press, New York.

Chapter 24
Pharmaceutical biotechnology

Miguel Cámara

1 Introduction: biotechnology in pharmaceutical sciences

The rapid developments in biotechnology and the applications of genetic engineering to practical human problems have allowed the advancement of pharmaceutical biotechnology at a staggering pace. Furthermore, the release of the human genome sequence has also been key for the identification of human genetic diseases and the design of revolutionary approaches for their treatment.

Genetic engineering involves altering DNA molecules outside an organism, making the resultant DNA molecules function in living cells. Many of these cells have been genetically engineered to produce substances that are medically useful to humans. Pharmaceutical biotechnology involves the use of living organisms such as microorganisms to create new pharmaceutical products, or safer and more effective versions of conventionally produced pharmaceuticals, more cost-effectively.

Since the manufacture of the first recombinant pharmaceutical, insulin, there has been a burst in the generation of new recombinant drugs, some of which will be covered later on in this chapter. Furthermore, the use of recombinant DNA technology has spread further allowing the development of not only subunit vaccines, such as the one used in the prevention of hepatitis B, but also attenuated vaccines, vector vaccines and DNA vaccines. One of pharmaceutical biotechnology's great potentials lies in gene therapy, which consists of the insertion of genetic material into cells to prevent, control or cure disease. It encompasses repairing or replacing defective genes and making tumours more susceptible to other kinds of treatment.

This chapter aims to describe some essential genetic manipulation techniques and illustrate, with some key examples, their use for the generation of recombinant pharmaceutical drugs. Applications of recombinant DNA techniques in the diagnosis of diseases also will be covered.

2 Enabling techniques

To understand how recombinant pharmaceutical products are manufactured we first need to review some of the essential DNA manipulation techniques used to generate these recombinant products. We will start by looking at ways to cut and join fragments of DNA and then examine step by step how these techniques can be exploited to clone and express any genes from eukaryotic and prokaryotic cells.

2.1 Cutting and joining DNA molecules

DNA isolated from any type of cell can be fragmented using restriction endonucleases. These are enzymes which cut DNA at specific points known as 'restriction sites' which are palindromic sequences (complementary sequences with identical nucleotide sequences when read in the direction 5′ to 3′) of various lengths (more frequently 4–6 base pairs (bp)), e.g. *Eco*RI has specificity for the sequence GAATTC. In general, the shorter the length of the restriction sites, the higher the probability of it appearing more frequently in DNA fragments.

There are two different types of DNA ends that can be generated using restriction enzymes; these are sticky ends and blunt ends (Table 24.1). DNA fragments that have been generated by restriction enzymatic digestion can be joined together using an enzyme called DNA ligase. There is a limitation, however, with regards to the type of ends this enzyme will be able to stick together. Only blunt ends generated by any restriction enzyme (e.g. *Dra*I and *Eco*RV) or sticky ends generated by either identical restriction enzymes (e.g. *Eco*RI) or enzymes that generate complementary overhanging ends (e.g. *Sau*3AI and *Bam*HI) will be joined by the DNA ligase (Table 24.1).

Table 24.1 Restriction enzymes and the compatibility of digested ends for ligation

Restriction enzyme	Restriction site		Digested ends	Compatibility for ligase	Ligation products
			Sticky		
*Sau*3A	5′-**GATC**-3′ 3′-**CTAG**-3′	5′-**GATC** 3′-	-5′ **CTAG**-3′	Compatible	5′-**GATC**C-3′ 3′-CTAGG-5′
			Sticky		
*Bam*HI	5′-GGATCC-3′ 3′-CCTAGG-5′	5′-GGATC 3′-C	C-3′ CTAGG-5′		5′-GGATC-3′ 3′-C**CTAG**-3′
			Sticky	Incompatible	
*Eco*RI	5′-**GAATTC**-3′ 3′-**CTTAAG**-5′	5′-**G** 3′-**CTTAA**	**AATTC**-3′ **G**-5′		5′-**G**AATTC-3′ 3′-**CTTAA**G-5′
			Sticky	Compatible	
*Eco*RI	5′-GAATTC-3′ 3′-CTTAAG-5′	5′-G 3′-CTTAA	AATTC-3′ G-5′		5′-G**AATTC**-3′ 3′-CTTAA**G**-5′
			Blunt	Incompatible	
*Dra*I	5′-**TTTAAA**-3′ 3′-**AAATTT**-5′	5′-**TTT** 3′-**AAA**	**AAA**-3′ **TTT**-5′		5′-**TTT**ATC-3′ 3′-**AAA**TAG-5′
			Blunt	Compatible	
*Eco*RV	5′-GATATC-3′ 3′-CTATAG-5′	5′-GAT 3′-CTA	ATC-3′ TAG-5′		5′-GAT**AAA**-3′ 3′-CTA**TTT**-5′

2.2 Cloning vectors

Genes present in DNA fragments that have been ex-cised with restriction endonucleases can be main-tained, i.e. replicated and expressed, by ligating them into different types of vectors. These vectors are relatively small DNA molecules that have the ability to replicate readily and independently from the chromosome. This allows them to be present in several copy numbers inside the host cell. The main type of vectors used for gene cloning are plasmids, cosmids and bacteriophages, which are normally used according to the size of the DNA fragments that need to be cloned into them.

2.2.1 Cloning of small fragments of DNA

To allow the cloning of small fragments of DNA, generally up to 8 kb in size, plasmids are the main vectors of choice.

2.2.1.1 Plasmids

Plasmids are small, circular extrachromosomal DNA molecules that replicate independently using their own origin of replication. There are a number of features generally found in plasmids that are used as cloning vectors:

Antibiotic resistance markers. These are genes that code for proteins that confer resistance to specif-ic antibiotics. These markers therefore allow the selection of hosts carrying them.

Multiple cloning sites (MCS). These are fragments of DNA that contain a number of unique differ-ent restriction sites, enabling the use of a choice of restriction enzymes for the cloning of DNA frag-ments.

Origin of replication. Required for plasmid replica-tion in a specific host. They can also determine the number of plasmid copies found in a cell. Plasmids having more than one different host-specific origin of replication are known as shuttle vectors.

Insertional inactivation markers. These allow selec-tion of recombinant plasmids from non-recombi-nants. The most commonly used is the *lacZ'* coding for β-galactosidase activity. This enzyme can cleave a substrate that mimics galactose known as X-Gal, which results in the generation

of a blue product. Insertion of a recombinant DNA fragment in the middle of *lacZ'*, results in the inactivation of the β-galactosidase and hence inability to cleave X-Gal. Hence colonies from bacteria carrying intact *lacZ'*, i.e. with non-recombinant plasmids, appear blue on agar plates containing X-Gal. In contrast, those with an insertion in this gene, i.e. harbouring recombi-nant plasmids, appear white.

Figure 24.1 shows all these features in a simpli-fied diagram of the cloning vector pUC18.

An ideal plasmid should have small size (2–10 kb), be conjugation-defective, i.e. non-mobiliz-able, and have a ready selectable phenotype on host cells. It should also contain a large number of single restriction sites and a high copy number (>10 copies per cell).

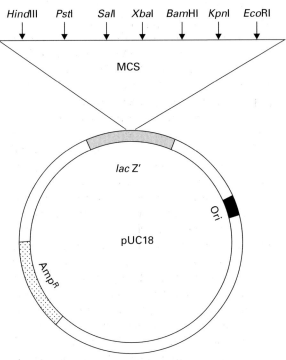

Fig. 24.1 Simplified diagram of the plasmid pUC18. *lacZ'* represents the insertional inactivation marker coding for β-galactosidase activity. A multiple cloning site (MCS) is present within the *LacZ'* gene to enable the cloning of DNA fragments. 'Ori' represents the origin of replication which, in this case, works in *Escherichia coli*. Finally, Amp^r represents an ampicillin resistance marker.

2.2.2 *Cloning of large fragments of DNA*

Sometimes there is a need to clone large fragments of DNA for the isolation of intact clusters of genes. An example would be the cloning of the genes responsible for the synthesis of a certain antibiotic. Sometimes the synthesis of an antibiotic requires more than 10 different genes. These genes are normally present in operons as they are co-transcribed in a single messenger RNA molecule of considerable length. To enable the cloning of intact operons, vectors such as bacteriophages and cosmids need to be used.

2.2.2.1 *Bacteriophages*

The most popular bacteriophage is the *Escherichia coli* λ (lambda) bacteriophage, which is made of a tubular protein tail and a protein head packed with approximately 50 kb of DNA. This phage has a complex cell cycle. After injection of the viral DNA into *E. coli* it can multiply and enter a lytic cycle leading to the lysis of the host cell and subsequent release of a large number of phage particles. Alternatively, injection of the DNA can lead to a lysogenic cycle in which the phage DNA is integrated into the *E. coli* chromosome where it is maintained until the environmental conditions change and is then excised, entering a lytic cycle. Out of the 50 kb that make the λ bacteriophage less than half are essential for the propagation of the phage and around 20 kb can be replaced for recombinant DNA, hence their name λ replacement vectors. Therefore, these vectors are very useful for the generation of genomic libraries. The structure of the λ bacteriophage and how it can be used as a cloning vector are shown in Fig. 24.2. λ Bacteriophages contain at each end small single-stranded complementary DNA fragments called 'cos ends'. Recombinant phages can be packed, in a test tube, into phage particles by enzymes which recognize and process the cos ends, provided that they are 35–45 kb apart. These enzymes, as well as the head and tails required for the packaging process, are commercially available as part of *in vitro* packaging kits. The *in vitro* packaging results in the formation of recombinant phages that can be transduced to *E. coli* cells. Transduced *E. coli* will be identified by the formation of plaques in agar plates seeded with a mixture of *E. coli* and recombinant λ bacteriophages.

2.2.2.2 *Cosmids*

Cosmids are cloning vectors that can carry up to 40 kb of cloned DNA and can also be maintained in *E. coli*. In essence, they are plasmids that have been engineered with the addition of cos ends. This allows them to be packed into λ phage particles using *in vitro* packaging extracts and then be transduced into *E. coli*. Once inside the bacterial host the DNA from the cosmid is circularized by the joining of the cos ends and thereafter behaves as a normal plasmid. This implies that *E. coli* carrying cosmids will grow in colonies and not plaques like the bacteriophages.

2.3 Introduction of vector into hosts

For the expression and maintenance of recombinant genes there is a need to introduce the recombinant vectors harbouring them into suitable hosts. The four main methods used to achieve this are transformation, electroporation, conjugation and transduction.

For *transformation* bacteria such as *E. coli* can uptake recombinant plasmid DNA by treating the cells with ice-cold $CaCl_2$ until they reach a 'competent' state in which they are ready to take up DNA. These cells are then presented with the recombinant plasmid and exposed briefly to a heat shock of 42°C which enables them to take up the DNA.

Electroporation, however is the most generalized way of introducing DNA not only in bacteria but also in eukaryotic cells. This technique is based on the induction of free DNA uptake by the bacterium after subjecting it to a high electric field. Electroporation allows the uptake of most sizes of plasmids.

In some cases *conjugation* can be used as a natural transmission of plasmid DNA from a donor cell to a recipient cell by direct contact through cell–cell junctions. Only plasmid cloning vectors containing conjugative elements can be transferred by conjugation. This procedure requires direct contact between the donor and the recipient cell. Conjugation is not as frequently used as electroporation as most plasmid vectors used for the cloning of recombinant DNA lack conjugative functions, pre-

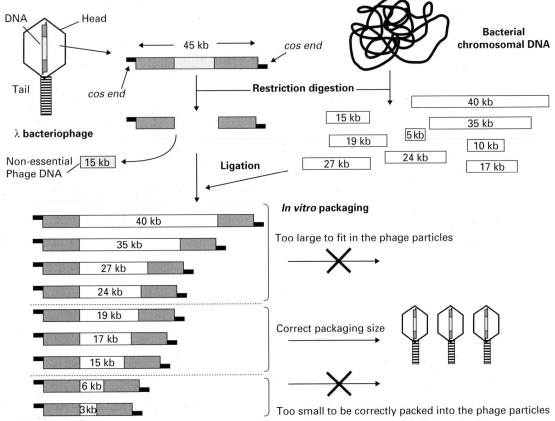

Fig. 24.2 Cloning of DNA into λ insertion vectors. The DNA from the λ bacteriophage can be purified from the phage particles and digested with restriction enzymes to remove an internal fragment of around 15 kb which is not required for the life cycle of the bacteriophage. This fragment can be replaced with other fragments of DNA such as those coming from digested bacterial chromosomal DNA. As the λ bacteriophage can only pack DNA fragments flanked by cos ends which are 35–45 kb apart, any recombinant fragments larger or smaller than that will not be successfully packed.

venting these plasmids from being passed to recipient cells accidentally.

Finally, in *transduction*, the transfer of recombinant non-viral DNA to a cell is achieved by a virus. This is the method of choice for the introduction of recombinant λ bacteriophages and cosmids into *E. coli* cells.

2.4 Construction of genomic libraries

Before we study how genomic libraries are made we first need to understand the differences between the genetic organization in eukaryotic and prokaryotic cells. Bacterial genes are uninterrupted sequences of

nucleotides encoding the genetic information required for the synthesis of a protein. These genes can sometimes be co-transcribed with adjacent genes of related function into the same mRNA molecule. This set of co-transcribed genes is called an operon (Fig. 24.3). The mRNA in bacteria does not generally need to be processed before translation.

In contrast, genes from eukaryotic cells contain non-coding sequences called introns and coding sequences called exons. The former are removed after transcription by a process called 'splicing' that occurs in the nucleus of the cell. In addition the mRNA is subjected to further processing involving the addition of a methylated guanine (M_7Gppp) called

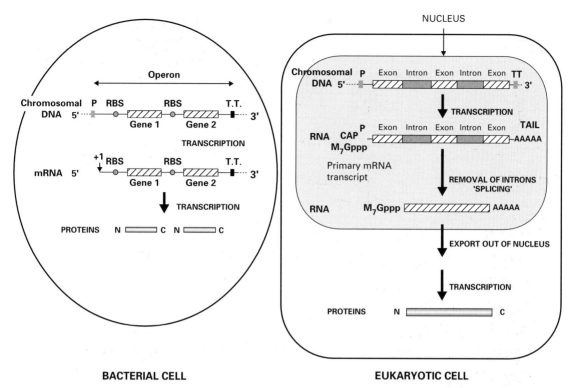

Fig. 24.3 Genetic organization in prokaryotes and eukaryotes. In prokaryotes genes can sometimes be grouped in operons and hence transcribed together in a single molecule of mRNA. In these organisms the whole process of transcription and translation takes place in the cytoplasm. In contrast, in eukaryotes, genes are organized in single transcriptional units interrupted by introns. Upon transcription in the nucleus, eukaryotic mRNA is firstly modified by the addition of a CAP and a polyA tail and then by the splicing of the introns. The mature mRNA is then exported into the cytoplasm where it is translated into proteins. P, promoter; T.T., transcriptional terminator; RBS, ribosome binding site.

CAP on its 5′ end, required for translation, and a poly-adenine tail on its 3′ end (Fig. 24.3). Mature mRNA is then exported from the nucleus into the cytoplasm. Eukaryotic genes are always transcribed individually, as operons have not been described in eukaryotes.

To enable the cloning and isolation of a specific gene(s) from a cell several steps are required. The first consists of choosing the source of genetic material which, in prokarotic cells, is normally the chromosomal DNA. In contrast, in eukaryotic cells this is the mature mRNA, as it is not interrupted by introns and consequently codes for full active proteins. The second step consists of the preparation of the purified DNA/RNA for cloning. This step is more straightforward when using prokaryotic DNA (section 2.4.1) than eukaryotic RNA (section 2.4.2). The result will be the construction of a collection of cloned DNA fragments propagated in bacteria that is called the genomic library. This library should contain representatives of every sequence in the chromosome of a prokaryotic cell and every expressed gene in the case of a eukaryotic cell. The final step consists of the screening of every recombinant clone to identify the required gene(s).

2.4.1 *Prokaryotic gene libraries: shotgun cloning*

The construction of a prokaryotic gene library can be achieved by a technique called 'shotgun cloning' (Fig. 24.4). This involves the purification and partial digestion of the genomic (chromosomal) DNA

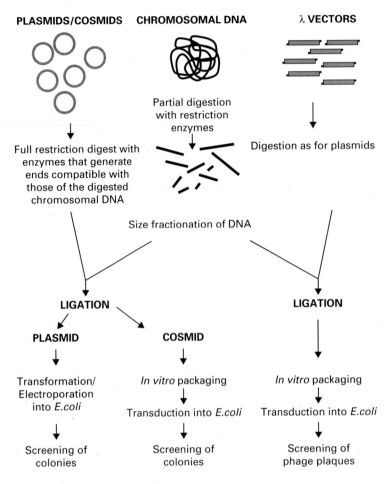

"SHOTGUN APPROACH"

PLASMIDS/COSMIDS   CHROMOSOMAL DNA   λ VECTORS

Partial digestion
with restriction
enzymes

Full restriction digest with
enzymes that generate
ends compatible with
those of the digested
chromosomal DNA

Digestion as for plasmids

Size fractionation of DNA

LIGATION   LIGATION

PLASMID   COSMID

Transformation/   *In vitro* packaging   *In vitro* packaging
Electroporation
into *E.coli*   Transduction into *E.coli*   Transduction into *E.coli*

Screening of   Screening of   Screening of
colonies   colonies   phage plaques

Fig. 24.4 Construction of prokaryotic genomic libraries by shotgun cloning. The shotgun approach for the construction of genomic libraries involves the purification and digestion of chromosomal DNA, from the prokaryotic organisms, followed by the cloning into a digested suitable vector using DNA ligase. The recombinant vector is then introduced into the host cell using the appropriate method and then the recombinant colonies or plaques are screened for the presence of the recombinant gene of interest.

from a prokaryotic organism with restriction endonucleases to produce a random mixture of fragments of different sizes. These fragments are then fractionated into different sizes and inserted into the appropriate vector similarly digested. The recombinant vectors are then transformed, in the case of plasmids, or transfected, in the case of bacteriophages and cosmids, into the host cell of choice. The resulting genomic library can then be screened for the presence of the recombinant gene of interest by a number of methods (see section 2.5).

2.4.2 Eukaryotic cDNA gene libraries

The shotgun approach cannot be applied for the construction of eukaryotic gene libraries due to the presence of introns in DNA, which prevents the direct cloning of intact genes from digested chromosomal DNA. Instead spliced RNA, from the cytoplasm of cells expressing the desired gene, is used as the source of genetic material. For example, to make a genomic library containing the insulin gene, RNA from pancreatic cells expressing this gene will have to be isolated. Remember that cells show distinct differentiation in different tissues and only express a low percentage of the whole genome according to their role in the tissue of which they form part. Consequently, it will not be possible to purify RNA coding for insulin from cells of the pituitary gland. Therefore, the cells expressing the gene of interest will have to be isolated and their mRNA purified. As mentioned earlier, virtually every eukaryotic mRNA has on its 3′ end a polyadenine tail. This provides a convenient way to isolate mRNA from total cellular RNA, the majority of which (98%) is ribosomal RNA (rRNA) and transfer RNA (tRNA). The total RNA purified from a cell can be passed through an affinity column packed with cellulose linked to oligonucleotides of deoxythymidine [oligo(dT)]. As the total RNA passes through the column, only the mRNA molecules will bind to the oligo(dT) by their polyadenine tails while the rest of the RNA will flow through the column. The purified mRNA then has to be converted into double-stranded cDNA (complementary DNA) to enable its cloning into any suitable vector.

2.4.2.1 Synthesis and cloning of cDNA

There are generally two main strategies used for the synthesis of cDNA from mRNA called the replacement synthesis and the primer adaptor synthesis. For both strategies the first strand cDNA synthesis is based on the priming of the mRNA with an oligo-dT which anneals to the poly(A) tail of the mRNA molecule and, consequently, with the action of the enzyme reverse transcriptase, in the presence of dNTPs, the synthesis of the first cDNA strand takes place. This results in the formation of a heteroduplex mRNA/cDNA hybrid. The second stage is different for the two strategies mentioned. The most commonly used is the replacement synthesis, which is based on the use of ribonuclease H (RNaseH), an enzyme that cleaves the RNA moiety of RNA/DNA hybrids and has 5′→3′ and 3′→5′ exonuclease activities. This results in partial digestion of the RNA in both directions. The resulting RNA fragments can serve as primers for DNA synthesis using DNA polymerase I. This enzyme, with its 5′→3′ exonuclease and polymerase activities will fill the nicks and effectively remove the RNA primers. The cDNA fragments synthesized will be joined using DNA ligase. This method potentially leaves the 5′ RNA cap region.

The primer adaptor method, for the synthesis of the second strand of cDNA, is based on the removal of the RNA strand, from the RNA/DNA hybrid, by treatment with alkali. This is followed by the addi-

tion of a polyC tail to the 3′ end of the DNA strand using an enzyme called terminal transferase. This enables the hybridization of a complementary polyG primer that will be the starting point for the synthesis of the second cDNA strand by the DNA polymerase (Fig. 24.5). This method, in contrast to the replacement synthesis, generates cDNA molecules with a complete 5′ DNA cap region. However, it requires more steps and the terminal transferase step is difficult to control.

Finally, the cloning of the resulting cDNA is aided by the addition of a polyC tail at the 3′ ends of the cDNA fragments using terminal transferase and the ligation of these to a linearized vector containing a complementary polyG tail also generated by the terminal transferase.

2.4.3 Comparison between libraries

There are a number of points to take into consideration when choosing a strategy to generate a genomic library. The larger the insert size, the lower the number of clones required to have full representation of an entire genome. To reduce the number of recombinant clones to be screened before the gene of interest is identified, cosmids and λ bacteriophages should be used, as they can take larger DNA insert sizes. Furthermore, if we want to isolate a large operon containing, for example, all the genes required for the biosynthesis of an antibiotic, plasmid libraries might not be the right choice. In contrast, if we are trying to isolate a single gene and the extent of the screening is not a problem, plasmid libraries are ideal as they reduce the subcloning steps required to single out the gene of interest. Table 24.2 shows a comparison between the insert sizes taken by different vectors, their hosts and the genomic libraries for which they can be suitable.

2.5 Screening of genomic libraries

Once the genomic library has been generated it is necessary to screen for the gene of interest within a population of thousands of recombinant clones. The choice of screening method will very much depend on the availability of reagents and the information on the target gene to be isolated.

423

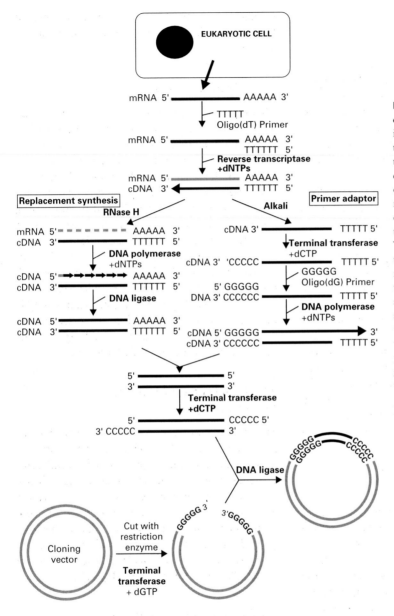

Fig. 24.5 Synthesis and cloning of cDNA. Cloning of eukaryotic genes involves the isolation of mRNA from the cytoplasm of the cells expressing the gene of interest. To allow the cloning of the mRNA the synthesis of double-stranded cDNA is first required. This involves the synthesis of the first cDNA strand by reverse transcriptase using an oligo(dT) primer. To generate the second strand of cDNA there are two main methods. The replacement synthesis method involves the generation of nicks in the mRNA strand by the RNaseH followed by the synthesis of the complementary strand, using the RNA fragments generated by the RNaseH as primers, by the DNA polymerase. The DNA fragments generated are then joined together by the DNA ligase. In contrast, the primer adaptor method requires the degradation of the mRNA strand by alkali followed by the addition of a polyC tail at the 3′ end of the cDNA strand by the terminal transferase. For the synthesis of the second strand of cDNA, addition of an oligo(dG) primer and DNA polymerase are required. The double-stranded cDNA generated by either method can be cloned into any vector upon addition of polyC sticky ends by the terminal transferase, provided that the vector has complementary polyG ends created by this enzyme.

Table 24.2 Comparison of vectors used for the construction of genomic libraries

Vector	Insert size (kb)	Host	Cloning method suitability
Plasmid	<10	Specified by origin of replication present on the plasmid	Shotgun cloning cDNA cloning
λ Bacteriophages (replacement only)	7–22	E. coli	Shotgun cloning
Cosmids	25–45	E. coli	Shotgun cloning

2.5.1 *Hybridization screening*

This technique is used when some of the DNA sequence for the gene we are screening for is known or when a fragment of this gene is available from previous cloning. Alternatively, a DNA fragment from a closely related gene can be used as a probe for the isolation of the gene of interest. The hybridization technique requires plating the library on a set of agar plates to generate a replica, on nitrocellulose or nylon membranes, of the plaques or colonies, each containing a different recombinant DNA fragment. This process transfers a portion of each plaque or colony to the membranes and is done in such a way that the pattern of plaques/colonies on the original plate is maintained on the filters. The membranes are then hybridized with a radio-labelled DNA probe containing part of the sequence to be isolated from the library. The probe will only bind/hybridize to the recombinant clones containing that sequence. After this process, the membranes are exposed to X-ray film (autoradiography). The presence of dark spots on the films represents the location of colonies containing the target gene. By orienting the film with the original agar plate, the colony/plaque carrying the complementary sequence can be identified and the desired clone isolated.

2.5.2 *Immunological screening*

This technique is used when we need to isolate a gene coding for a protein for which there are antibodies available. The success of this technique relies on the expression of the gene of interest, as it requires the synthesis of the target protein from the target recombinant gene. The screening steps are similar to those used for the hybridization screening with the difference that the membranes containing portions of plaques or colonies have to be incubated with the antibodies that will recognize the target protein. This antibody, called the primary antibody, will bind tightly to those colonies/plaques containing the recombinant gene of interest, provided that the protein encoded by this gene has been synthesized. The position of the bound antibody is revealed by incubating the membranes with a labelled antibody (secondary antibody) that recognizes the primary antibody. There are different types of labels for antibodies, all of which can easily be detected.

2.5.3 *Protein activity screening*

This type of screening is limited to proteins that have a specific activity that can easily be identified within a large population of recombinant clones. Needless to say, to detect a protein activity the gene coding for this protein must be expressed and an active protein must have been produced. Understanding of this technique can be helped by illustrating this screening with an example. Suppose we want to isolate a gene coding for a bacterial haemolytic toxin from a genomic library. As we know that this toxin lyses red blood cells, we could plate the library on plates containing agar mixed with these cells. Those colonies/plaques expressing the haemolytic toxin could easily be identified by the presence of a haemolytic halo around them resulting from the action of the toxin on the red blood cells.

2.6 Optimizing expression of recombinant genes

The primary objective of pharmaceutical companies involved in the production of recombinant drugs is the maximal expression of recombinant genes to generate large quantities of these drugs. Unfortunately, the cloning of a gene into a vector does not ensure that it will be highly expressed. Therefore to improve expression of a gene we have to optimize the different stages that lead to the synthesis of a protein. This is achieved by the use of so-called expression vectors (Fig. 24.6).

2.6.1 *Optimizing transcription*

To optimize transcription we must ensure that our recombinant gene is placed after a promoter (Fig. 24.6) that will be recognized by the RNA polymerase of the host cell where the gene is going to be expressed. There are two types of promoters that can be selected: (i) *constitutive promoters*, which are expressed all the time and (ii) *inducible promoters*, where expression is turned off during culture growth and turned on upon the addition of an inducible molecule to the culture, usually shortly before harvesting, when high numbers of bacteria are present in the culture. Inducible promoters are very useful when expressing genes coding for foreign toxic proteins as their premature expression could lead to growth impairments and consequently low yields of recombinant protein.

Furthermore, to ensure that transcription finishes after the 3′-end of the recombinant gene, a transcriptional terminator (Fig. 24.6) must be placed just downstream of this gene.

2.6.2 *Optimizing translation*

A key feature that determines whether a gene is going to be efficiently translated by a certain host is the nucleotide sequence of the ribosome binding site (RBS), located upstream of the gene (Fig. 24.6), which needs to be efficiently recognized by the ribosomes of this host. In addition, the distance between the RBS and the translation 'start' codon needs to be optimal to enable the right interactions between mRNA and ribosomes that lead to the start of protein synthesis. There are commercially available vectors carrying sequences for RBSs and translation start codons which are optimally recognized by the ribosomes of the host cells, ensuring that any recombinant genes cloned after the start codon will be maximally translated.

Small proteins are normally susceptible to proteolytic degradation when expressed in a foreign host. This degradation can be avoided by expressing them fused to a larger protein. This is normally achieved by cloning the small gene downstream of a gene coding for a protein such as β-galactosidase. To obtain the fusion protein (Fig. 24.6) it is essential to ensure that no translation stop codons are present between the β-galactosidase and the target gene, this enables the ribosome to read through, generating the fusion. Interestingly, there are affinity columns that can recognize the fused polypeptides, facilitating the purification of the recombinant protein by affinity chromatography.

2.6.3 *Post-translational modifications*

Although high levels of protein expression may be achieved by optimizing transcription and

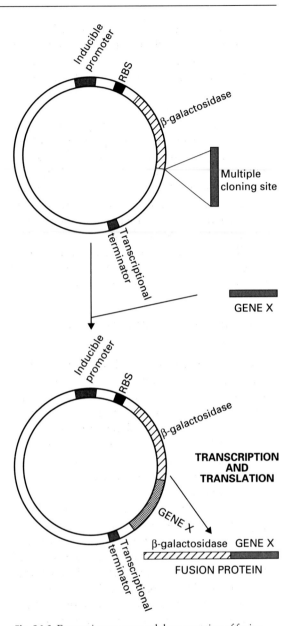

Fig. 24.6 Expression vectors and the generation of fusion proteins. Expression vectors have optimized all the signals required for transcription (inducible promoter and transcriptional terminator) and for translation (ribosome binding site). Some of them carry the gene for β-galactosidase with a multiple cloning site that allows the insertion of small genes for the generation of fusion proteins.

translation of a gene, the overexpressed protein may still need to undergo post-translational modifications before it can be active. Some of these modifications include correct disulphide bond formation, proteolytic cleavage of a precursor, glycosylation and additions to amino acids such as phosphorylation, acetylation, sulphation, acylation, etc. Unfortunately, the popular *E. coli* host, where most recombinant proteins are expressed, is unable to carry out some of these modifications. Hence, it is essential to select a suitable host for the expression of the target protein that can carry out the required post-translation modifications that will enable the synthesis of large amounts of a biologically authentic product. Table 24.3 shows a comparison of a selection of hosts currently used for the expression of recombinant proteins.

2.7 Amplifying DNA: the polymerase chain reaction (PCR)

This is an extremely simple and powerful technique that was devised by Kary Mullis in the mid-1980s and has revolutionized many studies in molecular biology, currently having applications ranging from forensic studies to the development of new recombinant drugs. This technique allows the generation of large amounts of copies of a specified DNA sequence from a single DNA molecule without the need for cloning.

The PCR exploits certain characteristics of DNA replication, as it uses single-stranded DNA as a template for the synthesis of complementary new strands in a 5′ to 3′ direction. The single-stranded DNA templates can be generated by heating double-stranded DNA to 90°C. DNA polymerase requires small fragments of double-stranded DNA to initiate DNA synthesis. Therefore the starting point of DNA synthesis can be specified by the addition of a synthetic oligonucleotide primer that anneals, due to complementarity of bases, to the template at that point. Hence the DNA polymerase can be directed to synthesize a specific region of DNA. The PCR reaction uses a special DNA polymerase (Taq DNA polymerase) that can withstand temperatures as high as 99°C, working optimally at 72°C and subsequently reducing the risk of mismatches that occasionally occur at lower temperatures.

In PCR both strands of DNA serve as template upon the addition of a pair of primers, one for each strand of DNA. A typical PCR amplification is shown in Fig. 24.7. Every PCR cycle is normally repeated up to 30 times. The net result of a PCR is that, at the end of n cycles, it will generate a maximum of 2^n double-stranded DNA copies of the DNA fragment located between the two primers.

2.7.1 Advantages and limitations of PCR

There are some obvious advantages of using PCR. The main one is specificity, as it allows, using the appropriate primers, the amplification of specific DNA fragments from a population of different cells. It is also a very rapid technique, as it only takes a few hours to amplify a fragment of DNA compared with days using conventional cloning methods. An important feature of PCR is its versatility, as it allows the incorporation of mismatches on the 5′ end of the primers provided that the 3′ end has perfect complementary with the sequence it needs to bind. This can be exploited to add restriction sites to enable subsequent cloning of the amplified DNA as well introducing specific mutations into genes. Furthermore, the equipment used for PCR is relatively inexpensive and allows the analysis of a large number of sequences at one time. Finally, PCR does not require pure template DNA and can amplify genes from whole cells or tissue samples.

Unfortunately, there are also a number of limitations to the use of PCR. The designing of primers for this technique requires partial knowledge of the DNA sequence to be amplified. Although there are new genetically engineered DNA polymerases that can synthesize large fragments of DNA there are still some restrictions with regards to the maximum length of DNA that can be amplified. Ideally, fragments of 0.1–3 kb can be easily amplified although this technique, under the appropriate conditions, would amplify larger fragments (up to 20 kb). In addition, the slightest sample contamination can lead to false positive results, which can have detrimental effects when this technique is used in diagnostics. Finally, sometimes there is a risk of non-specific amplification when the primers bind to closely related sequences, leading to the amplification of the wrong sequence.

Table 24.3 Comparison of different hosts used for the expression of recombinant genes

Prokaryotic hosts	Advantages	Disadvantages
Escherichia coli	Easy to grow in large-scale volumes Transcriptional and translational control well known Successfully used in the manufacture of insulin, interferon and human somatotropin	Difficult to achieve export of some proteins into growth medium Degradation of small proteins by proteases Unable to undertake most post-translational modifications, e.g. glycosylation Many proteins retained in the cytoplasm as insoluble aggregates
Bacillus subtilis	Many proteins can be exported into growth medium Easy to grow in large-scale volumes	Regulation of gene expression not very well known Lack of high level expression vectors Unable to carry out most post-translational modifications, e.g. glycosylation
Saccharomyces cerevisiae	Easy to grow in large-scale volumes Efficient protein glycosylation Good export of heterologous proteins into growth medium Wide range of high level expression systems available Recombinant proteins do not form insoluble aggregates in the cytoplasm	Gene expression still not well known Sometimes fails to achieve accurate post-translational modification of recombinant proteins

Eukaryotic hosts	Advantages	Disadvantages
Yeasts	Easy to grow in large-scale volumes Able to glycosylate. Improved glycosylating yeast: Pichia pastoris and Hansenula polymorpha Easy to achieve secretion of recombinant proteins into growth medium	Gene expression can be difficult to control Some post-translational modifications may not be correct
Insect cells	High expression levels Free of virus or prion-type agents Can produce accurate glycosylation	Difficult to scale up High mannose chains can be immunogenic
Mammalian cells	Precise post-translational modification of human proteins Good expression systems available High stability of recombinant proteins	Gene regulation not well known Low protein secretion levels They can harbour infectious agents such as viruses Difficult to scale up
Transgenic animals	Precise post-transcriptional modifications Easy to generate large amount of recombinant protein, e.g. one goat can generate 1 kg of recombinant protein in milk per year Relatively inexpensive	Risk of contamination with infectious agents Products can sometimes be unstable

2.7.2 Clinical applications of PCR

The discovery of PCR has revolutionized not only basic research but also different areas of medicine. Table 24.4 shows a list of some of the most important applications of PCR in the clinic. This type of analysis was not possible before the introduction of PCR owing to the large amount of samples that needed handling, the amount of time needed to obtain a result or the lack of sensitivity of the tests available.

428

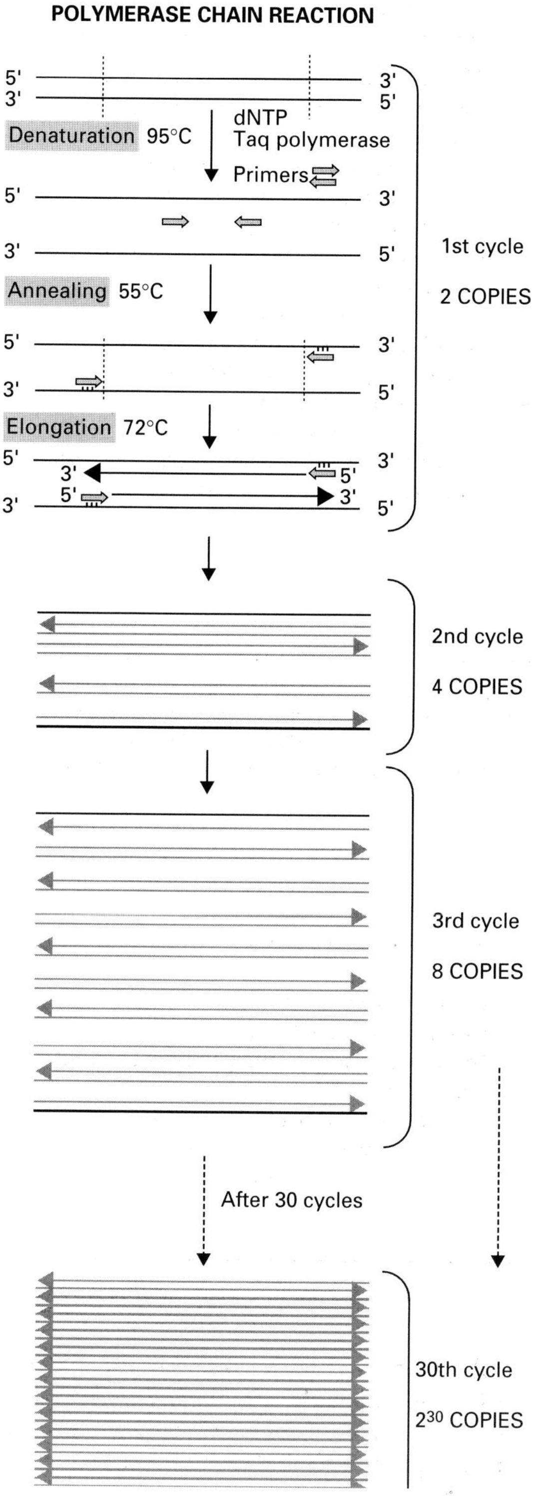

POLYMERASE CHAIN REACTION

5' —————————————— 3'
3' —————————————— 5'

Denaturation 95°C

dNTP
Taq polymerase
Primers

5' —————————————— 3'

⇒   ⇐

3' —————————————— 5'   1st cycle

Annealing 55°C   2 COPIES

5' —————————————— 3'

3' —————————————— 5'

Elongation 72°C

5' —————————————— 3'
    3' ◄————————— 5'
    5' ⇒————————► 3'
3' —————————————— 5'

2nd cycle

4 COPIES

3rd cycle

8 COPIES

After 30 cycles

30th cycle

2^{30} COPIES

3 Biotechnology in the pharmaceutical industry

One of the first and most important commercial applications of genetic engineering was the introduction of genes coding for clinically important proteins into bacteria. Because bacterial cells are cheap to grow on a large scale in fermenters, they can synthesize vast amounts of protein from the recombinant genes they carry. This results in a significant reduction in cost and increase in availability of these proteins. There are currently a large number of recombinant drugs available on the market. Table 24.5 shows examples of the most important ones. This chapter will only cover the genetic manipulation strategies used to produce some well-known recombinant drugs.

3.1 Recombinant human insulin

Recombinant human insulin was the first drug produced using genetic engineering in 1982. It is used for the treatment of diabetes. Before the development of recombinant human insulin, animals (notably pigs and cattle) were the only non-human sources of insulin. Animal insulin differs slightly from human insulin and, consequently, it can potentially elicit an immune response against it, when injected into humans, making this insulin ineffective. The use of recombinant insulin prevents problems generated through potential contamination of animal insulin with other hormones or viruses from animal sources. To understand how insulin is produced using recombinant DNA techniques we

Fig. 24.7 The polymerase chain reaction (PCR). A single PCR reaction involves the following steps. (1) Denaturation of the target double-stranded DNA by heating at 95°C and addition of a large excess of two oligonucleotide primers, each complementary to a different strand of the target sequence, Taq DNA polymerase and dNTPs. (2) Annealing of the primers to the DNA strands by decreasing the temperature to 55°C. (3) Elongation (or synthesis) of the new strand of DNA by the Taq DNA polymerase after increasing the temperature to 72°C. This cycle can be repeated up to 30 times. In each cycle the number of DNA copies is doubled, hence, at the end of a PCR reaction, we could have 2^{30} copies of the original target DNA.

Table 24.4 Clinical applications of PCR

Application	Examples
Diagnostics of inherited diseases	Duchenne muscular dystrophy
	Fragile X syndrome
	Lesch-Nyhan syndrome
	Tay-Sachs disease
	Kennedy disease
	Cystic fibrosis
	Haemophilia B
Infectious disease screening	HIV
	Measles virus
	Herpes virus
	Adenovirus
	Chlamydia trachomatis
	Lyme disease
Forensic examination	Identification of suspect criminals from samples of blood, tissue, hair, etc.
Prenatal screening	Haemophilia
	Sickle cell anaemia
	β-Thalassaemia
	Duchenne muscular dystrophy
	Batten disease
	Sex determination
HLA subtyping	Prevention of insulin-dependent diabetes mellitus
Susceptibility to cardiovascular disease	Mutations in gene coding for angiotensin-converting enzyme (ACE)
	Mutation in the angiotensinogen gene
	Mutation in the apolipoprotein CII gene
	Mutation in the LDL receptor
Susceptibility to cancer	Neoplastic disease
	Lymph node metastasis in melanoma
	Acute promyelocytic leukaemia
	Thyroid cancer
	Non-Hodgkin lymphoma

first need to review the structure of insulin. Figure 24.8 shows how insulin is initially synthesized as a single polypeptide called preproinsulin which, during export, gets processed into proinsulin and finally active insulin, once proteolytic cleavage of the connecting sequence for the two insulin chains (A chain and the B chain) has occurred. These two chains are joined through disulphide bridges.

Currently, different approaches are employed to produce recombinant insulin. Figure 24.8 shows one of them. First of all, two DNA fragments coding for the A or the B insulin chains are synthesized chemically. Each of these synthetic fragments is then individually inserted after the *E. coli* gene coding for β-galactosidase. This enables this bacterium to produce large fusion proteins with the insulin chains tacked onto the end of the β-galactosidase enzyme. These fusion proteins can then be purified from bacterial extracts and the insulin chains released upon treatment with cyanogen bromide, which cleaves peptide bonds following methionine residues. As methionine was inserted at the boundaries between the β-galactosidase and the insulin chains, and there are no methionines present internally within the insulin molecule, treatment with cyanogen bromide results in the cleavage of intact insulin chains from the fusion proteins. The purified A and B insulin chains can be mixed and reconstituted into an active insulin molecule. Currently there are also other methods used to produce recombinant insulin which are based on the generation of single β-galactosidase fusions to the full length insulin gene containing the genetic information for both A and B chains. These alternative methods can simplify the manufacturing of this drug.

3.2 Recombinant somatostatin

Somatostatin, also known as the 'antigrowth hormone', modulates the action of the growth hormone and is frequently used to treat acromegaly (uncontrolled bone growth). Being a very small peptide, the gene coding for it can easily be chemically synthesized and cloned into a suitable expression vector. As *E. coli* tends to degrade small peptides, the generation of a β-galactosidase–somatostatin fusion protein prevents this degradation. Furthermore, as with insulin, the absence of methionine residues in the somatostatin amino acid sequence allows the insertion of a methionine codon in the junction between β-galactosidase and the somatostatin gene. This enables the subsequent cleavage with cyanogen bromide of the recombinant hormone purified from *E. coli*. The strategy used to

Table 24.5 Examples of some commercial clinically important recombinant proteins

Protein	Size/structure	Commercial names/ Company	Expression host	Application
Human insulin	Two peptide chains: A = 21 amino acids B = 30 amino acids	Humulin (Eli Lilly) Humalog (Eli Lilly) Novolin (Novo Nordisk)	E. coli	Treatment of diabetes mellitus
Human somatotropin	191 amino acids	Protropin (Genentech) Genotropin (Pharmacia & Upjohn) Humatrope (Eli Lilly) Nutropin (Genetech) Biotropin (Bio-Technology General)	E. coli	Treatment of human growth hormone deficiency in children
Interferon α_{2a} and α_{2b}	166 amino acids	Roferon A (Hoffmann-La Roche) Actimmune (Genentech)	E. coli	Treatment of various cancers and viral diseases
Interferon γ_{1b}	143 amino acids — glycosylated	Actimmune (Genentech)	E. coli	Treatment of chronic granulomatous disease
Tissue plasminogen activator	530 amino acids — glycosylated	Activase (Genentech)	E. coli Yeast Animal cells	Treatment of acute mycocardial infarct and pulmonary embolism
Interleukin-2	133 amino acids	Proleukin (Chiron Corporation)	E. coli Animal cells	Treatment of kidney carcinoma and metastatic melanoma
Human serum albumin	582 amino acids with 17 disulphide bridges	Albutein (Alpha Therapeutic Corporation)	Yeast	Treatment of hypovolemic shock Adjunct in haemodialysis
Factor VIII	2332 amino acids	Recombinate (Hyland Immuno) Kogenate (Bayer) ReFacto (Wyeth)	Mammalian cells	Treatment of haemophilia
Factor IX	415 amino acids — glycosylated	BeneFIX (Hyland Immuno)	Mammalian cells	Treatment of haemophilia B
Erythropoietin	166 amino acids — glycosylated	Eprex (Jansen-Cilag) NeoRecormon (Roche)	Mammalian cells	Treatment of anaemia associated with dialysis and AZT/AIDS
Hepatitis B surface antigen	Monomer consists of 226 amino acids	Engerix B (SmithKline Beecham) HB-Vax II (Aventis Pasteur)	Yeast Mammalian cells	Vaccination

generate recombinant somatostatin is shown in Fig. 24.9.

3.3 Recombinant somatotropin

Somatotropin, also known as the 'human growth hormone' (hGH), is made of 191 amino acids; hGH is produced in the pituitary gland and regulates growth and development. Regular injections of hGH are given to children with dwarfism caused by the lack of this hormone so that they can reach near-normal heights. In this case, unlike with insulin, animal-derived hormones are ineffective and only the human protein works. Because of the lack of

A

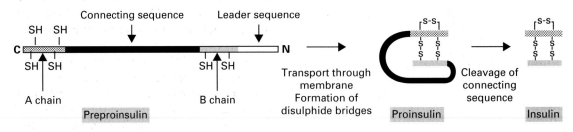

B

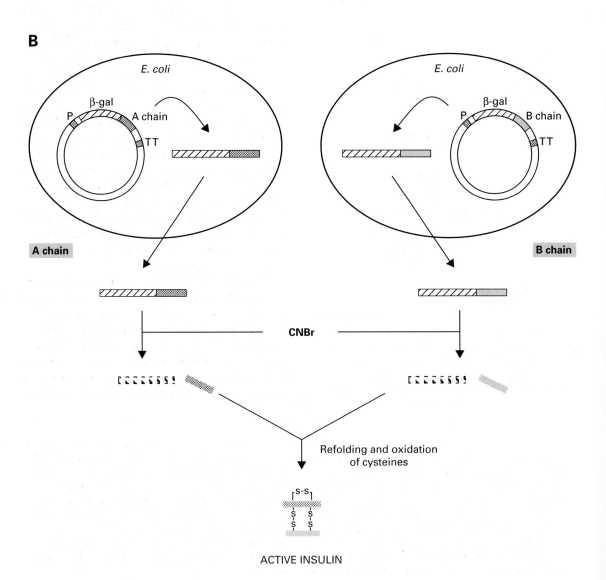

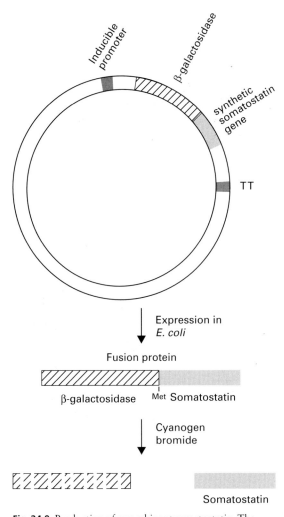

Fig. 24.9 Production of recombinant somatostatin. The small size of somatostatin allows the chemical synthesis of the gene coding for it. This gene can be cloned into an expression fused to β-galactosidase. The fusion protein generated in *E. coli* is then purified and the somatostatin polypeptide is released by treatment with cyanogen bromide.

pituitaries from human cadavers, the use of recombinant hGH has been imperative. Furthermore, the contamination of children with fatal viruses from the cadavers has been an additional reason for moving away from this source of hormone. As the gene for the hGH is 573 nucleotides long, it cannot be synthetically made to generate the recombinant hormone, as in the case of insulin and somatostatin. Hence there are two ways of generating recombinant hGH, one of which results in the generation of this hormone with an added methionine at the N-terminus. Figure 24.10 shows these two strategies.

Initially the coding region for hGH is isolated from a cDNA library. The DNA fragment coding for the mammalian signal peptide can then be excised by a restriction enzyme that also removes the first 24 nucleotides of the mature protein. A chemically synthesized DNA fragment containing a methionine codon, to enable translation in *E. coli*, followed by these first 24 nucleotides, is then ligated to the DNA fragment coding for the remaining 24–191 amino acids of the hGH (Fig. 24.10A). The resulting DNA is cloned into an expression vector and transformed into *E. coli* where the recombinant hGH will accumulate in the cytoplasm. The recombinant hormone can be isolated from bacterial cell extracts and, in contrast to the non-recombinant protein, carries a methionine residue on the N-terminus.

Figure 24.10B shows an alternative method consisting of the replacement of the mammalian signal peptide for a signal peptide that works in bacteria. This enables the purification of the recombinant hGH from the periplasm of the bacterial cell, reducing the difficulties associated with the purification of recombinant proteins from the cytoplasm. To achieve this, once the mammalian signal peptide

Fig. 24.8 Production of recombinant insulin. (A) Insulin is made of two polypeptide chains (A chain and B chain). It is initially synthesized as part of a larger peptide called 'preproinsulin'. The transport across the cell membrane of this peptide results in the cleavage of the signal peptide and the formation of disulphide bridges to generate 'proinsulin'. Finally, the connecting peptide is cleaved generating the mature 'insulin'. (B) One of the strategies used to make recombinant insulin consists of the cloning of the DNA fragment coding for the A chain and the B chain into two separate expression vectors as β-galactosidase fusions in *E. coli*. The fusion proteins are then purified and the insulin is cleaved with cyanogen bromide (CNBr) after a methionine incorporated in the intersection between β-galactosidase and insulin. The presence of several methionines in the β-galactosidase results in multiple cleavage of this molecule by CNBr. Finally, the resulting insulin A and B chains are refolded and the cysteines are oxidized for the generation of the active insulin.

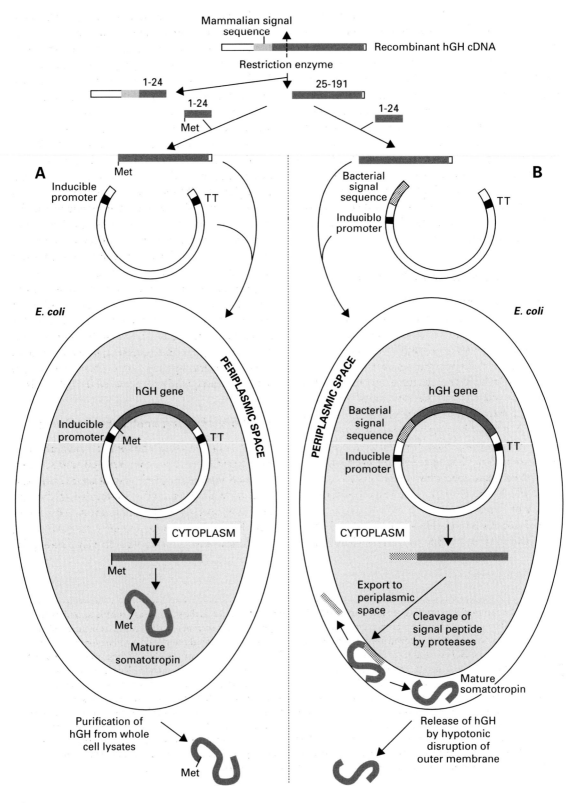

has been removed as above, a synthetic DNA molecule, containing the first 24 nucleotides of the hGH, without an added methionine, is ligated to the DNA fragment coding for the 24–191 remaining residues. The resulting DNA molecule is then fused to a DNA fragment contained within an expression vector, coding for a bacterial signal peptide. Once transformed into *E. coli*, the hGH is produced and the signal sequence will target the protein for secretion into the periplasmic space where it will accumulate. The periplasmic proteases release the signal peptide, leaving hGH without an extra methionine. The protein can then be easily purified from the periplasmic space after release by hypotonic disruption of the outer membrane.

3.4 Recombinant hepatitis B vaccine

Before the discovery of recombinant DNA technology there were two main strategies employed for vaccine production. These were the generation of *inactivated vaccines* consisting of chemically killed derivatives of the infectious agent, and *attenuated vaccines*, which are altered viruses and bacteria that no longer multiply in the inoculated organism. However, these vaccines were potentially dangerous as they could be contaminated with infectious organisms. To avoid these problems, recombinant DNA technology has enabled the production of *subunit vaccines* consisting solely of surface proteins, which can elicit immune responses without the risk of infection.

The hepatitis B virus (HBV) vaccine was the first successful subunit vaccine used. This virus infects the liver and can cause serious damage. This virus has a surface antigen HBsAg which is found in blood of infected patients and has been shown to elicit a significant immune response. The gene coding for this antigen has been isolated from the virus and cloned into a vector that allows high expression of this protein in yeast cells. Figure 24.11 shows the strategy currently used for the generation of recombinant HBV vaccine. The sequence of the 3.2-kb HBV genome is known and has allowed the isolation of the gene coding for the HBsAg. This gene has been cloned into a shuttle expression vector that replicates in both *E. coli* for the genetic manipulation steps, and in yeasts, such as *Saccharomyces cerevisiae*, for the production of the recombinant antigen. Transcription of the gene encoding HBsAg is driven from a strong yeast promoter and is stopped at a transcriptional terminator present in the vector. The vector also has a leucine marker for selection in yeasts and a tetracycline marker for selection in bacteria. The yeast harbouring this plasmid can grow in fermenters, in the absence of leucine, generating large amounts of the antigen that can subsequently be extracted from the cells.

3.5 Production of recombinant antibiotics

A large number of the antibiotics currently used have been isolated from the Gram-positive soil bacterium *Streptomyces*, although other bacteria and fungi have also been used as sources for antibiotics. The biosynthesis of an antibiotic can sometimes include 10–30 separate enzyme-catalysed steps, which makes the cloning of all the genes coding for

---

Fig. 24.10 Two strategies to produce recombinant hGH. These two strategies use as the starting material the recombinant cDNA for hGH which contains the mammalian signal sequence required for the secretion of this protein from mammalian cells. This signal peptide is first removed using a restriction enzyme that cleaves after the nucleotides coding for the first 24 amino acids of the hGH. From this stage two strategies can be followed. (A) A chemically synthesized fragment containing the genetic information for the first 24 nucleotides of the hGH, plus a methionine codon in the 5′ end, is ligated to the remaining cDNA fragment coding for amino acids 25–191 and introduced into an expression vector. The hGH expressed from this vector in *E. coli* accumulates in the cytoplasm and is extracted from whole cell lysates. (B) A chemically synthesized fragment also containing the genetic information for the first 24 nucleotides of the hGH, but without an added methionine codon, is ligated to the remaining cDNA fragment and cloned into an expression vector immediately after the sequence for a bacterial signal peptide. Consequently, when expressed in *E. coli*, the hGH is tagged on its N-terminus with this signal peptide that drives the export of this protein to the periplasm. Once in the periplasm, the signal peptide is cleaved by proteases and the mature hGH can be released and purified upon hypotonic disruption of the outer membrane.

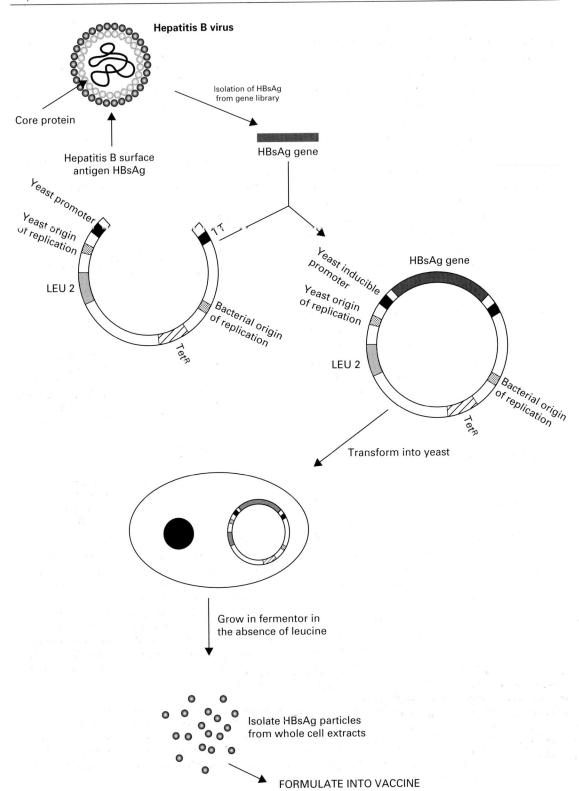

Hepatitis B virus

Core protein

Hepatitis B surface
antigen HBsAg

Isolation of HBsAg
from gene library

HBsAg gene

Yeast promoter

Yeast origin
of replication

LEU 2

Bacterial origin
of replication

Tet R

Yeast inducible
promoter

Yeast origin
of replication

HBsAg gene

LEU 2

Bacterial origin
of replication

Tet R

Transform into yeast

Grow in fermentor in
the absence of leucine

Isolate HBsAg particles
from whole cell extracts

FORMULATE INTO VACCINE

these enzymes very difficult. A strategy used to isolate the complete set of antibiotic biosynthetic genes consists of the transformation of a recombinant gene library, from an organism producing the antibiotic, into a mutant strain of the same organism unable to make this antibiotic. The transformants can be screened for the production of the antibiotic by plating them onto agar plates that have been seeded with a bacterium sensitive to this antibiotic. The appearance of halos of growth inhibition around the recombinant colonies indicates the successful cloning of the antibiotic biosynthetic gene cluster. This strategy has been successfully used for the cloning and production of the antibiotic undecylprodigiosin from *Streptomyces coelicolor* and is shown in Fig. 24.12.

In some instances, recombinant DNA technology has been successfully used to generate novel antibiotics by introducing in the same organism the genes responsible for the synthesis of two very closely related antibiotics. By cross-feeding antibiotic intermediates between two close pathways, novel antibiotics can be generated. This strategy has been very successful in the cross-feeding of antibiotic pathways between different *Streptomyces* spp.

4 New diagnostics using recombinant DNA technology

For many years clinical diagnostic laboratories had limitations in the detection of pathogenic bacteria and parasites due to time constraints in the identification of these agents, as they required to be cultured. Furthermore, these procedures were time-consuming and, consequently, detrimental to patients' health. In addition, many inherited genetic disorders could not be identified in advance owing to the lack of appropriate techniques and the unavailability of the human genome sequence. The rapid developments in molecular biology have enabled modern medicine to overcome some of

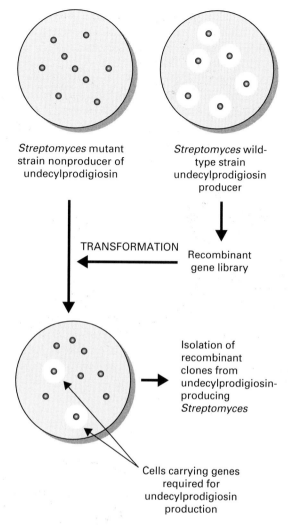

Fig. 24.12 Isolation of genes responsible for antibiotic production. For the isolation of the genes required for undecylprodigiosin biosynthesis a *Streptomyces* strain, unable to make this antibiotic, was transformed with a genomic library from a *Streptomyces* undecylprodigiosin-producing strain. The resulting cells were plated onto agar seeded with a bacterium sensitive to undecylprodigiosin. The recombinant genes required for undecylprodigiosin biosynthesis could be isolated from colonies showing a halo of cell lysis around them resulting from the production of this antibiotic.

Fig. 24.11 Production of hepatitis B subunit vaccine. The gene for the hepatitis B surface antigen (HBsAg) was isolated from a genomic library and cloned into a shuttle vector that promotes high expression levels of this gene in yeast cells. The presence of a LEU2 marker allows the selection of yeasts containing this plasmid by growing them in the absence of leucine. Recombinant yeast cells expressing the HBsAg are grown in large fermenters and the antigen is purified from whole cell extracts for further formulation into the hepatitis B subunit vaccine.

these problems. Currently, a good diagnostic test must be *specific* for the target molecule, *sensitive* enough to detect minute levels of the target molecule, *rapid* and technically *simple*.

This section will introduce some molecular diagnostic techniques, based on the detection of specific DNA sequences, currently used in the clinic.

4.1 Diagnosis of infectious diseases

Each microorganism contains genetic material that makes it distinct in features and characteristics from other microorganisms. This specific material is considered as a signature that allows scientists to identify one microorganism from a complex mixed population. In the diagnosis of infectious diseases, identification of specific sequences from microbial pathogens will allow appropriate treatment at an early stage as well as prevention of the spread of disease.

The two main techniques used for the diagnosis of infectious disease are hybridization and PCR amplification. There are currently primers and probes for the detection of more than 100 infectious disease. Table 24.6 shows just a few examples.

4.1.1 DNA hybridization techniques

Nucleic acid hybridization is based on the precise nucleotide base pairing and hydrogen bonding between one string of nucleotides and a complementary nucleotide sequence. Any diagnostic nucleic acid hybridization test has three essential elements: the DNA probe, the target DNA and the signal detection system. Recent developments in detection systems and improvements in safety have enabled

Table 24.6 Example of infectious diseases currently identified by PCR

Disease	Causative pathogen
Malaria	*Plasmodium falciparum*
Chagas disease	*Trypanosoma cruzi*
Respiratory failure	*Legionella pneumophila*
Food poisoning	*Salmonella typhi*
Gastritis	*Campylobacter intestinalis*
Gastroenteritis	Enterotoxigenic *Escherichia coli*

the use of highly sensitive non-radioactive detection methods rather than the radioactive methods frequently used in the past. Figure 24.13 shows the general steps required for DNA hybridization using chemiluminescent-based detection. This non-radioactive system achieves signal amplification by enzymatic conversion of a chemiluminescent substrate. First of all, the target DNA from the pathogen to be identified needs to be purified. A diagnostic biotin-labelled probe is then mixed with the target DNA bound to a membrane support. The biotin from the hybridized probe is then identified by incubation with streptavidin, which has several binding sites for biotin. Subsequent incubation with biotin-labelled alkaline phosphatase results in the recognition of the bound streptavidin. Finally, addition of a chemiluminescent substrate for the alkaline phosphatase results in the conversion of this substrate into a product with the generation of light which can be detected after exposure to an X-ray film or by using a luminometer.

4.1.2 PCR amplification using fluorescent primers

As in many other fields, the PCR has brought a revolutionary change in DNA-based diagnosis. In a clinical setting, PCR has many desirable features, such as the requirement for tiny amounts of DNA samples from blood or tissue to achieve a specific and significant amplification of target DNA sequences. Furthermore, the rapidity of this process, as explained previously in this chapter, provides a significant advantage in the early treatment of infectious diseases.

A PCR fluorescent-based technique has been used successfully in the diagnosis of infectious diseases. It consists of the labelling of the PCR primers with a fluorescent dye that is bound to the 5′ end of each primer. These primers will emit light of a longer wavelength after absorbing light of a shorter wavelength. Two main types of fluorescent dyes are normally used: one is fluorescein, which appears green under certain light wavelengths, and the other is rhodamine, which appears red. After PCR amplification of the target sequence with the fluorescent-labelled primers, the primers are removed by chromatographic separation, and the presence of

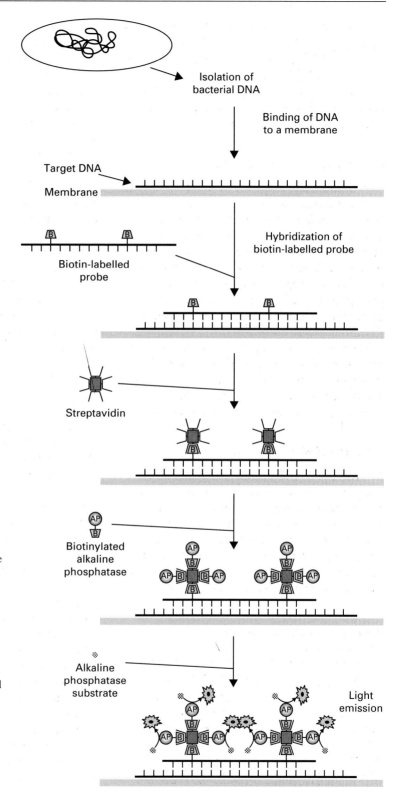

Fig. 24.13 Diagnosis using DNA hybridization with biotin-labelled probes. The DNA from the pathogen to be identified is first purified and bound to a membrane. The membrane is then incubated with a diagnostic biotinylated probe. The biotin from the probe will be recognized by streptavidin which has several biotin recognition sites. Hence, subsequent incubation with biotin-labelled alkaline phosphatase results in the recognition of the bound streptavidin. As several molecules of biotin-labelled alkaline phosphatase will bind to a single streptavidin molecule, incubation of the membranes with chemiluminescence substrate for this enzyme will lead to an amplified reaction and the generation of light-emitting products.

Isolation of bacterial DNA

Binding of DNA to a membrane

Target DNA

Membrane

Biotin-labelled probe

Hybridization of biotin-labelled probe

Streptavidin

Biotinylated alkaline phosphatase

Alkaline phosphatase substrate

Light emission

Table 24.7 Some of the inherited human diseases currently diagnosed by PCR

Haemophilia A and B	Gaucher's disease	Lesch-Nyhan syndrome
Cystic fibrosis	α_1-Antitrypsin deficiency	Maple syrup urine disease
Adenosine deaminase deficiency	β and δ Thalassaemia	Retinoblastoma
Fabry disease	Von Willebrand disease	Tay–Sachs disease
Familial hypercholesterolaemia	Sickle cell anaemia	Phenylketonuria

the labelled PCR product is detected. The absence of labelled PCR product is interpreted as the absence of the target DNA sequence.

4.2 Diagnosis of genetic disorders

The use of new diagnostic techniques has allowed individuals to discover whether they or their offspring are at risk of suffering from specific inherited diseases. DNA analysis using PCR has been used for the identification of carriers of hereditary disorders, for prenatal diagnosis of deleterious genetic conditions and for the early diagnosis of these disorders before the manifestations of any symptoms. Table 24.7 shows some examples of genetic human disorders that are currently identified by PCR.

5 Further reading

Bradley, J., Johnson, D. & Rubenstein, D. (1995) *Molecular Medicine*. Blackwell Science, Oxford.

Brookes, G. (1998) *Biotechnology in Heathcare*. Pharmaceutical Press. London.

Crommelin, D. J. A. & Sindelar, R. D. (1997) *Pharmaceutical Biotechnology: An Introduction to Pharmacist and Pharmaceutical Scientists*. Harwood Academic Publishers, Amsterdam.

Glick, B. R. & Pasternak, J. J. (1998) *Molecular Biotechnology: Principles and Applications of Recombinant DNA*. American Society for Microbiology, Washington, DC.

Madigan, M. T., Martinko, J. M. & Parker, J. (2003) *Brock Biology of Microorganisms*, 10th edn. Prentice Hall, London.

Mathews, C. K., van Holde, K. E. & Ahern, K. G. (2000) *Biochemistry*, 3rd edn. Benjamin/Cumming Publishing Company, Inc.

Old, R. W. & Primrose, S. B. (2001) *Principles of Gene Manipulation*, 6th edn. Blackwell Scientific Publications, Oxford.

Watson, J. D., Gilman, M., Witkowski, J. & Zoller, M. (1992) *Recombinant DNA*. WH Freeman & Co., Scientific American Books, New York.

Chapter 25
Additional applications of microorganisms in the pharmaceutical sciences

A Denver Russell

1 Introduction

There has long been a tendency, especially in medical and pharmaceutical circles, to regard microbes as harmful entities to be destroyed. However, as will be described in this chapter, the exploitation of microorganisms and their products has assumed an increasingly prominent role in the diagnosis, treatment and prevention of human diseases. Non-medical uses are also of significance, e.g. the use of bacterial spores (*Bacillus thuringiensis*) and viruses (baculoviruses) to control insect pests, the fungus *Sclerotinia sclerotiorum* to kill some common weeds, and improved varieties of *Trichoderma harzianum* to protect crops against fungal infections.

1.1 Early treatment of human disease

The earliest uses of microorganisms to treat human disease can be traced to the belief that formation of pus in some way drained off noxious humours responsible for systemic conditions. Although the spontaneous appearance of pus in their patients' wounds satisfied most physicians, deliberate contamination of wounds was also practised. Bizarre concoctions of bacteria such as 'ointment of pigs' dung' and 'herb sclerata' were favoured during the Middle Ages. Both early central European and South American civilizations cultivated various fungi for application to wounds. In the nineteenth century, sophisticated concepts of microbial antagonism were developed following Pasteur's experiments demonstrating inhibition of anthrax bacteria by 'common bacteria' simultaneously introduced into the same culture medium. Patients suffering with diseases such as diphtheria, tuberculosis and syphilis were treated by deliberate infection with what were then thought to be harmless bacteria such as staphylococci, *Escherichia coli* and lactobacilli. Following their discovery in the early part of this century, bacterial viruses (bacteriophages) were considered as potential antibacterial agents, an idea that soon fell into disuse. This idea has recently been revived but has been criticized because of the possibility of transferring antibiotic resistance genes from phage to host bacteria.

1.2 Present-day exploitation

Some of the most important and widespread uses of microorganisms in the pharmaceutical sciences are the production of antibiotics and vaccines and the use of microorganisms in the recombinant DNA industry. These are described in Chapters 22–24. However, there are a variety of other medicinal agents derived from microorganisms including vitamins, amino acids, dextrans, iron-chelating agents and enzymes. Microorganisms as whole or subcellular fractions, in suspension or immobilized in an inert matrix are employed in a variety of assays. Microorganisms have also been used in the pharmaceutical industry to achieve specific modifications of complex drug molecules such as steroids, in situations where synthetic routes are difficult and expensive to carry out.

2 Pharmaceuticals produced by microorganisms

2.1 Dextrans

Dextrans are polysaccharides produced by lactic acid bacteria, in particular members of the genus *Leuconostoc* (e.g. *L. dextranicus* and *L. mesenteroides*) following growth on sucrose. These polymers of glucose first came to the attention of industrial microbiologists because of their nuisance in sugar refineries where large gummy masses of dextran clogged pipelines. Dextran is essentially a glucose polymer consisting of $(1\rightarrow6)$-α-links of high but variable molecular weight (15 000–20 000 000; Fig. 25.1). Growth of the dextran producer strain is carried out in large fermenters in media with a low nitrogen but high carbohydrate content. The average molecular weight of the dextrans produced will vary with the strain used. This is important because

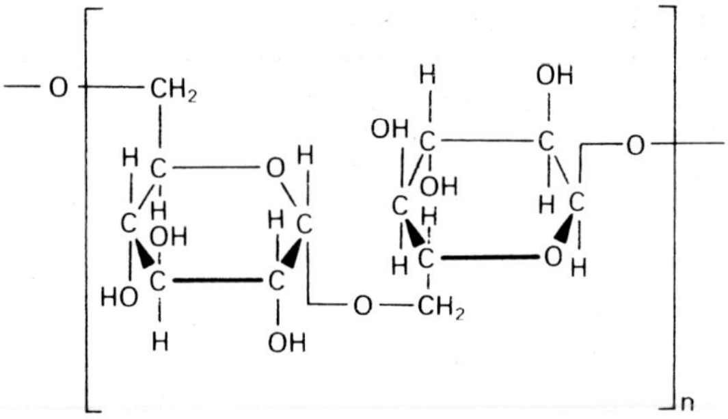

Fig. 25.1 Structure of dextran showing $(1 \rightarrow 6)$-α-linkage.

dextrans for clinical use must have defined molecular weights, which will depend on their use. Two main methods are employed for obtaining dextrans of a suitable molecular weight. The first involves acid hydrolysis of very high molecular weight polymers, while the second utilizes preformed dextrans of small size that are added to the culture fluid. These appear to act as 'templates' for the polymerization, so that the dextrans are produced with much shorter chain lengths. Once formed, dextrans of the required molecular weight are obtained by precipitation with organic solvents prior to formulation.

Dextrans are produced commercially for use as plasma substitutes (plasma expanders) which can be administered by intravenous injection to maintain or restore the blood volume. They can be used in applications to ulcers or burn wounds where they form a hydrophilic layer that absorbs fluid exudates.

A summary of the properties of the different types of dextrans available is presented in Table 25.1. Dextrans for clinical use as plasma expanders must have molecular weights between 40 000 (=220 glucose units) and 300 000. Polymers below the minimum are excreted too rapidly from the kidneys, while those above the maximum are potentially dangerous because of retention in the body. In practice, infusions containing dextrans of average molecular weights of 40 000, 70 000 and 110 000 are commonly encountered.

Iron dextran injection contains a complex of iron hydroxide with dextrans of average molecular weight between 5000 and 7000, and is used for the

Table 25.1 Properties and uses of dextrans

Type of dextran*	Molecular weight (average)	Product	Sterilization method	Clinical uses
Dextran 40	40 000	10% w/v in 5% w/v glucose injection or 0.9% w/v sodium chloride injection	Autoclave	IV infusion: improves blood flow and tissue function in burns and conditions associated with local ischaemia
Dextran 70	70 000	6% w/v in 5% w/v glucose injection or 0.9% w/v sodium chloride injection	Autoclave	IV: used to produce an expansion of plasma volume in conditions associated with loss of plasma proteins
Dextran 110	110 000	6% w/v in 5% w/v glucose injection or 0.9% w/v sodium chloride injection	Autoclave	IV: as for dextran 70
Iron dextran	5000–7500 (complex with ferric chloride)	Colloidal solution in 0.9% w/v sodium chloride injection	Autoclave	Deep IM: non-deficiency anaemia (oral therapy ineffective or impractical) IV (slow infusion): non-deficiency anaemia (oral therapy ineffective or impractical)
Dextran sodium sulphate		Powder for preparing solution	Autoclave	Anticoagulant (intravenous use of solution
Chemically cross-linked dextrans		—	—	Water-insoluble: chromatographic techniques (fractionation and purification

* In the USA, dextran injections with average molecular weights of about 75 000 are also available.
IV, intravenous; IM, intramuscular. The current *British Pharmacopoeia* and *British National Formulary* should be consulted for further information, including toxic manifestations.

treatment of iron deficiency anaemia in situations where oral therapy is ineffective or impractical. The sodium salt of sulphuric acid esters of dextran, i.e. dextran sodium sulphate, has anticoagulant properties comparable with heparin and is formulated as an injection for intravenous use.

2.2 Vitamins, amino acids and organic acids

Several chemicals used in medicinal products are produced by fermentation (Table 25.2).

2.2.1 Vitamins

Vitamin B_2 (riboflavin) is a constituent of yeast extract and is incorporated into many vitamin preparations. Vitamin B_2 deficiency is characterized by symptoms that include an inflamed tongue, dermatitis and a sensation of burning in the feet. In genuine cases of malnutrition, these symptoms will accompany those induced by other vitamin deficiencies. Riboflavin is produced commercially in good yields by the moulds *Eremothecium ashbyii* and *Ashbya gossypii* grown on a protein-digest medium.

Pernicious anaemia was a fatal disease first reported in 1880. It was not until 1926 that it was discovered that eating raw liver effected a remission. The active principle was later isolated and called vitamin B_{12} or cyanocobalamin. It was initially obtained from liver but during the 1960s it was noted that it could be obtained as a by-product of microbial metabolism (Table 25.2). Hydroxycobalamin is the form of choice for therapeutic use and can be derived either by chemical transformation of cyanocobalamin or directly as a fermentation product.

Biotin is a member of the vitamin B family and is an essential factor in the processes and maintenance of normal metabolism in human beings. It is an es-

Table 25.2 Examples of vitamins, amino acids, antibiotics and organic acids produced by microorganisms

Pharmaceutical	Producer organism	Use
Riboflavin (vitamin B$_2$)	Eremothecium ashbyii Ashbya gossypii	Treatment of vitamin B$_2$ deficiency disease
Cyanocobalamin (vitamin B$_{12}$)	Propionibacterium freudenreichii Propionibacterium shermanii Pseudomonas denitrificans	Treatment of pernicious anaemia
Amino acids, e.g. glutamate, lysine	Corynebacterium glutamicum Brevibacterium flavum	Supplementation of feeds/food; intravenous infusion fluid constituents
Antibiotics,* e.g. Benzylpenicillin	Penicillin notatum, P. chrysogenum	Antibacterial drug
Gentamicin	Micromonospora purpurea	Antibacterial drug
Nystatin	Streptomyces noursei	Antifungal drug
Organic acids, e.g. Citric acid	Aspergillus niger	Effervescent products; sodium citrate used as an anticoagulant; potassium citrate used to treat cystitis
Lactic acid	Lactobacillus delbrueckii, Rhizopus oryzae	Calcium lactate is a convenient source of Ca^{2+} for oral administration; constituent of intraperitoneal dialysis solutions
Gluconic acid	Gluconobacter suboxydans Aspergillus niger	Calcium gluconate is a source of Ca^{2+} for oral administration; gluconates are used to render bases more soluble, e.g. chlorhexidine gluconate

* For further information, see Chapters 10 and 22.

sential growth factor for some bacteria. Its chemical structure was established in the early 1940s and a practical, highly stereospecific, chemical synthesis enabled D-biotin, identical to that found in yeasts and other cells, to be produced.

2.2.2 Amino acids

Amino acids find applications as ingredients of infusion solutions for parenteral nutrition and individually for treatment of specific conditions. They are obtained either by fermentation processes similar to those used for antibiotics or in cell-free extracts employing enzymes isolated from bacteria (Table 25.2). Details of the many and varied processes reported in the literature will be found in the appropriate references in the Further reading section at the end of the chapter.

2.2.3 Organic acids

Examples of organic acids (citric, lactic, gluconic) produced by microorganisms, together with pharmaceutical and medical uses, are depicted in Table 25.2. Citric and lactic acids also have widespread

uses in the food and drink and plastics industries, respectively. Gluconic acid is also used as a metal-chelating agent in, for example, detergent products.

2.3 Iron-chelating agents

Growth of many microorganisms in iron-deficient growth media results in the secretion of low molecular weight iron-chelating agents called siderophores, which are usually phenolate or hydroxamate compounds. The therapeutic potential of these compounds has generated considerable interest in recent years. Uncomplicated iron deficiency can be treated with oral preparations of ferrous (iron II) sulphate but such treatment is not without hazard and iron salts are common causes of poisoning in children. The accidental consumption of around 3 g of ferrous sulphate by a small child leads to acidosis, coma and heart failure among a variety of other symptoms which, if untreated, are fatal. Desferrioxamine B (Fig. 25.2), the deferrated form of a siderophore produced by *Streptomyces pilosus*, is a highly effective antidote for the treatment of acute iron poisoning. Desferrioxamine owes its effectiveness both to its high affinity for ferric iron (its

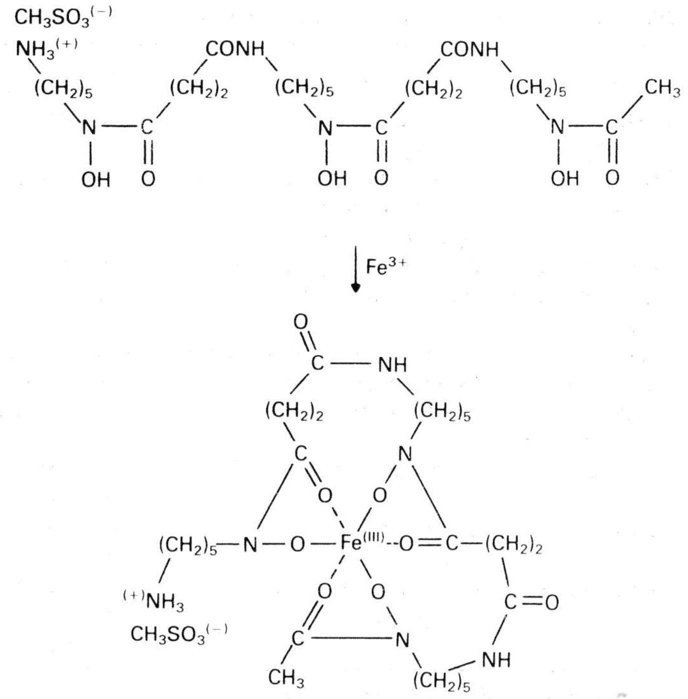

Fig. 25.2 Structure of desferrioxamine B (Desferal) and its corresponding iron chelate.

binding constant is in excess of 10^{30}) and because the iron–desferrioxamine complex is highly water-soluble and is readily excreted through the kidneys. In haemolytic anaemias such as thalassaemia, desferrioxamine is used together with blood transfusions to maintain normal blood levels of free iron and haemoglobin. Desferrioxamine is prepared as a sterile powder for use as an injection, but it is also administered orally in acute iron poisoning to remove unabsorbed iron from the gut. Patients with iron overload disorders treated with desferrioxamine may, however, have increased susceptibility to infections.

The important role played by iron availability during infections in vertebrate hosts has only been recognized relatively recently. The ability of the host to withhold growth-essential iron from microbial and, indeed, neoplastic invaders whilst retaining its own access to this metal has led to suggestions that microbial iron chelators or their semisynthetic derivatives may be of use in antimicrobial and anticancer chemotherapy. Preliminary work has shown some encouraging results.

The bacterial siderophores parabactin and compound II secreted by *Paracoccus denitrificans* have been shown to inhibit the growth of leukaemia cells in culture and in experimental animals. They also appear capable of inhibiting the replication of RNA viruses.

Siderophores like desferrioxamine may, therefore, find increasing applications not only in the treatment of iron poisoning and iron-overloaded disease states but also as chemotherapeutic agents, although the possible problems noted above cannot be ignored.

2.4 Enzymes

Several enzymes have important therapeutic and other medical or pharmaceutical uses (Table 25.3). In this section, those enzymes used therapeutically will be described, with section 4 discussing the applications of microbially derived enzymes for antibiotic inactivation in sterility testing and diagnostic assays.

445

Table 25.3 Clinical uses and other applications of enzymes

Enzyme	Source	Clinical and/or other use	Section(s)
Streptokinase	Certain streptococcal strains	Liquefying blood clots	2.4.1
Streptodornase	Certain streptococcal strains	Liquefying pus	2.4.1
L-Asparaginase	E. coli or Erwinia spp.	Cancer chemotherapy	2.4.2
Neuraminidase	Vibrio cholerae	Possible: increase immunogenicity of tumour cells	2.4.3
β-Lactamases	Bacillus cereus (or other bacteria, as appropriate)	Sterility testing, treatment of penicillin-induced allergic reaction	2.4.4, 4.5
Other antibiotic-modifying or -inactivating enzymes	Some AGAC-resistant bacteria		
	Some CMP-resistant bacteria	Sterility testing, assay	4.1.2, 4.5
		Sterility testing	4.5
Glucose oxidase	Aspergillus niger	Blood glucose analysis	4.6

AGAC, aminoglycoside-aminocyclitol antibiotics (see Chapter 10); CMP, chloramphenicol.

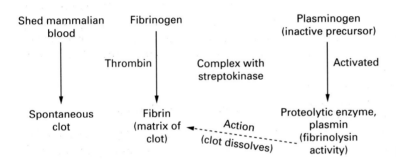

Fig. 25.3 Action of streptokinase.

2.4.1 Streptokinase and streptodornase

Mammalian blood will clot spontaneously if allowed to stand: however, on further standing, this clot may dissolve as a result of the action of a proteolytic enzyme called plasmin. Plasmin is normally present as its inactive precursor, plasminogen. Certain strains of streptococci were found to produce a substance which was capable of activating plasminogen (Fig. 25.3), a phenomenon that suggested a potential use in liquefying clots. This substance was isolated, found to be an enzyme and called streptokinase.

Streptokinase is administered by intravenous or intra-arterial infusion in the treatment of thromboembolic disorders, e.g. pulmonary embolism, deep vein thrombosis and arterial occlusions. It is also used in acute myocardial infarction.

A second enzyme, streptodornase, present in streptococcal culture filtrates, was observed to liquefy pus. Streptodornase is a deoxyribonuclease that breaks down deoxyribonucleoprotein and DNA, both constituents of pus, with a consequent reduction in viscosity. Streptokinase and streptodornase together have been used to facilitate drainage by liquefying blood clots and/or pus in the chest cavity. The combination can also be applied topically to wounds that have excessive suppuration.

Streptokinase and streptodornase are isolated following growth of non-pathogenic streptococcal producer strains in media containing excess glucose. They are obtained as a crude mixture from the culture filtrate and can be prepared relatively free of each other. They are commercially available as either streptokinase injection or as a combination of streptokinase and streptodornase.

2.4.2 L-*Asparaginase*

L-Asparaginase, an enzyme derived from *E. coli* or *Erwinia chrysanthemi*, has been employed in cancer chemotherapy where its selectivity depends upon the essential requirement of some tumours for the amino acid L-asparagine. Normal tissues do not require this amino acid and thus the enzyme is administered with the intention of depleting tumour cells of asparagine by converting it to aspartic acid and ammonia. While L-asparaginase showed promise in a variety of experimentally induced tumours, it is only useful in humans for the treatment of acute lymphoblastic leukaemia, although it is sometimes used for myeloid leukaemia.

2.4.3 *Neuraminidase*

Neuraminidase derived from *Vibrio cholerae* has been used experimentally to increase the immunogenicity of tumour cells. It appears capable of removing *N*-acetylneuraminic (sialic) acid residues from the outer surface of certain tumour cells, thereby exposing new antigens that may be tumour-specific together with a concomitant increase in their immunogenicity. In laboratory animals administration of neuraminidase-treated tumour cells was found to be effective against a variety of mouse leukaemias. Preliminary investigations in acute myelocytic leukaemia patients have suggested that treatment of the tumour cells with neuraminidase in combination with conventional chemotherapy may increase remission rates.

2.4.4 β-*Lactamases*

β-Lactamase enzymes, whilst being a considerable nuisance because of their ability to confer bacterial resistance by inactivating penicillins and cephalosporins (see Chapter 13), are useful in the sterility testing of certain antibiotics (see section 4.5) and, prior to culture, in inactivating various β-lactams in blood or urine samples in patients undergoing therapy with these drugs. One other important therapeutic application is in the rescue of patients presenting symptoms of a severe allergic reaction following administration of a β-lactamase-sensitive penicillin. In such cases, a highly purified penicillinase obtained from *Bacillus cereus* has been administered either intramuscularly or intravenously and in combination with other supportive measures such as adrenaline or antihistamines.

3 Applications of microorganisms in the partial synthesis of pharmaceuticals

Whole microbial cells as well as microbially derived enzymes have played a significant role in the production of novel antibiotics. The potential of microorganisms as chemical catalysts, however, was first fully realized in the synthesis of industrially important steroids. These reactions assumed increasing importance following the discovery that certain steroids such as hydrocortisone have anti-inflammatory activity, while derivatives of the steroidal sex hormones are useful as oral contraceptive agents. More recently, chiral inversion of non-steroidal anti-inflammatory drugs (NSAIDs) has been demonstrated.

3.1 Production of antibiotics

In the antibiotics industry, the hydrolysis of benzylpenicillin to give 6-aminopenicillanic acid by the enzyme penicillin acylase is an important stage in the synthesis of many clinically useful penicillins (see Chapters 10 and 22). The combination of genetic engineering techniques to produce hybrid microorganisms with significantly higher acylase levels, together with their entrapment in gel matrices (which appears to improve the stability of the hybrids), has resulted in considerable increases in 6-aminopenicillanic acid yields.

A second example is provided by the production by fermentation of cephalosporin C, which is used solely for the subsequent preparation of semisynthetic cephalosporins (Chapters 10 and 22).

Furthermore, antibiotics produced by fermentation of various moulds or, especially, *Streptomyces* spp., can be employed by medicinal chemists as starting blocks in the production of what might be more effective antimicrobial compounds.

3.2 Steroid biotransformations

As steroid hormones can only be obtained in small quantities directly from mammals, attempts were made to synthesize them from plant sterols, which can be obtained cheaply and economically in large quantities. However, all adrenocortical steroids are characterized by the presence of an oxygen at position 11 in the steroid nucleus. Thus, although it is easy to hydroxylate a steroidal compound it is extremely difficult to obtain site-specific hydroxylation, so that many of the routes used for synthesizing the desired steroid are lengthy, complex and consequently expensive. This problem was overcome when it was realized that many microorganisms are capable of performing limited oxidations with both stereo- and regio-specificity. Thus, by simply adding a steroid to growing cultures of the appropriate microorganism, specific site-directed chemical changes can be introduced into the molecule. In 1952, the first commercially employed process involving the conversion of progesterone to 11α-hydroxyprogesterone by the fungus *Rhizopus nigricans* was introduced (Fig. 25.4). This reaction is an important stage in the manufacture of cortisone and hydrocortisone from more readily available steroids. Table 25.4 gives several other examples of microbially directed oxidations employed in the manufacture of steroidal drugs.

More recent advances involving the employment of microorganisms in biotransformation reactions utilize immobilized cells (both living and dead). Immobilization of microbial cells, usually by entrapment in a polymer gel matrix, has several important advantages. Whole microbial cells contain complex multistep enzyme systems and there is therefore no longer a need to extract enzymes or enzyme systems which may be inactivated during purification procedures. It also increases the stability of membrane-associated enzymes that are unstable in the solubilized state, as well as permitting the conversion of water-insoluble compounds like steroids in two-phase water–organic solvent systems.

3.3 Chiral inversion

Several clinically used drugs, e.g. salbutamol (a β-adrenoceptor agonist), propanolol (a β-adrenoceptor antagonist) and the 2-arylpropionic acids (NSAIDs) are employed in the racemic form. In the

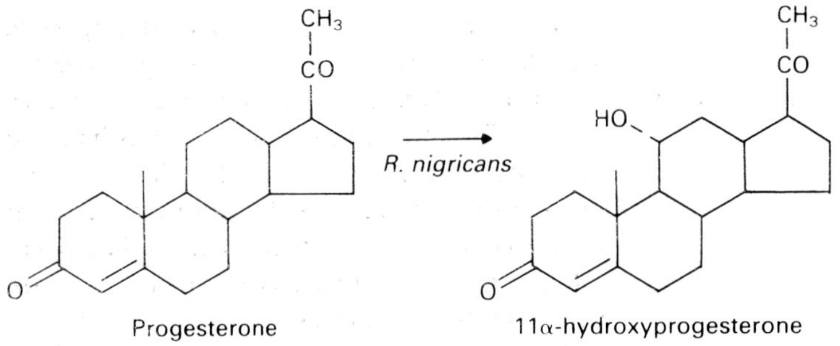

Fig. 25.4 Conversion of progesterone to 11α-hydroxyprogesterone by *Rhizopus nigricans*.

Progesterone → R. nigricans → 11α-hydroxyprogesterone

Table 25.4 Examples of biological transformations of steroids

Starting material	Product	Type of reaction
Progesterone	11α-Hydroxyprogesterone	Hydroxylation
Compound S*	Hydrocortisone	Hydroxylation
11α-Hydroxyprogesterone	Δ–11α-Hydroxyprogesterone	Dehydrogenation
Hydrocortisone	Prednisolone	Dehydrogenation
Cortisone	Prednisone	Dehydrogenation

* Derived from diosgenin by chemical transformation.

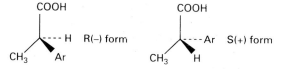

Fig. 25.5 Alternative isomeric forms of profens.

last series, e.g. ibuprofen, activity resides almost exclusively in the S(+) isomers. Chiral inversion, in the unidirectional manner R(−)→S(+) (Fig. 25.5) occurs *in vivo* over a 3-hour period. The S(+) form is a more effective inhibitor of prostaglandin synthesis, and enzymes from some fungal enzymes convert a racemic mixture into the S(+) isomer *in vitro*. It has thus been suggested that the enantiomerically pure S(+) form could be administered clinically to give a reduced dosage and possibly less toxicity.

4 Use of microorganisms and their products in assays

Microorganisms have found widespread uses in the performance of bioassays for:

1 determining the concentration of certain compounds (e.g. amino acids, vitamins and some antibiotics) in complex chemical mixtures or in body fluids;
2 diagnosing certain diseases;
3 testing chemicals for potential mutagenicity or carcinogenicity;
4 monitoring purposes involving the use of immobilized enzymes;
5 sterility testing of antibiotics.

4.1 Antibiotic bioassays

Antibiotics may be assayed by a variety of methods (see Chapter 8, pages 166–188, in *Pharmaceutical Microbiology*, 5th edition, 1992). Only microbiological and radioenzymatic assays will be considered briefly here: see Fig. 25.6 and sections 4.1.1 and 4.1.2.

4.1.1 *Microbiological assays*

In microbiological assays the response of a growing population of microorganisms to the antimicrobial

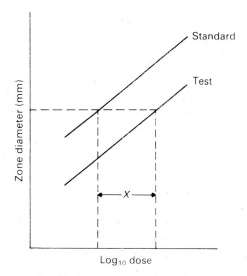

Fig. 25.6 Graphical representation of a two-by-two assay response. X is the horizontal distance between the two lines. The antilog of X gives the relative potency of the standard and test.

agent is measured. The usual methods involve agar diffusion assays, in which the drug diffuses into agar seeded with a susceptible microbial population and produces a zone of growth inhibition.

In the commonest form of microbiological bioassay used today, samples to be assayed are applied in some form of reservoir (porcelain cup, paper disc or well) to a thin layer of agar seeded with indicator organism. The drug diffuses into the medium and after incubation a zone of growth inhibition forms, in this case as a circle around the reservoir. All other factors being constant, the diameter of the zone of inhibition is, within limits, related to the concentration of antibiotic in the reservoir.

During incubation the antibiotic diffuses from the reservoir, and that part of the microbial population away from the influence of the antibiotic increases by cell division. The edge of a zone is formed when the minimum concentration of antibiotic that will inhibit the growth of the organism on the plate (critical concentration) reaches, for the first time, a population density too great for it to inhibit. The position of the zone edge is thus determined by the initial population density, growth rate of the organism and the rate of diffusion of the antibiotic.

In situations where the likely concentration

range of the tests will lie within a relatively narrow range (e.g. in determining potency of pharmaceutical preparations) and maximal precision is sought, then a Latin square design with tests and calibrators at two or three levels of concentration may be used. For example an 8×8 Latin square can be used to assay three samples and one calibrator, or two samples and two calibrators at two concentrations each (over a twofold or fourfold range), with a coefficient of variation of around 3%. Using this technique, parallel dose-response lines should be obtained for the calibrators and the tests at the two dilutions (Fig. 25.6). Using such a method, potency can be computed or determined from carefully prepared nomograms.

Conventional plate assays require several hours' incubation and consequently the possibility of using rapid microbiological assay methods has been studied. Two such methods are:

1 Urease assay. When *Proteus mirabilis* grows in a urea-containing medium it hydrolyses the urea to ammonia and consequently raises the pH of the medium. This production of urease is inhibited by aminoglycoside antibiotics (inhibitors of protein synthesis; Chapter 10). In practice, it is difficult to obtain reliable results by this method.

2 Luciferase assay. In this technique, firefly luciferase is used to measure small amounts of adenosine triphosphate (ATP) in a bacterial culture, ATP levels being reduced by the inhibitory action of aminoglycoside antibiotics. This method may find more application in the future as more active and reliable luciferase preparations become available.

4.1.2 Radioenzymatic (transferase) assays

These depend on the fact that bacterial resistance to aminoglycosides (Chapter 13), such as gentamicin, tobramycin, amikacin, netilmicin, streptomycin, spectinomycin, etc. and chloramphenicol is frequently associated with the presence of specific enzymes (often coded for by transmissible plasmids), which either acetylate, adenylylate or phosphorylate the antibiotics, thereby rendering them inactive (Chapter 13). Aminoglycosides may be susceptible to attack by aminoglycoside acetyltransferases (AAC), aminoglycoside adenylyltransferases (AAD) or aminoglycoside phosphotransferases

(APH). Chloramphenicol is attacked by chloramphenicol acetyltransferases (CAT). Acetyltransferases attack susceptible amino groups and require acetyl coenzyme A, while AAD or APH enzymes attack susceptible hydroxyl groups and require ATP (or another nucleotide triphosphate).

Several AAC and AAD enzymes have been used for assays. The enzyme and the appropriate radiolabelled cofactor ([1–^{14}C] acetyl coenzyme A, or [2–^{3}H] ATP) are used to radiolabel the drug being assayed. The radiolabelled drug is separated from the reaction mixture after the reaction has been allowed to go to completion; the amount of radioactivity extracted is directly proportional to the amount of drug present. Aminoglycosides are usually separated by binding them to phosphocellulose paper, whereas chloramphenicol is usually extracted using an organic solvent.

These types of assay are rapid, taking approximately 2 hours, show good precision and are much more specific than microbiological assays.

4.2 Vitamin and amino acid bioassays

The principle of microbiological bioassays for growth factors such as vitamins and amino acids is quite simple. Unlike antibiotic assays (see section 4.1) which are based on studies of growth inhibition, these assays are based on growth exhibition. All that is required is a culture medium that is nutritionally adequate for the test microorganism in all essential growth factors except the one being assayed. If a range of limiting concentrations of the test substance is added, the growth of the test microorganism will be proportional to the amount added. A calibration curve of concentration of substance being assayed against some parameter of microbial growth, e.g. cell dry weight, optical density or acid production, can be plotted. One example of this is the assay for pyridoxine (vitamin B$_6$) which can be assayed using a pyridoxine-requiring mutant of the mould *Neurospora*. Lactic acid bacteria have extensive growth requirements and are often used in bioassays. It is possible to assay a variety of different growth factors with a single test organism simply by preparing a basal medium with different growth-limiting nutrients. Table 25.5 summarizes some of the vitamin and amino acid bioassays currently available. In practice, high performance liquid chromatography (HPLC) has replaced bioassays as the method of choice for most amino acids and several B vitamins.

Table 25.5 Some examples of microorganisms used as bioassays for vitamins

Assay microorganism	Vitamin
Lactobacillus casei	Biotin
L. arabinosus	Calcium pantothenate
L. leichmannii	Cyanocobalamin
L. casei	Folic acid
Saccharomyces uvarum	Inositol
L. arabinosus	Nicotinic acid
Acetobacter suboxydans	Pantothenol
L. casei	Pyridoxal
Neurospora crassa or	Pyridoxine
S. carlsbergiensis	
L. casei	Riboflavine
L. viridans	Thiamine

4.3 Phenylketonuria testing

Phenylketonuria (PKU) is an inborn error of metabolism by which the body is unable to convert surplus phenylalanine (PA) to tyrosine for use in the biosynthesis of, for example, thyroxine, adrenaline and noradrenaline. This results from a deficiency in the liver enzyme phenylalanine 4-mono-oxygenase (phenylalanine hydroxylase). A secondary metabolic pathway comes into play in which there is a transamination reaction between PA and α-ketoglutaric acid to produce phenylpyruvic acid (PPVA), a ketone and glutamic acid. Overall, PKU may be defined as a genetic defect in PA metabolism such that there are elevated levels of both PA and PPVA in blood and excessive excretion of PPVA (Fig. 25.7).

Control of PKU can be achieved simply by resorting to a low PA-containing diet. However, failure to diagnose PKU will result in mental deficiency, and early diagnosis is essential. In 1968, the UK Medical Research Council Working Party on PKU recommended the adoption of the Guthrie test as a conve-

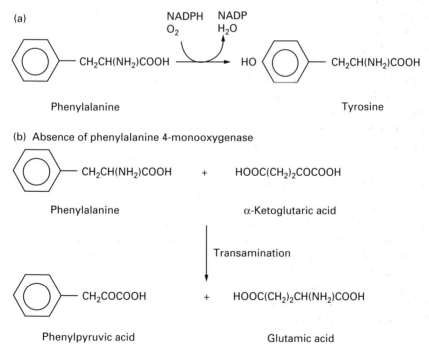

Fig. 25.7 (a) Normal metabolism, in which phenylalanine is converted by phenylalanine 4-mono-oxygenase to tyrosine. (b) Phenylketonuria, in which there is a transamination reaction between phenylalanine and α-ketoglutaric acid. Phenylalanine 4-mono-oxygenase is absent in about 1 in every 10 000 human beings because of a recessive mutant gene.

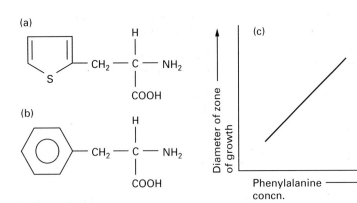

Fig. 25.8 (a) β-Thienylalanine, (b) phenylalanine, (c) standard curve in Guthrie test.

nient method for screening newborn infants. This assay employs *Bacillus subtilis* as the test organism. In minimal culture medium, growth of this bacterium is inhibited by β-2-thienylalanine (Fig. 25.8a) and its competitive reversal in the presence of PA (Fig. 25.8b) or PPVA. The use of filter-paper discs impregnated with blood or urine permits the detection of elevated levels of PA and PPVA. The test can be quantified by the measurement of the diameter of the growth zone around the filter-paper disc and comparing it with a calibration curve constructed from known concentrations of PA or PPVA (Fig. 25.8c).

If positive, the Guthrie test provides presumptive evidence for the presence of PKU. It should be confirmed by other, chemical, means.

4.4 Carcinogen and mutagen testing

A carcinogen is a substance that causes living tissues to become carcinomatous (to produce a malignant epithelial tumour). A mutagen is a chemical (or physical) agent that induces mutation in a human (or other) cell.

Mutagenicity tests are used to screen a wide variety of chemicals for their ability to cause a mutation in the DNA of a cell. Such mutations can occur at:
1 gene level (a 'point' mutation);
2 individual chromosome level;
3 chromosome set level, i.e. a change in the number of chromosomes (aneuploidy). Some compounds are only mutagenic or carcinogenic after metabolism (often in the liver). This aspect must, therefore,

be considered in designing a suitable test method (see section 4.4.2).

4.4.1 Mutations at the gene level

Forward mutation refers to mutation of the natural ('wild-type') organism to a more stringent organism. By contrast, reverse (backward) mutation is the return of a mutant strain to the wild-type form, i.e. it is a heritable change in a previously mutated gene that restores the original function of that gene.

There are two types of reverse mutation:
1 frame-shift: in these mutants, the gene is altered by the addition or deletion of one or more bases so that the triplex reading frame for RNA is modified;
2 base-pair: in these mutants, a single base is altered so that the triplex reading frame is again modified.

These principles of reverse mutation are utilized in one important method, the Ames test (section 4.4.2), which is used to detect compounds that act as mutagens or carcinogens (most carcinogens are mutagens).

4.4.2 The Ames test

The Ames test is used to screen a wide variety of chemicals for potential carcinogenicity or as potential cancer chemotherapeutic agents. The test enables a large number of compounds to be screened rapidly by examining their ability to induce mutagenesis in several specially constructed bacterial mutants derived from *Salmonella typhimurium*.

The test strains contain mutations in the histidine operon so that they cannot synthesize the amino acid histidine. Two additional mutations increase further the sensitivity of the system. The first is a defect in their lipopolysaccharide structure (Chapter 3) such that they are in fact deep rough mutants possessing only 2-keto-3-deoxyoctonate (KDO) linked to lipid A. This mutation increases the permeability of the mutants to large hydrophobic molecules. The second mutation concerns a DNA excision repair system, which prevents the organism repairing its damaged DNA following exposure to a mutagen.

The assay method involves treatment of a large population of these mutant tester strains with the test compound. Histidine-requiring mutants are used to detect mutagens capable of causing base-pair substitutions (in some strains) or frame-shift mutations (other strains). This can be carried out by incorporating both the test strain and test compound in molten agar (at 45°C), which is then poured onto a minimal glucose agar plate. Alternatively, the mutagens can be applied to the surface of the top agar as a liquid or as a few crystals. The medium used for the top agar contains a trace of histidine, which permits all the bacteria on the plate to undergo several divisions, as for many mutagens some growth is a necessary prerequisite for mutagenesis to occur. After incubation for 2 days at 37°C the number of revertant colonies can be counted and compared with control plates from which the test compound has been omitted. Each revertant colony is assumed to be derived from a cell which has mutated back to the wild-type and thus can now synthesize its own histidine: see Fig. 25.9 for a summary.

A further refinement to the Ames test permits screening of agents that require metabolic activation before their mutagenicity or carcinogenicity is apparent. This is achieved by incorporating into the top agar layer, along with the bacteria, homogenates of rat (or human) liver whose activating enzyme systems have been induced by exposure to polychlorinated biphenyl mixtures. This test is sometimes referred to as the *Salmonella*/microsome assay because the fraction of liver homogenate used, called the S9 fraction, contains predominantly liver microsomes.

It is important to realize that this test is flexible

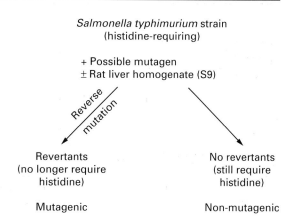

Fig. 25.9 Summary of the Ames test.

and is still undergoing modification and development. Almost all the known human carcinogens have been tested and shown to be positive. These include agents such as β-naphthylamine, cigarette smoke condensates, aflatoxin B and vinyl chloride, as well as drugs used in cancer treatment such as adriamycin, daunomycin and mitomycin C. Whilst the test is not perfect for the prediction of mammalian carcinogenicity or mutagenicity and for making definitive conclusions about potential toxicity or lack of toxicity in humans, it nevertheless represents a significant advance, providing useful information rapidly and cheaply. The Ames test forms an important part of a battery of tests, the others of which are non-microbial in nature, for detecting mutagenicity or carcinogenicity.

4.5 Use of microbial enzymes in sterility testing

Sterile pharmaceutical preparations must be tested for the presence of fungal and bacterial contamination before use (see Chapter 20). If the preparation contains an antibiotic, it must be removed or inactivated. Membrane filtration is the usual recommended method. However, this technique has certain disadvantages. Accidental contamination is a problem, as is the retention of the antibiotic on the filter and its subsequent liberation into the nutrient medium.

Enzymic inactivation of the antibiotic (see also Chapter 13) before testing would provide an elegant solution to this problem. Currently, the only pharmacopoeial method permitted is that of using an appropriate β-lactamase to inactivate penicillins and cephalosporins. Other antibiotics that are susceptible to inactivating enzymes are chloramphenicol (by chloramphenicol acetyltransferase) and the aminoglycosides, e.g. gentamicin, which can be inactivated by phosphorylation, acetylation or adenylylation. A method for acetylating and consequently inactivating aminoglycosides prior to testing and using 3-N-acetyltransferase (an enzyme with wide substrate specificity) in combination with acetyl coenzyme A has been described, but this method has yet to be adopted.

4.6 Immobilized enzyme technology

The therapeutic uses of microbially derived enzymes have already been examined (section 2.4). However, enzymes also form the basis of many diagnostic tests used in clinical medicine. For example, glucose oxidase, an enzyme used in blood glucose analysis, is obtained commercially from *Aspergillus niger*. Future development and improvement of such diagnostic tests is likely to involve the immobilization of enzymes in enzyme electrodes. Several types of glucose oxidase electrodes have been developed, although none is yet in clinical use. One basic system employs glucose oxidase layered over a platinum electrode. As the reaction proceeds and oxygen is consumed, i.e. glucose + oxygen producing gluconic acid + hydrogen peroxide, the reduction in oxygen levels is detected by the underlying electrode. However, problems of enzyme inactivation *in vivo*, competition between glucose and oxygen in body fluids and calibration have prevented the adoption of this system as an implantable glucose monitor in diabetic patients. Nevertheless, there are currently a number of major research efforts in this area and it is likely that biosensors employing immobilized enzymes which are potentially useful for monitoring many substances of clinical importance will become readily available in the not-too-distant future.

5 Use of microorganisms as models of mammalian drug metabolism

The safety and efficacy of a drug must be exhaustively evaluated before its approval for use in the treatment of human diseases. Investigations of the manner in which a drug is metabolized are extremely valuable as they provide information on its mode of action, why it exhibits toxicity and how it is distributed, excreted and stored in the body. Traditionally, drug metabolism studies have relied on the use of animal models and, to a lesser extent, liver microsomal preparations, tissue culture and perfused organ systems. Each of these models has certain advantages and disadvantages. Animals in particular are expensive to purchase and maintain and there is considerable pressure from animal welfare groups to curb the use of animals in scientific research.

The use of microbial systems as *in vitro* models for drug metabolism in humans has been proposed, as there are many similarities between certain microbial enzyme systems and mammalian liver enzyme systems. The major advantages of using microorganisms are their ability to produce significant quantities of metabolites that would otherwise be difficult to obtain from animal systems or by chemical synthesis, and the considerable reduction in operating costs compared with animal studies.

Microbial drug metabolism studies are usually carried out by firstly screening a large number of microorganisms for their ability to metabolize a drug substrate. The organism is usually grown in a medium such as peptone glucose in flasks which are shaken to ensure good aeration. Drugs as substrates are generally added after 24 hours of growth and are then sampled for the presence of metabolites at intervals up to 14 days after substrate addition. Once it has been determined that a microorganism can metabolize a drug, the whole process can be scaled up for the production of large quantities of metabolites for the determination of their structure and biological properties.

As an example of this the metabolism of the antidepressant drug imipramine can be considered. In mammalian systems, this is metabolized to five major metabolites: 2-hydroxyimipramine, 10-

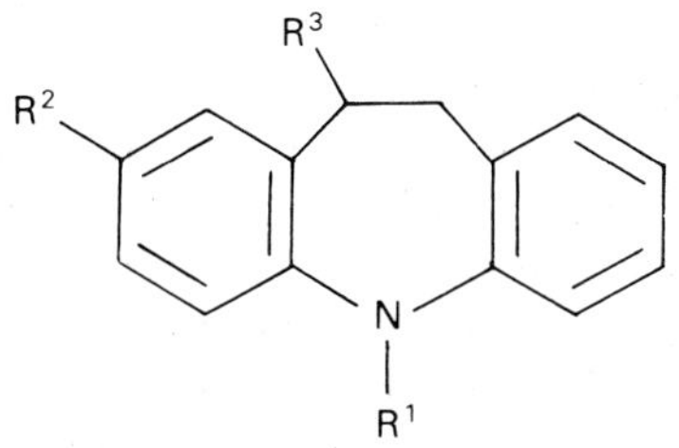

Imipramine	$R^1=(CH_2)_3N(CH_3)_2;R^2=R^3=H$
Desipramine	$R^1=(CH_2)_3NHCH_3; R^2=R^3=H$
2-hydroxyimipramine	$R^1=(CH_2)_3N(CH_3)_2;R^2=OH;R^3=H$
10-hydroxyimipramine	$R^1=(CH_2)_3N(CH_3)_2;R^2=OH;R^3=H$
Iminodibenzyl	$R^1=R^2=R^3=H$
Imipramine-*N*-oxide	$R^1=(CH_2)_3N(CH_3)_2; R^2=R^3=H$

Fig. 25.10 Structure of imipramine and its metabolites.

hydroxyimipramine, iminodibenzyl, imipramine-*N*-oxide and desipramine (Fig. 25.10).

For microbial metabolism studies, a large number of fungi are screened, from which several are chosen for the preparative scale production of imipramine metabolites. *Cunninghamella blakesleeana* produces the hydroxylated metabolites 2-hydroxyimipramine and 10-hydroxyimipramine; *Aspergillus flavipes* and *Fusarium oxysporum* f. sp. *cepae* yield the *N*-oxide derivative and iminodibenzyl, respectively; while the pharmacologically active metabolite desipramine is produced by *Mucor griseocyanus* together with the 10-hydroxy and *N*-oxide metabolites. By scaling up this procedure, significant quantities of the metabolites that are formed during the mammalian metabolism can be obtained.

Microorganisms thus have considerable potential as tools in the study of drug metabolism. Whilst they cannot completely replace animals they are extremely useful as predictive models for initial studies.

6 Insecticides

Like animals, insects are susceptible to infections, which may be caused by viruses, fungi, bacteria or protozoa. The use of microorganisms to spread diseases to particular insect pests offers an attractive method of biological control, particularly in view of the ever-increasing incidence of resistance to chemical insecticides. However, any microorganism used in this way must be highly virulent, specific for the target pest but non-pathogenic to animals, man or plants. It must be economical to produce, stable on storage and preferably rapidly acting. Bacterial and viral pathogens have so far shown the most promise.

Perhaps the best studied, commercially available insecticidal agent is *B. thuringiensis*. This insect pathogen contains two toxins of major importance. The δ-endotoxin is a protein present inside the bacterial cell as a crystalline inclusion within the spore case. This toxin is primarily active against the larvae of lepidopteran insects (moths and butterflies). Its mechanism of action is summarized in Fig. 25.11. Commercially available preparations of *B. thuringiensis* are spore-crystal mixtures prepared as dusting powders. They are used primarily to protect commercial crops from destruction by caterpillars and are surprisingly non-toxic to man and animals. Although the currently available preparation has a rather narrow spectrum of activity, a variant *B. thuringiensis* strain has recently been isolated and found to produce a different δ-endotoxin with activity against coleopteran insects (beetles) rather than lepidopteran or dipteran (flies and mosquitoes) insects.

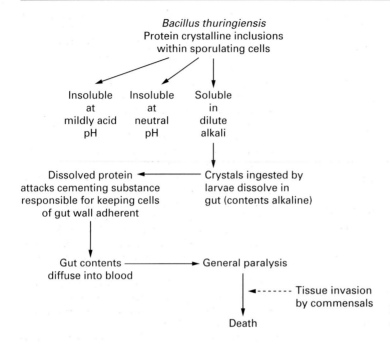

Fig. 25.11 Mechanism of action of δ-endotoxin form *B. thuringiensis*.

7 Concluding remarks

The second *B. thuringiensis* toxin, the β-exotoxin, has a much broader spectrum encompassing the Lepidoptera, Coleoptera and Diptera. It is an adenine nucleotide, probably an ATP analogue which acts by competitively inhibiting enzymes which catalyse the hydrolysis of ATP and pyrophosphate. However, this compound is toxic when administered to mammals, so commercial preparations of the *B. thuringiensis* δ-endotoxin are obtained from strains that do not produce the β-exotoxin.

Strains of *B. sphaericus* pathogenic to mosquitoes were isolated several years ago. More recently, strains of this organism with increased toxicity to mosquitoes have been isolated and might have considerable potential as control agents.

Other insect pathogens are currently being evaluated for activity against insects that are vectors for diseases such as sleeping sickness, as well as those that cause damage to crops. Viruses may well have the greatest potential for insect control as they are host-specific and highly virulent, and one infected insect can release vast numbers of virus particles into the environment. They have already been used with considerable success against the spruce sawfly and pine moth.

Microorganisms are not always the killers they are made out to be. In fact, mankind has been remarkably adept at harnessing microbes for a variety of purposes. In many instances — e.g. antibiotics by whole or partial synthetic production (Chapter 22) and various forms of vaccines — products have been obtained to turn the tables on infecting organisms. Other products have been used for a variety of purposes (including many non-pharmaceutical or non-medical ones, outside the scope of this chapter). Microorganisms have also been employed for specific assay purposes and different types of chemical transformations, as well as in genetic engineering (Chapter 24). Immobilized microorganisms have now been used with considerable success in the partial synthesis of steroids and antibiotics and in the production of the antiviral compound adenine arabinoside (Chapter 5).

Bacteriophages with specific activity against bacteria have been claimed to be effective chemotherapeutic agents in Russia. Several bacteriophages are currently being investigated in the UK and elsewhere to determine the validity of this contention.

Probiotics (literally, replacing 'bad' germs with 'good' ones) have been studied. For example, lactic acid-producing bacteria such as *Lactobacillus acidophilus*, which acidifies the intestinal contents and is a normal inhabitant of the human intestine, have been used in the treatment of vaginal and gastrointestinal disorders.

There are reports of the benefits of botulinum toxin in the treatment of cerebral palsy in children. The toxin, produced by *Clostridium botulinum*, is a powerful and deadly poison, but is also an effective muscle relaxant. It is not licensed for use as such in the UK but is undergoing clinical trials. Current evidence suggests that repeat injections are necessary some 4–6 months after the first.

Recent studies on the therapeutic uses of toxins have also demonstrated that:

1 Botulinum toxin can be used to study synapse remodelling and enzyme-inactivated toxin can be employed to deliver other molecules into motor nerve endings.

2 *Pseudomonas* cytotoxin hybrids destroy cancer cells and have given promising results in tumour destruction.

3 Cholera toxin and related toxins act as immune modulators, with potential use as adjuvants and as therapeutic agents in the treatment of immunologically mediated human disease.

A cautionary note must still be added, however: problems of toxicity remain and these must be overcome before widespread therapeutic usage is feasible.

The beneficial harnessing of microbes is likely to continue for many years.

8 Further reading

Ames, B. N., McCann, J. & Yamasaki, E. (1975) Methods for detecting carcinogens and mutagens with the *Salmonella*/mammalian microsome mutagenicity test. *Mutat Res*, **31**, 347–364.

Breeze, A. S. & Simpson, A. M. (1982) An improved method using acetyl-coenzyme A regeneration for the enzymic inactivation of aminoglycosides prior to sterility testing. *J Appl Bacteriol*, **53**, 277–284.

Clark, A. M., McChesney, J. D. & Hufford, C. D. (1985) The use of microorganisms for the study of drug metabolism. *Med Res Rev*, **5**, 231–253.

Conference (1973) Streptokinase in clinical practice. *Postgrad Med J*, **49**, 3–142.

Data, J. L. & Nies, A. S. (1974) Dextran 40. *Ann Intern Med*, **81**, 500–504.

Davis, G., Green, M. J. & Hill, H. A. O. (1986) Detection of ATP and creatinine kinase using an enzyme electrode. *Enzyme Microb Tech*, **8**, 349–352.

Demain, A. L., Somkuti, G. A., Hunter-Cevera, J. C. & Rossmore, H. W. (1989) *Novel Microbial Products for Medicine and Agriculture*. Elsevier, Amsterdam.

Doenicke, A., Grote, B. & Lorenz, W. (1977) Blood and blood substitutes. *Br J Anaesth*, **49**, 681–688.

Fukui, S. & Tanaka, A. (1982) Immobilized microbial cells. *Annu Rev Microbiol*, **36**, 145–172.

Harvey, A. (1993) *Drugs from Natural Products. Pharmaceuticals and Agrochemicals*. Ellis Horwood, Chichester.

Hewitt, W. & Vincent, S. (1989) *Theory and Application of Microbiological Assay*. Academic Press, London.

Hutt, A. J., Kooloobandi, A. & Hanlon, G. W. (1993) Microbial metabolism of 2-arylpropionic acids: chiral inversion of ibuprofen and 2-plienylpropionic acid. *Chirality*, **5**, 596–601.

Jones, R. L. & Grady, R. W. (1983) Siderophores as antimicrobial agents. *Eur J Clin Microbiol*, **2**, 411–413.

Kier, D. K. (1985) Use of the Ames test in toxicology. *Reg Toxicol Pharmacol*, **5**, 59–64.

Mackowiack, P. A. (1979) Clinical uses of microorganisms and their products. *Am J Med*, **67**, 293–306.

Priest, F. G. (1992) Biological control of mosquitoes and other biting flies by *Bacillus sphaericus* and *Bacillus thuringiensis*. *J Appl Bacteriol*, **72**, 357–369.

Queener, S. W. (1990) Molecular biology of penicillin and cephalosporin biosynthesis. *Antimicrob Agents Chemother*, **34**, 943–948.

Reid, E. & Wilson, D. (eds) (1990) *Analysis for Drugs and Metabolites including Anti-infective Agents. Methodological Surveys in Biochemistry and Analysis*, vol. 20. Royal Society of Chemistry.

Scientific American (1981) Issue on industrial microbiology, vol. 245, No. 3. [An excellent series of papers describing the manufacture by microorganisms or products useful to mankind.]

Smith, R. V. & Rosazza, J. P (1975) Microbial models of mammalian metabolism. *J Pharm Sci*, **64**, 1737–1759.

Turner, A. P. F. & Pickup, J. C. (1985) Diabetes mellitus: biosensors for research and management. *Biosensors*, **1**, 85–115.

Verall, M. S.(1985) *Discovery and Isolation of Microbial Products*. Ellis Horwood, Chichester.

Weinberg, E. D. (1984) Iron withholding: a defence against infection and neoplasia. *Physiol Rev*, **64**, 65–107.

White, L. O. & Reeves, D. S. (1983) Enzymatic assay of aminoglycoside antibiotics. In: *Antibiotics: Assessment of Antimicrobial Activity and Resistance* (eds A.D. Russell & L.B. Quesnel), pp. 199–210. Society for Applied Bacteriology Technical Series No. 18. Academic Press, London.

White, R. J. (1982) Microbiological models as screening tools for anticancer agents: potentials and limitations. *Annu Rev Microbiol*, **36**, 415–433.

Index

Page numbers in *italics* indicate figures and those in **bold** indicate tables.